Lecture Notes in Electrical Engineering

Volume 269

For further volumes:
http://www.springer.com/series/7818

Shaozi Li · Qun Jin · Xiaohong Jiang
James J. (Jong Hyuk) Park
Editors

Frontier and Future Development of Information Technology in Medicine and Education

ITME 2013

Volume 4

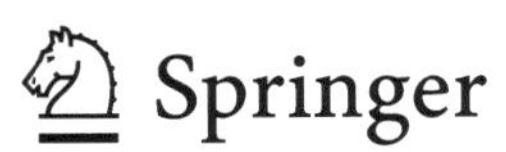

Editors
Shaozi Li
Cognitive Science
Xiamen University
Xiamen
People's Republic of China

Qun Jin
Networked Information Systems Lab,
Human Informatics and Cognitive Sciences
Waseda University
Waseda
Japan

Xiaohong Jiang
School of Systems Information Science
Future University Hakodate
Hakodate, Hokkaido
Japan

James J. (Jong Hyuk) Park
Department of Computer Science and Engineering
Seoul National Universityof Science and Technology (SeoulTech)
Seoul
Korea, Republic of South Korea

ISSN 1876-1100 ISSN 1876-1119 (electronic)
ISBN 978-94-007-7617-3 ISBN 978-94-007-7618-0 (eBook)
DOI 10.1007/978-94-007-7618-0
Springer Dordrecht Heidelberg New York London

Library of Congress Control Number: 2013948373

Printed on acid-free paper

Springer is part of Springer Science+Business Media (www.springer.com)

Message from the ITME 2013 General Chairs

ITME 2013 is the 5th International Symposium on IT in Medicine and Education. This conference took place in July 19–21, 2013, in Xining, China. The aim of the ITME 2013 was to provide an international symposium for scientific research on IT in Medicine and Education. It was organized by Qinghai University, Future University Hakodate, Xiamen University, Shandong Normal University. ITME 2013 is the next event in a series of highly successful international symposia on IT in Medicine and Education, ITME-12 (Hokkaido, Japan, August 2012), ITME-11 (Guangzhou, China, December 2011), ITME-09 (Jinan, China, August 2009), ITME-08 (Xiamen, China, December 2008).

The papers included in the proceedings cover the following topics: IT Application in Medicine Education, Medical Image Processing and compression, e-Health and e-Hospital, Tele-medicine and Tele-surgery, Standard in Health Informatics and cross-language solution, Computer-Aided Diagnostic (CAD), Health informatics education, Biomechanics, modeling and computing, Digital Virtual Organ and Clinic Application, Three Dimension Reconstruction for Medical Imaging, Hospital Management Informatization, Construction of Medical Database, Medical Knowledge Mining, IT and Biomedicine, IT and Clinical Medicine, IT and Laboratory Medicine, IT and Preclinical Medicine, IT and Medical Informatics, Architecture of Educational Information Systems, Building and Sharing Digital Education Resources on the Internet, Collaborative Learning/ Training, Computer Aided Teaching and Campus Network Construction, Curriculum Design and Development for Open/Distance Education, Digital Library, e-Learning Pedagogical Strategies, Ethical and Social Issues in Using IT in Education, Innovative Software and Hardware Systems for Education and Training, Issues on University Office Automation and Education Administration Management Systems, Learning Management Information Systems, Managed Learning Environments, Multimedia and Hypermedia Applications and Knowledge Management in Education, Pedagogical Issues on Open/Distance Education, Plagiarism Issues on Open/Distance Education, Security and Privacy issues with e-learning, Software Agents and Applications in Education. Accepted and presented papers highlight new trends and challenges of Medicine and Education. The presenters showed how new research could lead to novel and innovative applications. We hope you will find these results useful and inspiring for your future research.

We would like to express our sincere thanks to Steering Chair: Zongkai Lin (Institute of Computing Technology, Chinese Academy of Sciences, China). Our special thanks go to the Program Chairs: Shaozi Li (Xiamen University, China), Ying Dai (Iwate Prefectural University, Japan), Osamu Takahashi (Future University Hakodate, Japan), Dongqing Xie (Guangzhou University, China), Jianming Yong (University of Southern Queensland, Australia), all program committee members, and all the additional reviewers for their valuable efforts in the review process, which helped us to guarantee the highest quality of the selected papers for the conference.

We cordially thank all the authors for their valuable contributions and the other participants of this conference. The conference would not have been possible without their support. Thanks are also due to the many experts who contributed to making the event a success.

June 2013

Yongnian Liu
Xiaohong Jiang
James J. (Jong Hyuk) Park
Qun Jin
Hong Liu

Message from the ITME 2013 Program Chairs

Welcome to the 5th International Symposium on IT in Medicine and Education (ITME 2013), which will be held on July 19–21, 2013, in Xining, China. ITME 2013 will be the most comprehensive conference focused on the IT in Medicine and Education. ITME 2013 will provide an opportunity for academic and industry professionals to discuss the recent progress in the area of Medicine and Education. In addition, the conference will publish high-quality papers which are closely related to the various theories and practical applications on IT in Medicine and Education. Furthermore, we expect that the conference and its publications will be a trigger for further related research and technology improvements in these important subjects.

For ITME 2013, we received many paper submissions, after a rigorous peer review process; only very outstanding papers will be accepted for the ITME 2013 proceedings, published by Springer. All submitted papers have undergone blind reviews by at least two reviewers from the technical program committee, which consists of leading researchers around the globe. Without their hard work, achieving such a high-quality proceeding would not have been possible. We take this opportunity to thank them for their great support and cooperation. We would like to sincerely thank the following keynote speakers who kindly accepted our invitations, and, in this way, helped to meet the objectives of the conference: Prof. Qun Jin, Department of Human Informatics and Cognitive Sciences, Waseda University, Japan, Prof. Yun Yang, Swinburne University of Technology, Melbourne, Australia, Prof. Qinghua Zheng, Department of Computer Science and Technology, Xi'an Jiaotong University, China. We also would like to thank all of you for your participation in our conference, and also thank all the authors, reviewers, and organizing committee members.

Thank you and enjoy the conference!

Shaozi Li, China
Ying Dai, Japan
Osamu Takahashi, Japan
Dongqing Xie, China
Jianming Yong, Australia

Organization

General Conference Chairs

Prof. Yongnian Liu (QHU, China)
Prof. Xiaohong Jiang (FUN, Hakodate, Japan)
Prof. James J. (Jong Hyuk) Park, Seoul National University of Science and Technology, Korea
Prof. Qun Jin (Waseda, Japan)
Prof. Hong Liu (SDNU, China)

General Conference Co-Chairs

Prof. Yu Jianshe (GZHU, China)
Prof. Ramana Reddy (WVU, USA)
Dr. Bin Hu (UCE Birmingham, UK)
Prof. Dingfang Chen (WHUT, China)
Prof. Junzhong Gu (ECNU, China)

Program Committee Chairs

Prof. Shaozi Li (XMU, China)
Prof. Ying Dai (Iwate Prefecture University, Japan)
Prof. Osamu Takahashi (FUN, Hakodate, Japan)
Prof. Dongqing Xie (GZHU, China)
Dr. Jianming Yong (USQ, Australia)

Organizing Committee Chairs

Prof. Mengrong Xie (QHU, China)
Prof. Gaoping Wang (HAUT, China)

Dr. Jiatuo Xu (SHUTCM, Shanghai, China)
Prof. Zhimin Yang (Shandong University)

Local Arrangement Co-Chairs

Prof. Jing Zhao (QHU, China)
Prof. Peng Chen (QHU, China)

Publication Chairs

Prof. Hwa Young Jeong, Kyung Hee University, Korea
Dr. Min Jiang (XMU, Xiamen, China)

Program Committee

Ahmed Meddahi, Institute Mines-Telecom/TELECOM Lille1, France
Ahmed Shawish, Ain Shams University, Egypt
Alexander Pasko, Bournemouth University, UK
Angela Guercio, Kent State University
Bob Apduhan, Kyushu Sangyo University, Japan
Cai Guorong, Jimei University, China
Cao Donglin, Xiamen University, China
Changqin Huang, Southern China Normal University, China
Chaozhen Guo, Fuzhou University, China
Chensheng Wang, Beijing University of Posts and Telecommunications, China
Chuanqun Jiang, Shanghai Second Polytechnic University, China
Cui Lizhen, Shandong University, China
Cuixia Ma, Institute of Software Chinese Academy of Sciences, China
Feng Li, Jiangsu University, China
Fuhua Oscar Lin, Athabasca University, Canada
Hiroyuki Mituhara, Tokushima University, Japan
Hongji Yang, De Montfort University, UK
Hsin-Chang Yang, National University of Kaohsiung, Taiwan
Hsin-Chang Yang, National University of Kaohsiung, Taiwan
I-Hsien Ting, National University of Kaohsiung, Taiwan
Jens Herder, University of Applied Sciences, Germany
Jian Chen, Waseda University, Japan
Jianhua Zhao, Southern China Normal University, China
Jianming Yong, University of Southern Queensland, Australia
Jiehan Zhou, University of Oulu, Finland

Yuichi Fujino, Future University, Japan
Yujie Liu, China University of Petroleum, China
Zhang Zili, Southwestern University, China
Zhao Junlan, Inner Mongolia Finance and Economics College, China
Zhaoliang Jiang, Shandong University, China
Zhendong Niu, Beijing Institute of Technology, China
Zhenhua Duan, Xidian University, China
Zhongwei Xu, Shandong University at Weihai, China
Zonghua Zhang, Institute Mines-Telecom/TELECOM Lille1, France
Zongmin Li, China University of Petroleum, China
Zongpu Jia, Henan Polytechnic University, China

Contents

Volume 1

Volume 2

Volume 3

Volume 4

Chapter 338
Research and Practice of University Statistics Sharing Scheme

Suping Xie, Huaichu Chen, Shixue Yin and Zou Xiangrong

Abstract With the deepening of the University Electronic platform, various business systems achieve close sharing of data, but data sharing is generally limited in basic business data. We lack the understanding of shared statistical data. The sharing process of statistical data is limited to verbal or one-time providing and lack the supporting of effective information technology, which is not conducive to an authorized history dating back. In order to solve the above problems, the author proposed and designed a statistical data sharing scheme for college management, which unify the approval of statistical data applying, archive working mechanism of the application and authorization of statistical data and facilitate data authorization, history traced, management and sharing of statistical data.

Keywords University · Statistics · Sharing scheme

338.1 University Data Sharing Status and Demand

With the deepening of the electronic school platform of universities and the continuous expansion and Cross-fusion of the functions of all departments, the university business management system establish close data sharing. Data sharing and fusion can be helpful for breaking up information silos and improve the general efficiency and level of the university information service. The status is that each type of business data is in charge of corresponding department. Other departments who want to share other data need to apply to the competent departments. After the competent departments agree and make sure the sharing data fields and Update frequency, the technology department completes the

S. Xie (✉) · H. Chen · S. Yin · Z. Xiangrong
Technology Center of the Information Technology, Tsinghua University,
Beijing 100084, China
e-mail: xsp@cic.tsinghua.edu.cn

S. Li et al. (eds.), *Frontier and Future Development of Information Technology in Medicine and Education*, Lecture Notes in Electrical Engineering 269,
DOI: 10.1007/978-94-007-7618-0_338, © Springer Science+Business Media Dordrecht 2014

sharing implement. Such as the personal data is in charge of the HR department and research project data is in charge of research management department. The common problem of all colleges and universities in the information system data sharing are as follows.

338.1.1 Data Sharing is Generally Limited to Basic Business Data, Lack of Understanding to Statistical Data Sharing

In daily work, when some departments need the statistic information which is based on the basic data, they always need to get help from corresponding department too. Such as there were how much teachers who having the Senior title, how much projects which were in research and etc. These statistics can not be simply calculated from the basic data or the calculated diameter is not clear, inconsistent, and the caliber of these definitions can be accurately calculated by counterpart management department in the business systems. In demand for data sharing, in addition to the basic detail data sharing, statistics data is also a very important and can not be replaced by the basic detail data.

338.1.1.1 Statistical Data Sharing Process is Limited to Verbal or One-Time Provision, Which is in Lack of Effective Information Support

The statistics data is shared by phone, mail and etc. Sometimes different person in the same department may apply various types of statistical data to the same or different person in another business department. Different departments may apply for the same statistical data to the same business department, However, due to the randomness of the data application time, the person who provide the data may be different person, which results in that statistical data are often one-time check and one-time providing, and wasting so much time. Otherwise this application of statistical data is inevitable in the day-to-day work.

338.1.1.2 Existing Data Sharing is Not Standardized and is Not Conducive to the Authorized History Dating Back

Existing data sharing modes include the three ways such as real-time, periodic synchronization and one-time. The business department applying data fill out the data grant application form, after approval of the competent business department, the data sharing will be implemented by the technical department. From a management point of view, the application departments, the competent departments, technical departments will tripartite retain data application form, which will be conducive to management and can be the authorization historical retrospective. But over the years, due to the time span of various departments applying for data is wide and the number of applications is so much. The paper application form is not as good as electronic application which is easy to store. It is not impossible for the major department who is in charge of business data or the technology department to grasp all the authorization details to other departments.

In order to solve the above problems and to meet the common statistical data sharing requirements in the university, we propose a statistical data sharing scheme for the university management requirements and the status.

338.2 Statistical Data Sharing Scheme

Statistical data, as a separate shared resources, needs the information technology to achieve norms and effective management. Statistics data has the characteristics such as relatively simple, Requiring high accuracy. In view of the above characteristics, our preliminary design solutions are as below.

We design and Implement a statistics publishing and sharing system. It's main users include data the data applying department, the data authorities departments and the technical departments. It is mainly used to collect and publish all kinds of business statistics based on the business systems and basic data. The authorized user get the specified statistics data by the account designated in the system.

The business process of the statistics publishing and sharing system are as follows (Fig. 338.1).

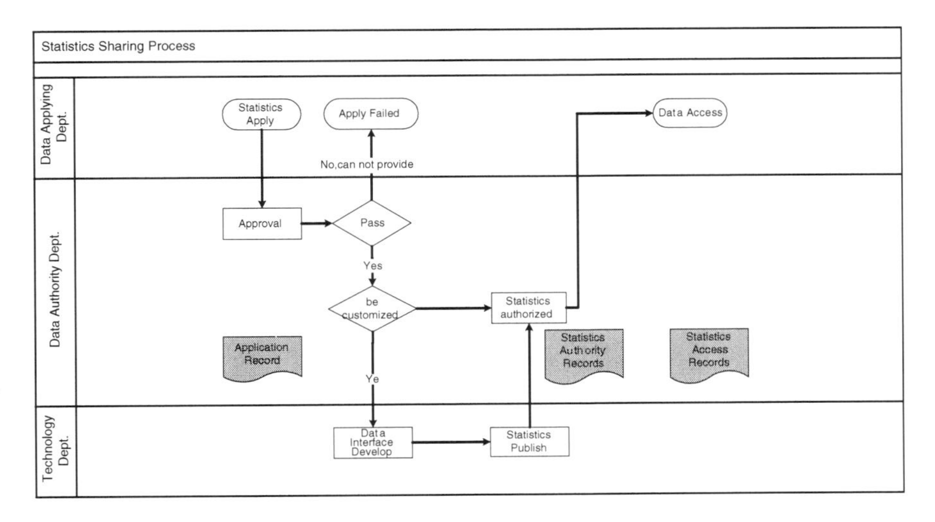

Fig. 338.1 Statistics sharing Process

After the data application department put forwards the data application, the data authorities departments will verify the application. If there is this kind of statistical data and the data authorities department confirm that the data sharing is valid, it will complete the authorities in the system. If there is not the kind of statistical data, the authorities department will firstly define the data interface in the system, then complete the publishing and sharing of this statistical data. Users who get the authorization can log on the system and get the statistical data.

In this process, the system will automatically record the process of data application, approval, authorization and accessing operation and facilitate the follow-up history traced.

During the implementation of the system, you should firstly research on commonly used statistical data, and regularly publishing this statistics. In addition, in the statistics updating mechanism, you can use the Webservice technology. When the department applying data access the system, it can call the corresponding method to update the statistics automatically, obtain the corresponding statistics system and ensure the accuracy of the data.

338.3 Summary

By constructing the system, the application and approval of statistical data will be unified. The authorization, access history traced and management will be easier. It will facilitate the accumulation and sharing of statistical data. The advantages of the statistical data sharing scheme are as follows:

1. It can be helpful for establishing the application and approval process of statistics, achieving a unified data application, approval and authorization mechanism. It will change the original application mode by telephone and mail. The data applying department complete thee data approval in the information system and the authorization department can complete Online approval and authorization. The process of data application and approval is standardized.
2. The application, authorization, access control of statistics will be monitored, which can facilitate the data authorized, access history dating back and management. The system automatically records the data application, approval, authorization and accessing records and the form the data authorized records. The major department can master all the competent authority history.
3. The statistics publishing and sharing system will facilitate the accumulation and sharing of statistical data. By the construction of the system, we realize the accumulation of statistical data. Under the original operating mode, if the data application department apply the same statistical data for the same or different person in the same department at different times, then each time the major department needs to recalculate to obtain the newer statistics. In the publishing and sharing system, we can not only solve the problems of duplication work in

the competent authorities department and also provide the sharing between different data application departments.

4. The ancestry dates back will be established between statistical data and basic data. When the basic data changes, we can timely adjust the rules of the statistics and ensure the accuracy of the statistics. For example, there are ten departments who have the same data sharing demand for the same department, then nine person number of times will be saved. And with the wider the sharing range, statistical sharing data will be relatively aggregated, so that the labor costs we saved will increase exponentially and the data accuracy and continuity will be insured.

In addition, we can improve the existing business systems in our daily work to cover the common statistical data so as to feedback rapidly when users put forward the application form. On the other hand, on the statistics providing modes, we can also use a link in the user mail. When the user clicks the link, he can see the data. The link will lose effectiveness after a few clicks or a period of time.

References

1. Tu Y (2012) Data sharing design based on webservice. Science Mosaic, pp 36–38
2. Xu Y (2012) Research on storage security mechanism of trans-departmental data sharing. Academic Research, pp 84–87
3. Luan X-D, Xie Y-X, Wu L-D, Mao C-L, Lao S-Y (2005) Information assistant: a novel initiative topic search engine. In: Proceedings of 2005 international conference on machine learning and cybernetics, vol 4, pp 2363–2367
4. Cakir E, Bahceci H, Bitirim Y (2008) An evaluation of major image search engines on various query topics. In: ICIMP '08. the third international conference on internet monitoring and protection, pp 161–165
5. Li Y, Mo Q, Wang F (2010) An interactive mathematics education platform based on topic-based deep search. In: 2010 second international workshop on education technology and computer science (ETCS), vol 2, pp 163–169
6. Uluhan E, Badur B (2008) Development of a framework for sub-topic discovery from the web. In: PICMET 2008. Portland international conference on management of engineering and technology, pp 878–888

Chapter 339
A Formal Framework for Domain Software Analysis Based on Raise Specification Language

Yuanzheng Zhao, Tie Bao, Lu Han, Shufen Liu and Qu Chen

Abstract This paper presents domain software formal analysis method based on the specification language, and establishes the corresponding framework. A variety of products were collected from software development process, through standard evidence file, formal description based on feature, formal description based on model, and so on stages, they were translated into Raise specification language (RSL) description by formal methods, so that the analysis and verification work can be done through formal tools to analyze domain software. This framework is able to transform all products in the life cycle of domain software into the formal description, to establish solid foundation for formal analysis and construct high reliability software.

Keywords Software engineering · Formal analysis · Domain software · RSL

Y. Zhao
Navy Equipment Department, Vessel Office, Beijing, China
e-mail: zyzlll@yahoo.com.cn

T. Bao (✉) · L. Han · S. Liu · Q. Chen
College of Computer Science and Technology, Jilin University, Changchun, China
e-mail: baotie@jlu.edu.cn

L. Han
e-mail: hanlu@jlu.edu.cn

S. Liu
e-mail: liusf@jlu.edu.cn

Q. Chen
e-mail: chenqu12@mails.jlu.edu.cn

S. Li et al. (eds.), *Frontier and Future Development of Information Technology in Medicine and Education*, Lecture Notes in Electrical Engineering 269,
DOI: 10.1007/978-94-007-7618-0_339,

339.1 Introduction

During the development of information society and the increasing degree of information, software system dependence of all social domains is increasing day by day. Domain software plays a more and more important role in various industries of the national economy and social development. Many software systems play a vital role as a control system of large equipment or the core software of industry production. With the increasing demand of domain, the domain software system is becoming large, complex, unstable and difficult control, even appear different kinds of fault and failure to cause huge losses to the user. With these problems highlighting, domestic and overseas related researchers are highly valued construction technology and reliability research of domain software, and the formal method became the most powerful tool. How to analyze the domain software reliability through the formal tool, how to ensure their reliable operation, and how to continuously improve the running quality become the problems urgent need to be solved.

On account of the importance of domain software, people began to research from different angles and levels of domain software and its development process. Metayer and others [1] proposed an accurate formal method without ambiguity to define software capacity, and provided tools in order to reduce the uncertainty. Pena [2] modeled the NASA cluster through the software project based on agent and formal method. Fallah-Seghrouchni [3] discussed the problem aimed at the multi-agent system selecting formal methods and tools. Brosch and others [4] proposed a reliability modeling and forecasting technique considering the relevant structure factors of software system. Si Guannan [5] proposed the method calculating components and system of the internetware bottom-up approach layer by layer based on Bayesian network. Dai Fei [6] proposed software evolutionary process meta-model algebra to reason and validate the behavior of the software evolution model based on equation. Wu Caihua [7] proposed a method to build the markov chain usage model by UML model, and provided the verification algorithm of UML model generating Markov chain usage model. Above research lacks the domain software formal analysis framework with good operability, they can't clear description each stage of domain software. So this paper mainly researches and establishes the framework of formal analysis for domain software.

339.2 Formal Analysis Framework for Domain Software

The formal method is the most powerful tool to ensure the software reliability, so we adopted formal method to analysis products in each phase of domain software lifecycle, and establish the corresponding framework. The framework of formal analysis for domain software is shown in Fig. 339.1. The analysis process of domain software should be processed by evidences. The evidences comes from all

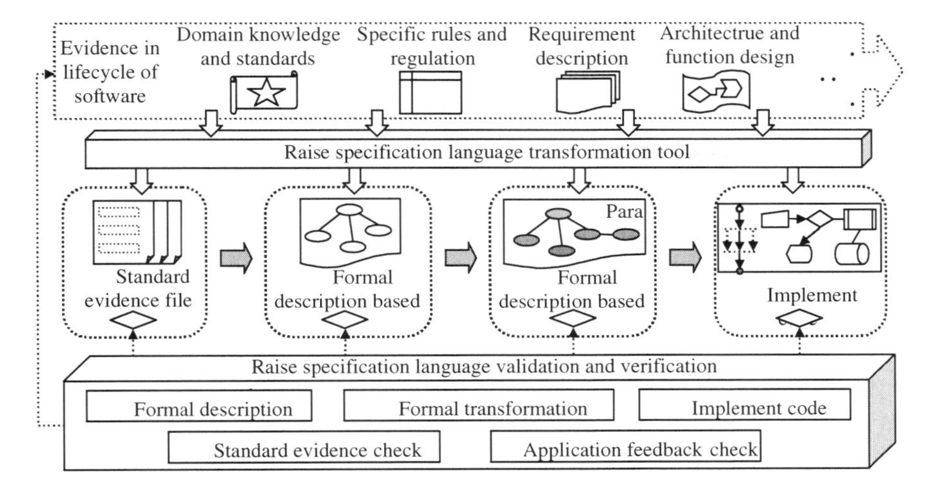

Fig. 339.1 Formal framework for domain software analysis

kinds of products of software development life cycle, such as: knowledge and unified standard of domain, specific rules and regulations of domain, requirement information of domain expert and user, software function analysis, software structure design, and so on. The form of evidence is multiple, and it can be a document, questionnaire, UML files. The evidences can be processed by RSL transformation tool, and to generate the formal description or model.

The domain software analysis evidence experienced a series of formal conversion process: First, standard evidence document would be generated through the transformation, the document extracted the various of formal described elements; standard evidence document generated formal description based on feature by formal transformation, it mainly represented the characteristics and application functions of domain; formal description based on feature generated formal description based on model by formal transformation, it mainly included the concrete mathematical model and parallelism; formal description based on model generated specific implement code by formal transformation, it depends on the concrete platform and language. The analysis evidence and formal description would be analyzed and validated by validation and verification tools. It mainly including: the completeness and correctness of the standard evidence should be checked to ensure the effectiveness of analysis source; formal description check, the check to the elements, expresses and the logical relation of formal description; formal transformation check, the check to different stages of conversion process of formal description; in addition, the validation and verification process also need to compare some original evidence.

339.3 Formal Transformation of Analysis Evidence

The key part of formal analysis framework for domain software is the formal transformation of evidence. The formal conversion process was completed by the formal method through standard evidence file, formal description based on feature, formal description based on model, and so on stages. The transformation process need be checked by verification tools used, and compared the different formal description. Formal description based on model included model and implementation details, it can be easily converted into the implement code relying on platform and language, RSL also provides such tool. The formal conversion process is illustrated through the example of a simple power domain information management system. The conversion process is shown in Fig. 339.2.

The concept, role, behavior were analyzed and extracted through the collection of domain application characteristics, the rules and regulations of the enterprise, the user requirement and so on original evidence, to be able to form standard evidence file. As the top left file in Fig. 339.2, the first part of the text explains the system application of electric domain software in the power generation enterprises. The second part explains the specific provisions of night watch in the power generation enterprises. The third part explains the fault information records needed a fault

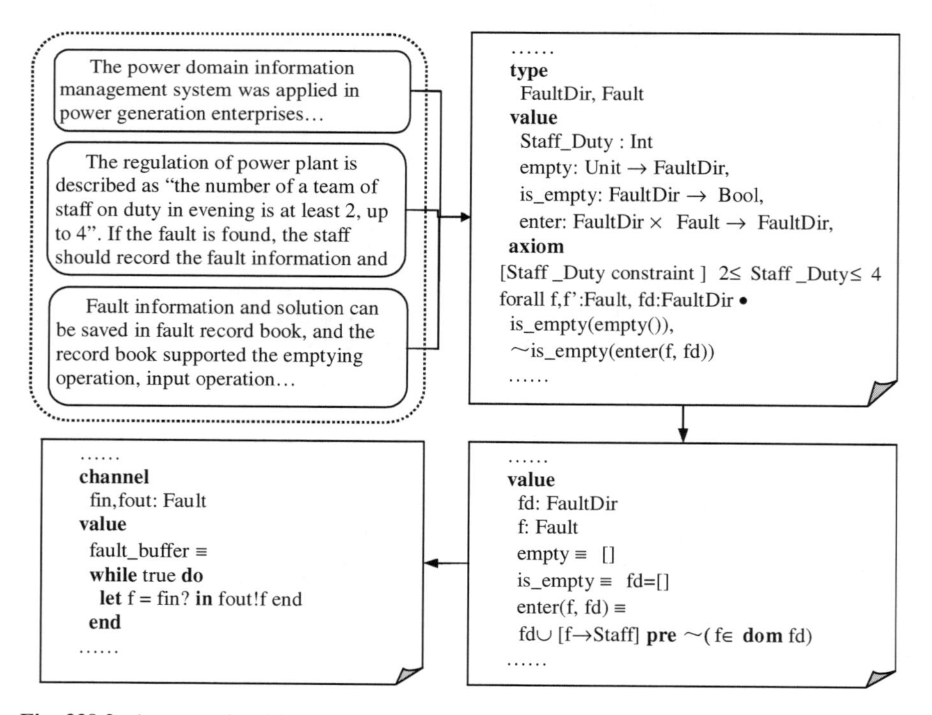

Fig. 339.2 An example of formal transformation process to evidence

record book, and part functions of the record book. Standard evidence file had a clear description, and it should be the basic of formal description transformation.

The characteristics and functions were mainly expressed by formal description based on feature which can be transformed from standard evidence file, and not contained specific implementation details. The formal description was generated according to the left side standard of evidence as the upper right of Fig. 339.2. The type part defined identifiers of fault record book and fault types, the value part defined the main function of fault record book. The fault record book currently supported the emptying operation, input operation and empty distinguishing operations, the axiom part mainly described domain properties.

The formal description based on feature converted formal description based on mode, it was mainly focused on implementation model, contained the specific implementation details. As the lower right Fig. 339.2 showed, the formal description was generated according the above file, and it defines the implement model of fault records book. Mapping was adopted in this paper, and the three kinds operation of fault record book was based on mapping. As the lower left Fig. 339.2 showed, the model included the parallel properties of the actual operation, and it defined the buffer channel for the parallel run of the fault input function to implement the buffer memory of unit fault information, and to support the parallel operation of multi-users.

339.4 Application in the Construction of Domain Software

Various kinds of models and formal description in analysis process can be saved to the formal analysis resource library after analysis to domain software by formal framework, so that they can be used in the construction process of domain software. The formal framework we established can played an important role in the construction process of domain software, it can speed up the development of domain software, reduced the work complexity, and can provided formal foundation to ensure the domain software reliability in a certain extent. Application is showed in Fig. 339.3.

The existing formal analysis resources were stored in the resource library. Firstly, the appropriate requirement model extracted in the resource was amended through the differentiation requirement analysis when the software system need be developed for specific domain application. The function and structure design of software is based on the modified requirement model, and then entering the specific coding stage. The software can extract some application data and user feedback in the application stage. These data will also be analyzed as evidence to improve existing model. The whole developed and applied process of domain software can refer to the existing formal model, analyzed and modified by framework tools.

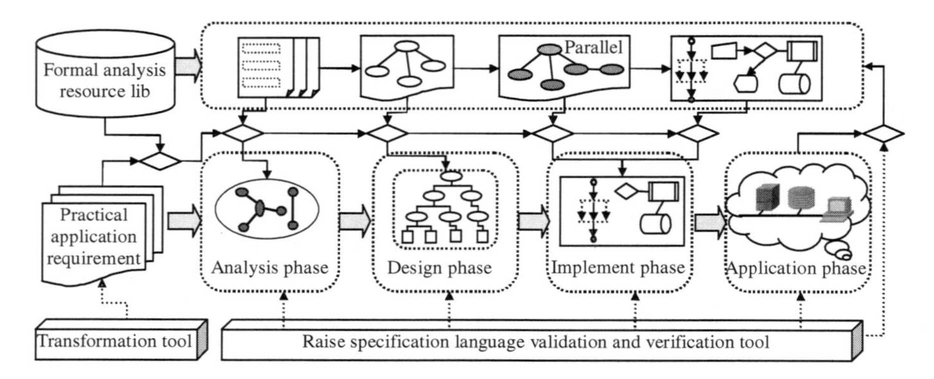

Fig. 339.3 Construction of domain software based on formal framework

339.5 Conclusion

This paper presents a practical domain software formal analysis method with a good operation, and established the corresponding framework. Based on a variety of evidence in the domain software life cycle, through formal translation in standard evidence file, formal description based on feature, formal description based on the model and such as multiple phases, the formal description which can be analyzed and verified will be generated. This is expressed by RSL, so that domain software can be further analyzed and verified through formal tool, thus domain software reliability can be analyzed and verified from the angle of formal. This framework provides good domain software formal analysis method with good operation and low complexity, it is able to transform all products in the life cycle of domain software into the formal description, to establish solid foundation for formal analysis and construct high reliability software.

References

1. Le Metayer D, Maarek M, Mazza E (2011) Liability issues in software engineering the use of formal methods to reduce legal uncertainties. Commun ACM 54(4):99–106. doi:10.1145/1924421.1924444
2. Pena J, Rouff CA, Hinchey M, Ruiz-Cortes A (2011) Modeling NASA swarm-based systems: using agent-oriented software engineering and formal methods. Softw Syst Model 10(1):55–62. doi:10.1007/s10270-009-0135-2
3. El Fallah-Seghrouchni A, Gomez-Sanz JJ, Singh MP (2011) Formal methods in agent-oriented software engineering. Agent-Oriented Softw Eng 6038:213–228
4. Brosch F, Koziolek H, Buhnova B, Reussner R (2012) Architecture-based reliability prediction with the Palladio component model. IEEE Trans Softw Eng 38(6):1319–1339. doi:10.1109/TSE.2011.94
5. Si G, Ren Y, Xu J (2012) A dependability evaluation model for internetware based on Bayesian network. Comput Res Dev 49(5):1028–1038

6. Dai F, Li T, Xie Z (2012) Towards an algebraic semantics of software evolution process models. J Softw 23(4):846–863. doi:10.3724/SP.J.1001.2012.04160
7. Wu C, Liu J (2012) Deriving Markov chain usage model from UML model. Comput Res Dev 49(8):1811–1819

Chapter 340
Video Feedback Teaching Method in Teaching of Abdominal Physical Examination

Huihao Ma, Wang Bo, Juju Liu, Daoling Jian and Yuanlong Xie

Abstract To explore effects of video feedback teaching method on clinical skill teaching of abdomen physical examination in undergraduate clinical medicine specialty students. The 100 students of two small class, being selected from 09 grade clinical medicine specialty of China Three Gorges University, were randomly divided into observation group (video feedback teaching method, N = 50) and the control group (traditional teaching methods, N = 50). Three time video of abdomen physical examination completed by observation group students were collected. First video is primary ones taken by each other during 1st experimental skill trains, second video is the most satisfactory ones after repeated self practice within 3 weeks since the 1st train class, and final video is test ones taken by at the fifth weeks since the 1st training class and meanwhile, questionnaires for the students to be completed. In control group, only test video is taken and questionnaires to be completed at the same time. According to score evaluation criterion of the abdomen physical examination, the scores of first video is significantly lower than the most satisfactory ones in observation group. The students' numbers of after-class abdomen physical examination exercise is more in observation group than in control group. The scores of the test video is significantly higher in observation group than in control group. Questionnaires investigation of students show three major factors promoting video feedback teaching method are to promote students' self-control ability, improve the training equipment, renew education idea. Video feedback teaching method is a practical and

H. Ma · W. Bo · J. Liu · D. Jian (✉) · Y. Xie
The Second Clinical Medical College of China Three Gorges University,
Yichang 443001 Hubei, China
e-mail: 976760430@qq.com

H. Ma
e-mail: 502182322@qq.com

S. Li et al. (eds.), *Frontier and Future Development of Information Technology in Medicine and Education*, Lecture Notes in Electrical Engineering 269,
DOI: 10.1007/978-94-007-7618-0_340,

more effective teaching method in the clinical skills training for medical students compared with the traditional teaching method, it is worth to popularize in clinical skills teaching in medical college.

Keywords Video feedback teaching method · Clinical skills · Teaching reform

340.1 Introduction

Mastering basic clinical skills not only is one of the main contents for medical education of clinical medicine specialty students in China, but also is the basal demand of global minimum essential requirements in medical education (GMER) [1]. Therefore, teaching management and clinical teachers have given more and more attention to the teaching method of clinical skill drills and its effect for the students. In other countries' medical education, it has been confirmed that video feedback teaching method is a very effective and practical teaching method for improving cognitive competence, communication skills and clinical skills [2–4]. However, Video feedback teaching method is rarely used in the clinical skills training of medical schools in China. We use the video feedback teaching method in practice or experimental class of abdominal examination skills train among 09th grade clinical medical students, so as to investigate effect of the video feedback teaching method and feasibility to study the teaching effects and investigation analysis of video feedback teaching method for the clinical skills and analyze the possibility of applying this method in clinical skill training in Chinese medical education.

340.2 Object of Study and Method

340.2.1 Objects of Study

Two classes, 100 students, from 09th grade of clinical medicine specialty of the China Three Gorges University, were selected and divided into observation group and control group. Each group included equally 50 students and both groups have almost similar average age, class performance and gender proportion.

340.2.2 Method

340.2.2.1 Contents and Steps

We selected abdominal examination as investigation content and observed possible benefits induced by video feedback teaching method for the students. Teaching standards about abdominal examination are based on abdomen physical examination skills in textbook Diagnostics (Unified national medical colleges textbook, 7th version, People's Medical Publishing House).

Observation group applied video feedback teaching method. The research steps were as followed: 50 students were randomly divided into 8 learning groups, of which each at least equipped with a kind of video recording equipment. Teachers were required to teach standard abdominal physical examination skills, demonstrated these and played video of standard examination skills. Students should submit a first video of full operation after first experimental training lesson. Teachers choose randomly two pieces for videos submitted by the students, and teachers and students together review, analyze and point out deficiency of students' examination. Every student should keep their own operation video and practice the operation. Students were required to submit a most satisfactory video of abdomen physical examination 3 weeks after first experimental training lesson. A test was carried out 5 weeks after the first training. On the test, the students, who were randomly chosen and must completed item of the abdominal physical examination operation, were required to take a complete video of operation by each other, and anonymous questionnaires survey were given.

Control group apply traditional teaching method. Fifty medical students were also divided in 8 learning groups. In the first class, teachers taught the standard examination and demonstrated it. Students practiced in the learning groups, and teachers corrected their mistakes in their groups. The students randomly chosen and must completed the abdominal physical examination operation, were also required to take a complete video of the operation on the test, and anonymous questionnaires survey were also carried out as the same as those of observation group.

340.2.2.2 Score Assessment

Operation Assessment score standards were made according to unified national medical colleges textbook Diagnostics and assessment of certified doctors. Total scores is 50 points and details were as followed: communication (1 point), abdomen visual examination (5 points), abdomen palpation (basic skill 8 points, viscera palpation 14 points), abdomen percussion (basic skill 3 points, shifting dullness 3 points, and viscera percussion 8 points) abdomen auscultation (basic skill 3 points, bowel sound auscultation 3 points, abdomen vascular murmur auscultation 2 points).

Research members were trained to be familiar with score standards before assessing video. Blind method was used during score assessment of the videos.

Questionnaires of observation group is mainly concerned with application of video feedback teaching method, including evaluation of video feedback teaching method, matters needing attention for furthermore promoting video feedback teaching method, advantages and shortcomings of video feedback teaching method. Control group mainly focus on the feedback of traditional teaching method. In observation group 21 and in control group 16 Questionnaires were given and all of them were retrieved.

340.2.2.3 Statistical Processing

Comparison of final video scores between control and observation group was processed by randomized t-test. Scores comparison between first video and the most satisfactory video was also processed by paired t-test.

340.3 Results

340.3.1 Operation Scores

Scores of the first video was significantly higher than that of most satisfactory video in observation group ($p < 0.01$) (Table 340.1).

Final scores of observation group on the teat is significantly higher than that of control group ($p < 0.01$) (Table 340.2).

340.3.2 Questionnaires Survey

Numbers of after-class-practice times. Numbers of training after class were significantly more in the students of observation group (2.79 ± 0.787 times) than those in control group (1.50 ± 1.317 times), P = 0.002.

Satisfaction and evaluate about video feedback teaching method. Here are these four questions for answer with only yes or no. First, are you satisfied with video feedback teaching method? Second, are you interested in video feedback teaching method? Third, do you think video feedback teaching method can supervise and urge you to practice after class? Finally, do you think it is worthy to promote video feedback teaching method in clinical skill teaching? All the answers of 21 students for four questions are yes.

Table 340.1 Scores comparison between first video and most satisfactory video in observation group ($\bar{x} \pm s$)

	First video (N = 50)	Satisfying video (=50)	t	P
Grade	23.58 ± 6.968	35.14 ± 3.736	−11.060	0.000

Table 340.2 Comparison of final video scores between control group and observation group ($\bar{x} \pm s$)

	Observation group (N = 21)	Control group (n = 16)	t	P
Scores	34.275 ± 3.6759	23.094 ± 7.9040	5.225	0.000

Table 340.3 advantages and disadvantages of video feedback teaching method in clinical skill teaching(N = 21)

Advantages	Disadvantages
To improve proficiency of clinic skills (18 students)	A waste of too much time and energy (15 students)
To improve initiative and enthusiasm in learning (15 students)	Lack of resources and being inconvenient to shoot videos (14 students)
To help us find out our mistakes and defects (10 students)	Direction instruct from teachers decrease (7 students)

About some matters of needing to be solved for better spreading video feedback teaching method. In questionnaires, there were three questions. First, Should students and teachers renew their teaching concept about self-learning oriented method? Twelve students answered yes. Second, Should students have a better ability of self-control to adapt to video feedback teaching method? Fifteen students answered yes. Third, Should the college have better camera equipment? Thirteen students answered yes.

About advantages and disadvantages of video feedback teaching method in clinical skill teaching (The results of questionnaires are as followed Table 340.3).

340.4 Discussion

Video feedback teaching method is a practical and effective method in clinical skill teaching [5]. In our investigation, the scores of most satisfactory video was higher in the observation group than that of first video. Students' operation video could record their operation process and the students can review it can find their mistakes and deficiency of their examination, and then improve it [6, 2]. At the same time, students within a group can point out other members' mistakes interactively. Thus, students can have a deeper understanding of not only their own examination skills, but also their common mistakes. This deep understanding can improve proficiency of clinic skills, and at the same time help others by pointing out the similar mistakes exist in other students' examination. Thus, it enhances students' consciousness of learning and team work, which lead to a result of improvement in learning and collaboration [7].

Because of lacking of accuracy when students recall their operation procedures in traditional teaching method, video feedback is better comparative to traditional teaching method [8]. All these effects work together to get a great effect of helping students in learning and training clinical skills [9].

Video feedback teaching method is a promoted-worthy method in clinic teaching. The method is a method that students love very much, and inspire students' interesting in learning clinic skill, and is well-accepted by them. In a survey about satisfaction, interesting, and whether it is worthy of promoting the method, all 21 students hold a positive opinion. But most importantly, when submitting examination video and assessing, not only is it convenient for students to develop a habit of analyzing feedback video and makes teachers have an overall evaluation of their student and have an improvement in teaching. So video feedback teaching method is promoted-worthy in clinical education.

The results showed that most students said the ability of self-control was an important matters in promoting video feedback teaching method because this method is mainly about self-control and it helps students in reviewing, feeding back, analyzing, correcting [6], which need students have a good ability of self-control. Moreover, camera device function is popular, which provide a good situation for promotion. Suggestions were also given to clinic skill teaching center and teachers about paying more attention to students' skill training and their initiative, enthusiasm, their ability of learning and upgrade of camera devise provided by clinic center. Thus, this method can become a more easily accepted and loved one.

There are still some matters needing attention for furthermore promoting video feedback teaching method. Questionnaire survey showed that video feedback teaching method was good for students to find out their mistakes and improve proficiency of abdomen examination skills. However, some students pointed out some disadvantages of video feedback teaching method. For example, some students wasted too much time in taking videos rather than practicing. It can be believed that with promotion of this teaching method, students can understand the main objective of the video is applicable for reviewing, feedback, analysis, correction, which means video itself is just a medium and it is accuracy of recording operation process that matters.

In short, video feedback teaching method is a well-accepted teaching method and especially suitable for clinical skills teaching. Therefore, it is worth to popularize in clinical skills teaching in medical education in China.

References

1. Wang X, Li J, Li L (2009) Current situation of medical education evaluation. Explor Med Educ 8(9):1150
2. Scherer LA, Chang MC, Meredith JW et al (2003) Videotape review leads to rapid and sustained learning. Am J Surg 185(6):516–520
3. Olsen JC, Gurr DE (2000) Video analysis of emergency medicine residents performing rapid-sequence intubations. J Emerg Med 18(4):469–472
4. Minardi HA, Ritter S (1999) Recording skills practice on videotape can enhance learning: a comparative study between nurse lecturers and nursing students. J Adv Nurs 29(6):1318–1325
5. Zick A, Granieri M, Makoul G (2007) First-year medical students' assessment of their own communication skills: A video-based, open-ended approach. Patient Educ Couns 68(2):161–166

6. Crook A, Mauchline A, Maw S et al (2012) The use of video technology for providing feedback to students: can it enhance the feedback experience for staff and students. Comput Educ 58(1):386–396
7. Li L, Li H, Zhang Q (2009) Applications of video feedback teaching method in nurse clinical training. J Nurs Sci 24(2):23–24
8. Gage M, Polatajko H (1994) Enhancing occupation performance through an understanding of perceived self-efficacy. Am J Occup Ther 48:452–461
9. Xeroulis GJ, Park J, Moulton C et al (2007) Teaching suturing and knot-tying skills to medical students: a randomized controlled study comparing computer-based video instruction and (concurrent and summary) expert feedback. Surgery 141(4):442–449
10. Chetwynd F, Dobbyn C (2011) Assessment, feedback and marking guides in distance education. Open Learn 26(1):67
11. Wieling MB, Hofman WHA (2010) The impact of online video lecture recordings and automated feedback on student performance. Comput Educ 54(4):992–998

Chapter 341
Evaluation of EHR in Health Care in China: Utilizing Fuzzy AHP in SWOT Analysis

Ying Xiang and Jinchang Li

Abstract EHR has been introduced into China for years. Many cities are leaping into adopting EHR while some others are lagging behind in the use of it or in efficiently use of it, not to mention backward rural areas. In order to find out the reasons, Strengths, Weaknesses, Opportunities and Threats (SWOT) analysis is utilized in this paper. As SWOT analysis possesses deficiencies in the measurement and evaluation steps, the fuzzy AHP is utilized. The results were presented in an illustrative way by utilizing the quantitative information achieved by the hybrid method. The results indicated that EHR could be adopted and the most important factors in the EHR are Growing Demand for Medical and Health, The growth of health care spending, Personalized Service and Quality of Care.

Keywords Electronic Health Record (EHR) · SWOT · Fuzzy AHP

341.1 Introduction

Although the concept of EHR is not fixed, its characteristics of electronic storage and instant availability of information to authorized practitioners are widely accepted by scholars around the world. With technology being used in every walk of life, more and more countries are looking into implementing EHR in health management. EHR offers potential advantages over paper for the storage and retrieval of patients' data and one of the studies indicated the systems could save

---

Y. Xiang (✉) · J. Li
School of Statistics, Zhejiang Gongshang University, Hangzhou 310018, People's Republic of China
e-mail: yingxiang0571@hotmail.com

J. Li
School of Management, Zhejiang Chinese Medical University, Hangzhou 310053, People's Republic of China

S. Li et al. (eds.), *Frontier and Future Development of Information Technology in Medicine and Education*, Lecture Notes in Electrical Engineering 269,
DOI: 10.1007/978-94-007-7618-0_341,

up to $81 billion in healthcare costs annually [1]. The overall status and the effects of EHR systems are topics of growing interest to researchers. Minal Thakkar and Diane C Davis [2] found out the risks, barriers and benefits of EHRs by the investigation in hospitals in the USA. A recent study conducted by Nahid Tavakoli, Maryam Jahanbakhsh [3] divided the opportunities of EHR implementation into two categories: clinical opportunities and financial opportunities. Knut Bernsteina, Morten Bruun-Rasmussena et al. [4] analyzed the challenges of using different information models and integration platforms in EHR.

EHR has been introduced into China for years. In order to identify the strengths, opportunities, weaknesses and threats of using EHR systems in China, SWOT analysis was used. And fuzzy AHP was utilized in this paper to provide an analytical means to determine the relative importance of the factors.

341.2 Outline for Applying Fuzzy AHP in SWOT Analysis

Fuzzy analytic hierarchical (Fuzzy AHP) process is able to solve uncertain 'fuzzy' problems and to rank excluded factors according to their weight ratios. The advantages and disadvantages between different fuzzy AHP methods can be seen from Mahammad Haghighi, Ali Divandari and Masoud Keimasi [5]. In this paper, we prefer Chang's extent analysis method [6]. The method introduced proceeds as follows:

341.2.1 SWOT Analysis is Carried Out

Our case study communities are in Zhejiang province, which is situated in eastern China. As one of the dominant economic provinces in China, health care has been paid more attention by the public and EHR is introduced to Zhejiang province rather earlier than many other provinces of the nation (Fig. 341.1).

Until the end of 2011, 12,000,000 citizens' electronic health records have been set up in Zhejiang province [7] Although EHR develops fast in Zhejiang, there are still weaknesses and threats when applying EHR in health care. We organized an investigation from July 22th to August 10th 2012. In the course of which a SWOT analysis was performed and the key factors concerning the strategic option were collected on the basis of 150 responses.

341.2.2 The Weight of Each Factor is Determined

Step 1 Establish the comparison matrix.

Step 2 Let the evaluation system including n indicators, 6 scholars participated the assessing: $m_i = \prod_{j=1}^{n} a_{ij}$, i = 1, 2,..., n

STRENGTHS	OPPORTUNITIES
+ Personalized Service +Exchanging Patient Information Electronically with Hospitals or other Medical Institutions +Quality of Care +Work Efficiency and Time Management +Saving Cost of Care	+Growing Demand for Medical and Health + The growth of health care spending +Self-Awareness of Health Care and Health Management +Development of Health Care Industry
WEAKNESSES	**THREATS**
- Technological backwardness - Lack of Medical Information Talent -Shortage of Financial Support - Over Reliance on EHR System	-Security of data -Privacy of data (access control) - Imperfect Standards and Legal issues

Fig. 341.1 A result of SWOT analysis for EHR in China

Step 3 Get the quartic root of Mi: $w_i = \sqrt[n]{m_i}$

Step 4 The weights $\bar{W} = (\bar{w}_1, \bar{w}_2, \cdots, \bar{w}_n)^T$ could be obtained by the following formula: $\bar{w}_i = w_i \Big/ \sum_{i=1}^{n} w_i$,

Step 5 Calculate the eigenvalue of $\lambda_{\max}$ as: $\lambda_{\max} = \frac{1}{n}\sum_{i=1}^{n} (A\overline{W}/\overline{w_i})$

Step 6 To keep the consistency of the judgment matrix, its consistency should be tested. Defining CI as: $CI = (\lambda_{\max} - n)/(n-1)$.

The bigger CI was, the worse consistency the matrix had. Then, the consistency ratio (CR) is calculated as follows: $CR = CI/RI$.

When CR was less than 0.10, the matrix had a reasonable consistency. Otherwise the matrix should be changed.

The values of weights with respect to SWOT group are calculated as below:

$W_g = (0.28\ 0.16\ 0.46\ 0.10)^T$

$\lambda_{g\max} = 4.04$; CIg $= 0.011$; CRg $= 0.01 < 0.1$

In a similar way, the weights of SWOT Factors are calculated as follows:

$\bar{W}_s = (0.32\ 0.14\ 0.32\ 0.06\ 0.16)^T$ $\lambda_{s\max} = 5.30$; CIs $= 0.08$; CRs $= 0.07$

$\bar{W}_w = (0.49\ 0.16\ 0.29\ 0.06)^T$ $\lambda_{w\max} = 4$; CIw $= 0$; CRw $= 0$

$\bar{W}_o = (0.48\ 0.25\ 0.18\ 0.09)^T$ $\lambda_{o\max} = 4.20$; CIo $= 0.07$; CR0 $= 0.08$

$\bar{W}_t = (0.65\ 0.23\ 0.12)^T$ $\lambda_{t\max} = 3.04$; CIt $= 0.018$; CRt $= 0.03$

All of the SWOT factors' CI are less than 0.10. To make comparisons among factors within the same hierarchy more convenient Table 341.1 shows all of the priority weights driven from the calculations explained above (see Table 341.1).

Positive factors predominated: all the five of the biggest global priorities represented strengths or opportunities (Table 1.3). The whole situation is easily observed by referring to Fig. 341.2.

Table 341.1 Priorities of the SWOT groups and factors carried out in a session by 6 scholars

SWOT group	Weights	SWOT factors	Local weights	Global weights
Strengths	0.28	Personalized service	0.32	0.090
		Exchanging patient information Electronically with hospitals or other medical institutions	0.14	0.039
		Quality of care	0.32	0.090
		Work efficiency and time management	0.06	0.017
		Saving cost of care	0.16	0.045
Weakness	0.16	Technological backwardness	0.49	0.078
		Lack of medical information talent	0.16	0.026
		Shortage of financial support	0.29	0.046
		Over reliance on EHR system	0.06	0.010
Opportunities	0.46	Growing demand for medical and health	0.48	0.221
		The growth of health care spending	0.25	0.115
		Self-awareness of health care and health management	0.18	0.082
		Development of health care industry	0.09	0.041
Threats	0.10	Security of data	0.65	0.065
		Privacy of data (access control)	0.23	0.023
		Imperfect standards and legal issues	0.12	0.012

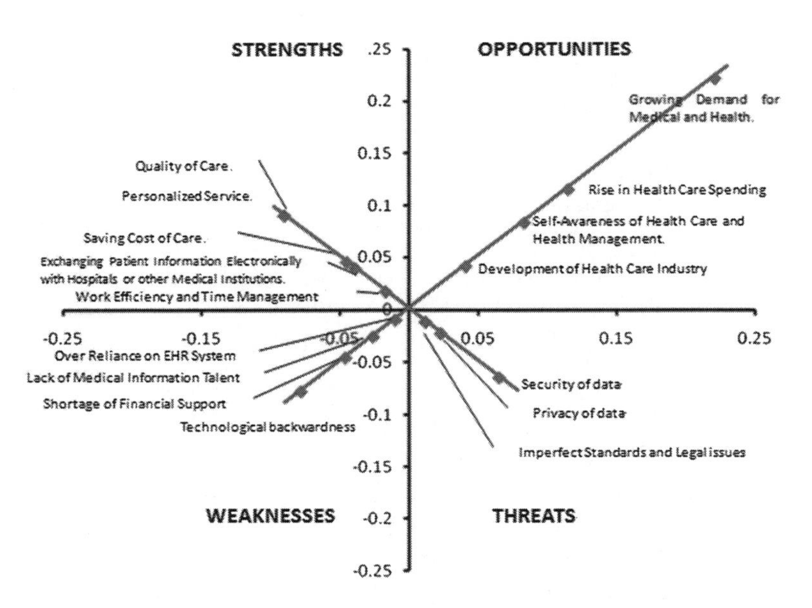

Fig. 341.2 A result of SWOT analysis for EHR in China graphical interpretation of the results of utilizing fuzzy AHP in SWOT groups and factors (the factors are arranged in such a way that the factor possessing the highest global priority is the outermost point)

The lengths of the lines in the different sectors point out that the strengths and opportunities predominate. The implemented analysis suggests that based on factors that significantly describe the health care in China, EHR could be adopted. It points out the most important factors in the EHR are Growing Demand for Medical and Health, The growth of health care spending, Personalized Service and Quality of Care.

341.3 Conclusions

In this study, a common strategic planning tool, SWOT, was used in the study concerning evaluation of EHR in health care in China. Although SWOT is in common use as a planning tool, it is not capable of quantitatively determining the weights and effects of the factors. In this study, we linked SWOT with a decision analysis method (fuzzy AHP), which can avoided SWOT's weaknesses and help to use SWOT more effectively.

According to the experiences of this study, the results of the combined use of fuzzy AHP and SWOT analysis were promising. The results of our study were presented in an illustrative way, which is often needed to clarify the interactions of numerous and contradictory factors.

References

1. Hillestad R, Bigelow J, Bower A, Girosi F, Meili R, Scoville R, Taylor R (2005) Can electronic medical record systems transform health care? Potential health benefits, savings, and costs. Health Aff 24(5):1103–1117
2. Thakkar M, Davis DC (2006).Risks, barriers, and benefits of EHR systems: a comparative study based on size of hospital. Perspect Health Inf Manage (Published online 14 Aug 2006) PMCID:PMC2047303
3. Tavakoli N, Jahanbakhsh M, Mokhtari H, Tadayon HR (2011) Opportunities of electronic health record implementation in Isfahan. Procedia Comput Sci 3:1195–1198
4. Bernstein K, Bruun-Rasmussen M et al (2005) Modelling and implementing electronic health records in Denmark. Int J Med Inform 74:213–220
5. Haghighi M, Divandari A, Keimasi M (2010) The impact of 3D e-readiness on e-banking development in Iran: a fuzzy AHP analysis. Expert Syst Appl 37:4084–4093
6. Chang D-Y (1996) Applications of the extent analysis method on fuzzy AHP. Eur J Oper Res 95:649–655
7. Sheng J, Zhang Z (2012) The history and current situation of electronic health records of Zhejiang province. Chin J Health Inform Manage 9(3):84–87 (in Chinese)
8. Yuksel I, Dagdeviren M (2007) Using the analytic network process (ANP) in a SWOT analysis: a case study for a textile firm. Inf Sci 177:3364–3382

Chapter 342
A Method of Computing the Hot Topics' Popularity on the Internet Combined with the Features of the Microblogs

Yongqing Wei, Zhen Zhang, Shaodong Fei and Wentao Du

Abstract The article puts forward a new formula of computing the popularity of the topics, which is based on the stream of the news on the internet. What's more, the features of the microblogs should be also considered and combined. The hot topics are sorted by the values of them, so the information of the topics is convenient and accurate to be acquired for the public. It is beneficial to the government to supervise the public opinion as well. The experiments are based on both news and the microblogs. Our system could figure out the value of the hot topics by the popularity among users, after that the topics will be sorted automatically. The results of the experiments have shown that the system worked well.

Keywords Hot topic · Topic popularity · Microblogging-features · The formula of computing the topic popularity

Y. Wei (✉)
Basic Education Department, Shandong Police College, Jinan 250014, China
e-mail: weiyongqing1963@126.com

Z. Zhang · W. Du
School of Information Science and Engineering, Shandong Normal University, Jinan 250014, China

Z. Zhang · W. Du
Shandong Provincial Key Laboratory for Novel Distributed Computer Software Technology, Jinan 250014, China

S. Fei
Shandong University of Finance and Economics, Jinan 250014, China

S. Li et al. (eds.), *Frontier and Future Development of Information Technology in Medicine and Education*, Lecture Notes in Electrical Engineering 269,
DOI: 10.1007/978-94-007-7618-0_342,

342.1 Introduction

With the rapid development of the internet, the influence of the internet media is becoming more and more important to guide the public opinion and affect the public in turn. The large impact of the internet is reflected by its widely raged applications. Until the end of the June, 2012, the number of the Chinese net users has risen to 538 millions, the penetration of the internet is 39.9 % [1]. Especially with the arrival of the web 2.0 technology, the participatory role of the users is fully embodied. At the present stage, Chinese web users have reached an unprecedented level of speech activity, a number of hot topics are sourced from the internet, the power of the participated users cannot be overlooked [2].

The hot topics detection is the practical application of the topic detection and tracking. TDT is an technology of the information processing that aims at the streaming media information to recognize the unknown topics and track the known [3]. Its target is to find the hot topics from the news report streaming information in order to provide convenience for the government to monitor and guide the public opinion in the internet.

342.2 Related Research

There are many studies on the hot topics currently, but how to get the measure of topic popularity is a unique work for the hot topics detection [4, 5].

The research studied on abroad is relatively earlier and more mature. Martijin raised the approach based on language model to find the topics, the representation and the similarity computing of the document are both based on the language model [6]. David put the named entities to the system to help determine whether the sub-topics belong to the same conversation [7].

The research studied in our country started relatively later. Ting ting He analyzed the graph of the popular words trend, concluded the feature of the popular words, made quantity by this and got the formula of making quantity of the popular words popularity. Make use of the formula to get the popularity of every candidate's words and finally get the popular words [8]. In the research of the hot topic detection written by Ya ping Luo, the model considered not only the attention of the media but also the attention combination of the users. It mostly pointed at the news reports and the feedback of the users. The system of hot event detection designed by Xing xing Liu is towards the reports flu of the internet. The corpus is divided into different groups by the time, getting the micro class through agglomerative clustering, selecting all the micro classes of some period of time, making single-pass clustering to get the event list, calculating the candidate events to get the popularity values though formula of events popularity, finally sorting the values. It can find the hot events on the internet at any time [9].

342.3 Problem Analysis

Considering the considerable research and the feature of the hot topics detection, the hot topics detection is facing the following problems:

(1) The definition of the hot topics mainly involves the news corpus. However, the important role the users play in the formation of the hot topics is obvious at present, which deserves our consideration. So judging a hot topic in the hot equation needs the consideration about the user attitude, which is neglected almost in relevant research.
(2) The hot topics of the different period of time are clearly different. And the popularity values are also dynamic, which requires us to design a system to automatically discover the hot topics of the different time periods and the popularity sorting according to user needs, so as to facilitate users to understand the hot topic in a different time.

In this paper, we consider both from the media and users, and propose a method of automatically discovering the hot topic of the arbitrary time period according to news reports and microblogs. We use the popularity calculation formula to assess hot topics and get the popularity value. Next, sort the topics according the popularity value. Finally, we get the sorting of the hot topics within any period of time, which is easy for people to keep abreast of the latest, and hottest topics. Meanwhile, it is beneficial for government departments to monitor and guide network public opinion.

342.4 Hot Topic Detection and the Method of Topic Popularity Calculation

342.4.1 Basic Ideas and Processes of the Hot Topic Detection

The discovery process of the hot topic must take into account the behaviors of the user. The user's behaviors to some extent reflect their potential psychological state, and at present, the twitter is the best way which can reflect the user's behavior. In this section, we firstly overview of the basic ideas and processes of public opinion monitoring system, focusing on the popularity calculation and making selective analysis and elaboration.

The specific steps of the hot topic detection are stated as followed:

Step 1 Collect the news reports from the portal site. Next, classify them with the field of headline, content, publish time, resource, etc. And put into the news table of the database; Likewise, the microblogs gathered from the Web site Sina.com are classified similarly then to be kept in the Weibo table.

Step 2 Processing of the corpus: deal with the acquisition of the news content as followed: segmentation, text preprocessing, feature extraction and so on. What's more, the topic models are adopted the vector representation.

Step 3 Topic clustering: the method of the topic clustering is adopted the Single-pass incremental clustering algorithm to calculate the similarity of documents and models.

Step 4 After the cluster, make the topic category of news table, the reports number of topic category, the each report of each category, the release time and the links of the site to display in the textbox window.

Step 5 Extraction of the subject terms: extract the topic whose field of Hot-if is one, then save the topic number. For each topic, match the topic number with the point of news table. Save the corresponding text and title of the successful matched news for segmentation and count the word frequency. Considering the representation of nouns, extract the five nouns of the higher frequency of the news title as the subjects.

Step 6 News tracking: extract the whole news whose tracking field is NULL, compute the similarity with the hot news model (adopting the cosine similarity computing of the vector space model). For the topic whose similarity value is highest, set the Hot-if field as one. The Topic ID field is set as the topic number of the biggest similarity, and the Tracked field as one. If all the similarity values are less than or equal to the threshold which is tentative 0.3, just set the Tracked field as one.

Step 7 Topics' popularity calculation: calculate the popularity of the topics gathered from the previous steps through the formula of topics popularity.

342.4.2 Calculation of the Topics Popularity Value

Considering the network news coverage and the amount of the twitter users comprehensively, firstly, generalize the characteristic that can affect the topic popularity, and then to get the computing formula of the topic popularity.

The news report ratio of the subject is divided into the proportion of reporting time and reporting accounts. The proportion of reporting time is defined as followed: in some period of time (such as the period the users selected), making the day as the unit, the ratio is the result of the valid days dividing the total days about some topic. In that definition, the valid days of some topic are referred to the reporting accounts about which one topic is bigger than a specific value which is given by the actual situation. The bigger the proportion of reporting time is, the more attention the accounts of the topic get. The proportion of the reporting accounts is defined as followed: in some period of time, the value is equal to the accounts of one topic' reports divided by the accounts of all the topics' reports. The bigger the value is, the more likely to be a hot one the topic becomes.

The microblog is also dealed in the same method. The microblogging proportion of the publishing time is defined as followed: In some period of time, making the day as the unit, the ratio is equal to the value of the valid accounts of the days divided by the total accounts of the days about the same topic. The bigger the value is, the more attention the relative topic get. So the relative topic is more likely to be the hot topic. The proportion of the publishing accounts of the microblog is defined as followed: in some period of time, the value is equal to the accounts of one topic' relative microblog divided by the accounts of all the topics' relative microblogs. The bigger the value is, the more likely to be a hot topic the relative topic is.

Thus, we conclude the formula to get the two value of the ratio. We use Ratio_1 and Ratio_2 to represent respectively the ratio of time and the ratio of accounts. According to the aforementioned statement, we get the following two formulas:

$$\mathrm{Ratio}_1 = \frac{n_1}{N} \tag{342.1}$$

$$\mathrm{Ratio}_2 = \frac{\sum_{j=1}^{n} df_{ij}/df_j}{n} \tag{342.2}$$

In the formula 342.1, n_i represents the valid days and the N represents the total days. In the formula 342.2, df_{ij} represents the accounts of the topic i in the day of j. df_j represents the accounts of the total topics.

Based on the two above factors, we assume that the day i viewed as the valid reporting day when the number of the reporting number of the event i is bigger than the threshold. Likely, the day is viewed as the valid when the number of the relative microblog is bigger than the threshold. For the different hot topics, we conclude the formula of computing the hot value of the topic i, and the formula is:

$$T_i = a \times \mathrm{newstdi} \times \mathrm{newsddi} + b \times \mathrm{weibotdi} \times \mathrm{weibddi} \tag{342.3}$$

In that formula, the newstdi represents as the proportion of the reporting accounts of the event i in the period time when the users are selected, and the newsddi represents as the proportion of the reporting time of the event i. Equally, the weibotdi is represented as the proportion of the weibo' publishing time of the relative topic and the weiboddi is represented as the proportion of the weibo' publishing number of the relative topic. The a and b are the adjustment coefficient. Tested by some experiments, the a is selected as 0.7 and the b is selected as 0.3.

342.5 Hot Topic Detection and the Method of Topic Popularity Calculation

342.5.1 The Experimental Resource

In order to evaluate the performance of the system accurately, resource is gathered from the portal sites, and the microblogs ones from the sina blogs. In the experiment, we gather partial news and microblogs of the ones from the time between the Aug 3 to the Aug 9 2012. Rately, the resources of the experiments included the news resource and the microblogs resource.

342.5.2 The Procedure of the Experiment

According the resources gathered, we select one day and one week to conduct the experiments.

The experimental results of one day are showed in the Tables 342.1 and 342.2.

The experimental results of one week are showed in the Tables 342.3 and 342.4.

342.5.3 Analysis of the Experimental Results

For the hot topics detected automatically by the system, there hasn't a unified testing standard. In the paper, we compare the hot topics detected by the system

Table 342.1 Hot topics from web sites in one day

Order	Hot topics
1	Effect of typhoon on the country and response measures
2	The incident of He bei train hit and cause 9 death and 4 injuries
3	Central invited experts and representatives of grass roots talent to Beidaihe vacation
4	Around dealing with storm disaster in Beijing
5	The case of Hunan Yong zhou young girls forced into prostitution

Table 342.2 Hot topics towards news and microblogs in one day

Order	Hot topics	Popularity value (%)
1	Effect of typhoon on the country and response measures	23.63
2	Around dealing with storm disaster in Beijing	20.03
3	The incident of Hebei train hit and cause 9 death and 4 injuries	18.95
4	The case of Hunan Yongzhou young girls forced into prostitution	15.66
5	A plant explosion in Wenzhou	12.53

Table 342.3 Hot topics from web sites in one week

Order	Hot topics
1	Typhoon anemones
2	The Liu Zhijun corruption case
3	13 provinces and cities in the effectiveness of medical reform: the dilemma of "see a doctor expensively"
4	China was not represented at the commemoration of the atomic bombings in Japan
5	Yunnan Qiaojia bombings: Zhao Teng used be used to act as suicide bombers

Table 342.4 Hot topics towards news and microblogs in one week

Order	Hot topics	Popularity value (%)
1	Typhoon anemones	22.51
2	The Liu Zhijun corruption case	13.5
3	The yong girl of Hunan forced into prostitution case continued	12.26
4	13 provinces and cities in the effectiveness of medical reform: the dilemma of "see a doctor expensively"	10.20
5	More than 450 people were trapped in Benxi high-speed rail tunnel	10.12

with the ones gathered from the main portal sites. Through contrasting the results of the experiments, we can find some advantages of our system.

The hot topics are ordered by the popularity value, then the users can get the information of the topics clearly. Comparing with the hot information got from other portal sites, it is more specific for the users to grasp.

The hot topics detected by the system are more comprehensive. They are based on both web news and microblogs, the data source of which contains web medias and users. Combing the two main factors, the hot topics in your system are more exact and persuade.

342.6 Conclusion

The article is based on the news and combined the features of the microblogs, considering the effect of the hot topics from both the media and the users. The system can get the order of the values of the hot topics by the topic popularity computing formula in any period of time. It is convenient for the audience to get the hot topics. Meanwhile, it is useful for the government to grasp the hot topics and know the public opinion and correctly control that.

Acknowledgments This research was supported by the National Natural Science Foundation of China (No. 60873247), National Social Science Fund (12BXW040) and the Natural Science Foundation of Shandong Province of China (No. ZR2012FM038).

References

1. CNNIC (2012) 30th China internet development statistics report. Beijing
2. Li H, Zhang H (2009) The network hot topic detection based on the subject. In: Fifth national conference on information retrieval
3. The 2004 Topic Detection and Tracking (TDT2004) (2004) Task definition and evaluation plan. version 1.0, 5 August 2004
4. Ye H, Chen W, Dai GZ (2006) Design and implementation of on-line hot discovery model. Wuhan Univ J Nat Sci 11(1):21–26
5. Allan J (2002) Introduction to topic detection and tracking: event-based information organization. Kluwer Academic Publishers, Boston, pp 1–16
6. Spitters M, Kraaij W (2001) TNO at TDT2001: language model-based topic detection. In: Proceedings of TDT 2001 workshop
7. Smith DA (2002) Detecting and browsing events in unstructured text. In: The 25th annual ACM SIGIR conference, Finland
8. He T, Yi Z, Yong Z (2006) Study on computer-aided popular words and prases extraction based on words' attributes. J Chin Inf Process 20(6):38–45
9. Liu X, He T, Gong H, Chen L (2008) The design of the system of the network hot events detection. J Chin Inf Process 22(6):80–85

Chapter 343
The Value of CBL Autonomous Learning Style for the Postgraduate of Medical Imageology: Promoting Professional Knowledge Learning Based on the PACS

Peng Dong, Ding Wei-yi, Wang Bin, Wang Xi-zhen, Long Jin-feng, Zhu Hong and Sun Ye-quan

Abstract *Aims* This thesis is to explore the new mode which improves medical imaging masters' professional knowledge acquisition through the application of CBL autonomous learning mode based on PACS teaching system. *Methods* 12 full-time postgraduates of medical imageology from level 2004 to 2005 are selected as experimental group. The research platform is PACS in campus teaching system. The professional knowledge teaching and studying process is realized through the CBL teaching method combined with independent teaching studying mode. The evaluation index is based on questionaries and quizes. *Results* Through this mode of learning, the postgraduate students' professional knowledge scores of theory and practice are higher than the control group's obviously. The difference was statistically significant ($P < 0.05$). *Conclusion* The CBL autonomous learning mode based on PACS teaching system does well to postgraduates of medical imageology in grasping professional knowledge better, and it can effectively improve the postgraduate students' self-study ability and the ability of using knowledge comprehensively.

Keywords Postgraduates' education · PACS · CBL · Autonomous learning

P. Dong (✉) · W. Bin · W. Xi-zhen · L. Jin-feng · S. Ye-quan
Imaging Center of Affiliated Hospital, Weifang Medical University, Weifang, People's Republic of China
e-mail: dongpeng98021@sina.com

D. Wei-yi · Z. Hong
Department of Foreign Languages, Weifang Medical University, 261031 Weifang, People's Republic of China

S. Li et al. (eds.), *Frontier and Future Development of Information Technology in Medicine and Education*, Lecture Notes in Electrical Engineering 269,
DOI: 10.1007/978-94-007-7618-0_343,

343.1 Introduction

The professional knowledge teaching to postgraduate is different from that to the undergraduate. Most of the postgraduates of medical imageology have certain knowledge of clinical medicine and medical imaging. Study at post graduate level is the extension and expansion of undergraduate course education. The learning of professional knowledge on medical imageology is more systematic. In addition to the traditional methods such as lectures, seminars, various new teaching methods constantly emerges in recent years. In order to improve the postgraduate students' self-study ability and their ability to use knowledge comprehensively, it is wise to apply CBL autonomous learning mode based on campus PACS teaching system. It has been proved that it greatly enhanced the professional knowledge learning of the postgraduates of medical imageology.

343.2 Materials and methods

We respectively picked up 12 full-time professional postgraduates of medical imageology from level 2004 to 2005 as research objects. The 2005 level is treated as experimental group using the CBL autonomous learning group while 2004 level treated as the control group. Specific plans are arranged to make sure the theoretical study and clinical practice of experimental group do not conflict with CBL autonomous learning. With the help of the school teaching of PACS system, the autonomous learning group has CBL lectures to learn independently once a week. Post-graduate students are required to make teaching courseware independently. Firstly, the postgraduates make preparations of 3–5 correlated issues aiming directly at a case/group or some kind of/set diseases, then they are given time to discuss with other students. Secondly, after the film reading of a case or group or some kind/set of diseases, the postgraduates introduce and summarize the basic types, imaging findings and physiopathology and other related knowledge, clinical manifestations, and the latest research dynamic, etc. Through the supplemental discussions and expanding exercises on PACS in campus teaching system, students can discuss questions and communicate with each other freely. It is high recommended to arrange a tutor to take responsibility for error correction, guidance and comment on the performance of all postgraduate students every time. At the same time in different classrooms or labs, students of the control group learn and read in a traditional way. This process of different study goes on for four semesters.

We evaluate the teaching result by undertaking expertise integration testing during the intermediate stage and before graduation respectively. We use statistical software SPSS 13.0 to do statistics analysis. At the same time, questionaires are distributed to students, teachers and tutors to analyse and evaluate the pros and cons of this kind of teaching method.

343.3 Result

Through the CBL autonomous learning, the postgraduate students' professional knowledge scores of theory and practice are higher than the control group's obviously. The difference was statistically significant ($P < 0.05$). Through the result of questionnaire, it is found that the teachers and students who support this teaching mode accounted for 100 and 98.75 %. All the teachers and students believe that this teaching mode is beneficial to the learning of professional knowledge. It is conducive to improve the postgraduate students' self-study ability. It is effective to urge the students to consult literature initiatively and it is beneficial to review the knowledge about the medical imaging. Learning becomes more targeted and practical by the help of this method (Table 343.1).

343.4 Discussion

343.4.1 PACS CBL Autonomous Learning Mode Promotes Postgraduates' Study

CBL autonomous learning mode based on PACS can improve the utilization rate of resources. Based on PACS PBL teaching network, autonomous learning models do not take up the hospital equipment and working hours and don't conflict with clinical work. Postgraduates majoring clinical imageology can apply the teaching resources of PACS system to make the courseware production, to expand the practice, to carry on the comparison to cases, to carry on post-processing and retrospective analysis and to make full use of the existing teaching facilities and resources.

CBL autonomous learning model based on PACS can improve postgraduate students' self-learning ability. First of all, students in the process of learning are more likely to prepare the problem of preparation. In preparation, postgraduate students will actively review related clinical intelligence and the basis of professional knowledge. Students need to consult relevant literature focused on the latest developments in research. At the same time, in order to prepare questions and film reading expansion, students have to take the initiative to examine the correlated

Table 343.1 The comparison in theoretical test and practice skill performance between two groups

Group	Results of theoretical test			Results of clinical skill examination		
	$\bar{x} \pm s$	T	P	$\bar{x} \pm s$	t	P
CBL autonomous learning group	94.03 ± 5.46	4.33	<0.05	97.35 ± 10.24	6.52	<0.05
Control group	88.71 ± 8.53			90.06 ± 12.95		

cases of particular disease to carry out comparison and differential diagnosis. According to the questionnaire, postgraduate students in the process of preparing will actively turn to students or teachers for guidance and help. This model can fully mobilize the postgraduate student's subjective motility, and can also improve their learning initiative and subsequent learning ability.

CBL autonomous learning mode based on PACS can improve postgraduate student's ability to use knowledge comprehensively. In the process of teaching preparation, the main speakers tend to acquire the elementary knowledge, the latest research development of the diseases consulting textbooks and references. Then they are likely to analyze and make courseware which can greatly improve students' understanding of professional intelligence and understanding. Students who are asked to answer specific questions are more likely to acquire knowledge in the process of answering and thinking. The students as audience in reflecting process will of course have the chance to grasp related knowledge. In the progress of questioning and film reading, we use theory to guide practical reading effectively, which has greatly improved their ability of clinical practice. Discussions among students and teachers may also be helpful to promote the professional skills on all sides.

CBL autonomous learning mode based on PACS is more likely to elevate and promote students' computer proficiency and also promote the ability of expressing and adopting. The result of PBL questionnaire indicates that at the time of graduation thesis oral defense, the answers of autonomous learning postgraduate students are much more professional. Due to the professional training at the postgraduate stage, postgraduates of clinical imageology are confident on thesis oral defense and this is especially helpful in the future work and study for them.

343.4.2 PACS CBL Autonomous Learning Mode Promotes Teaching Skills

In teaching process, the CBL autonomous learning mode based on PACS puts forward a higher request to the existing PACS teaching system. CBL autonomous learning mode based on PACS puts forward a higher request for existing teaching resources. Some rare cases, typical and non-typical cases comparison of performance are still needed in addition to the common diseases and frequently-occurring diseases. It is safe to say that students promote us to add, update and improve unceasingly in the practical application.

The CBL autonomous learning mode based on the PACS also puts forward higher request to the teacher and mentor. In order to give postgraduate students better guidance, the teachers need to consolidate knowledge and update knowledge continuously, which enable them to guide and comment effectively. At the same time, they give guidance to the professional learning of the postgraduates and can they also give guidance for the postgraduate's courseware situation, knowledge situation, level of language expression, reading and problem analysis and so on. Depending on the comment and guidance, the goals of comprehensively improving the postgraduates' overall quality can be achieved.

Now, it is safe to conclude that the CBL autonomous learning mode is useful to help students to further consolidate professional knowledge of medical imaging, review the related basic and clinical knowledge, reinforce the basic training of image-reading, consolidate and expand the professional knowledge of learning and improve the level of the actual reading and language skills. Simultaneously, it puts forward higher request on teaching equipment, teaching resources and teachers' ability which requires teachers' innovative power continuously.

343.4.3 PACS CBL Autonomous Learning Mode Promotes Postgraduates' Study

Acknowledgments This study was supported by Research topic of innovation program in graduate education in Weifang Medical University (YY0601); Research topic of innovation program in graduate education in Shandong Province (SDYC11085); Shandong provincial natural science foundation of china (ZR2010HM078).

References

1. Wang X-F, Chen J-H, Zhong Y-H et al (2010) The application of CBL teaching method in the teaching of medical microbiology. China High Med Educ 4:13–14
2. Wang H-H, Liang S-H, An S et al (2012) The application of CBL teaching method in the experiment teaching of clinical microbiology. Basic Med Educ 5:344–345
3. Wang B, Dong P, Zhang S-Z et al (2008) The application of PACS teaching method in the teaching of medical imageology. Res Med Educ 7:665–666
4. Wang X-H, Meng X-C, Kong Q-C et al (2007) The value of autonomous teaching and learning style in the clinical practice of medical imageology. Suppl J Sun Yatsen Univ 27:54–56
5. Dong P, Wang B, Sun Y-Q et al (2008) To explore the relationship between the construction of department of molecular imageology and the fostering the ability of postgraduate of medical imageology. China High Med Educ 6:117–118

Chapter 344
Web-Based Information System Construction of Medical Tourism in South Korea

Yinghua Chen and Jaekwang Lee

Abstract This paper aims to find the weak points of South Korea's medical tourism websites construction by relevant websites' situation analysis. Customer attraction, customers' information gathering, medical treatment plan design service, support service, and aftercare feedback are selected as first evaluation standards. And several secondary evaluation items are included under each item. The weak points of South Korea's web-based information system in medical tourism are shown through the compassion analysis with tourism information sites in the conclusion part.

Keywords Web-based information system · Medical tourism · South Korea tour information sites

344.1 Introduction

With the rapid growth of globalization and increased requirement of health service supply, the trend of increased reliance upon individual health and wellbeing emerged in many countries in recent decades. More and more people prefer to go abroad to receive medical treatments for higher medical service quality, less cost, shorter waiting time. This kind of phenomenon is called medical tourism, which is defined as "the organized travel outside one's natural healthcare jurisdiction for

Y. Chen (✉)
School of Management, Jiangsu University, 301 Xuefu Road, Zhenjiang 212031
Jiangsu, China
e-mail: touchstones8@yahoo.com

J. Lee
School of Humanities, Inha University, 100 Inha-ro, Nam-Gu, Incheon 402751, Korea
e-mail: ray@inha.ac.kr

S. Li et al. (eds.), *Frontier and Future Development of Information Technology in Medicine and Education*, Lecture Notes in Electrical Engineering 269,
DOI: 10.1007/978-94-007-7618-0_344,

the enhancement or restoration of the individual health through medical intervention" (Carrera and Bridges 2006).

"With these trends, interest in developing tourism related to the medical industry has increased globally, and medical tourism is now marketed as a niche product that encompasses both medical services and tourism packages [1]. Following the developed countries in medical tourism, such as European countries, Singapore, and Thailand, South Korea began to pay more attention on medical tourism industry based on Korea's high medical technology both on selected surgeries and on cosmetic surgeries. As the most important information channel of medical tourism when the customers do their decisions, web-based information system plays a great role. The internet research we done for this study shown that Korea is still short of internet information system for medical tourism, which will be a big barrier for the development of Korea's medical tourism.

344.2 Literature Review

344.2.1 Medical Tourism

The quarrel about the definition of medical tourism first comes from the scope of medical tourism and the difference between medical tourism and health tourism, which includes two completely different opinions. Smith and Puczko (2009) argued that medical tourism is a subset of health and the health tourism is composed of medical tourism and wellness tourism. Yu and Ko [1] agreed with it. Some scholars argued that the distinction must be made between medical tourism and health tourism. But also some scholars insisted that the medical tourism should be a synthesis of medical service and tourism industry. Hyeony Jun, Kim (2009:7–9) defined the medical tourism as a kind of combination of medical and tourism. The patients can receive medical treatment, while enjoying leisure by travelling to the destination with high medical technique and lower medical service cost. The degree of synthesis between medical service and tourism service is also a debate point. Most of the scholars points out that the key contents of medical tourism should be on medical service supply, rather than tourism service supply.

344.2.2 Web-Based Information System

Internet website is a common channel to be used for information gathering to leisure travellers. Patterson (2007) concluded that the internet was the second important channel after friends as a information source to get necessary travel information. But toward medical tourism, the internet potentially serves an even more important role. Wolfe, Hsu, and Kang (2004) indicated a desire by travellers for "one-stop shopping".

344.2.3 Contents of Web-Based Information System

Cormany and Baloglu [2] set two sets of criteria for contents items. The following 12 items should be included in web-sited information system: email contact, telephone number, mailing address, information request form, maps of destinations served, hospital selection, notation of hospital accreditation, listing of medical procedures available, estimated treatment costs, past traveller testimonials, links to informational websites, and whether the date of the last web page update was provided. The second set of criteria includes the following services offered by the firm: air travel, ground transportation, hotel accommodations, translation service, concierge service, site-seeing options, arrangement of medical appointments, transfer of medical records, provision of aftercare support service(during recuperation while still in the country of the medical treatment), and provision of an international cell phones. Kil-lae Kim gave out xix basic steps and set secondary indexes by analyzing the service process of medical tourism. The basic steps are composed of Customer attraction, information gathering, treatment design, supporting service, treatment, and aftercare feedback.

344.3 Methodology

Literature Review and internet retrieval are mainly used in this study. The basic concepts and developmental situation of medical tourism in South Korea are searched. The data gathering are done by internet retrieval through the typical search site "naver" (http://www.naver.com) in South Korea. The search key words are "provincial location name + medical tourism". Fourty four related websites are found in 14 provincial locations in Korea. But only 14 effective websites left after excluding the invalid pages. And 8 pages are managed by public government, 6 pages are run by private companies or hospitals (Table 344.1).

Customer attraction, members' information gathering, medical treatment plan design service, support service, and aftercare service are set as the evaluation framework in this study. We use foreign language usage, telephone number, email address, and Information about hospital or treatment to judge step 1. Whether the Registration function is supplied in website is the second step. The step 3 checks online consulting function. The visa procedure, transportation, translation service, and hotel accommodation can be regarded as the secondary standards of step 4. And in step 5, tour information and aftercare feedback are the secondary items.

Table 344.1

Location	Name of website	Language	Public/ private	Total
Seoul	Medical Korea Gangnam	5	Public	13
	Lime Medical Korea	5	Private	
	Lyle Services Corporation	5	Private	
Busan	Busan Medical Tourism	5	Public	11
	Seomyeon Medical Street	4	Private	
	Medina Medical Tour Consulting Firm	4	Private	
	Medical Tour Mast	4	Private	
Daegu	Colorful Taegu	4	Public	5
	Wit Medical Tour	3	Private	
Incheon	Incheon Medical Tourism Foundation	7	Public	4
Daejeon	Daejeon Medical Tourism	6	Public	3
Gyeonggi-do	Gyeonggi International Medical Toruism Association	3	Public	4
Gangwon-do	Gangwon Medical Tourism Support Center	1	Public	4
	Gangwon Medical Tour	5	Public	

344.4 Result and Discussion

344.4.1 Customer Attraction

All the 14 websites use several foreign languages in their websites. Besides Korea, at least two kind foreign languages are used. English, Chinese, and Japanese are supplied nearly in all the sites. Some websites even can supply Russian and Thailand Language. Telephone number is shown in most of the websites. And 8 pages supplied e-mail address. This can be explained that the online consulting function can take the place of e-mail. 12 pages have information of treatment or hospitals.

344.4.2 Members' Information Gathering

In the 14 pages, 6 pages did not supply the registration function. That means customer information gathering are done in 40 % of the pages.

344.4.3 Medical Treatment Plan Design Service

Whether the medical treatment plan or design services are supplied can be evaluated by consultation function. Five pages have not this function in their sites. Nine pages supplied treatment plan design service.

Table 344.2

Steps	Secondary items	Locations													
		Seoul			Busan				Daegu		Incheon	Daejeon	Gyeonggi-do	Gangwon-do	
		S1	S2	S3	B1	B2	B3	B4	DG1	D2	I1	DJ1	GGD1	GWD1	GWD2
Step 1	Languages	O	O	O	O	O	O	O	O	O	O	O	O	O	O
	Telephone	O	O	X	O	O	O	O	O	O	O	O	O	O	O
	Email	O	O	O	X	O	O	O	O	O	X	X	X	X	X
	Information	O	O	X	O	O	X	O	O	O	O	O	O	O	O
Step 2	Registration	X	O	X	O	O	O	X	O	O	O	X	O	X	X
Step 3	Consultation	O	X	X	X	X	O	O	X	O	O	O	O	O	O
Step 4	Visa	X	X	X	O	X	O	X	X	X	O	O	X	X	X
	Transportation	X	X	X	O	X	O	O	O	O	O	O	X	O	X
	Translation	X	X	X	O	X	O	X	O	X	X	O	X	X	X
	Hotel	X	X	X	O	X	O	O	O	O	O	O	X	O	O
Step 5	Tour information	O	X	X	O	X	O	O	O	O	O	O	O	O	O
	Feedback	X	X	X	O	X	X	X	X	X	O	X	X	X	X

344.4.4 Support Service

Ten pages did not supply any information of visa apply. Six pages did not supply transportation information or service. And translation service or information is supplied in four sites. Only five sites did not supply any information about hotel.

344.4.5 Aftercare Feedback

Only three pages did not supply any tour information. But only two sites have the item of feedback from the customers (Table 344.2).

344.5 Conclusion

As a result, the relevant contents of step 1, step 2, and step 3 are provided by most of the web pages. It means that the secondary items in these 3 steps are in general common items in tour sites. It can be easily removed to medical tourism sites. And as basic items supplied in tour sites, the transportation, hotel information in step 4, tour information in step 5 are also supplied in medical tourism sites. The weak points in medical tourism websites include visa applying service, translation service, and aftercare feedback.

Through the above analysis, we found that all three items not been provided in most of the medical tourism web pages are not common items provided in tour information system. It shows that the main contents of medical tourism come from common tourism web sites. Furthermore, the items with more characteristic of medical tourism should be strengthened in the future for Korean medical tourism industry. Thirdly, the contents of medical tourism websites showed no clear distinction between the websites run by public government or by private companies. The explanation is to be done in the future study.

References

1. Yu JY, Ko TG (2012) A cross-cultural study of perceptions of medical tourism among Chinese, Japanese and Korean tourists in Korea. Tourism Manage 33:80–88
2. Cormany D, Baloglu S (2011) Medical travel facilitator websites: an exploratory study of web page contents and services offered to the prospective medical tourist. Tourism Manage 32(2011):709–716
3. Choi C-H (2011) A study on the development of the Korean traditional medicine tourism industry. Northeast Tourism Study 14:227–248 (Korean Version)
4. Byeon H (2011) Users' cognitive absorption and satisfaction on intention to system use in trabel agency websites. Tourism Study 26(2):163–179 (Korean Version)

5. Hazarika I (2009) Medical tourism: its potential impact on the health workforce and health systems in India. Health Policy Planning 25:248–251
6. Kim K (2010) The configuration of medical tourism information system by analyzing medical tourism service process. Tourism Study 81:311–329 (Korean Version)
7. Lunt N, Haardey M, Mannion R (2010) Nip, tuck and click: medical tourism and the emergence of web-based health information 4:1–11. http://www.ncbi.nlm.nih.gov/pmc/articles/pmc2874214 (27th March 2013)
8. Lunt N, Carrera P (2010) Medical tourism: assessing the evidence on treatment abroad. Maturitas 66:27–32
9. Yu TG (2009) Healthcare system's governance construction type in medical tourism advanced. Korean Public Manage Rev 23(4): 257–280 (Korean Version)
10. Heung VCS, Kucukusta D, Song H (2011) Medical tourism development in Hong Kong: an assessment of the barriers. Tourism Manage 32:995–1005

Chapter 345
Quantitative Modeling and Verification of VANET

Jing Liu, Xiaoyan Wang, Shufen Liu, Han Lu and Jing Tong

Abstract As VANET become more mission- and even safety–critical, the need for guarantees on adaptive behaviours increases dramatically. It is therefore timely to study the application of formal verification to VANET development, in particular to guarantee that a system demonstrates the correct behavioural adaptations in all circumstances. In recent years, a complementary technique of probabilistic model checking, an automated verification technique for probabilistic models has been developed. In this paper, we focus on the formal quantitative verification of the probabilistic behaviors of VANET which can be expressed quantitatively and require quantitative verification.

Keywords VANET · Quantitative modeling · Quantitative verification · Interval probabilistic timed automata

345.1 Introduction

Software is surreptitiously becoming the backbone of modern society, how to assure the correctness and reliability of software system is one of the most important tasks for computer researcher and developer. Automated verification is a

J. Liu
China State Shipbuilding Corporation, Beijing, China

X. Wang (✉) · S. Liu · H. Lu
College of Computer Science and Technology, Jilin University, Changchun, China
e-mail: wangxy@jlu.edu.cn

S. Liu
e-mail: liusf@jlu.edu.cn

H. Lu
e-mail: hanlu@jlu.edu.cn

J. Tong
College of Automotive Engineering, Jilin University, Changchun, China

S. Li et al. (eds.), *Frontier and Future Development of Information Technology in Medicine and Education*, Lecture Notes in Electrical Engineering 269,
DOI: 10.1007/978-94-007-7618-0_345,

powerful way to uphold it, which is a technique for establishing certain properties, usually expressed in temporal logic, and verify if these properties hold for a system model [1]. When people want to model and analysis complex systems, some factors such as non-determinism of event occurring, time constraint of event occurring and cost of finishing jobs should be considered. These properties are expressed in temporal logic extended with probabilistic and reward operators. Quantitative verification is an analogous technique for establishing quantitative properties of a system model. In recent years, a complementary technique of probabilistic model checking, an automated verification technique for probabilistic models has been developed [2–4].

Vehicular Adhoc Network (VANET) is a promising approach for future intelligent transportation system (ITS) [5]. With the development of VANET, more requirements are raised up according to the properties of VANET, such as its capacity for information system confidentiality (the prevention of unauthorized disclosure), availability (the prevention of unauthorized suppression of data or resources). However, as VANET become more mission- and even safety–critical, the need for hard guarantees on adaptive behaviours increases dramatically. It is therefore timely to study the application of formal verification to VANET development, in particular to guarantee that a system demonstrates the correct behavioural adaptations in all circumstances.

In this paper, we focus on the formal quantitative verification of the probabilistic behaviour of VANET which can be expressed quantitatively and require quantitative verification. Moreover, the requirements that software must guarantee are expressed in terms of these properties.

345.2 Interval Probabilistic Timed Automata

Probabilistic Timed Automata (PTA) [6] constitutes an expressive model for real-time behaviors with both probabilistic and nondeterministic parts. Interval Probabilistic Timed Automata (IPTA) [7] has been recently introduced as an extension of PTA and additionally allowed to explicitly model an uncertainty for probabilities. In IPTA, probabilities for events are not given as fixed values, but as intervals. An important aspect of this model is that the actual probability for an event may change over time. In this paper we use the IPTA model to describe the components in VANET.

Definition 1 (Interval Probabilistic Distribution) Let S be a finite set. An interval probability distribution on S is a pair of functions $\rho = (\rho^l, \rho^u), 0 \leq \rho^l \leq \rho^u \leq 1$, such that $\rho^l(s) \leq \rho^u(s)$, for all s ∈ S and furthermore: $\sum_{s \in S} \rho^l(s) \leq 1 \leq \sum_{s \in S} \rho^u(s)$

The set of probability interval distributions over S is denoted by IDist(S).

Definition 2 (Interval Probabilistic Timed Automata) An interval probabilistic timed automaton (IPTA) is a tuple $IPTA = (L, L^0, \mathbf{X}, Act, inv, enab, prob, \mathbf{L})$

- a finite set of locations L with $L^0 \subseteq L$ the set of initial locations,
- a finite set of action A,
- a finite set of clocks X,
- a clock invariant assignment function inv: L → CC(X),
- an interval probabilistic edge relation $prob \subseteq L \times CC(X) \times IDist(2^X \times L)$
- a labeling function $\mathbf{L} : L \longrightarrow 2^{AP}$assigning atomic propositions to locations.

Definition 3 (Interval Probabilistic Timed System) An interval probabilistic timed system (IPTS) is a dual tuple $IPTS = (S, Steps, \mathbf{I})$, where S is the set of states, $Steps \subseteq S \times R_+ \times IDist(S)$. For $(s, d, \rho_{s' \in S}) \in Steps$, real number $d \in R_+$denotes the time for system staying in state s and means there is a point distribution $\rho = 1$; while $d = 0$ means system takes a state transition to next state and the transition probability distribution is $\rho_{s'}$, with $0 < \rho_{s'} \leq 1$. For a IPTS, a path ω can be denoted as $\omega = s_0 \longrightarrow d_0, \rho_0 s_1 \longrightarrow d_1, \rho_1 s_2 \longrightarrow d_2, \rho_2 \ldots$. The probability calculation on a finite path of IPTS is $P(\omega) = \rho_0(s_1) \cdot \rho_1(s_2) \cdot \rho_2(s_3) \cdot \ldots \cdot \rho_{n-1}(s_n)$. On IPTS, an adversary is denoted by a function, which maps every finite path ω to a (d, u) to let $(last(\omega), d, u) \in Steps$. The set of adversaries on IPTS is denoted as Adv_{IPTS}. Semantically, an IPTA can be denoted as an IPTS.

345.3 Modeling with IPTA in VANET

VANET is a type of wireless networks which are expected to support a large number of mobile applications in the roads. There are three primary components of the VANET: on board unit (OBU), roadside unit (RSU), and the backhaul network. VANET tries to transmit useful information about road and traffic conditions as well as other information. There are two main types of VANET, one is V2V (Vehicle to Vehicle) in which Communication establish between two or more vehicles, the other is V2R (Vehicle to Roadside) in which Communication establish between roadside equipment and available vehicles in the range of equipment.

We assume a base station (RSU) with an omni-directional antenna that covers a certain area (within say 1 km radius), providing contents and services to one or more cars, equipped with a VANET 802.11p interface (OBU). These cars (clients), when approach the coverage area of the RSU can start a message exchange with the RSU in order to access to the provided services. We use this scenario to describe the quantitative modeling and verification.

Normally, vehicles will keep on changing their positions while travelling along the road. A vehicle needs to periodically exchange data with RSU and its neighbors so that they are aware of any changes to the surrounding vehicles. When the vehicle approaches the coverage area of the RSU, it will receive a message from RSU. Then an algorithm is computed if the vehicle needs the handoff from the RSU_1 to the RSU_2. If it does, a service channel will be allocated to it and the vehicle can connect with the RSU_2. This work should be done in 50 ms. In the next

50 ms, the vehicle will receive messages from RSU_2. We build these two phases in Fig. 345.1.

When the OBU calculate the handoff, it uses interval distribution to describe the relationship between RSSI and β, where RSSI represents the received signal strength indication and β is the threshold value.Because the perceived value of RSSI depends on the accuracy of the sensors and the distance between OBU and RSU, the result must be a value between the interval probability. When OBU needs handoff from RSU_1 to the RSU_2, RSU_2 will allocate a service channel for OBU first, the result is not accurate value because it depends on the capacity of RSU_2.

RSUs are important part of a VANET infrastructure. Every RSU is connected by wired links to other RSUs. In this paper, we only consider its main function to send message to OBU as shown in Fig. 345.2. If the message is emergent, then the control channel is used to send the messages to all the vehicles in this RSU group, otherwise the message will be sent to the designated vehicles using socket protocol.

345.4 Quantitative Verification for VANET

The formal specification of quantitative properties of PTA is PCTL [8], a probabilistic extension of the logic CTL which has been proposed for specifying properties of both MDPs and discrete-time Markov chains. Apart from the usual operators from classical logic such as $\wedge(and), \vee(or) and \Rightarrow (imples)$, PCTL has the probabilistic operator $p_{\sim p}[.]$, where p $\in$ [0, 1] is a probability bound and $\sim$ is one of $<$, $\leq$, $\geq$,or $>$.

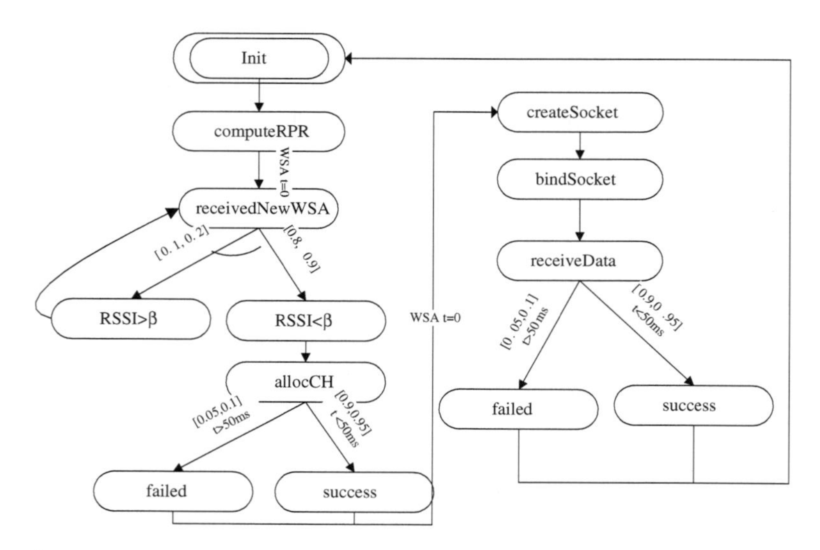

Fig. 345.1 The OBU model

Fig. 345.2 The RSU model

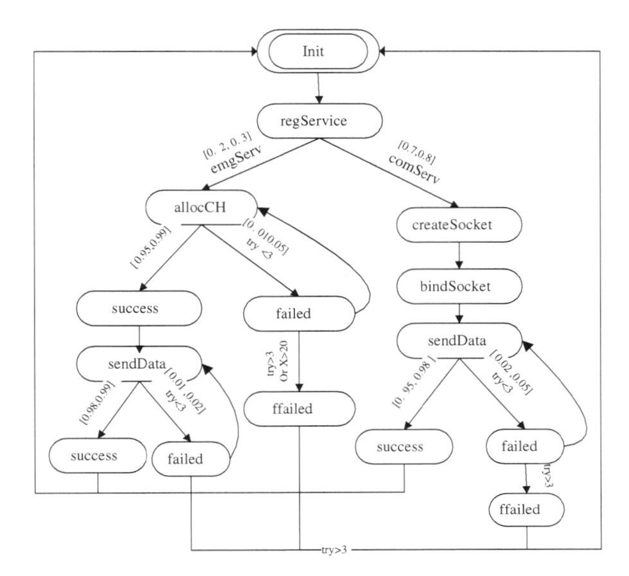

The different messages (emergent message or common message) can be sent from RSU to OBU with different probability as seen in Figs. 345.1 and 345.2, but we want to know what's the biggest and smallest of this probability. We can use PCTL expression to describe them as follows:

(1) the maximum probability of a failure occurring before message transmission is complete.

$$P_{\max=?}[\neg sent \cup fail]$$

(2) the minimum probability that the message successfully received by OBU.

$$P_{\min=?}[sent \cup success]$$

(3) the probability of the emergent message failing within 50 ms is strictly less than 0.1

$$P_{<0.1}[emerMessage \cup fail]$$

345.5 Conclusion

Verification of probabilistic real-time systems is an active field of research. In this paper, the concept of IPTA and IPTS are introduced, and one specific example which describes how to model OBU and RSU in VANET with IPTA is proposed. In the future, we will extend this method to build the models of the other scenarios in VANET, and improve the verification algorithm.

References

1. Baier C, Katoen J-P (2008) Principles of model checking. MIT Press
2. Forejt V, Kwiatkowska M, Norman G, Parker D (2011) Automated verification techniques for probabilistic systems. In: Bernardo M, Issarny V (eds) Formal methods for eternal networked software systems (SFM'11), vol 6659 of LNCS, pp 53–113
3. Zhang C, Pang J (2012). An algorithm for probabilistic alternating simulation. In: Bielikov′a M, Friedrich G, Gottlob G, Katzenbeisser S, Tur′an G (eds) Proceedings of the 38th conference on current trends in theory and practice of computer science (SOF-SEM'12), vol 7147 of LNCS, pp 431–442
4. Chen T, Forejt V, Kwiatkowska M, Parker D, Simaitis A (2012). Automatic verification of competitive stochastic systems. In: Flanagan C, Konig B (eds) Proceedings of the 18th international conference on tools and algorithms for the construction and analysis of systems (TACAS'12), vol 7214 of LNCS, pp 315–330
5. Papadimitratos P, La Fortelle A, Evenssen K, Brignolo R, Cosenza S (2009). Vehicular communication systems: enabling technologies, applications, and future outlook on intelligent transportation. IEEE Commun Mag 47:84–95
6. Kwiatkowska M, Norman G, Segala R, Sproston J (2002) Automatic verification of real-time systems with discrete probability distributions. Theoret Comput Sci 282:101–150
7. Zhang J, Zhao J, Huang Z, Cao Z (2009) Model checking interval probabilistic timed automata. In: Proceedings of the IEEE computer society ICISE'09, pp 4936–4940
8. Bianco A, de Alfaro L (1995) Model checking of probabilistic and nondeterministic systems. In: Thia-garajan P (eds) Proceedings of the 15th conference foundations of software technology and theoretical computer science (FSTTCS'95), vol 1026 of LNCS, pp 499–513

Chapter 346
Study on the Financial Change of the Primary Health Care Institutions After the Implementation of Essential Drug System

Changchun Zhan and Yasai Ge

Abstract The implementation of essential drug system can reduce the burden of medical expenses, guarantee the supply of essential drug. And it also affects the financial situation of primary health care institutions. This paper analyzes the financial change of the primary health care institutions after the implementation of essential drug system by the case analysis of Dantu district, Zhenjiang city, Jiangsu province from the aspects of financial income, financial expenditure, and the balance of financial income and expenditure. The result shows that their financial income and expenditure increase simultaneously, and maintain a financial balance in most primary health care institutions by receiving financial assistance at all levels.

Keywords The essential drug system · Primary health care institutions · Financial change

346.1 Introduction

In order to effectively reduce the burden of medical expenses, and guarantee the supply of essential drug, in August of 2009 the Ministry of health and other relevant departments jointly issued "the implementation opinions on establishing a essential drug system." To require primary health care institutions which is owned by the government should equip with national essential drugs and use them gradually. In 2011, the national essential drug system is established initially. By 2020, it will implement standardized, covering urban and rural essential drug system fully.

C. Zhan (✉) · Y. Ge
College of Administration, Jiangsu University, XueFu Road, Zhenjiang 212013, China
e-mail: zcc1973@ujs.edu.cn

S. Li et al. (eds.), *Frontier and Future Development of Information Technology in Medicine and Education*, Lecture Notes in Electrical Engineering 269,
DOI: 10.1007/978-94-007-7618-0_346,

At the beginning of 2010, all primary health care institutions in Zhenjiang city begin to implement the essential drug system. The new system requires all the primary health care institutions should be equipped with essential drugs and use them. Purchasing essential drugs will realize open invite tenders and unified distribution through the provincial online, and implement zero profit sales. These provisions will affect the operation of primary health care institutions, causing the change in finance.

346.2 Methods and Data Sources

In 2012, from June to July field investigation of all the 13 community health service centers in Dantu district was conducted. Through questionnaire survey we collected annual financial statements of thirteen community centers in 2009–2010. We use Excel 2007 to establish the data base and analyze relevant data.

346.3 Results

Financial income of 13 community health service centers in Dantu district is from the business income and financial assistance at all levels. Among them, business income includes medical service income, drug income and other income. Financial expenditure includes business expenses, special financial expenditure, management fees and other costs.

346.3.1 The Change of Financial Income

From a general overview, since the implementation of the essential drug system in 2010 the financial income of 11 community centers has showed different growth and only two declined slightly. The average rate of increase in financial income is 16.10 %. From the view of the composition of financial income, business income has increased slightly, the average increase rate is 8.38 %. But the financial assistance at all levels increased substantially. The financial assistance of thirteen community centers amounted to an increase of 6.15 million Yuan, the growth rate is 91.29 % (see Table 346.1).

Table 346.1 The change of financial income of the 13 community centers in 2009–2010

Community center	Total financial income (ten thousands)			Financial assistance (ten thousands)			Business income (ten thousands)		
	2009	2010	Growth (%)	2009	2010	Growth (%)	2009	2010	Growth (%)
A	548.85	570.86	4.01	100.40	97.89	–2.50	448.45	472.97	5.47
B	449.52	494.82	10.08	81.93	77.01	–6.01	367.59	417.81	13.66
C	660.36	1013.13	53.42	14.98	202.50	1251.80	645.38	810.63	25.61
D	339.14	351.42	3.62	6.19	28.53	360.90	332.95	322.89	–3.02
E	627.50	650.24	3.62	67.87	76.40	12.57	559.63	573.84	2.54
F	943.99	933.16	–1.15	74.31	125.22	68.51	869.68	807.94	–7.10
G	419.74	536.10	27.72	8.90	82.32	824.94	410.84	453.78	10.45
H	673.62	759.16	12.70	69.88	83.36	19.29	603.74	675.80	11.94
I	320.51	421.29	31.44	45.52	78.56	72.58	274.99	342.73	24.63
J	1210.48	1537.32	27.00	51.21	253.52	395.06	1159.27	1283.80	10.74
K	611.00	641.00	4.91	77.00	89.00	15.58	534.00	552.00	3.37
L	187.68	178.12	–5.09	51.06	27.58	–45.99	136.62	150.54	10.19
M	240.00	310.00	29.17	24.00	66.00	175.00	216.00	244.00	12.96
Total	7232.39	8396.62	16.10	673.25	1287.89	91.29	6559.14	7108.73	8.38

346.3.2 The Change of Financial Expenditure

Since the implementation of the essential drug system in 2010, the financial expenditure of thirteen community centers has increased substantially. The total financial expenditure rises 15.53 million Yuan than 2009, the average increase rate is 23.24 %. The increase of central financial expenditure was mainly caused by the increase in its business expenditure. Business expenditure of 13 community centers increase 30.71 % than 2009. However, special financial expenditure, management fees and other costs have fallen, which is 16.21 % than 2009 (see Table 346.2).

346.3.3 The Balance of Financial Income and Expenditure

Before the implementation of essential drug system in 2009, four of thirteen community centers occurred gap in business income and expenditure. After financial assistance at all levels, only one occurred gap in financial income and expenditure. Since the implementation of essential drug system in 2010, there has been a gap in business income and expenditure in 9 community centers. Through financial assistance at all levels, four still exist gap, which is 2.69 million Yuan. The financial income and expenditure of other community centers maintain a balance basically (see Table 346.3).

Table 346.2 The change of financial expenditure of the 13 community centers in 2009–2010

Community center	Total financial expenditure (ten thousands)			Business expenditure (ten thousands)			Special financial expenditure, management fees and others (ten thousands)		
	2009	2010	Growth (%)	2009	2010	Growth (%)	2009	2010	Growth (%)
A	464.04	601.52	29.63	424.04	601.52	41.85	40.00	0.00	–100.00
B	430.00	459.49	6.86	316.75	338.62	6.90	113.25	120.87	6.73
C	612.15	920.53	50.38	524.79	833.47	58.82	87.36	87.06	–0.34
D	323.52	323.45	–0.02	276.46	275.41	–0.38	47.06	48.04	2.08
E	571.47	707.92	23.88	571.47	705.82	23.51	0.00	2.10	-
F	882.82	1026.31	16.25	642.12	852.28	32.73	240.70	174.03	–27.70
G	396.09	623.54	57.42	269.29	524.54	94.79	126.80	99.00	–21.92
H	665.93	750.21	12.66	498.93	583.40	16.93	167.00	166.81	–0.11
I	347.25	415.27	19.59	336.68	349.64	3.85	10.57	65.63	520.91
J	1063.38	1318.83	24.02	881.30	1209.91	37.29	182.08	108.92	–40.18
K	515.00	620.00	20.39	502.00	605.00	20.52	13.00	15.00	15.38
L	184.16	158.81	–13.77	152.07	156.82	3.12	32.09	1.99	–93.80
M	226.00	309.00	36.73	222.00	307.00	38.29	4.00	2.00	–50.00
Total	6681.81	8234.88	23.24	5617.90	7343.43	30.71	1063.91	891.45	–16.21

Table 346.3 The balance of financial income and expenditure of 13 community centers in 2009–2010

Community Center	Financial balance (ten thousands)		Business balance (ten thousands)	
	2009	2010	2009	2010
A	84.81	–30.66	24.41	–128.55
B	19.52	35.33	50.84	79.19
C	48.21	92.60	120.59	–22.84
D	15.62	27.97	56.49	47.48
E	56.03	–57.68	–11.84	–131.98
F	61.17	–93.15	227.56	–44.34
G	23.65	–87.44	141.55	–70.76
H	7.69	8.95	104.81	92.40
I	–26.74	6.02	–61.69	–6.91
J	147.10	218.49	277.97	73.89
K	96.00	21.00	32.00	–53.00
L	3.52	19.31	–15.45	–6.28
M	14.00	1.00	–6.00	–63.00
Total	550.58	161.74	941.24	–234.70

346.4 Conclusions

346.4.1 The Implementation of Essential Drug System Significantly Affects Business Income of the Primary Health Care Institutions

Since the implementation of essential drug system, business income of the community centers has increased slightly, but business expenditure has increased substantially, which leads to the gap in financial income and expenditure in most primary health care institutions.

346.4.2 Financial Assistance Ensures the Normal Operation of the Primary Health Care Institutions

Since the implementation of essential drug system at the beginning of 2010 in Dantu district, the government has increased financial assistance to the primary health care institutions. Because of the government finance assistance in time 13 community centers in this paper have made up for the gap which was caused by the drugs zero profit sales.

346.5 Suggestions

346.5.1 Ensure the Stable and Effective Financial Assistance

At present, Zhenjiang city has established a funds compensation mechanism and method which is used to examine the quality and quantity of service in primary health care institutions. The government gives different level financial assistance according to the examination result. The government finance assistance in time in 2010 made up for the gap which was caused by the drugs zero profit. In addition, from the second half of 2011, primary health care institutions began to carry out the wage reform by performance. After the reform, the staff obtain wage and benefit according to the results of performance appraisal, and their welfare treatment get obviously improved, which further increase the operating pressure in primary health care institutions. Therefore, it is particularly important to ensure the stability of government financial assistance and increase the amount of compensation according to the actual situation [1–3].

346.5.2 Establish Evaluation and Supervision System on the Essential Drug System

From the above analysis, the implementation of essential drug system has produced some effect. However, it also has brought some problems, such as the rapid rise of medical service charge. Therefore we suggest that an evaluation and supervision department should be established, which includes finance, medical insurance, health and other departments [4]. At the same time, evaluation and supervision methods should be established in order to ensure the effective implementation of the system and reduce the irregularities [5].

References

1. Xie W (2012) The phenomenon of drug income subsidized medical service income tends to the end. China Hospital CEO 3:30–35
2. Zhou L-L (2013) Analysis on impact of national essential medicine system on primary health institutions. Chongqing Med 5:532–535
3. Zhan C-C (2011) Effects of national essential drugs system on drug income in primary medical institutions. China Pharm 36:3374–3375
4. Peng L (2010) Effects of essential drug system on primary medical institutions. China Pharm 32:2998–2999
5. Chen X-Z (2008) Discussion on the problem of drug income subsidized medical service income. Chine Health Econ 9:8–9

Chapter 347
Construction of a Recombinant Plasmid for Petal-Specific Expression of HQT, a Key Enzyme in Chlorogenic Acid Biosynthesis

Yuting Bi, Wei Tian, Wen Zeng, Yushan Kong, Yanhong Xue and Shiping Liu

Abstract The flower buds of *Lonicera japonica* are widely used in Chinese medicine due to the anti-inflammatory properties. Chlorogenic acid (CGA) may be one of the most critical components in *L. japonica*. Previous studies suggest that *HQT* gene play a very important role in the synthesis of CGA. In order to overexpress *HQT* gene specifically in the petals, we successfully isolated the full-length cDNA of *HQT* gene from *L. japonica*. Then from *Lilium orential* 'Sorbonne', we cloned an 896-bp promoter (*PLoCHS*) which can drive *chalcone synthase gene* (*CHS*) specifically expression in flowers. After sequencing and bioinformatical analysis, two constructs based on pCAMBIA2300 were obtained, one was a constituently expression vector driving *HQT* by 35S promoter, and the other fused *HQT* and *PLoCHS* promoter. In the further research, we will transform the constructs into *L. japonica* callus. This study provides a means of improving the CGA content in *L. japonica* flowers, and will be helpful in understanding the expression pattern of *HQT* related with CGA and development of the plants.

Keywords HQT · PLoCHS · CGA · Construction · Petal

347.1 Introduction

Chlorogenic acid (CGA), an important polyphenol compound in fruits and vegetables, has various bioactivities such as heat-clearing, detoxifying, antioxidant, anti-inflammatory, and so on [1, 2]. Therefore, it is widely used as a prodrug in fever, influenza, sores, swellings, arthritis, pneumonia, infections, and diabetes

---

Y. Bi · W. Tian · W. Zeng · Y. Kong · Y. Xue · S. Liu (✉)
College of Chemistry and Life Science, China Three Gorges University, Yichang 443002, People's Republic of China
e-mail: liuspain@ctgu.edu.cn

S. Li et al. (eds.), *Frontier and Future Development of Information Technology in Medicine and Education*, Lecture Notes in Electrical Engineering 269,
DOI: 10.1007/978-94-007-7618-0_347,

mellitus [3, 4]. In the flower buds of *Lonicera japonica*, a traditional Chinese medicine, CGA is one of the most abundant ingredients, which ranged 5–10 % [3].

CGA is formed by esterification of caffeic and quinic acids in vivo [1–3]. It is generally admitted that HQT, a hydroxycinnamoyl-CoA quinate hydroxycinnamoyl transferase, is a key enzyme for CGA biosynthesis [5–9]. Many evidences suggest that overexpression *HQT* lead to high CGA contents in plants, and knockdown would decrease correspondingly [5]. Gene silencing proved HQT to be the principal route for accumulation of CGA in *Solanaceous* species [5]. Overexpression of *HQT* in tomato caused plants to accumulate higher levels of CGA, with no side-effects on the levels of other soluble phenolics [5]. Transgenic tobacco plants overexpressing *AtPAL2* showed two and five times increases of CGA and rutin levels than the wild-type (WT) plants, respectively [6]. Overexpression of *NtHQT* further increases the accumulation of CGA in the *AtPAL2* plants to about three times than that of the WT level, while silencing of *NtHQT* in *AtPAL2* plants results in 12 times increase in rutin level than that of the WT plants [6].While all these data were acquired from *Solanaceae* or other plants with middle or low CGA, hence, we can not help wonder that how about the plants with high CGA? A recent study involving isolated *HQT* gene from *L. japonica* demonstrated that the expression of *HQT* showed a positive correlation with CGA synthesis [1].

In order to enhance the CGA content in the flower of *L. japonica*, here, we construct two recombinant plasmids to overexpress *HQT* gene. One was carrying *HQT* gene and CaMV35S promoter, the other carrying a petal-specific promoter named *PLoCHS*, of which the downstream *Chalcone synthase* gene in *Lilium orential* 'Sorbonne' is predominantly expressed in flowers and under developmental control [10]. All these attempts would enrich the knowledge about the relationship between CGA accumulation and the expression of HQT.

347.2 Materials and Methods

347.2.1 Plant Material and RNA Isolation

The flower buds of *L. japonica* were collected from botanical garden in China Three Gorges University. All samples were immediately frozen in liquid nitrogen during the field collection and stored at −80 °C. Total RNA was extracted from approximately 100 mg young leaves using the Trizol reagent, according to the manufacturer's instructions (Takara). Final RNA integrity was examined by electrophoresis in 1 % (w/v) agarose gel.

347.2.2 cDNA Preparation and RT-PCR

The first-strand cDNA was synthesized from 2 μg of total RNA using Oligo d (T) 18 and M-MLV reverse transcriptase (Takara) in 10 μL reactions, following the manufacturer's instructions. PCR was carried out using a pair of gene-specific primers designed using *L. japonica HQT* open reading frame recorded in Genebank (JF261014). The primers used for amplification of *HQT* were HQT-XP-U and HQT-XP-L (Table 347.1), which contained additional protective bases and restriction sites, respectively, *Xba* I (TCTAGA, 5′-end) and *Pst* I (CTGCAG, 3′-end). The cycling parameters were as follows: 94 °C for 5 min; 35 cycles of 94 °C for 30 s, annealing at 55 °C for 30 s, extension at 72 °C for 1.5 min; a final extension at 72 °C for 10 min. The PCR products were loaded on 1.0 % agarose gels and photographed. Reactions were carried out in 20 μL mixtures containing DNA (10 ng), 2 μL PCR buffer, 200 nM of each primer, 0.2 mM of each dNTP and LA Taq DNA Polymerase (Takara Bio. Dalian, China). The amplified fragments were cloned into pMD18-T Easy vector (Takara) and sequenced.

347.2.3 Cloning PLoCHS Promoter

Genomic DNA of *Lilium orential* 'Sorbonne' was isolated from young leaves using a small-scale DNA isolation method. 896 bp of the *PLoCHS* promoter were amplified from the genomic DNA using two specific primers CHS-U and CHS-L, added two restriction sites *Nco* I (CCATGG, 5′-end) and *Bam*H I (GGATCC, 3′-end) (Table 347.1). A total of 1.5 U of enzyme together with 2 mM $MgCl_2$ were used. The PCR parameters is as follows: 94 °C for 5 min to denature the DNA template and then 35 cycles of 30 s at 94 °C, 30 s at an appropriate annealing temperature 50–60 °C for the primers used to hybridize to the target sequence, and the extension step for polymerization at 72 °C for 1 min. The amplified fragments were reprepared and ligated with pMD18-T Easy vector (Takara), and then sequenced for verification.

Table 347.1 Primers used in the experiments

Name	Sequence
HQT-XP-U	CAG**TCTAGA**ATGGGAAGTGAAGGAAGTGTGAA
HQT-XP-L	CCG**CTGCAG**TCAGAACTCGTACAAACACTTCTCAAA
CHS-U	CATG**CCATGG**CATGAGTCGTGGTTTGTGAGCT
CHS-L	CGC**GGATCC**GCGTGGTTGGATGGGAGG

347.2.4 Construction of pCAMBIA 2300::HQT Vector

The recombinant plasmid pMD18-T::*HQT* was digested with *Xba* I and *Pst* I restriction endonucleases (3 h at 37 °C). After digestion, the fragments were ligated into the cloning site of *Xba* I and *Pst* I digested pCAMBIA 2300 plasmid to create constitutive vector pCAMBIA 2300::*HQT*. The resulting plasmid was confirmed by sequencing and enzyme digestion.

347.2.5 Construction of pCAMBIA 2300::PLoCHS::HQT Vector

The recombinant plasmid pMD18-T::*PLoCHS* was digested with *Nco* I and *Bam*H I restriction endonucleases (3 h at 37 °C). After digestion, the fragments were ligated into the cloning site of *Nco* I and *Bam*H I digested pCAMBIA 2300 plasmid to create petal-specific vector pCAMBIA 2300::*PLoCHS*. The next processing followed the construction of pCAMBIA 2300::*HQT* vector as the above mentioned. All vectors were confirmed by PCR, sequencing and restriction enzyme digestion.

347.3 Results and Discussion

347.3.1 Amplification of HQT Gene

Using a pair of primers, HQT-XP-U and HQT-XP-L, the 1320 bp full-length ORF encoding a 439-residue protein was isolated (Fig. 347.1). It shares 99 % identity and owns three bases different from the template. It causes three amino acids different (Fig. 347.2). The amino acids Ala, Gln, Tyr at codon 80, 145, 148, respectively, change to Thr, Arg, His. Arg and Gln are similar in structure as well as His to Tyr. It is maybe that the differences in species lead to the amino acids diversity for adapting to different environments.

347.3.2 Cloning and Sequence Analysis of PLoCHS Promoter

A PCR product of the PLoCHS promoter of 896 bp was amplified (Fig. 347.2a, b). Besides some typical promoter elements, such as the TATA and CCAAT boxes, many cis-acting elements associated with flower-specific expression were found in the PLoCHS promoter region (Fig. 347.2c). For example, the G-box, P-box, and

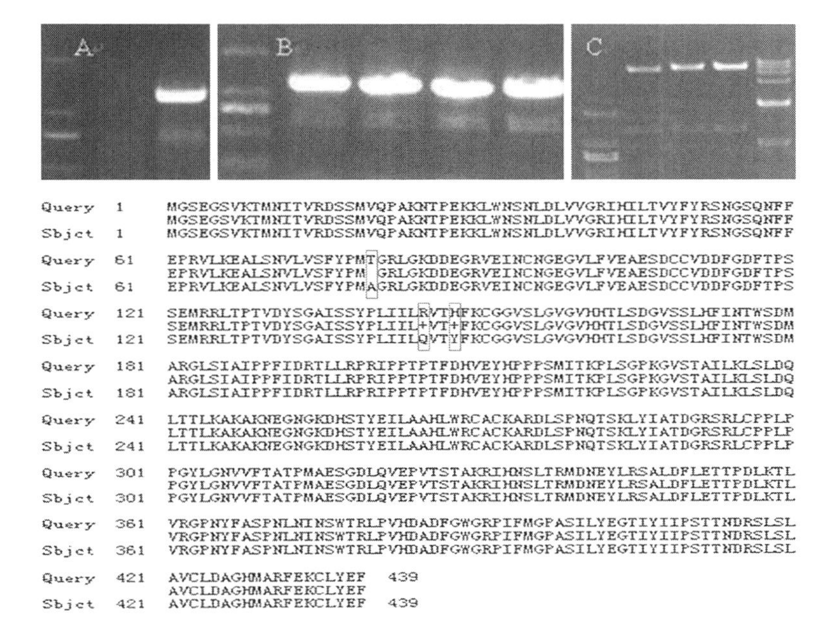

Fig. 347.1 **a** PCR products of the *HQT* gene approximate 1320 bp. **b** Colony PCR to confirm *HQT* ligation in pMD18-T. **c** Confirmation of *HQT* ligation in pMD18-T with the digestion of enzymes *Xba* I and *Pst* I. **d** The comparison results of amino acids sequence translated from *HQT* gene to the published sequence in NCBI

TACPyAT motifs are thought to make major contributions to flower-specific expression [11]. The P- and G-boxes form a very common cooperative unit and have been identified in a variety of flower-specific promoters in plants, including *Gentiana triflora* [12], *Pisum sativum* [13], and *Phalaenopsis Orchid* [11]. However, a constituent of this cooperative unit, the P-box, was not identified in the *PLoCHS* promoter. Only three G-boxes were located in this promoter at positions -849 (sequence GTCGTG), -819 (sequence GTCGTG), -525(sequence TACGTG) and, respectively, TACPyAT elements (TACCCT or TACCAAT), act as dom-inant *cis*-elements in controlling flower-specific expression of the CHSA and DFRA genes [14, 15].

347.3.3 Construction of pCAMBIA 2300::HQT Vector

By the function of restriction enzymes *Xba* I and *Pst* I, *HQT* gene was isolated from pMD18-T::*HQT*. With the same restriction enzyme, pCAMBIA 2300 was opened and shared the same sticky ends. The fragment of *HQT* gene was fused with pCAMBIA 2300 injured by ligase. To confirm *HQT* ligation in pCAMBIA 2300, colony PCR and restriction enzyme digestion were done (Fig. 347.3).

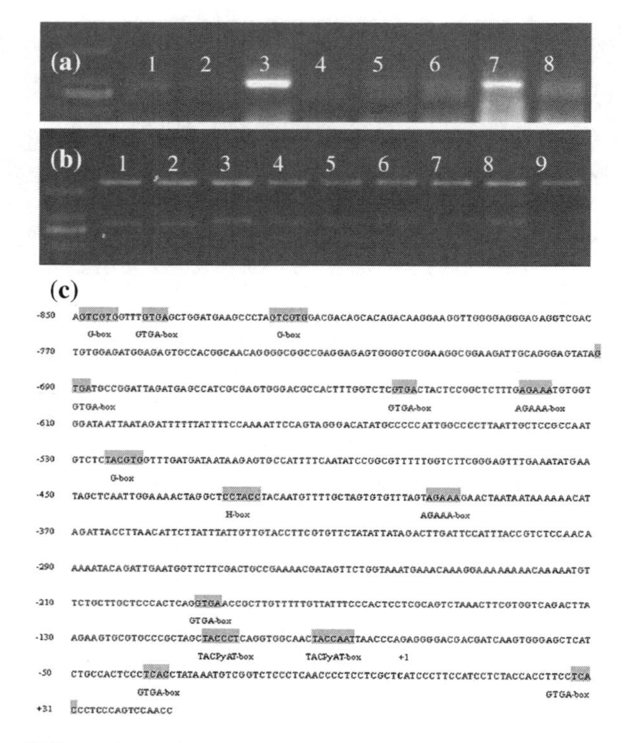

Fig. 347.2 **a** PCR product of the *PLoCHS* promoter approximate 896 bp. Number *1–8* represented for eight different temperatures from 60 to 50 °C. Number *3* and *7* standed for 58 and 50.7 °C, respectively. The study followed choosed the product at 58°C in consideration of that higher temperature can make higher fidelity. **b** Confirmation of *PLoCHS* promoter ligation in pMD18-T with the digestion of enzymes *Nco* I and *Bam*H I. **c** Nucleotide sequence of the 896-bp upstream region of the chalcone synthase gene (*CHS*) in *Lilium orential* 'Sorbonne'. The putative transcription site is in *bold* and designated as +1. All putative *cis*-elements related to flower-specific expression are indicated and their names are given below each element

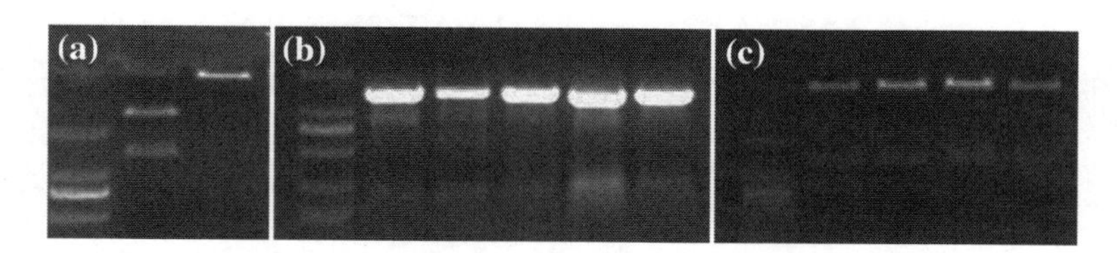

Fig. 347.3 **a** Restriction enzyme digestion for pMD18-T::*HQT* and pCAMBIA 2300 by *Xba* I and *Pst* I to obtain *HQT* gene and pCAMBIA 2300 with the same cohesive ends. **b** Colony PCR to confirm *HQT* ligation into pCAMBIA 2300. C. Confirmation of *HQT* ligation in pCAMBIA 2300 with the digestion of enzymes *Xba* I and *Pst* I

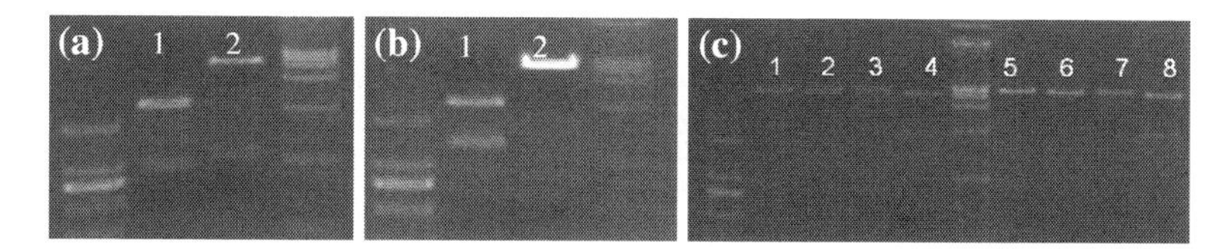

Fig. 347.4 **a** Restriction enzyme digestion for pMD18-T::*PLoCHS* (*1*) and pCAMBIA 2300 (*2*) by *Nco* I and *Bam*H I to acquire *PLoCHS* promoter which shared the same sticky ends with pCAMBIA 2300 without CaMV35S promoter. **b** Restriction enzyme digestion for pMD18-T::*HQT* (*1*) and pCAMBIA 2300::*PLoCHS* (*2*) by *Xba* I and *Pst* I. **c** Confirmation of relative position of *HQT* gene and *PLoCHS* promoter in the finished vector. The fragments at number *1–4* were *PLoCHS* promoter (896 bp), *HQT* gene (1320 bp), small fragments (approximate 10 bp), *PLoCHS* promoter:: *HQT* gene (approximate 2200 bp) as well as *5–8,* respectively

347.3.4 Construction of pCAMBIA 2300::PLoCHS::HQT Vector

The imported *PLoCHS* promoter fragment was cleaved from vector pMD18-T::*PLoCHS* using the enzymes *Nco* I and *Bam*H I and successfully incorporated pCAMBIA2300 without CaMV35S promoter by the same way. Then the *HQT* gene extracted from vector pMD18-T::*HQT* by the action of *Xba* I and *Pst* I was successfully ligated into pCAMBIA2300:: *PLoCHS*. To confirm the relative position of *HQT* gene and *PLoCHS* promoter, four groups of restriction endonuclease assemblies were designed: *Nco* I and *Bam*H I (Fig. 347.4c*1* and c*5*), *Xba* I and *Pst* I (Fig. 347.4c*2* and c*6*), *Bam*H I and *Xba* I (Fig. 347.4c*3* and c*7*), *Nco* I and *Pst* I (Fig. 347.4c*4* and c*8*). Respectively, four kinds of different results were obtained in accordance with expectation. Sequencing the two kinds of vectors, the

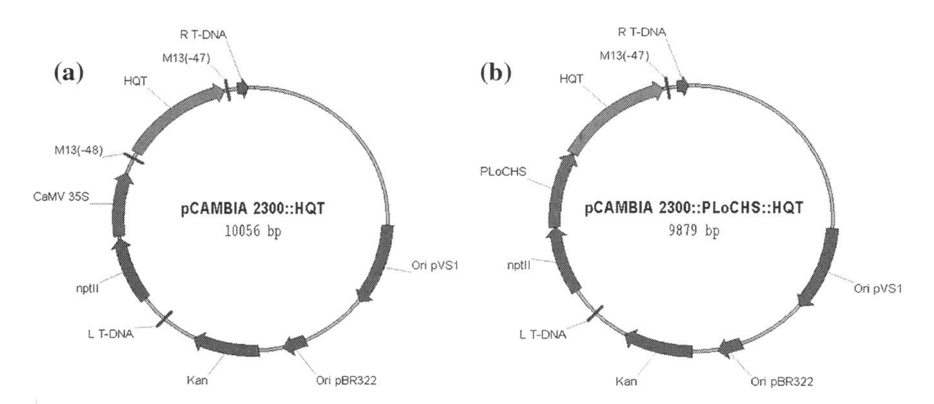

Fig. 347.5 **a** Schematic map of vector *pCAMBIA 2300::HQT* carrying CaMV35S promoter, *HQT* gene. **b** Schematic map of vector *pCAMBIA 2300::PLoCHS::HQT* carrying petal-specific promoter *PLoCHS*, *HQT* gene

result showed they shared the same *HQT* gene. It makes sure that the different phenotypes brought by them are due to the different promoters in the future. The schematic maps of two constructs were displayed in Fig. 347.5.

347.4 Conclusion

In conclusion, in these experiments a cDNA coding an HQT involved in chlorogenic acid biosynthesis in *L. japonica* has been obtained the first time. Then we successfully cloned an 896-bp promoter (*PLoCHS*) from *Lilium orential* 'Sorbonne'. After sequencing and bioinformatical analysis, two constructs based on pCAMBIA2300 were obtained, one was a constituently expression vector driving *HQT* by 35S promoter, and the other fused *HQT* and *PLoCHS* promoter. Further work need to be done so as to improve the CGA content in *L. japonica* flowers. This study will be helpful in understanding the expression pattern of *HQT* related with CGA and development of the plants.

Acknowledgments Thanks to the support of China Three Gorges University for the preliminary study. This project was supported by the National Natural Science Foundation of China (31270389) and Natural Science Research of Hubei Education Department (D20121301).

References

1. Peng XX, Li WD, Wang WQ, Bai GB (2010) Cloning and characterization of a cDNA coding a hydroxycinnamoyl-CoA quinate hydroxycinnamoyl transferase involved in chlorogenic acid biosynthesis in *Lonicera japonica*. Planta Med
2. Zang LY, Cosma G, Gardner H, Castranova V, Vallyathan V (2003) Effect of chlorogenic acid on hydroxyl radical. Mol Cell Biochem 247:205–210
3. State Pharmacopoeia Committee (2005) Pharmacopoeia of China, Part 1. Chemical Industry Press, Beijing, pp 152–153
4. Teng HL (2007) Synthetically study on medicinal materials of *Lonicera japonica*. J Chin Med Mat 30:744–748
5. Niggeweg R, Michael AJ, Martin C (2004) Engineering plants with increased levels of the antioxidant chlorogenic acid. Nat Biotechnol 22:746–754
6. Chang JL, Luo J, He GY (2009) Regulation of polyphenols accumulation by combined overexpression/silencing key enzymes of phyenylpropanoid pathway. Acta Biochim Biophys Sin 41(2):123–130
7. Comino C, Hehn A, Moglia A, Menin B, Bourgaud F, Lanteri S, Portis E (2009) The isolation and mapping of a novel hydroxycinnamoyltransferase in the globe artichoke chlorogenic acid pathway. BMC Plant Biol 9:30
8. Ulbrich B, Zenk MH (1979) Partial purification and properties of hydroxycinnamoyl-CoA: quinate hydroxycinnamoyl transferase from higher plants. Phytochemistry 18:929–933
9. Lofty S, Fleuriet A, Macheix JJ (1992) Partial purification and characterization of hydroxycinnamoyl CoA: transferases from apple and date fruits. Biochemistry 13:767–772

10. Liu YL, Lou Q, Xu WR, Xin Y et al (2011) Wang Characterization of a chalcone synthase (CHS) flower-specific promoter from *Lilium orential* 'Sorbonne'. Plant Cell Rep 30:2187–2194
11. Han YY, Ming F, Wang JW, Ye MM, Shen DL (2006) Molecular characterization and functional analysis of a novel chalcone synthase gene from *Phalaenopsis Orchid* in transgenic tobacco. Plant Mol Biol Rep 23:193a–193m
12. Kobayashi H, Oikawa Y, Koiwa H, Yamamura S (1998) Flower-specific gene expression directed by the promoter of a chalcone synthase gene from *Gentiana triflora* in *Petunia hybrida*. Plant Sci 131:173–180
13. Uimari A, Strommer J (1997) Myb26: a MYB-like protein of pea flowers with affinity for promoters of phenylpropanoid genes. Plant J 12:1273–1284
14. Van der Meer IM, Spelt CE, Mol JNM, Stuitje AR (1992) Promoter analysis of the chalcone synthase (*CHSA*) gene of *Petunia hybrida*: a 67 bp promoter region directs flower-specific expression. Plant Mol Biol 15:95–109
15. Huits HSM, Gerats AGM, Kreike MM, Mol JNM, Koes RE (1994) Genetic control of dihydroflavonol 4-reductase gene expression in *Petunia hybrida*. Plant J 6:295–310

Chapter 348
Explorations on Strengthening of Students' Programming Capabilities in Data Structure Teaching

Song Yucheng, Jin Shaoli and Xu Fasheng

Abstract This paper considers some common problems in data structure teaching. The paper elaborates how to stimulate students' interest and strengthen their programming capabilities. We mainly discuss in three aspects of developing the second class to train students' programming skills, improving the proficiency of C language, and constructing a multi-level experiment teaching mode.

Keywords Programming capabilities · Data structure teaching · Practice teaching

348.1 Introduction

Data structure is an important basic course of the information and computational science specialty in University of Jinan. This course discusses various basic data structures and the methods of searching and sorting. The purpose of this course is to make students understand the logical features, storage methods and fundamental operations of several common data structures, and grasp the principles and technology methods of common searching and sorting. In addition, the another purpose of this course is to enable students to choose appropriate structures to write clear programs according to the specific problems, which lays a good foundation for students to learn lessons afterwards and improve software designing.

As a highly practical course, the learning process of data structure is also the training process of complex program design, which requires students to write correct programs with clear structure and good readable. Therefore, the teaching of this course should not only focus on the student's understanding of basic theories, but also on the cultivation of their programming capabilities [1–4].

S. Yucheng (✉) · J. Shaoli · X. Fasheng
School of Mathematical Sciences, University of Jinan, Jinan, China
e-mail: ss_songyc@ujn.edu.cn

S. Li et al. (eds.), *Frontier and Future Development of Information Technology in Medicine and Education*, Lecture Notes in Electrical Engineering 269,
DOI: 10.1007/978-94-007-7618-0_348,

As we know, there are a lot of algorithms in data structure. All algorithms are given in similar C language in all kinds of textbooks based on C language, which purpose is to help students to get rid of tedious source programs so as to focus on algorithm ideas [2]. On the other hand, C language programming is a prerequisite for data structure. The level of students' mastering C language directly determines the teaching effect of data structure. Actually, during our teaching process, we find that although students had 1earned the main C language programming in their first college year, they have only a bit of conceptual knowledge and understanding of the program design. Most students only know four simple data types and three basic structures in structured programming. They have a superficial understanding of structural body and pointer which are the most frequently used in data structure. According to statistic data and feedback information from the class teachers, more than 70 % students of the year 2008 who major in information and computing science specialty never mastered programming, and more than 50 % students of the year 2009 did not fully grasp C language programming. Students felt very difficult in understanding algorithms in similar C language. They didn't know how to transform algorithms to complete source programs. Therefore, it is very difficult for students at the initial phase of doing experiment on computer. Most students lost interests and confidence in learning data structure after several experiments.

In order to help students better learn this course and master algorithm design theories and techniques, while explaining theoretical knowledge, we take appropriate measures to enhance students' programming skills.

348.2 Improving Students' Programming Skills

In order to enable most students to skilled master programming, and part of students to have the high programming skills so as to fulfill relatively difficult project development, we make full use of extra-curricular time to develop the second classroom to train students' programming skills. Detailed training plan has been established for this purpose.

348.2.1 Reasonable Time Arrangement

We practice programming training in the third term and the fourth term according to curriculum provision. The subjects are sophomores who have finished learning C language in the second term. So the training will lay the foundation for their learning data structure in the fifth semester.

348.2.2 Training Steps

There are three steps involved in the training skills. Firstly, at the beginning of the third term, teachers make training mobilization of students and introduce the purpose and significance of training to them. All participants take part in the training activity voluntarily. And then, teachers test participants on C language knowledge. Students are divided into two groups based on the test results, which are basal group and improved group. Secondly, teachers introduce the basic grammar of C language and programming training to the basal group. While advanced content of C language is introduced to the improved group. Two groups adjust at any time according to how students master the knowledge. Thirdly, teachers provide some small projects for students to complete in order to improve their programming level.

348.2.3 Training Content

The basal group's training contains data type, variable, operator, expression, program structures and statements, as well as modular programming technique and the use of array. The improved group's training contains the use of pointer, the operations and use skills of file. And the training contents of projects are decided by the study situation of students.

348.2.4 Training Method

Because the goal of training is mainly to improve students' self-practicing ability, we asked students to be in the laboratory and carry out practical operation on computer. In training, teachers explain a part of content, and then students write programs under the guidance of teachers. In addition, in order to inspire students' learning interests, teachers will provide some small games which are popular with students to students for use in programming training.

348.3 Paying More Attention to Proficiency of C Language

In the teaching of basic theory, teachers will connect knowledge point with array, pointer, structure body and function as much as possible. And at the beginning of learning the firstly several algorithms, teachers will give corresponding source programs of algorithms, and explain them in detail, so as to let students understand the relationship between algorithms and source programs. For example, while explaining the operation of sequence table initiating, teachers will give the initialization algorithm in similar C language after the algorithm idea is introduced. And then, teachers explain in detail how to transform the algorithm into source program. Through teachers' explanation and demonstration, students have a further understanding of the difference and connection between algorithms and source programs. They will practically grasp the transformation method step by step with proper exercises. So it not only deepens students' comprehension for algorithms but also strengthens their programming ability, and also lays a good foundation for the experiment on computer.

348.4 Constructing a Multi-level Experiment Teaching Mode

Data structure is a professional basic course with strongly practical. Experiment teaching is the important part of this course teaching. Experiments should not only take account into the depth of students' understanding of the algorithms, but also focus on the combination of principle and application, which aim to make students solve practical problems with learned knowledge. For this purpose, we build multi-level practice teaching system. That is, the practice content is divided into three layers, including basic experiment, course design, and extracurricular scientific activities.

348.4.1 Basic Experiment

Basic experiment is that, while learning theory, students debug algorithms in C compiler to realize various data structures and basic operations. According to the theory teaching, we carefully set eight basic experiments, 2 h each experiment and total 16 h. The major contents include: the basic operations of linear list, the operations of sequence stack and linked queue, traversing binary tree, creating and traversing graphs, the operation of searching binary sort trees, and so on.

In order to help students to form correct idea and prevent them from writing programs with unreasonable structure, we have made strict criteria for each experiment, and given a unified format, which consists of five parts: experiment purpose, preparative knowledge, experiment content, experiment process, as well as thinking and suggestion. In addition, considering the difference of students' programming ability, we provide reference programs. That is, teachers provide students with source program related to the first algorithm for each experiment. For example, teachers will give the initialization source program while making experiment on the basic operations of sequence table. Before experiment class, teachers will make experiment content arrangements. Meanwhile, students are required to analyze the subject and design algorithms. We encourage students with good school record and good capability of programming to accomplish the preparation independently. On the other hand, we suggest students with poor programming ability write algorithms into the given reference program. Thus, they can focus on understanding and debugging algorithms. Students debug and test programs on computer. Teachers guide students timely and inspire them to be independent and effective learners. Practice proves that these measures not only improve the success ratio of debugging program but also enhance students' confidence and interest in learning.

348.4.2 Course Design

As an important practical teaching process, course design is set up as subsequent supporting practice curriculum after theory teaching, which aims to realize the combination of theory and practice, improve students' ability of organization data and programming, as well as train their ability of relationship and cooperation.

In this stage, students are required to solve some larger scale problems combining with practical application. We design some more difficult and strong application projects to be chosen by students, such as sparse matrix calculator, parking management system, the problem of minimum spanning tree, and so on [4–6]. During this process, we take in the form of grouping, 3 students each group. Each group randomly selects a project. Group members cooperate to finish the project. With aspects of analysis, design, coding and debugging, students can understand deeply and master the logical features and physical storage as well as the algorithm design and software implementation.

In order to give students the basic training of the strict but good program design, we formulate the request of the standardization for course design steps: Firstly, requirement analysis. In this stage, the main job is to demand recognition analyze problems. Secondly, overall design. The main job is to define the data types and the basic function models of system. Thirdly, design in detail. The design task mainly is to refine the specification of data structure and basic operations, define the data stored structure, and determine the main procedure of algorithms. Fourthly, design realization. The job is to make students master the basic technique of error-detecting by coding and debugging. Fifth, completing the course design report is the last stage.

348.4.3 Extracurricular Scientific Activities

In order to broaden students' knowledge and improve their integrated competence, we encourage students to take part in all kinds of extracurricular scientific activities, such as university students innovation fund project, teachers' scientific research, mathematical contest in modeling, and so on. These activities contain many basic theoretical issues of data structure. By resolving these problems, it can arouse students' study enthusiasm, enhance their programming skills, and raise their ability to analyze and solve problems.

348.5 Practical Effect

We have taken those measures mentioned above in students of grade 2010 majored in the information and computer sciences, and found that, by being trained systemically step by step, during the fifth semester at the end of the data structure course, most students' programming ability was obviously improved. More than 80 % students could skillfully master the common algorithms in teaching materials. The successful experiments rate had been increased sharply. Students' interesting and confidence in learning was increased. And students' fear of difficulty in this course was also overcome. Practice proves that it is not only popular with students but also helpful to teachers to improve their teaching quality effectively.

Acknowledgments This work is supported by the teaching and research project of university of Jinan (J1121) and (J1123). The authors are grateful to Zhang Huaqing, College of Science, China University of Petroleum, and Chen Zhaoying, School of Mathematical Sciences, University of Jinan, for their suggestions. The authors are grateful for the anonymous reviewers who made constructive comments.

References

1. Yan W, Wu W (2003) Data structure. Tsinghua University Press, Beijing
2. Chen Y (2004) Attention to the importance of the source program in the course of data structre. Higher Edu Forum (1):73–75
3. Geng X (2007) Research and exploration of data structure teaching. J Changchun Norm Univ (Nat Sci) 26(3):104–105
4. Yan W (1999) Exercises set data structure. Tsinghua University Press, Beijing
5. He C (2003) Teaching innovation in data structure. J Sichuan Teachers College (Nat Sci) 2(1):19–21
6. Chen C (2003) Training students' logical thinking ability and innovative thinking ability in the data structure Course. J Zhejiang Shuren Univ 3(5):49–5

Chapter 349
A Study of the Effect of Long-Term Aerobic Exercise and Environmental Tobacco Smoke (ETS) on Both Growth Performance and Serum T-AOC, Ca^{2+}, BUN in Rat

Xiao Xiao-ling, Huang Wen-ying, Wu Tao, Yu Chun-lian and Xu Chun-ling

Abstract The purpose of this study was to examine the interaction and possible mechanism between long-term swimming program and exposed by Cigarette smoke in rats,on calcium concentration and the T-AOC and BUN's level. Methods:Thirty-two healthy Sprague–Dawley rats were randomly divided into 4 groups (n = 8/group): Exercise-Smoke (SD-Es), passive smoking (SD-S), exercise (SD-E), the control group (SD-C).SD-E and SD-Es group performed moderate-intensity swimming training for 12 weeks, More specifically, the exercise groups were progressively swim trained for 25 min, 6 days/week increasing from 25 to 70 min/day by the end of 12 weeks. SD-S exposed 8 cigarettes per day. Results: After regular swimming training and ETS stimulation for 12 weeks, the body weight showed a rising trend, and the average weight and thymus index of each group haven't significant difference ($P > 0.05$); But for spleen index terms, SD-Es and SD-S showed significant increase compared with group SD-C ($P < 0.05$), especially SD-S increased very significantly ($P < 0.01$); Serum T-AOC activity of SD-Es, SD-E were significantly lower than SD-C ($P < 0.05$); Serum Ca^{2+} concentration and BUN level of SD-S, SD-E and SD-Es were significantly lower ($P < 0.05$)compared with SD-C,but SD-Es and SD-S had a greater change. Results and conclusion Antioxidant adaptations associated with exercise training or an elevated fat diet individually reduced basal lipid per oxidation levels in the plantaris muscle. However, the combination of exercise plus a monounsaturated fat diet increased lipid peroxidation levels above that with either treatment alone. This suggests an exhaustion of the antioxidant capacity in the plantaris muscle when both exercise and increased dietary fat diet are combined.

X. Xiao-ling (✉) · H. Wen-ying · W. Tao · Y. Chun-lian · X. Chun-ling
Institute of Physical Education, Jiang xi Normal University, Zi yang Avenue No.99, Nanchang, China
e-mail: 624544378@qq.com

S. Li et al. (eds.), *Frontier and Future Development of Information Technology in Medicine and Education*, Lecture Notes in Electrical Engineering 269,
DOI: 10.1007/978-94-007-7618-0_349,

Keywords Aerobic exercise · Environmental tobacco smoke · T-AOC · Ca^{2+} · BUN

Many studies have shown that environmental tobacco smoke more dangerous for several times of harmful substances than active smoke. A national epidemiological survey in 1996 points out that about 71.2 % of people was plagued by environmental tobacco smoke in China. Tobaccos has been the focus of attention all the time, but studies very rarely related to effect and prevention of aerobic exercise on harm of environmental tobacco smoke. This article highlights the effects of ETS and aerobic exercise on oxidation resistance in rats through compared thymus, spleen index and serum T-AOC, Ca^{2+} and BUN's level each group,for a forward to provide a reference for public physical training.

349.1 Materials and Methods

349.1.1 Grouping[1]

32 two-month-old healthy male Sprague–Dawley rats were randomly divided into four groups after adjustment period for 1 week. Namely Eexercise-Smoke (SD-Es, n = 8), passive smoking group (SD-S, n = 8), exercise group (SD-E, n = 8) and the control group (SD-C, n = 8). Temperature was kept at 20–23 °C, Air relative humidity (RH) was 45 ~ 55 %, SD rats can feeding freely when total diet was controlled in clean cage at natural light room.

349.1.2 Methods

349.1.2.1 Experimental Method

(1) smoking protocol
 The ES, S groups were placed in semi-hermetic homemade glass box (60 × 40 × 40 cm), which has ventilation on both sides, through burning cigarette motionlessly to make rats in environmental tobacco smoke. Cigarette is made in Jiangxi province, in which there are 10 mg tar, 0.8 mg nicotine, 14 mg carbon monoxide. Smoking stimulation at 7:00 a.m.for 1 h, 6 days a week, over a 12-week period.

[1] [Fund project] In 2012, the Jiang xi provincial graduaande to student innovation fund project (project number YC2012 - S034), Jiang xi normal university graduate student innovation fund project (project number YJS2012040).

(2) Aerobic exercise protocol
ES and E group performed moderate-intensity swimming training in 7:00 p.m, rats swam without load in the white translucent plastic bucket which diameter is 75 cm in pairs,controlling water temperature at about 33 ± 6 °C, depth of water was 40 cm. Rats were progressively swim trained for 25 min at the first time after adjustment period, 6 days/week increasing from 25 to 70 min/day by the end of 12 weeks.
(3) Laboratory Equipment, Supplies and and index test
Rats were dissected at the end of day of the 12th week, heart blood was dispose with anticoagulant, leaved it rest for 30 min for testing index(T-AOC, BUN). Skeletal muscle tissue homogenate is used for testing calcium concentration. All test methods in this experiment is Colorimetry,and all of laboratory testing reagent were provided by the Nanjing Jiancheng Bioengineering Institute.

Laboratory Equipment and Supplies and : semi-autobiochemical analyzer (made in Italy), homemade glass boxes, homemade swim pool high speed and large capacity centrifuge machine (Centrifuge TDL-5), CS202B type electric dry oven (made in Chong Qing)

1.2.2 Mathematical Statistics Act

Data were analyzed by a factorial 2 × 2 (smoking x exercise) ANOVA performed using SPSS for Windows, version 18.0.

349.2 Results

349.2.1 Growth Performance of Rats

349.2.1.1 Body Weight and Organ Index

Dissection data shows body weight, index of thymus and spleen in Table 349.1.

The results in Table 349.1 shows that, all groups showed a growth trend in body weight during 12 weeks, average weight and thymus index was no significant

Table 349.1 Thymus, spleen index, and weight

Group N	Weight (unit g)	The thymus index (mg/g)	The spleen index(mg/g)
ES 6	296.37 ± 39.76	1.28 ± 0.42	2.42 ± 0.54*
S 7	317.90 ± 62.71	1.27 ± 0.76	2.76 ± 0.66△#
E 7	277.51 ± 11.92	1.35 ± 0.33	2.07 ± 0.40
C 8	313.61 ± 32.96	1.51 ± 0.68	1.73 ± 0.32

Note Significantly different of spleen index from SD-Es compared with SD-C, $^*p < 0.05$; significantly different of spleen index from SD-S, $^*p < 0.01$; significantly different of spleen index from SD-S compared with SD-C, $^{\#}$ $P < 0.05$

difference ($P > 0.05$); But spleen index is significantly different each group, compared with group SD-C, three groups' spleen index was significantly increased ($P < 0.05$), S group were very significant increase in spleen index ($P < 0.01$); S, E rat spleen index increased significantly ($P < 0.05$).

349.2.2 Impact of Taerobic Exercise and Smoking on Calcium Concentration and the T-AOC and BUN's Level

Laboratory testing results is showed in Table 349.2

349.3 Discussions

349.3.1 The Effects of Aerobic Exercise and Environmental Tobacco Smoke on Body Weight and Organ Index

Exposed to ETS has been shown to be associated with increased prevalence of upper respiratory tract infections, wheeze, asthma, lower respiratory tract infections,cancer and cardiovascular disease risk,especially in the fetus, youth and gravid as [1]. WANG Ai-ping [2], found a negative correlation between environmental tobacco smoke and height, body mass of children. They believe that ETS threaten growth and development of children. Experimental method is close to the actual environment, in which used semi-hermetic box imitate environmental tobacco smoke, and based on that, this result could be a reference for human experiments. It is well known that organ index is one of the signs that used to estimate nutrition status and pathological changes, and index of thymus and spleen are the most immediate and extensive sign to reflect the body's immune function.

Table 349.2 4 groups of rat's serum T-AOC, BUN level and Ca^{2+} concentration

Group N	T-AOC(U/mg port)	Ca^{2+}(m mol/L)	BUN(m mol/L)
ES 6	1.12 ± 0.76*	1.95 ± 0.27	9.61 ± 6.53*
E 7	0.92 ± 0.44*	$1.67 \pm 0.41\triangle^{\#}$	$2.92 \pm 1.81^{\star}$
S 7	1.45 ± 1.14	2.57 ± 0.48	5.93 ± 4.65
C 8	2.84 ± 1.89	2.14 ± 0.28	3.46 ± 2.58

Note Table 349.2 The results showed that compared with the ES group, serum T-AOC level of SD-ES, SD-E group were significantly lower activity ($p < 0.05$); rats serum Ca^{2+} concentration of SD-S group was significantly lower compared with SD-C ($\triangle P < 0.05$), SD-S, SD-E reduced significantly compared with SD-C ($P < 0.05$); SD-ES serum BUN levels were significantly increased, the difference was significantly ($P < 0.05$), SD-ES, SD-S group changed significantly compared, significant differences ($P < 0.05$)

The results of this study showed that the average weight and thymus index were not significantly different among all of groups, but there are significantly differences of spleen index from SD-Es, SD-S compared with SD-C and SD-E, indicating that long-term ETS exposure on rats impede growth. It has identical views with Li chen-Hao's [3]. Although aerobic exercise mitigated negative effect of ETS on growth and development of rats,it was not completely compensatory compare to negative effect harmfulness。 Plausible mechanisms of these differences is that ETS lead to gastric emptying delayed, duodenal fluid reflux and reduction in stomach blood flow which affect the digestion and absorption functions. It thus appears that ETS causes the metabolic disorder, that is increasing of physiological burden,then affects body weight, growth and development of tissues and organs.

349.3.2 Effect of Aerobic Exercise and ETS on Serum T-AOC Level

Cigarette smoke contains nicotine, tar, nitrosamines, carbon monoxide, radioactive substances and other Chemical hazards that can make the body produce free radicals or transformer into themselves which these Chemical hazards enter the body. It is generally known that free radicals is a common unstable intermediate that has strong the chemical activity. Free radical scavenging capacities of rats in this experiment are reflected by resting T-AOC serum level. Zhang Yi-ling, etc. [4] discussed the role of inflammation under ETS, studies show that ETS can induce lot of NO, thus forming a large number of free radicals, lead to inflammation at last. Li Qiyun, etc. [5] proved smoke (nicotine, etc.) weakened body antioxidant abilities and damaged DNA. Aerobic exercise can not only improve the body's antioxidant capacity, but also reduce the formation of free radicals. Chen Cai-zhen, etc. [6] suggest that low-intensity aerobic exercise can increase the body's activity of antioxidant enzymes in resting state, bind effectively free radicals that produce during exercise or after exercise. The results of this study have shown that exposured to long-term ETS cause a significantly difference in serum T-AOC level. T-AOC activity of SD-E was higher than SD-Es, but still lower than SD-C。 This illustrates that ETS bind activity of antioxidant enzymes, whereas aerobic exercise enhance it.

349.3.3 Effect of Aerobic Exercise and ETS on the Serum Ca^{2+} Concentration

Ca^{2+} plays an important role in development of life, it involves in the regulation of nerve conduction, muscle contraction, secretion and cell growth, etc. Exercise can cause imbalance of free radicals and Ca^{2+} concentration, with which cause significant mechanical damage and inflammatory response, then may lead to necrosis or apoptosis of cells [7, 8]. This study showed that ETS stimulation cause decrease of Ca^{2+} concentration for increase and transformation of Free radical. This indicating that aerobic exercise can reduce oxidative damage to improved functional disorders situation, thereby release free radicals damage, enhance the anti oxidant system.

349.3.4 Effect of Aerobic Exercise and ETS on the Serum BUN level

Urea is the end product of protein metabolism in human body that constitutes most of NPN. Blood Urea comes from liver, going through kidneys out of body with urine. In 1994,researchers have reported that smoking stimulate blood pressure and tachycardia, What does it cause by? The reason is smoking can affect amount of neurological effects of catecholamine by increasing it or decreasing clearance of it. As a result, it activates sympathetic, vasoconstriction of the system and slow down skin, and coronary blood flow.In daily life, BUN is usually used as monitoring induce in sport training [9]. This study showed that all groups have significant difference that serum BUN level is increasing clearly under stimulation of ETS and aerobic exercise. The result indicate that energy balance in rat muscle was destructed cause significant loss of glycogen in the body, thereby delaying protein and amino acid metabolism.

349.4 Conclusions

349.4.1 ETS Cause Increased Spleen Index

Spleen index of SD-ES and SD-group have increased significantly means metabolism disorder that caused by smoking which increases the body's physiological burden, then affects body weight, growth and development of tissues and organs.

349.4.2 Long-Term Exposed to ETS Decrease Antioxidant Capacity

Serum T-AOC level of SD-ES and SD-S decreased significantly, this indicating that ETS stimulation Inhibit activity of serum antioxidant enzyme. T-AOC activity of SD-E was higher than SD-Es, but lower than SD-C。 This illustrates that ETS bind activity of antioxidant enzymes, whereas aerobic exercise enhance it and maintain metabolic balance.

349.4.3 ETS Causes Decreased Serum Ca^{2+} Concentration, Aerobic Exercise Increases Serum Ca^{2+} Concentration

Increasing free radicals caused by ETS lead to Serum Ca^{2+} concentration decreased, in contrast, aerobic exercise make a increase in Serum Ca^{2+} concentration. Aerobic exercise decreases free radical transformation, improves functional disorder, and boost body's immune System.

349.4.4 Aerobic Exercise and ETS Increased Serum BUN Level Significantly

Stimulation of ETS and aerobic exercise cause significant difference that serum BUN level is increasing clearly. This indicates that energy balance in rat muscle was destructed, Aerobic exercise play an even greater role in load ability than ETS.

References

1. Guli, (2006) Acrylic wooden aspen wood, guli bahr, CARDS, nur guli, etc. Passive smoking for 7 to 12 years old children's lung capacity Ring. J Sch Health Chin 27(8):704–705
2. Wang A-P (2005) Passive smoking effect on preschool children's growth and development. Mod Combine Tradit Chin West Med J 14(7):974–975
3. Li C-H, Lai L-F, permission, etc. (2009) The influence of passive smoking in rat's growth and development level. J Jilin Med Coll 30(3)1127–1129
4. Zhang Y-L, Zhang X-H (2011) Passive smoking in rat lung tissue, alveolar larvae fluid, the influence of NO and NOS in serum. Guangdong Med 32(3):296–298
5. Li Q-Y, Zou D-Q, Xu Y-Y (2003) Smoker's lymphocyte DNA and serum SOD, LPO detection [D]。 Chin Public Health 12(7):832–833
6. Chen C-Z, Lu J, Xu H-W, etc. (2000) Aerobic exercise effect on antioxidant capacity in elderly mice skeletal muscle. J Sports Med Chin (3):273–274
7. Yang H-P, Wang J-M, Xiao-Lin (2009) Low oxygen, exhaustion exercise on skeletal muscle of rats, SOD, MDA, and the effects of mitochondria calcium. J Shan Dong Sports Inst 25 (5):24–28
8. M. de Paula Brotto, SA van Leyen, LS Brotto et. al. (2001) Hypoxia/fatigue- induced degradation of troponin I and troponin C:new insights into physiologic muscle fatigue. Folgers Arch- Eur Phys L 42: 738–744
9. Gao B-H, Ma G-J, Cui D-R (2006) 8 weeks practice (LoHi) low living high serum CK, BUN for a swimmer changing law. The Influence Sports Sci 26(5):48–52

Chapter 350
Research on Multimedia Teaching and Cultivation of Capacity for Computational Thinking

Yongsheng Zhang, Yan Gao, Jiashun Zou and Aiqin Bao

Abstract Computational thinking is a keenly concerned and important concept in current international computer community. The training of computational thinking capability is also an important issue of the current education community. With the further reform in education and the rapid development of information technology, the teaching media with computer multimedia technique at the core has been widely used in education and teaching. The paper introduces characteristics of multimedia teaching and the concept of computational thinking. in addition, on the basis of previous work, try to permeate computational thinking into multimedia teaching to enhance the students' computational thinking capability.

Keywords Education · Multimedia teaching · Computational thinking

350.1 Introduction

The computational thinking refers to the use of the basic concepts of computer science to solve problems, designing systems and understanding human behavior, which is an approach of thinking, a type of analytical thinking. Computational

Y. Zhang · Y. Gao (✉) · J. Zou
School of Information Science and Engineering, Shandong Normal University,
Jinan 250014, China
e-mail: zise0705@163.com

Y. Zhang
e-mail: zhangys@sdnu.edu.cn

J. Zou
e-mail: 1010336028@qq.com

A. Bao
School of Historical Culture and Social Development, Shandong Normal University,
Jinan 250014, China
e-mail: zkzkzhang@yahoo.com.cn

S. Li et al. (eds.), *Frontier and Future Development of Information Technology in Medicine and Education*, Lecture Notes in Electrical Engineering 269,
DOI: 10.1007/978-94-007-7618-0_350,

science has been side by side with the theoretical science and experimental science, to jointly be the three means to push forward the progress of social civilization and promote technological development. Strengthening the research in the teaching course system which cultivation of capacity for computational thinking as the core, optimize the structure of courses, improve the curriculum system, has become an important task of today's information technology education. Meanwhile, with the rapid development of multimedia technology and network technology, putting multimedia technology in traditional teaching has become the mainstream of the modernization development of education [3].

350.2 Multimedia Teaching and its Development

350.2.1 Multimedia and Multimedia Teaching

Multimedia has had a profound impact on many aspects of education. In multimedia teaching, utilize multimedia computer, synthesize word, sound, image, video and other multimedia information, complete the teaching process by means of the human–computer interaction between teacher and multimedia computer.

350.2.2 The Advantages of Multimedia Teaching

When using multimedia, situations and environment can be created, abstraction can be changed into concreteness, the teaching points will be highlighted to help students understand concepts and methods [5].

Multimedia teaching exploits dynamic presentation, to make up for the lack of experiment, to promote the development of the students' association and reasoning ability.

Multimedia teaching also facilitates students' self-learning and personalized training. Taking advantage of the network instructional videos, courseware and other resources, students' learning speed can be adjusted. For example, Web-based E-learning education model, it can maximize the use of existing educational resources.

350.3 Computational Thinking

350.3.1 Characteristics of Computational Thinking

Computational thinking is a kind of recursive thinking. Computational thinking using abstraction and decomposition to meet numerous and jumbled tasks or design. Computational thinking seeks answers by means of heuristic reasoning, which has the following characteristics: conceptual, not procedural; fundamental, not rigid skills; human, not a computer's way of thinking; complementarity and integration of mathematics and engineering thinking; thought, not a human creation; for all, be used in all places [2].

350.3.2 Importance of Cultivation of Capacity for Computational Thinking

Using basic concepts of computer science to solve problems, design systems and understand behavior, that is the establishment of computational thinking [2]. Professor Zhou Yi-Zhen, who believes computational thinking should be the basic skill essential for everyone, not only belong to computer scientists. Not only reading, writing and arithmetic (3R) but also computational thinking should be mastered when we cultivate children's analytical capability. Just like the printing and publishing to promote popularity of 3R, computing and computer is in a similar positive feedback to promote the spread of computational thinking. As a problem-solving tool, computational thinking truly integrates human activity, which everyone should master, everywhere will be used [6]. The prominent computational thinking ability will become an integral part of the creative talents' quality.

350.4 Multimedia Teaching and Cultivation of Capacity for Computational Thinking

350.4.1 Integrate Computational Thinking into Multimedia Teaching

With all the advantages and resources of multimedia teaching, penetrate computational thinking throughout all aspects of multimedia teaching to enhance students' computational thinking ability. During multimedia teaching process based on computational thinking, when teachers developing instructional objectives, providing instruction, and evaluating student performance, as well as the learners setting up right objective, finishing the task, sharing and exchanging learning content cultivation of capacity for computational thinking always be regarded, so that students can grasp the learning content with high efficiency [3]. The following is a multimedia teaching process which is integrated into computational thinking, the process is briefly given in Fig. 350.1.

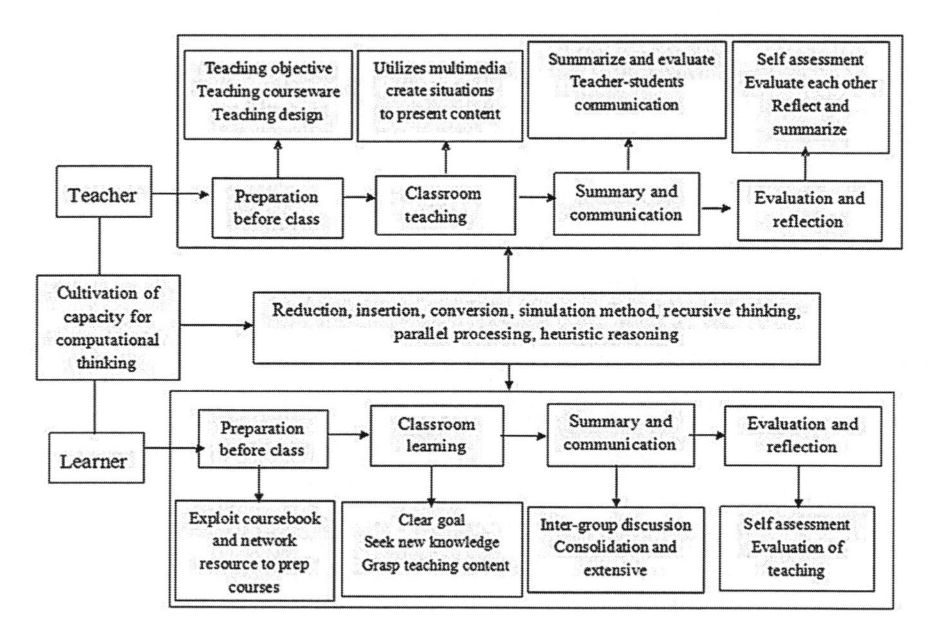

Fig. 350.1 The process of multimedia teaching which is integrated into computational thinking

350.4.2 The Process of Multimedia Teaching Which is Integrated into Computational Thinking

The first step of the implementation is preparation. Teacher takes full use of multimedia teaching resources which based on the idea of computational thinking, decomposes the difficult point of knowledge. Namely, teacher adopts computational thinking to achieve the decomposition of complex problems, takes separation of concerns (SOC) approach to convert a large and complex problem into small problems, when solve small problems, the complex issues are complete at the same time [1].The learner can take advantage of network teaching resources, to have general understanding of the course.

The second step of the implementation is classroom teaching. Teacher will present the multimedia courseware vividly to the students in the classroom, so that students can be impressed with the teaching content to learn efficiently and explore an in-depth solution of the problem, feel and improve the computational thinking ability. In addition to the traditional classroom teaching, teachers also can adopt class projects, regular seminars and exchange experiences in the network learning platform so that achieve the aim of cultivation of capacity for computational thinking.

The third step of the implementation is summary and communication. After classroom teaching, the teacher should analyze and summarize to determine whether the students' computational thinking ability was improved or not, leading students to summarize the knowledge point of the whole learning process.

In addition, guide the students to demonstrate the learning results of this stage, exchange and share their own learning experience. Learners can take advantage of Web 2.0 personal learning platform to achieve the share and communication: learners use blog to organize individual learning records and feelings, use RSS, tag technology to get a quick access to the resources needed, and then achieve the sharing and exchange of resources between the different individual platforms [4]. The use of multimedia teaching network platform can make teachers and students easily exchange learning problems, also improve computational thinking ability.

The fourth step of the implementation is evaluation and reflection. After the teaching activities, teachers' self-evaluation and their interactive evaluation is needed, to evaluate whether the teaching process contribute to students' mastery of the knowledge system and cultivation of computational thinking ability. Learner can use the network platform to evaluate teaching, the learner also need to evaluate their own learning process and share on the network. According to the evaluation of the various aspects from the teachers and students, they can explore how to better cultivate the computational thinking ability.

350.5 Conclusions

Making good use of multimedia can assist teaching. On how to cultivate computational thinking capacity during multimedia teaching, the paper carried out some bit of exploration, further study is needed, related theory and technology should be further gone into. Every IT teacher needs to pay attention to the advantages of multimedia teaching in the teaching process, vigorously develop students' computational thinking ability.

Acknowledgments This research was supported by Natural Science Foundation of Shandong Province of China under Grant No. ZR2011FM019. It was also supported by the Project of Shandong Province Higher Educational Science and Technology Program under Grant No. J12LN61. In addition, the authors would like to thank the reviewers for their valuable comments and suggestions.

References

1. Chen G-L (2012) Computational thinking. Commun CCF (Chin Comput Fed):31–34
2. Wing JM (2006) Computational Thinking. Commun ACM 49(3):33–35
3. Li S-J, Wei X-F, Jiang S-Z (2008) Study on the application of Web 2.0 in education technology ability training of normal university students. Mod Educ Technol:98–101
4. Mou Q, Tan L, Zhou X-J (2011) Research of task-driven teaching pattern based on computational thinking. Mod Educ Technol:44–49
5. Zhang Q-Z, Yu X-H (2011) Computer based education. Higher Education Press, Beijing
6. Zhou Y-Z (2007) Computational thinking. Commun CCF (Chin Comput Fed):83–85

Chapter 351
The Algorithm of DBSCAN Based on Probability Distribution

Ma Yu, Gao Yuling and Song Shaoyun

Abstract Data cluster is an important area of data mining and this technology has been vastly applied in many fields like data mining, statistical data analysis, mode recognition and image processing. Up to now, many cluster calculation methods that are applied to large-scale datbase have been put forward. The algorithm of DBSCAN is the spatial cluster method based on density with the advantages of fast-speed, effectiveness in dealing with noise and finding out clusters of any shape. Aimed at the limitations of DBSCAN in dealing with non-core object, this paper puts forward the algorithm of DBSCAN based on probability distribution. The results shows that the improved algorithm has improved the quality of cluster.

Keywords The algorithm of DBSCAN · Cluster algorithm · Probability · Data mining

351.1 Introduction

Spatial database stores plenty of data about space, like the map, the remote sensing or medical graphical data after the data preprocessing. Spatial data mining means to extract the non-obvious knowledge, spatial relation or other meaningful modes of the spatial data base. Data clustering is one of important subjects in the field of data mining and it divides data into subclasses, making the data of different subclasses different,, the data of the same subclasses is the same [1]. Up to now, many calculation methods of data clustering has been put forward, which all try to deal with the problem of data clustering in the large-scale data.

M. Yu (✉) · G. Yuling · S. Shaoyun
School of Information Technology and Engineering, Yuxi Normal University, Yuxi, Yunnan, China
e-mail: yxmy@yxnu.net

S. Li et al. (eds.), *Frontier and Future Development of Information Technology in Medicine and Education*, Lecture Notes in Electrical Engineering 269,
DOI: 10.1007/978-94-007-7618-0_351,

The algorithm of DBSCAN [2] is the spatial clustering method based on density, which uses the conception of cluster based on density. That is to say, it requires that the number of the objects (points or other spatial objects) in a certain area in the required clustering space is not less than a certain threshold. The algorithm of DBSCAN is representative of the spatial clustering method, which divides the areas dense enough into clusters, and finds out clusters of any shape in the noisy spatial database. In order to solve the problems of the rather large internal memory support, lack of IO consumption, and the poor quality of cluster resulting from non-average distances between the data density and cluster, ZhouShuigeng [3–5] puts forward some solutions. This paper brings up the algorithm of DBSCAN based on probability distribution to deal with the imprudent phenomenon existing in the boundary objects. That is to say, the method calculates the function value of the non-core objects based on the probability density function and deals with the non-core objects again according to the probability. The result shows that the improved method has improved the quality of cluster.

351.2 Related Knowledge

351.2.1 The Algorithm of DBSCAN

The algorithm of DBSCAN put forward by Ester Martin, et al. is a spatial clustering method based on density. Its main idea is: as for the every object in a certain cluster, the number of data objects in the neighborhood whose radius (Eps in the paper) is made certain must be more than a certain number. That is to say, the neighborhood density must surplus a certain threshold (MinPts in the paper). The cluster process of the DBSCAN is based on the fact that a cluster could be made certain by any core objects. Equivalently, it could be shown like this:

(1) make the data object p certain which meets all the requirements of a core object, then the data objects o which could be reached from p in the database D form an assemblage O,
$O = \{o|o \in D, \text{and the density about Eps and MinPts from o to p isreachable}\}$
the assemblage forms a complete cluster C, and $p \in C$;
(2) make the cluster C and any of its core objects p, C equals to assemblage O;

In order to find out such a cluster, p needs be found out from D, then find out all the objects that could reach p as regards to density in D. if p is the core object, that is to say, the number of objects in the neighborhood whose radius p is Eps is not less than MinPts, the cluster about Eps and MinPts could be found. If p is a boundary point, the number of objects in the neighborhood whose radius p is Eps is less than MinPts, to wit, no density could be reachable from p, p is to be marked as temporarily. Then, use the DBSCAN to analyze another object in the process

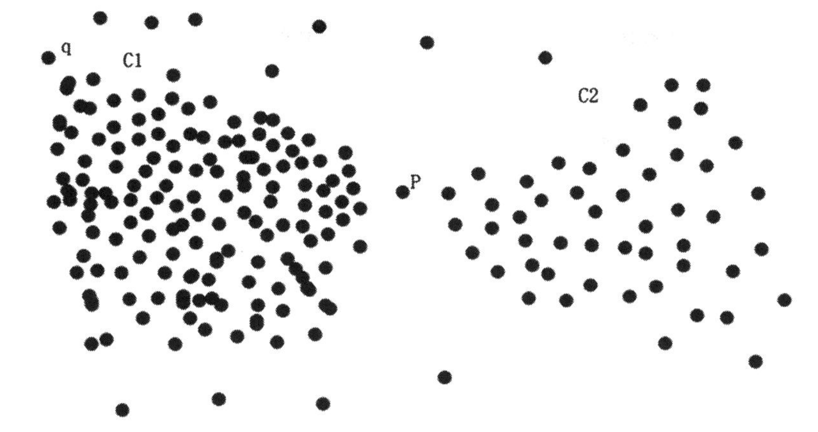

Fig. 351.1 Clusters of different densities

database, from what has been analyzed, it shows that there exist 2 problems in the process of dealing with boundary point.

(1) Some boundary points in the boundary of two clusters may link with the density of the two clusters at the same time, and the algorithm places the cluster that is to be dealt with first. When the DBSCAN is applied, these boundary points may be divided into different clusters if the sequence of the core points is not the same. Therefore, the results are likely to be different because of the different sequences. As the point p in the Fig. 351.1, if the first core point to be used belongs to cluster, p is to be arranged C_1 in cluster C_1; If the first core point to be used belongs to cluster p, is to be arranged C_2 in cluster C_2;

(2) The method arranges all the non-core points that have a distance of less than Eps from the core point to the cluster that the core point belongs to and make them the boundary points of the cluster. But, there exist some problems in the method, because it may include those points surrounding the real boundary points into the cluster. In the real data, every cluster has different density, some more dense, and others less dense, but this calculation method uses the global parameter Eps and MinPts. So, the boundary points of the denser cluster may be core points, and the boundary points of the less dense cluster may not be core points. If the distance between the denser cluster and the points surrounding it is not more than Eps, the points may be included into the cluster as boundary points and some points may also be included. Point p in the Fig. 351.1 could be arranged into cluster C_1 as its boundary points.

351.2.2 The Algorithm of the Expectation Maximization [6]

Make certain the conjecture of the parameter values and use the algorithm of the Expectation Maximization to calculate the probability of every point belonging to every layout. Then use the probability to calculate new conjectures of the parameter values which are maximum likelyhood. Repeat this process again and again until the conjecture of the parameter values does not change or has little change [7]. The algorithm of the Expectation Maximization is shown as the following:

Choose the initial set of the model parameter:

Expectation step: for every object, calculate the probability of every object belonging to every layout, namely calculate $prob(\text{layout j}|\text{x}_\text{i}, \theta)$.

Maximum step: use the probability gotten in the expectation step and find out the maximum to estimate the new parameter.

(Replace the conditions, and if the changes of the parameter are less than pre-supposed threshold stop replacing the conditions.)

The algorithm of EM uses the probability as the measurement of similarity. Suppose the data in the clusters obey the specific layout, evaluate the layout function system of every cluster and use the probability to determine the object's belonging to which cluster. Then, use the algorithm of EM to adjust the layout function system of every cluster. Finally, arrange these points based on the new layout function system. Repeat this process until the cluster results form [8]. For example, if the layout of cluster C_i obeys the probability function $f_{C_i}(v)$, the probability of points belonging to this cluster is:

$$P(C_i|v) = \frac{P(v|C_i) \times P(C_i)}{P(v)} = \frac{P(C_i)}{P(v)} f_{C_i}(v)$$

If $P(C_i|v) > P(C_j|v)$, the points in the place of v are more likely to belong to cluster C_i than C_j; then this object is to be arranged in the cluster C_i.

351.3 The Algorithm of DBSCAN Based on the Probability Distribution of Objects

351.3.1 The Main Idea of the Algorithm of DBSCAN Based on the Probability Distribution of Objects

Because of the above problems exist in the method of DBSCAN when dealing with boundary points, this paper uses probability distribution to judge the belonging of boundary points. The improvement method deals with the boundary points as the following: calculate the density value of boundary points according to the density function value of every cluster in the whole data base and make it

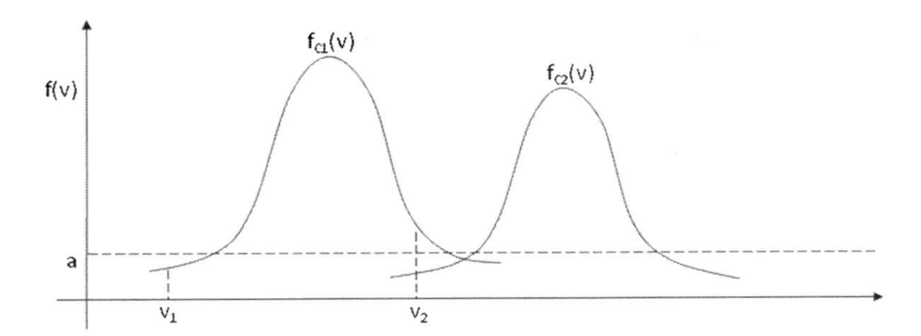

Fig. 351.2 Density processing examples of boundary points

belong to the cluster with larger density value. If all the density function value are less than a given threshold, the threshold is the noise. Thus, as far as the first problem is concerned, the function value belongs to the cluster with larger density value; as far as the boundary points in the second problem is concerned, the boundary point and the noise could be classified based on the function value. As the Fig. 351.2 shows, $f_{C_1}(v)$ is the probability density function of cluster C_1, $f_{C_2}(v)$ is the probability density function of cluster C_2, a is the threshold, the points in v_1 are considered as noises because their function values are less than a, v_2 belongs to the cluster C_1 because of $f_{C_1}(v) > f_{C_2}(v)$.

The processing of algorithm is as the following: use the algorithm of DBSCAN to get the cluster result of the whole database, in the process of which mark the data object as core point, boundary point and noise. Then, calculate the probability density function of every cluster based on the layout of core points in every cluster. Finally, based on the layout function results, calculate the layout function of the every layout function of the boundary points and make it the cluster that has the largest probability. If the largest probability is less than a given threshold, mark it as a.

Generally, the layout function could be estimated in the constant time range [9]. This paper presupposes that the core object in every cluster is placed according to multivariate normal distribution, namely, $V \sim N_d(\mu, \psi)$, in which d is the spatial dimension, μ is the mean vector, ψ is the covariance matrix, and the distribution function is

$$f(v) = (2\pi)^{-\frac{d}{2}}(\det\psi)^{-\frac{1}{2}}\exp[-\frac{1}{2}\Delta^2(\upsilon)] \tag{351.1}$$

$$\Delta^2(\upsilon) = (\upsilon - \mu)^t\psi^{-1}(\upsilon - \mu)$$

In this formula(1), the place v of a cluster and the mean vector, μ are both dimensional vector and define covariance matrix ψ as d*d dimension. The mean vector and covariance matrix are unknown, so in practice the value of (μ, ψ) is estimated at its maximum and name a cluster that has n points at the place of

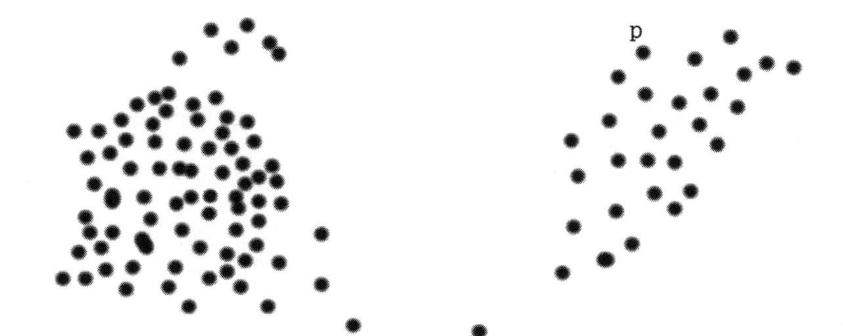

Fig. 351.3 An example

$(v_1, v_2, \ldots, v_n)$. So, the value of (μ, ψ) could be calculated according to the following formula:

$$\hat{\mu} = \frac{1}{n}\sum_{i=1}^{n} v_i \text{ and } \psi = \frac{1}{N}\sum_{i=1}^{n} (v_i - \hat{u})(v_i - \hat{u})^T$$

Noise is the object that is different from other data or that does not belong to any cluster. The number of the objects in the neighborhood Eps of the data object p is less than Minpts. And the data object q does not exist in any cluster. So, the density of and p are linked with each other about Eps and Minpts and p is marked as noise in the method of DBSCAN. If the problems are dealt with like this, the points arranged in the cluster have the chance of being marked as noise because every cluster has different density in the practical situation. Also, this method uses the global parameter Eps and Minpts, so the boundary points of the more dense clusters may be core points and the boundary points of the less dense clusters may not be core points. As for the points of the less dense clusters, they are regarded as noise because the boundary points are not core points. As the Fig. 351.3 shows, p may be looked as noise because its surrounding data objects may be boundary points.

The improvement algorithm deals with the noise point like this: calculate every function value of points based on the probability density function of every cluster. If the function value is more than the given threshold, classify it into the corresponding cluster, if the function value is less than the given threshold; mark it as the noise points. The p in the Fig. 351.3 may be classified into cluster after calculating the probability density function value.

351.3.2 Description of the Calculation

The algorithm is as the following:

Input: object assemblage DB in spatial database to be dealt with; Minimum neighbor Minpts to the core points; distance of neighbor object Eps; probability density function threshold a;

Output: objects in the spatial data base that has been cluster-marked or noise-marked;

Step1: cluster using the algorithm of DBSCAN and classify the data objects into core points, boundary points and noise points;

Step2: calculate the probability density function system $(\mu_1, \psi_1), (\mu_2, \psi_2), \cdots (\mu_n, \psi_n)$ of the cluster calculated in the step 1';

Step3: calculate the probability density function value of every non-core points; if the largest function value is more than a given threshold, it belongs to the cluster that is gotten by the largest value; Or, it is the noise point

351.3.3 *Analysis of the Algorithm of DBSCAN and Experimentation*

The extra added by the improved algorithm: the first is the calculation of the probability density function system of every cluster. Hypothesize that there are *m* clusters and the job of calculating the probability density function system could be done within the constant time, so the complexity of the added time is *O(m)*. The second is value of non-core points. Hypothesize that there are *k* non-core points in the database, so the time complexity of probability density function system is *O(km)*. Therefore, the final time complexity is $O(n \log n + m + km) = O(n \log n + km)$, and $k, m << n$. The added space complexity *O(m)* is the probability density function of the memory clusters. Because *k*, *m* is not more than *n*, the added time and spatial complexity is not that much. The improved algorithm based on the simulated data could get better results in dealing with non-core points.

351.4 Conclusion

Spatial cluster is a vital part in the data mining and it divides the object assemblage of the spatial database into many a meaningful clusters that are formed by similar objects. The algorithm of DBSCAN based on density has the advantages of fast-speed, effectiveness in dealing with points and finding out clusters of any shape. Also, it is not prudent enough in dealing with boundary objects of clusters. Aimed at its shortcoming, this paper puts forward the algorithm of DBSCAN based on probability distribution. The experimentation based on the simulated data shows the improved DBSCAN is superior to the former one as regards to the quality of clustering.

References

1. Han J, Kamber M (2001) Concept and technology of data mining translated by fang ming, meng xiaofeng. Machine Press, Beijing
2. Ester M, Kriegel HP, Sander J, Xu XA (1996) Density-based algorithm for discovering clusters in large spatial databases with. In: Proceedings second international conference knowledge discovery and data mining, AAAI Press, Portland
3. Zhou S, Fangye, Zhou A (2000) DBSACAN algorithm based on the data extraction. Micro-Comput Syst 21(12):1270–1274
4. Zhou S, Zhou A, Caojin (2000) DBSACAN algorithm based on the data distribution. Comput Res Dev 37(10):1153–1159
5. Zhou S, Zhou A, Caojin, Hu Y (2000) Algorithm of speedy cluster based on density. Comput Res Dev. 37(11):1287–1292
6. Dempster AP, Larid NM, Rubin DB (1997) Maximum likelihood from incomplete data via the EM algorithm. J R Stat Soc B 39(1):1–38
7. Tan P-N, Steinbach MC, Kumar V (2006) Introduction of data mining translated by fangming, fang Jianhong. People's Post Press, Beijing
8. Lin C-R, Chen M-S (2005) Combining partitional and hierarchical alorithms for robust and efficient data clustering with cohesion self-merging. IEEE Trans Knowl Data Eng 17(2):145–159
9. Gen S, Zhang L (2001) Probability statistics (second version). Beijing University Press, Beijing

Chapter 352
Exploration and Practice on Signal Curriculum Group Construction of Instrument Science

Wang Rui, Liang Yu, Li Hui and Zhou Hao-min

Abstract Instrument science and technology is the source of information. Based on the target of cultivating high-quality talented personnel in the field of instrument science, the School of Instrument Science and Optoelectronic Engineering in Beihang University has integrated the signal curriculum resources for undergraduates in order to realize the teaching purpose of "Building a knowledge system to foster innovative thinking". A signal curriculum group that consists of core course "signal analysis and processing", elective course "DSP Technology" and optional course "Virtual Instrument" is built. The teaching contents of the signal curriculum group are organized by the curriculum relevance in order to form functional coupling among the various programs. The non-additively effect of the courses is generated and it promotes the integration and interaction between the undergraduate teaching and the discipline construction for instrument science.

Keywords Signal processing · Curriculum integration · Signal curriculum group construction · Instrument science · High-quality talented personnel

Instrument science and technology is an important means to provide detection and monitoring for objective things. With the penetration of high technology, instrument science and technology has gradually developed as a comprehensive discipline of knowledge-intensive and technology-intensive, which intersects with Precision Instrument, Measurement Technology and Instrument and Photoelectric Engineering. Therefore, instrument science and technology is not only an

W. Rui (✉) · L. Yu · L. Hui · Z. Hao-min
The School of Instrumentation Science and Opto-Electronics Engineering, Laboratory of Precision Opto-Mechatronics Technology, Ministry of Education, Beihang University, Beijing 100191, China
e-mail: wangr@buaa.edu.cn

L. Yu
e-mail: lybuaa@yeah.net

S. Li et al. (eds.), *Frontier and Future Development of Information Technology in Medicine and Education*, Lecture Notes in Electrical Engineering 269,
DOI: 10.1007/978-94-007-7618-0_352,

important part of information science and technology but also the source of information. The school of Instrument Science and Optoelectronic Engineering was reconstructed by four departments, which are Department of measurement and control system and information technology, Department of inertial navigation technology and instrument system, Department of optoelectronic engineering, Department of remote sensing science and technology. In order to catch up with the continuous development of cross subject and to promote the professional construction of the universities [1], the school defined its professional training target for the cultivation of undergraduate students. The principles are:

1. To meet the basic demand of society for the students majoring in instrument science and technology and to cultivate students with the ability of sustainable development.
2. To have the characteristic of the fusion of aeronautics, astronautics and information.

Considering the research contents of each subject are closely related to the theory and technology of signal sensing and detection, signal conversion and processing, information management and application, the school has established a training target of cultivating advanced application-oriented talents with high-level, high-quality in the field of precision photo-mechanic-electronic integration. Based on the guiding ideology that undergraduate teaching should intersect with discipline construction and the fact that our direction is mainly for photoelectric sensor test and detection guidance, we think it necessary for students to understand effective technologies related, thus they can fully experience the application of signal analysis and processing in the instrument science. From the perspective of being conducive to the interdisciplinary integration, we construct the signal curriculum group which was made up of core course "signal analysis and processing" (48 h), elective course "DSP Technology" (16 h) and optional course "Virtual Instrument" (36 h) in a logically integrated way.

352.1 Integration of Teaching Content to form the Core Course –"Signal Analysis and Processing"

In order to make undergraduate course of signal processing play a role of improving the undergraduates' innovative quality, the curriculum conformity is conducted based on the idea of adjusting the structure of courses, adopting advanced contents and reforming the management. The Beijing Higher Education High-quality Teaching Material "Measurement Signal Processing Technology" coauthored by ZHOU Hao-min and WANG Rui is adopted as teaching material for the core course, whose contents combine "signals and systems" and "digital signal processing" together. This teaching material is not only beneficial to the requirements of wide professional, thick foundation and high quality teaching, but also groundwork to achieve the teaching aim of compressing class hours.

"Signal analyzing and processing" is an extremely theoretical subject. Two methods (Continuous signal analysis, Discrete signal analysis) and three transformations (Fourier transform, Laplace transform, Z transform) have occupies an important position. Therefore, we have conducted a series of educational reforms with an innovation education mode that is "The physical concept is clear, mathematical methods combine with the engineering application". We first embark on perfecting teaching materials by compiling lab handout with three experiments and supplementing the materials about the Laplace transform on the "signal analysis and processing" website. The main characteristics of our educational reforms are summarized as the following:

1. The method of scientific metaphor teaching. We compare the function of the Fourier transform to a glass prism light decomposition (as shown in Fig. 352.1a) so that students have a thorough understanding of Fourier transform, which has core status in signal analysis and linear filtering. The Fourier transform is considered to be a "mathematical prism" and the function accordingly can be decomposed into different frequency components by the "prism". Teaching in this way is not only concrete and easy to understand, but also illustrating the mutual association of different curriculum knowledge.
2. Using symmetry and visualize format. When lecturing the concept about time shift and frequency shift of Fourier transform, circle convolution (as shown in Fig. 352.1b), as well as the relationship of signals' periodicity and continuity in both time domain and frequency domain, we summarize their crossing symmetry peculiarity and demonstrate them in a classified contrast way to make students understand the basic concepts clearly.
3. "Teaching by doing, learning by doing" [2]. Targeted at improving students' ability in comprehension, we developed the dynamic virtual simulation software and combined it with the multimedia. It was used in the signal processing teaching [3, 4] to strengthen the understanding of the important contents of the course (as shown in Fig. 352.1c, d). The use of the software in the signal teaching preliminarily realizes the virtual demonstration teaching method of "teaching and learning while doing". The real-time dynamic demonstration [5] causes strong resonance among students.

Consequently, "Signal analysis and processing" was rated as Beijing High-quality Course in 2007.

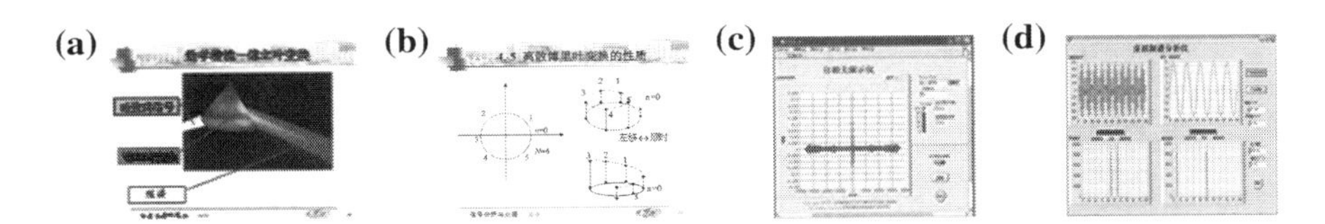

Fig. 352.1 Scientific metaphor teaching method in class

352.2 The Construction of Undergraduate Curriculum Group of Signal Analysis and Processing

High-quality course construction and educational reforms is characterized by incorporating the teaching idea of “fewer but better; the more profound, the more proficient” into curriculum reform [6]. Theoretical teaching and practical teaching not only have their own emphasis respectively, but also have cross-hybridization. Besides, practice teaching is not simply auxiliary and complementary to theory teaching, but an extension and a major link of the cultivation of creative quality [7].

Optional course “Virtual Instrument” uses virtual instrument graphical programming software LabView [8] for its lectures and experiments. Thus, students can understand that the core feature of virtual instrument technology is reconfiguration. They can also learn that virtual instrument technology is composed of three main parts, namely, modular hardware, hardware integration platform and software development platform. Signal processing is one of the important research points. Actually, the functions of the virtual instrument can be reflected in signal processing set, so the construction of the signal processing module library is the basis of the realization of its functions. The virtual instrument assists students to achieve the goal of cultivating the ability of developing virtual instruments.

“DSP technology” begins next term after the completion of the core course “signal analysis and processing”. With the support of the company MOTOROLA (now Free scale) and the school, we have developed 13 sets of “DSP56311 embedded experimental platform” (as shown in Fig. 352.2) for the course [9]. Through the platform, students will be able to get the configuration of the DSP chip and acquaint the development flow of signal processing and measurement control system. This course adopts the “Motorola 24-bit DSP theory and application”, edited by Zhou Hao-min professor, aiming at fostering the students’ abilities to apply DSP technology preliminarily to analyse and solve practical problems. At present, we have developed nearly 20 experiments on the “DSP56311EVM embedded experimental platform” for students’ alternatives.

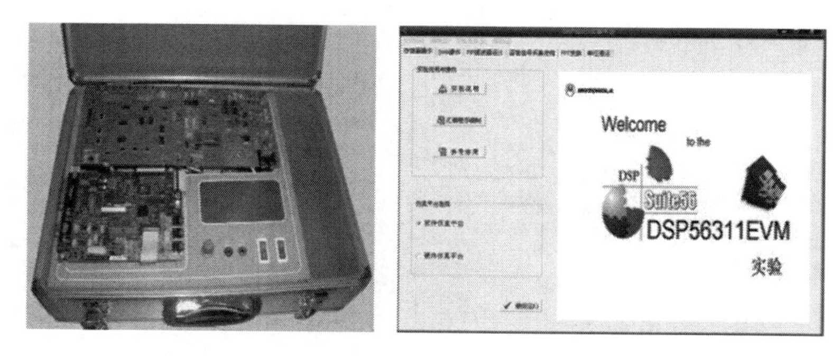

Fig. 352.2 DSP56311EVM Embedded system platform and main interface

"DSP technology" benefits students in understanding resource environment, unique Harvard bus structure and pipelining technology.

The signal curriculum group that consists of "signal analysis and processing", "DSP Technology" and "Virtual Instrument" dilutes the boundary between the software and hardware experiments, furthermore, strengthens practical teaching of specialized courses of signal. Throughout the courses, the contents of them have inheritance relationship longitudinally and have internal relations laterally. On the other hand, they are self-contained.

352.3 Conclusion

Teaching practice has proven that integration scheme has not only strengthened the fundamental theory of the signal processing, but also stimulated students' learning interest, above all, cultivated students' innovation consciousness and ability by the reasonable span among the course contents. The integrated teaching mode trinity of "teaching, learning, doing" is in favor of cultivating comprehensive qualities for the high-level instrumental science talents, and corresponds to the three training objectives of undergraduate education, namely, knowledge, ability and quality with the logic structure of "upside-down 品" [10]. Our next research direction is to effectively reduce class hours, combine the characteristic construction with curriculum group construction, and strengthen bilingual teaching to make the course in line with international standards.

Acknowledgments This work is financed by Beijing High-quality Course Construction project and Beihang University teaching reform project of "signal analysis and processing platform course construction".

References

1. Lei Q, Zhao N (2007) The analysis on the training objectives of engineering programs. J High Educ 28(11):11–15(Ch)
2. Wang R, Li B, Zhou H (2008) Research and realization of dynamic demonstration system for signal processing course. Exp Technol Manage 25(1):30–33(Ch)
3. Wang R, Li B (2008) Signal processing of dynamic virtual simulation software for teaching V1.3(Abbreviation: SigLaSim). Software copyright publication no. 2008SRBJ5389
4. Wang R, Liu Y, Zhao Y (2011) Kill two birds with one stone: boosting graduate students' abilities in simulation by realization dynamic demonstration experiments. The 6th international conference on computer science and education, ICCSE 2011, SuperStar Virgo, Singapore, 3–5 August 2011
5. Castro IP (1990) Computer aided teaching of digital signal processing[J]. Comput Educ 14 (5):433–443
6. Lu J, Feng J (2009) Exploration on integral teaching reform of curriculum for majors in science and engineering. Res High Educ Eng (2):137–139(Ch)

7. Fan X, Chen L, Qi H (2008) Create high-quality teaching resources with the main line of course group construction. Chin Electron Educ (3):40–44(Ch)
8. Wang R, Xu R, Li H (2012) Design and application of LabVIEW courseware in the signal processing teaching. In: Proceedings of computer science and education (ICCSE), 2012 7th international conference on Melbourne, VIC, pp 1365–1368
9. Yan L, Zhou H (2006) Design of DSP56311EVM teaching experiment platform microcontrollers and embedded systems. 29–34(Ch)
10. Yang Z (2005) A search on chinese undergraduate training objective. Higher Education Press, Beijing(Ch)

Chapter 353
On Improving the E-learning Adaptability of the Postgraduate Freshmen

Ruan Jianhai and Deng Xiaozhao

Abstract The learning adaptability is the psychological tendency of learner who strives to overcome the difficulties in the learning process, be consistent with the learning environment, so as to obtain good learning efficiency. Due to the change of learning environment and learning goals, the postgraduate freshmen face the problems of the learning adaptability at the first semester, so it is essential to explore the learning adaptability. This paper aims to improve the e-learning adaptability of the postgraduate freshmen. The problems, influencing factors and the significances of e-learning adaptability of the postgraduate freshmen are discussed, and the strategies of improving their learning adaptability are provided.

Keywords E-learning adaptability · Postgraduate freshmen · Influencing factors · Improving strategy

353.1 Introduction

With the rapid development of China's higher education, the postgraduate education achieves great-leap-forward developments, and the number of postgraduate enrollment is growing on a large scale. Due to the change of learning environment and learning goals, the postgraduate freshmen will face many learning disabilities at the first semester. These learning barriers lead to the problems of learning adaptability about the postgraduate freshmen. Therefore, to improve the learning

R. Jianhai (✉)
Library, Southwest University, Chongqing 400715, China
e-mail: rjh@swu.edu.cn

D. Xiaozhao
School of Computer and Information Science, Southwest University, Chongqing 400715, China
e-mail: dxz@swu.edu.cn

S. Li et al. (eds.), *Frontier and Future Development of Information Technology in Medicine and Education*, Lecture Notes in Electrical Engineering 269,
DOI: 10.1007/978-94-007-7618-0_353,

adaptability of the postgraduate freshmen becomes the focus of attention. The learning adaptability refers to the behavioral process of learner who strives to adjust oneself to achieve the balance with the learning environment according to the need of the environment and learning. With the continuous development of Information Technology, e-learning has become a main way of learning for learners. Therefore, the learning adaptability in the article refers to the e-learning adaptability.

353.2 The Problems of E-learning Adaptability of the Postgraduate Freshmen

The problems of e-learning adaptability of the postgraduate freshmen are as follows:

353.2.1 Lacking of Self-Regulated Learning Ability

The study of postgraduate is different from the learning of undergraduate. Besides the mandatory classes and elective classes, self-study is the main way of learning for the postgraduate students. Self-regulated learning is the indispensable ability for postgraduate students. However, a number of the postgraduate freshmen are lack of the self-regulated learning ability. For example, the postgraduate freshmen don't know how to do the self-regulated learning online.

353.2.2 Lacking of Information Consciousness

Information Consciousness refers to the level of the conscious awareness on Information value understanding, the urgency of Information Need, the sensitive degree of capturing information, and the information ability of analysis, judgment and absorb. If there is not the necessary training in undergraduate study stage, the postgraduate freshmen will not have the Information Consciousness. The postgraduate freshmen do not realize the information, for example, how important it is for their studies and research.

353.2.3 Lacking of Information Literacy

Information literacy is a kind of comprehensive ability which person acquires by integrating one's Information consciousness, Information need, Information tools and Information sources, and the skill of Information evaluation, Information absorption, and Information utilization organically. Because of the lack of professional training in undergraduate study stage, the postgraduate freshmen tend to show a lack of information literacy. For example, the postgraduate freshmen didn't realize the importance of reading academic papers and monographs.

353.2.4 Lacking of Information Ability

Information ability refers to the ability to collect information, or the information processing ability which a person can improve one's ability to work and study better by analyzing and understanding information to absorb new knowledge. If there is not the specialized training in undergraduate study stage, the postgraduate freshmen will not know how to choose a specialized databases and how to retrieve the information what they need by themselves.

353.2.5 Lacking of Academic Communication Ability

Academic communication is an important part of scientific research work. The nature of academic communication is the information exchanges. The ultimate goal of academic communication is to make scientific information, thoughts and ideas get communication and exchanges. The postgraduate freshmen often didn't realize the importance of academic exchanges, as a result, they rarely participate in academic seminars and lectures in the first semester.

353.3 The Influencing Factors of Learning Adaptability of the Postgraduate Freshmen

The influencing factors of learning adaptability of the postgraduate freshmen mainly include two aspects: the environmental factors and the postgraduate students' personal factors.

353.3.1 The Environmental Factors of Learning Adaptability

353.3.1.1 The Curricula Registration is Unreasonable

Almost all colleges and universities require the postgraduate freshmen to register all of the courses (the compulsory courses and the optional courses) in the first semester. In the case of don't understand the curriculum system and the course content, the course registration has the nature of objective blindness for the postgraduate freshmen. Besides, once registered, it is difficult for the postgraduate students to change the registered courses later.

353.3.1.2 The Guidance of Supervisor is Non-Individuality

The supervisor of postgraduate students in China are busy, they are busy with teaching, and engage in scientific research. If the freshman of postgraduate student is not communicates with the supervisor actively and timely, the study goals and research interests of the freshman of postgraduate student will be unclear. The situation of non-individuality guidance is very much conspicuous when the supervisor has several postgraduate students in the same year.

353.3.2 The Postgraduate Students' Personal Factors of Learning Adaptability

353.3.2.1 Learning Objectives are Unclear

Because of unclear learning goals, some of the postgraduate students lack of learning motivation. The purpose for some of the postgraduate students is just to get the master's degree, rather than to accumulate knowledge and to improve ability. Learning is just to deal with the examinations. The utilitarian purpose is becoming more and more serious.

353.3.2.2 Learning Methods are Improper

Many postgraduate freshmen still follow the learning methods at the undergraduate level. They do not realize the importance of self-regulated learning, and do not know how to do the research-based learning. They rely too much on the guidance of supervisor or classroom teaching, and do not know how to actively explore or to make a thorough inquiry. Some postgraduate freshmen are to focus only on books knowledge, while ignoring the psychological health and the ability of problem-solving from experiment. Some postgraduate freshmen pay attention to the accumulation of knowledge, while ignoring the improvement of scientific research ability.

353.4 The Significances of Improving the Learning Adaptability of the Postgraduate Freshmen

To improve the learning adaptability of the postgraduate freshmen has special impact and roles for the postgraduate students. The significances of improving the learning adaptability of the postgraduate freshmen are as follows:

353.4.1 To Enhance the Postgraduate Freshmen to Achieve Their Goals

The learning adaptability is the psychological tendency of learner who strives to overcome the difficulties in the learning process, be consistent with the learning environment, so as to obtain good learning efficiency. To improve the learning adaptability of the postgraduate freshmen will help the postgraduate freshmen contribute to make the postgraduate freshmen aware of value of learning, to familiar with the method of self-regulated learning, to develop science skills and processes, to promote self-regulating capacity and learning ability, to build their own learning goals, and to lay a good foundation of achieving their learning goals.

353.4.2 To Empower the Postgraduate Freshmen and Expand their Knowledge Structure

To improve the learning adaptability of the postgraduate freshmen will help the postgraduate freshmen contribute to stimulate the learning motivation, to reinforce and develop the natural love of learning of the postgraduate freshmen, and expend the knowledge scope of the postgraduate freshmen, and the ways that the post-graduate freshmen acquire knowledge. It also can play a vital role in changing the postgraduate freshmen's experience and knowledge structure, and in creating and developing attitudes and skills such as information skills and critical thinking skills. These experiences, attitudes and skills will empower the postgraduate freshmen to navigate in the ocean of knowledge and will be useful for lifelong learning.

353.5 The Strategies of Improving the Learning Adaptability of the Postgraduate Freshmen

In order to promote the postgraduate freshmen to achieve their goals, the following strategies or measures will help to improve the learning adaptability of the post-graduate freshmen and to maximize the effectiveness of the learning adaptability.

353.5.1 To Carry Out the Learning Adaptability Education

The learning adaptability education, as the priority of the entrance education of postgraduate freshmen, should closely combined with professional features, and give full play to the role of experts, scholars, supervisors, the senior postgraduate students and outstanding graduates, and take various educational ways to help the postgraduate freshmen to understand the postgraduate training schemes and various teaching management rules and regulations as soon as possible, and facilitate the postgraduate freshmen timely to generate professional interest in learning and self-confidence, and change the learning attitude from passive learning to active learning.

353.5.2 To Stimulate Continuously the Learning Motivation

Instructors and administrators should actively to help the postgraduate freshmen to establish the correct world outlook, outlook on life and values, and to set clear goals in life. Supervisors should actively to help the postgraduate freshmen to design the study projects and career planning, and to stimulate their sense of responsibility, to develop academic quality, and to promote their strong interests of the professional training program, and build clear learning goals, and strengthen constantly the learning motivation.

353.5.3 To Improve the Ability of Self-Regulated Learning

The self-regulated learning refers to the learning process or ability which learners set the learning goals, develop the learning plans, select the learning methods, control the learning process, and evaluate the learning outcomes. The learning behaviors of self-regulated learning are mainly the continuous cycle of self-planning, self-management, self-monitoring and self-evaluation. The self-regulated learning is a learning method that the postgraduate student must master. Therefore, instructors and administrators must allow the postgraduate freshmen have the apparent direction and the target, and know what should be done and what is the right way. To improve the ability of self-regulated learning will help the postgraduate freshmen to stimulate the self-motivated and to enhance their capabilities and quality.

353.5.4 To Create a Good Learning Atmosphere

Education practice shows that the study style or school climate is the key factor of influencing student's learning behavior. Good style of study will establish good study habits. To create a good learning atmosphere is the historical mission of colleges and universities, and is the needs of students' growth and development. Therefore, colleges and universities must attach great importance to the construction of good style of study, and establish and improve the regulations and long-term mechanism of the construction of study style. Instructors and administrators should help the postgraduate freshmen to set up the correct learning value orientation, and to establish the positive learning behavior.

353.6 Conclusion

To improve the learning adaptability of the postgraduate freshmen will help the postgraduate freshmen to familiar with the method of self-regulated learning, to promote self-regulating capacity and learning ability, and to lay a good foundation of achieving their learning goals. It is essential and important to improve the e-learning adaptability of the postgraduate freshmen.

References

1. Total number of Postgraduate Students (Master's Degrees) http://www.moe.edu.cn/publicfiles/business/htmlfiles/moe/s7255/list.html
2. Feng T, Li H (2002) The preliminary research on the learning adaptability of the contemporary college students. Explor Psychol 22(1):44–48
3. Wei X (2013) Thinking about strengthening the learning adaptability education of college students. http://www.cnki.net/kcms/detail/11.3776.G4.20130321.1156.095.html
4. Lu X (2012) Literature review of domestic research on learning adaptability. J HuBei Adult Educ Inst 18(3):3–5,17
5. Lin X (2004) Analysis of environmental factors influencing e-learning adaptability. Open Educ Res 51(5):61–63
6. Deng X, Ruan J (2008) Empowering internet users to use 6 W-based learning. In: Proceedings of 2008 IEEE international symposium on IT in medicine and education (ITME 2008), Dec 2008

Chapter 354
Construction of a Network-Based Open Experimental Teaching Management System

Yan-Rong Tong and Peng-Bo Song

Abstract Constructing an open college physical experiment management system based on Browse/Server architecture has a lot of function such as experiment preparation, experiment booking, score managing and mutual communing between teachers and students, as well as improving the students' independency and the ability of select during the process of studying experiment. It has a promoted effect to the information standardization of the experimental management. And it can effectively improve the utilization efficiency and quality of the lab. So opening lab is the main form of implementing the open experiment teaching mode, and networked experiment teaching platform is the foundation of the opening experiment teaching.

Keywords College physics experiment · Network · Open teaching mode

354.1 Introduction

The college physics experiment is the compulsory course for science and engineering students in the college and university. It's of vital importance for cultivating students' innovative spirits and improving students' practical ability. There are about 3,000 students who take part in the college physics experiment in our school each semester, meanwhile, 30 experiments need to be completed timely by each student. For quite some time, the teaching mode is schemed uniformly with fixed experiment projects, fixed experiment time and fixed experiment places, as

Y.-R. Tong (✉)
School of Physics and Technology, University of Jinan, Jinan, China
e-mail: hztyr@163.com

P.-B. Song
School of Physics and Electronics, Shandong Normal University, Jinan, China

S. Li et al. (eds.), *Frontier and Future Development of Information Technology in Medicine and Education*, Lecture Notes in Electrical Engineering 269,
DOI: 10.1007/978-94-007-7618-0_354,

well as unified arranged grouping list of students because of the lack of support of relevant information management platform. Although it can guarantee the complement of the students' studying tasks, it also performed less than satisfaction in bringing students' subjective initiation into play in the aspects of giving them adequate learning time and abundant free content. But as time passes, it is not conducive to cultivating students' practical and innovative ability. Therefore, It's of primary importance to building an open experiment teaching system for college physics experiments [1].

354.2 Design the Open Management System of College Physics Experiment

By using PHP technology, we made full use of campus network to design and develop the teaching management system of college physics experiments which is based on B/S architecture. Its main function is experiment booking and score managing. Users are divided into three categories according to their access to modifying the permissions: students, teachers and administrators. Students can finish experimental inquiring, experiment booking and experiment changing, appointment querying, score inquiring and experiences exchanging through any terminal connected to the network. Teachers can also see about students' information, confirm the experimental reservation, release the experimental information, input, dispose and correct the experimental score. Administrators can complete many schedules such as: the announcement of the experiment information, the management of the teachers' information, browsing and modifying of the experimental information, the information of the reservation, the development of the experiment and the summarizing and printing of the experimental score. Moreover, the platform can also be used to manage laboratory devices, to resource the experimental teaching and to discuss the experimental technique as well. Rich teaching resources such as electronic courseware, experimental videos, device images, simulation experiments are included in the physical experimental teaching database, students can browse these resources through the Internet, they can preview before classes and review after classes. The content of the experimental teaching was extended in both space and time [3].

354.3 Realization of the Open Experimental Teaching Management System

The system chosen the scheme which is based on multimedia and network technology, that is to say, that the whole system was installed on a dedicated server who uses the WWW mode to realize a visit. This pattern broke the limit of time and space, students can preview, book, inquiry and communicate while teachers can upload experimental information, query the background situation of the reservation system, manage the experiment score, answer questions and communicating with students at the same time whenever and wherever the computer and the Internet are available. The development environment of the System is based on the B/S structure, the database server adopts the Windows 2003 operating system, the database management system adopting the Mysql technique, the Web server adopting the Apache server and the scripting environment adopting the PHP script for development [4].

The system is divided into five modules with every mode connected with each other according to different design requirements. The system's security management module lies upon four other modules (the users' and experimental information management module, the students' course selection module, the teachers' experiment operation module and the system's process management module) and the system sets different permissions for different users. Administrators are allowed to use the whole functions offered by the system while other users are only permitted to use part of the functions. The adoption of the modular design is beneficial to the functional improvement of each part and the design is advantageous to the expansion of the system owning to the reserved room for new increased modules.

354.3.1 The System's Security Management Module

The system adopts double limits to ensure the secure operation on the system. First of all, the function of setting different permissions according to different users is added to the management webpage; Second, limitations of power for different users is also added to every management operating web. At the same time, the function of file backups and data updating is provided in the database as well, which ensured the fundamental protection of the system.

354.3.2 The Users' and Experimental Information Management Module

Users' information management module includes information management of the students, teachers and the administrators. The information management of the teachers is relatively simple for the number and data quantity are less when compared with students. Considering this situation, for student's data, the system carried out the classified management method, that is, to classify the students into several groups according to their different schools, professions, classes, and the classification, when we need read the data, there is no need to open the database for the classification. We can reach easily and directly. Furthermore, when the students' data changes, such as the adding of a new profession or a new class, the only thing need to do is just to regenerate the students' classification file in the interface.

The experimental information management module is used by administrators to conduct many operations such as: adding, modifying and deleting. First, it is the setting of the basic information of the experiment; and then the class time of the experiment. Management of the experimental projects itself including two items: modifying the experimental information and deleting the experimental projects, of which the latter operation would delete the relevant experimental time at the same time.

Management of the experimental class time, including two other items: checking the list of the students who are scheduled in this experiment and modifying the information of this experiment. For some special cases, such as the temporary change of the experimental class site, the temporary change of the class time and the sudden canceling of the experiment can also be modified just through a separate modification of the experimental time information.

354.3.3 The Students' Course Selection Module

Students' course selection module is the uppermost function of the system, for most of the data inputed in the selective system platform obtained by large number of students' course selection operation. Although the design of the course selection module is not complicated, it does have quite strict requirements for security and stability, which lies in the fact that hundreds of people always login at the same time, and this requires the system occupying the resources as few as possible by the designing of delicate algorithm to prevent the case of abnormal operation due to the server's insufficient system resources.

Several questions should be taken into consideration when we book the experiment: ①the class time; ②the accommodation and saturation of the laboratory; ③the denunciation of the students. Students are asked to cancel the appointment a week prior to the experimental time according to fact of the school.

354.3.4 The Teachers' Experiment Operation Module

The main operations of the teachers are attendance registering and score inputed. In the experimental class time interface, teachers are able to know the experimental condition very clearly: whether the attendance has been resorted or not, whether the grades has been inputted or not, thus they are able to arrange the next procedure according to the current situation.

354.3.5 The System's Process Management Module

System management module is the most important part of the system, which includes management of experimental projects, management of teaching resources, management of report printing, experiment information releasing, online message replying and management of fundamental configuration. Administrators use the experimental projects management module to carry out many operations such as: adding, modifying and deleting experiments. The management is divided into two levels: one is management of the experimental projects itself and the other management of the experimental class time, at the same time, experimental courses with few students can be canceled timely and classes can be changed easily.

354.4 Conclusion

Information management is an inevitable trend in the college and university. This paper introduce the open network experiment teaching management system of college physics experiment which is an important component of the instruction reformation project in our school. The system is based on B/S mode and developed by PHP And MYSQL technology. Being a solid platform for realization of modernization, informationization and scientization of the experiment teaching management, The system promote the standardization of the experiment teaching management and make the experiment teaching more flexible and diverse and as well improved quality of the experiment teaching management and utilization of the experiment resources effectively. The platform has been in successful operation on campus network for many years and has won broadly popularity among teachers and students in our school, which made the teaching of college physics experiment extend on both time and space. The platform constitute an important part of experiment methods of open mode and courses reformation of credit teaching.

References

1. Wan G (2011) Construction of a network-based open experimental education resources management system. Res Explor Lab
2. Wang K (2006) Scientific management of opening physics experimental teaching. Chin Adult Educ 163
3. Song G, Gai G (2010) Research and practice of the open experimental teaching mode. Res Explor Lab 92
4. Xu B, Fan J (2007) A network-based opening experiment teaching management system. Opt Techn 339

Chapter 355
Prediction of Three-Dimensional Structure of PPARγ Transcript Variant 1 Protein

Cong Sun, Qiang Wu, Ye-chao Han, Ting-ting Tang and Li-li Wang

Abstract To predict three-dimensional structure and binding site of ligand from amino acid sequence of peroxisome proliferator-activated receptor gamma (PPARγ) transcript variant 1 protein. The secondary structure and surface properties of PPARγ transcript variant 1 protein such as hydrophilicity, physical and chemical properties, surface probability, flexible regions, motif, transmembrane domain, signal peptide and secondary structure were analyzed to predict its binding site of ligand by bioinformatics methods and means. Many potential binding sites of ligand were identified. *Conclusion* The secondary structure and binding site of ligand of PPARγ transcript variant 1 protein were predicted successfully by multiparameter. This study provided a foundation for identification of its advantage binding site of ligand and understanding its biological functions on the basis of protein structure.

Keywords PPARγ · Transcript variant 1 protein · Binding site of ligand · Motif

C. Sun · T. Tang · L. Wang
Changchun University of Chinese Medicine, Changchun 130117, China
e-mail: suncong7097@sina.com

Q. Wu (✉)
Department of Chinese Medicine, China-Japan Union Hospital Jilin University, Changchun 130033, China
e-mail: zap1210@163.com

Y. Han
Jilin Institute for Veterinary Drug and Feed Control, Changchun 130062, China
e-mail: hyc7097@sina.com

S. Li et al. (eds.), *Frontier and Future Development of Information Technology in Medicine and Education*, Lecture Notes in Electrical Engineering 269,
DOI: 10.1007/978-94-007-7618-0_355,

355.1 Introduction

PPARs is a kind of nuclear ligand-activated transcription factor found by Issemann in 1990. PRARs family contains three subtypes which are PPARα, PPARβ(or PPARδ) and PPARγ. The current research on PPARγ subtype was the most advanced which has many biological effects [1–3] including anti-inflammatory response, anti-oxidative stress, protection to endothelial cells and regulation of lipid metabolism. This study analyzed the structure of PPARγ transcript variant 1 protein and predict binding site of ligand in theory by internet and software such as DNA star.

355.2 Materials and Methods

355.2.1 Amino Acid Sequence

Amino acid sequence of PPARγ transcript variant 1 protein used to predict is from GeneBank (accession number: NM_138712.3).

355.2.2 Prediction to Secondary Structure

Conducted by the Protean module provided by DNA Star Protein software. Predicted secondary structures by the crystal structure of the sequence of amino acid residues raised by Chou–fasman. Analyzed and predicted secondary structures by Gamier-Robson method that is calculating the possibility of specific amino acid residues in specific structure.

355.2.3 Analysis of Hydrophilicity, Accessibility and Plasticity

Analyzed hydrophilicity by hydrophilic standard in Kyte-Doolittle scheme. Analyzed surface accessibility by Emini scheme. Analyzed plasticity by Karplus-Schultz scheme.

355.2.4 Analysis of Hydrophilicity, Accessibility and Plasticity

Predicted antigen index by antigen index analysis module provided by DNA Star Protean software and Anthe Prot software. The module adopted Jameson-Wolf' method that is a kind of integrated prediction method including prediction scheme of hydrophilicity, surface characteristics, plasticity and secondary structure.

355.2.5 Prediction of Signal Peptide and Transmembrane Region

Predicted signal peptide and cleavage site by Neural network and hidden Markov model methods on the internet (http://www.cbs.dtu.dk/services/Signal/). Predicted region of transmembrane structure of PPARγ transcript variant 1 protein utilizing Tampm method.

355.2.6 Confirmation of Binding Site of Ligand

Screened out the site with good quality in hydrophilicity, accessibility and plasticity according to the prediction results of protein in hydrophilicity, surface accessibility, plasticity, signal peptide, transmembrane region and secondary structure. Excluded the sequence of α-helix, β-pleated sheet, signal peptide and transmembrane region, confirmed the sequences located at the corner and random coil especially the regions that can form special domains as dominant binding site of ligand.

355.3 Results

355.3.1 Whole Protein Composition Analysis

The length of protein: 477; Molecular Weight: 54680.20 Daltons; Isoelectric Point: 6.45; Charged amino acids's number count is 164; Acidic amino acids's number count is 64; Basic amino acids's number count is 58; Polar amino acids's number count is 123; Hydrophobic amino acids's number count is 160.

355.3.2 Prediction to the Secondary Structure

The secondary structures of protein gotten from different prediction methods were not exactly the same. The number and location of α-helix, β-pleated sheet and β-turn is difference. The calculation results show that predicted structural class of the whole protein belongs to α-helix protein according to the prediction to secondary structure. Chou–Fasman scheme displays that α-helix accounted for 68.2 %, β-pleated sheet accounted for 4.39 %, β-turn accounted for 9.41 %, random coil accounted for 18 %. β-helix of small interval was crowded in the complete sequence. There were structures of random coil and few structures of turn in the septal area. Most structures of random coil and turn located on the protein surface. There were the regions with flexibility and easy to deformation. Most α-helix with large fraction located in transmembrane region. Garnier-Robson scheme displays that α-helix accounted for 45.6 %, β-pleated sheet accounted for 24.1 %, β-turn accounted for 28.5 %, random coil accounted for 1.8 % (Fig. 355.1).

355.3.3 Analysis of Hydrophilicity, Accessibility and Plasticity

Hydrophilicity is the inherent characteristics of 20 kinds of amino acids. It is one of important factors to decide the final three-dimensional conformation of protein. Analyzed hydrophilicity of protein by Kyte-Doolittle method. Hydrophilic region were more than hydrophobic regions obviously on the whole. It means the protein is soluble in water. Predicted the analysis curve of surface accessibility by Emini scheme. Located at the molecular surface in high accessibility areas, buried in the interior of the molecule in low accessibility. Predicted plasticity by Karplus-Schultz scheme. There was a piece of region with high plasticity at the N terminal (47 ~ 104). There were many pieces of region with high plasticity at the N terminal in intermediate peptides (154 ~ 163; 184 ~ 194; 238 ~ 245; 269 ~ 275; 458 ~ 463). The regions were flexible and easy to combine with ligands (Fig. 355.2).

355.3.4 Analysis of Antigen Index

Predicted ligand binding site of PPARγ transcript variant 1 protein by Jameson-Wolf method and software such as DNAstar, AnthePro t. It showed that that there were many potential ligand binding sites (Fig. 355.3). Potential ligand binding domains were 35 ~ 45; 47 ~ 53; 55 ~ 66; 76 ~ 110; 126 ~ 135; 138 ~ 152; 158 ~ 173; 179 ~ 194; 209 ~ 216; 229 ~ 249; 251 ~ 256; 263 ~ 270; 281 ~ 290; 292 ~ 315; 317 ~ 328; 330 ~ 351; 356 ~ 361; 371 ~ 376; 387 ~ 395; 400 ~ 413; 418 ~ 425; 429 ~ 442; 446 ~ 457; 461 ~ 476; 482 ~ 492.

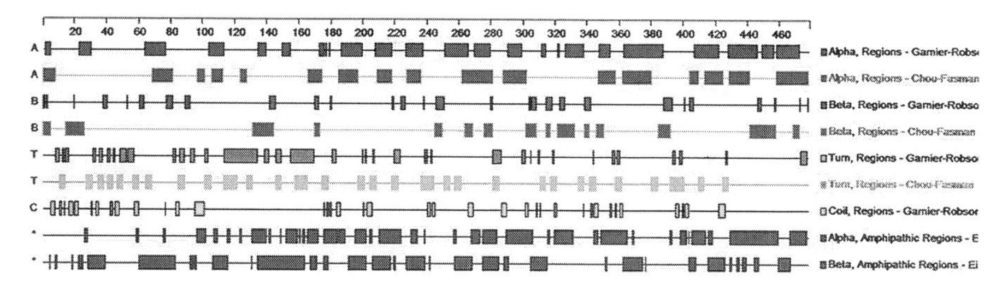

Fig. 355.1 Prediction of secondary structure

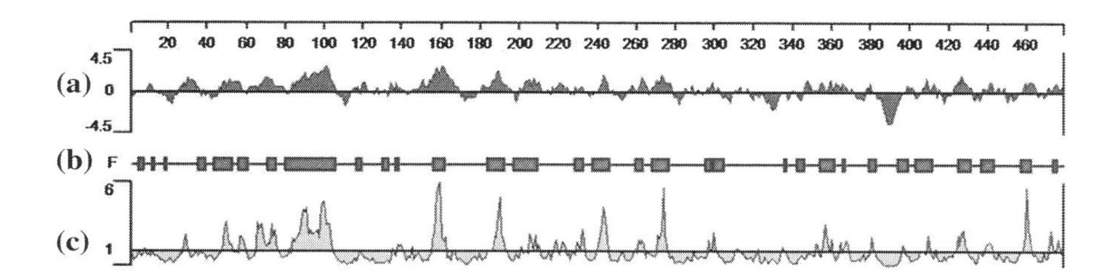

Fig. 355.2 Analysis of hydrophilicity, surface probability and flexible regions. **a** Hydrophilicity plot-Kyte Doolittle. **b** Flexible regions-Karplus-Schulz. **c** Surface probability plot-Emini

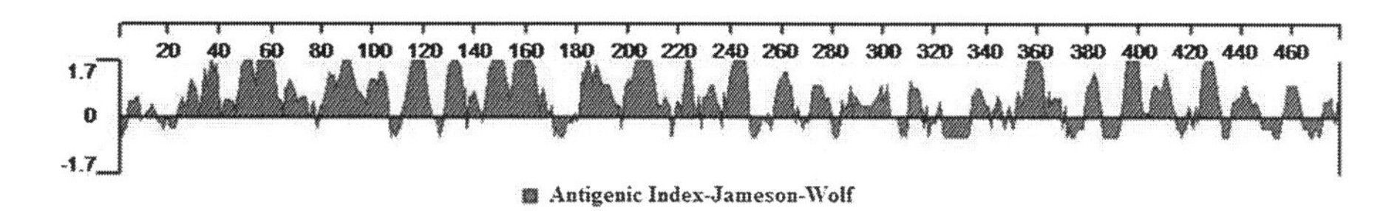

Fig. 355.3 Analysis of antigenic index of PPARγ transcript variant 1 protein

355.3.5 Prediction of Signal Peptide and Transmembrane Region

The transmembrane region is major position where protein combines with lipid in membrane. In general it is comprised by 20 hydrophobic amino acid residues. Forms α-helix to fix on the cell membrane. The prediction results showed 3 transmembrane regions which were $97 \sim 132$, $164 \sim 195$, $394 \sim 420$; PPARγ transcript variant 1 Protein has no signal peptide.

355.3.6 Comprehensive Evaluation on Ligand Binding Site

Predicted signal peptide and cleavage site by Neural network and hidden Markov model methods on the internet (http://www.cbs.dtu.dk/services/Signal/). Predicted region of transmembrane structure of PPARγ transcript variant 1 Protein utilizing Tampm method.

355.4 Discussions

Bioinformatics is a cross subject which formed gradually at the end of 1980s along with genome sequencing data increases rapidly. With the continuous improvement of protein database, research and development of algorithm to predict of structural domain provide simple and fast method to predict ligand binding sites for us. The method is applied to the prediction of ligand binding sites of protein or peptide whose primary structure are known. We can utilize the correlation of binding sites and the physicochemical properties or secondary structures to predict through the calculation of the protein sequence of physicochemical properties and secondary structures on the basis of phenomenological theory. This method can enhance the purpose in the late function experiment, improve the rate of success, decrease the workload, save time and research funding.

More and more experts and scholars pay attention to the study on PPARγ [4, 5]. This study adopts bioinformatics technology to predict and analyse the secondary structure structure, ligand binding sites, transmembrane region and three-dimensional structure of PPARγ transcript variant 1 protein. Dominant ligand binding region are chosen from the regions of strong hydrophilicity, good flexibility, β-turn on the protein surface and random coil. β-turn and random coil are flexible construction, most of them are located on the protein surface, easy to deformation. Although α-helix and β-turn are not easy to deformation,they can form specific motif to combine with the ligand. In addition, four or more contiguous hydrophobic residues in the sequence should be avoided. The more the charged amino acids have, the better [6]. Signal peptide and transmembrane sequence should also be excluded. Based on the above factors, predicted and got 6 dominant ligand binding sites that are amino acid sequences between 76∼110, 158∼173, 229∼249, 263∼270, 292∼315, 330∼351. The main structure between 76∼110; 292∼315 were αα. The main structure between 330∼351 were α β α, formed specific motif.

References

1. Brown J, Plutzky J (2007) Peroxisome Proliferator-activated receptors as transcriptional nodal points and the rapeutietargets. Circulation 115:518–533
2. Glass CK, Ogawa S (2006) Combinatorial roles of nuclear receptors in inflammation and immunity. Nat Rev Immunol 6:44–55
3. Lehrke M, Lazar MA (2005) The many faces of PPARgamma. Cell 123(6):993–999
4. Jing K, Bei CH, Lei J (2010) PPAR signal transduction pathway in the foam cell formation induced byvisfatin. Acta Physiol Sin 62:27–432
5. Heikkinen S, Auwerx J (2007) Argmann CA.PPARgamma in human and mouse physiology. Biochim BioPhys Acta 1771:999–1013
6. Tu S, Chen K, Zhong L-P et al (2010) Structural analysis and antigenic epitope prediction of snake venom C type lectin family proteins. Chin J Immunol 50:963–972

Chapter 356
Interactive Visualization of Scholar Text

Ming Jing and Xueqing Li

Abstract Text visualization method depends on the contents of documents to analyze patterns and abstract characters. Words set or semantic relationships often get involved. However, visualizing the large scholar text as an understandable view for users is a challenging. We propose an interactive model to describe the scholar information by statistical work and clustering results. The users' diverse interests are concerned by customizing the parameters. And the interface is designed to access data easily. Our conception comes from our experiences designing the Scholar Browser for a university which displays the contribution of departments and topic similarity between them.

Keywords Information visualization · Scholar text · Statistical model

356.1 Introduction

Information Visualization is arguably the fastest-growing branch of the visualization discipline in the last decade. The main goal of visual character analytics research is to augment human cognition by devising new methods of coupling data modelling and interactive visualization [12]. The word interaction is often used in different situation, always with animation, which often concerns navigation, making choices, animated transitions.

Text is an important attribute in infovis datasets. This information can be structured into three categories: content, structure, and metadata. And the methods are diverse for different categories of interest. A scholarly article or book generally is based on original research or experimentation. It is written by a researcher or

M. Jing (✉) · X. Li
The department of Computer Science and Technology, Shandong University, 250101 Shandong, China
e-mail: jingming@sdu.edu.cn

S. Li et al. (eds.), *Frontier and Future Development of Information Technology in Medicine and Education*, Lecture Notes in Electrical Engineering 269,
DOI: 10.1007/978-94-007-7618-0_356,

expert in the field who is often affiliated with a college or university. Most scholarly writing includes footnotes and/or a bibliography and may include graphs or charts as illustrations as opposed to glossy pictures. Find a method to analysis the relationships or connections between those scholar texts is important to abstract the required information from the growing mass.

There are many algorithms to visualize text related to scholar or academy. But the most scenes of visualization are static displays of specific parts. They lack interaction and transitions, as well as flexibility.

In this paper we introduce an interactive method to visualize scholar texts, which includes published papers and thesis. We concern the users' diverse interests by customizing the parameters. Meanwhile, our interactive design does not only focus on the visual interface but also on modelling choices. Our conception comes from our experiences designing the Scholar Browser and research on text visualization.

We first discuss the prior work on text visualization and other related work in Sect. 356.2. Then describe our story of setting up the Scholar Browser. In this process, we discuss the model and metadata for this project and the method to compute word and topic similarity of publication from departments. Also, we provide the visualization and interaction details of the browser. We will give a conclusive text and future work.

356.2 Related Works

Text visualization method depends on the types of information contained in a text document, which can be structured into three levels: content, structure and metadata. The content includes the details in the text itself. The basic way to visualize a document is to show the content via a document's interface such as PDF viewer. Meanwhile, some interface also display the structure and metadata.

The most text visualization involves all these three level simultaneously. The tag clouds [13] or word clouds, which are found both in analysis tools and across the web, are a common method to visualize unstructured text. It mainly focuses on the semantic relationships but structures by summary or statistics tools [4]. The words in the cloud are expected to cover all the terms according to the language or document contents to get the ideal results [5]. For some situations, more than one word needs to anticipate to get in-depth analyses especially for the words have diverse meanings. Other methods are proposed to solve vague text, such as WordTree [14], DocuBurst [6].

Topic modeling research attempts to understand document text. Latent Dirichlet allocation (LDA)[1] is a popular method to discover latent topics, which are often proposed to analysts as a set of probable items [2], via intelligently learning distributions of words. An analysis of "topical concepts" can generate an outline of a collection [7]. However, if the analysis project becomes specific, the value of the topic model degrades. The issues of trust arise to improve the confidence of model on latent topics [3, 8].

Based on entity-relation models exhibit clearly-defined units of analysis, which may include location, people, data, time and connections between them. They have strong ability to verify and modify model and have support for progressive disclosure of model abstractions.

Some issues are often concerned in interactive research. Interactive navigation is to change either the viewpoint or the position of an object in a scene. In non-navigational settings, making choices is common, for example through radio buttons on a control panel or menu choices that affect the display. Viewers have a much easier time retaining their mental model of an object if changes to its structure or its position are shown as smooth transitions instead of discrete jumps [10]. Many studies of multimedia applications have compared user performance between still imagery and prescript animations where the user has start, pause, and stop controls [9].

356.3 The Design of a Scholar Browser

The Scholar Browser is to display the quantity and quality of the university-wide publications ordered by time. Manually numerate all the document is impossible due to not only the number of documents but also the expertise required to understand especially when the cross-topic occurs. Our goal is to design a model-driven visualization browser to help the university administrators to acquaint the situation of university-wide publication.

356.3.1 Metadata

The dataset we use here contains full-text Ph.D. dissertations, graduate thesis and all published papers from an university from 2007 to 2013. For each document, the advisor, department, year and type of publication, and Impact factor for each paper are included as metadata. Here the type of publication is divided to journal, conference, and others. We abstract the keywords from each document as the input data to compare and analysis the similarity between two departments based on keyword and topic. To compute the word similarity of departments, we use the cosine similarity of TF-IDF vectors representing each department, a standard approach used in information retrieval [11] as follows.

$$\cos(v_{D_1}, v_{D_2}) = \frac{v_{D_1} \cdot v_{D_2}}{||v_{D_1}||\,||v_{D_2}||}$$

where v_D is the vector for a department made up of combination topic catalog SC_D.. Here combination subject catalog is a transition of IC which is the index of the Chinese Library Classification (CLC). We apply latent Dirichlet allocation (LDA) [1] to infer latent topics in the corpus, and represent documents as a lower-dimensional distribution over the topics. We compute the topic similarity of two departments D_1 and D_2 as the cosine similarity of their expected distribution over the topics θ_d learned by LDA. This expectation is the average distribution over latent topics for dissertations in that department as follows.

$$\mathbb{E}|\theta_D| = \frac{1}{|D|}\sum\nolimits_{d \in D} \theta_d$$

Meanwhile, for each department, we compute the publication contribution by weighted combination of impact factor which is devised by Eugene Garfield, the founder of the Institute for Scientific Information. The impact factor is a measure reflecting the average number of citations to recent articles published in the journal. It is frequently used as a proxy for the relative importance of a journal within its field, with journals with higher impact factors deemed to be more important than those with lower ones. That would be impartial to evaluate the achievement of department.

356.3.2 Timeline

We summarize the data by a year to show the state of publications organized by departments. Comparing to the nearby years, it is easy to discover the trend of publications including the subject movement and quantity. Along this time line, each department has a depiction according to the quantity and quality of publication. Also, the position shows the topic similarity between any two departments.

356.3.3 Interactive

It is inflexible to observe micro and macro features simultaneously with complex graphs. If all interfaces zoom in for details, the graph is too big to view entirety. If you zoom out to see the overall structure, small details are lost. Focus + context [] techniques allow interactive exploration of an area of interest (the *focus*) in greater detail, while preserving the surrounding environment (the *context*). For our browser, the data is organized by year sequentially which is logical and understandable. The interested region will extend to show more details as users wish. To show the trend of changes for a chosen department such as subject movement, all relevant data will be displayed in one page expressly. To focus the plot, other irrelevant visualization will fade and bedim until the captured department is released.

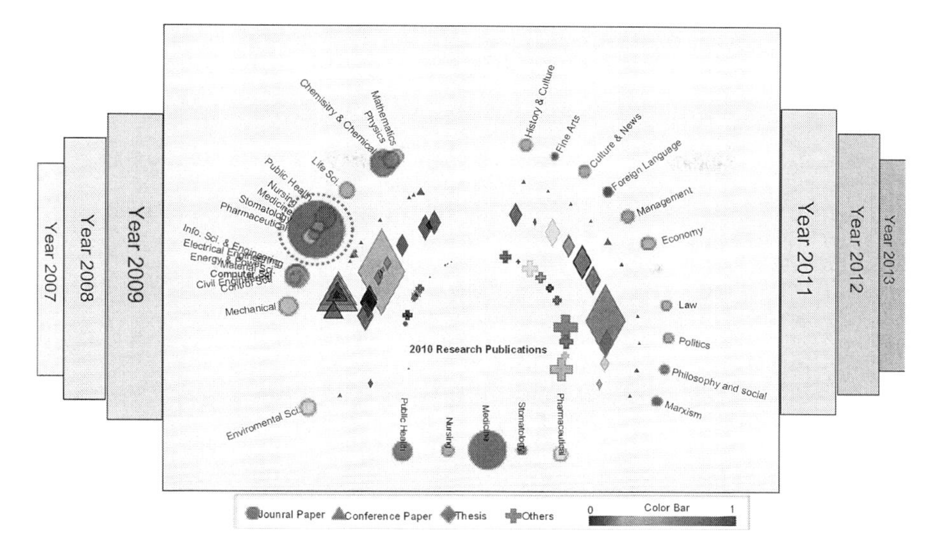

Fig. 356.1 Interactive interface of scholar browser

356.3.4 Visualizations

In the interface, we project departments to 2D views to show the summary of publications which is structured into four catalogs: journal paper, conference paper, thesis and others. We encode them as circles, triangles, rectangles and cross respectively, with areas proportional to the number of them in a given year. On the other hand, the contributions of them are encoded as color from 0 to 1, as the color bar in Fig. 356.1 shows. Distance between two items encodes as the similarity measure. Time axis passes through the year block as a flexible way to access a specific year. Some departments are so close to overlap in the inter face, for example, the school of medicine and the school of nursing circling in the Fig. 356.1. For this case, we introduce an active board to show the details.

356.4 Conclusion

In this paper, we offered a method to visualize scholar text, which comes from the university-wide publication database, to display the quantity and quality of research achievements grouped by departments. We discussed the design details of the Scholar Browser and described the method to abstract metadata. The data was structured to four catalogs to analyze and visualize separately. The approach to compute contribution of publications involved impact factor which a fair criteria to measure the quality. The topic similarity was computed based on the CLC and LDA. With the interactive interface, the region of interested could be accessed freely. More features will be introduced as the future work.

References

1. Blei DM, Ng AY, Jordan MI (2003) Latent Dirichlet allocation. J Mach Learn Res 3:993–1022
2. Chang J, Boyd-Graber J, Wang C, Gerrish S, and Blei DM (2009) Reading tea leaves: how humans interpret topic models. In: NIPS, pp 288–296
3. Chuang J, Ramage D, Manning C, et al. (2012) Interpretation and trust: designing model-driven visualizations for text analysis[C]. In: Proceedings of the 2012 ACM annual conference on human factors in computing systems. ACM, pp 443–452
4. Clough PD, Sen BA (2008) Evaluating tagclouds for health-related information research. In: Health Info Management Research
5. Collins C, Carpendale S, Penn G (2009) DocuBurst: visualizing document content using language structure. Comput Graph Forum 28:3
6. Collins C, Viegas FB, Wattenberg M (2009) Parallel tag clouds to explore and analyze faceted text corpora. In: VAST, pp 91–98
7. Cutting DR., Karger, DR, Pedersen JO (1993) Constant interaction-time scatter/gather browsing of very large document collections. In: SIGIR
8. Hall D, Jurafsky D, Manning CD (2008) Studying the history of ideas using topic models. In: EMNLP, pp 363–371
9. Morrison JB, Tversky B, Betrancourt M (2000) Animation: does it facilitate learning? In: Proceedings of smart graphics AAAI Spring Symposium, pp 53–60. AAAI Press Technical Report SS-00-04
10. Robertson GG, Card SK, Mackinlay JD (1993) Information visualization using 3D interactive animation. Commun ACM 36(4):57–71
11. Salton G, Wong A, Yang C (1975) A vector space model for automatic indexing. Commun ACM 18(11):613–620
12. Thomas J, Cook K, Eds (2005) Illuminating the path: the research and development agenda for visual analytics. IEEE Press, Los Alamitos
13. Viegas FB, Wattenberg M (2008) TIMELINES: tag clouds and the case for vernacular visualization. Interactions 15:49–52
14. Wattenberg M, Viegas FB (2008) The word tree, an interactive visual concordance. In InfoVis, pp 1221–1228

Chapter 357
Date-driven Based Image Enhancement for Segmenting of MS Lesions in T2-w and Flair MRI

Ziming Zeng, Zhonghua Han, Yitian Zhao and Reyer Zwiggelaar

Abstract This paper proposed a data-driven based image enhancement scheme to segment Multiple Sclerosis (MS) lesions. It utilizes a class-adaptive Gaussian Markov random field modelling (HMRF) and mutual information to automatic enhance the MS lesions. Then an alpha matting technique is used to refine the segmentation results. The advantages of the approach lies in its date-driven processing. It can automatically enhance the density of MS lesions, which is guided by calculating the mutual information value of the segmentation results in the successive steps. In addition, the partial volume effects are considered and the regions of interests are segmented in a sub-pixel precision. The experiments on real MR images show the proposed segmentation method can effectively segment MS lesions.

Keywords Date-driven · Enhancement · MS lesions · Segmentation · Mutual information

357.1 Introduction

MS is characterized by the destruction of proteins in the myelin surrounding nerve fibers. The region demonstrating clearly destroyed myelin is called a lesion. The loss of myelin can lead to short-circuits or transmission blocks of the nerve impulses which may result in the gradual decline of movement, visual, sensory and

Z. Zeng (✉) · Z. Han
Information and Control Engineering Faculty, Shenyang Jianzhu University, Liaoning, China
e-mail: zengziming1983@gmail.com

Z. Zeng · Y. Zhao · R. Zwiggelaar
Department of Computer Science, Aberystwyth University, Aberystwyth, UK

S. Li et al. (eds.), *Frontier and Future Development of Information Technology in Medicine and Education*, Lecture Notes in Electrical Engineering 269,
DOI: 10.1007/978-94-007-7618-0_357,

cognitive functions. Accurate and robust segmentation methods for segmenting and measuring MS lesions are much needed. In clinical, T2-w and Flair MR images are commonly used to recognize the MS lesions. Manual segmentation for MS lesions is difficult for human expert because of the complicated shape, size and inhomogenity of the MS lesions. Therefore, many semi- or fully- automatic segmentation methods are proposed instead of the manual segmentation. Dugas-Phocion et al. [1] applied a multi-sequence MRI (T1-w, T2-w, Flair, PD-w) within an EM based probabilistic framework to segment MS lesions. Zeng et al. [2] proposed a two dimensional joint histogram modelling for MS lesions which can recognise the small lesions. Souplet et al. [3] combined EM and morphology post-processing of resulting regions of interest to extract MS lesions. However, the segmentation results can be easily affected by noise, density in- homogenity, and partial volume effects. In addition, the accuracy of the above segmentation results is too depend on the segmentation rules which should be specified before segmenting. As a partial solution, an unsupervised date-driven based image enhancement technique is proposed to segment the MS lesions.

357.2 The Proposed Method

As the preprocessing, a mutual information based method [4] is used to registrate T2-w and Flair MR images. Then the brain skull in T2-w MRI is removed by using the BET toolkit [5]. Subsequently, the segmented brain region is used as a binary mask to extract the corresponding pixels in Flair. Finally, the two different modalities are fused into one image I by using $(1/2)T2 + Flair$ in order to enhance the density of MS lesions. Our segmentation method including three steps are shown below.

357.2.1 Date-driven Based Image Enhancement

In the first step, the MS lesion is enhanced in an iteration processing which is driven by the image density information. Specifically, the class-adaptive Gaussian Markov modeling [6] is used to segment the brain tissues with four groups which corresponding to background (BG), cerebrospinal fluid (CSF), grey matter (GM), and white matter (WM), respectively. Then the group centers of WM and GM defined as C_{WM} and C_{GM} can be estimated. Subsequently, the MS lesions are enhanced by using an enhancement function $E(x)$ which is defined as:

$$E_k(x) = \left(\frac{1}{2}\left[1 + \frac{2}{\pi}\arctan\left(\frac{x - T_k}{\varepsilon}\right)\right] \times I_k(x)\right) * K_\sigma \qquad (357.1)$$

where I is the fusion MR image, K_σ is a Gaussian kernel, ε is a constant value, T is defined as $(C_{wm-}C_{gm})/2$, k is the iteration number. As the iteration number increasing, the mutual information value (*MI*) which is calculated by using two enhanced images ($E_k(x)$ and $E_{k-1}(x)$) which are obtained in successive iterations (k iteration and $k-1$ iteration ($k \geq 2$)) is utilized as the iteration stopping criteria. The iteration will be stopped when *MI* is convergent (*MI* is below an small threshold value δ). With each iteration, the enhanced slice is segmented again, and the new parameter T is estimated by using the new group centers. Finally, the potential MS lesions are obtained by using the segmentation group which has the highest group center in the last iteration. An example of this step is shown in Fig. 357.1 Step 1.

357.2.2 False Positive Reduction

In the second step, due to the gray level of MS lesions in the fusion image has overlap with the other tissues, false positives should be removed from the previous results. Specifically, since 95 % of MS lesions occur within white matter tissue [7], we only

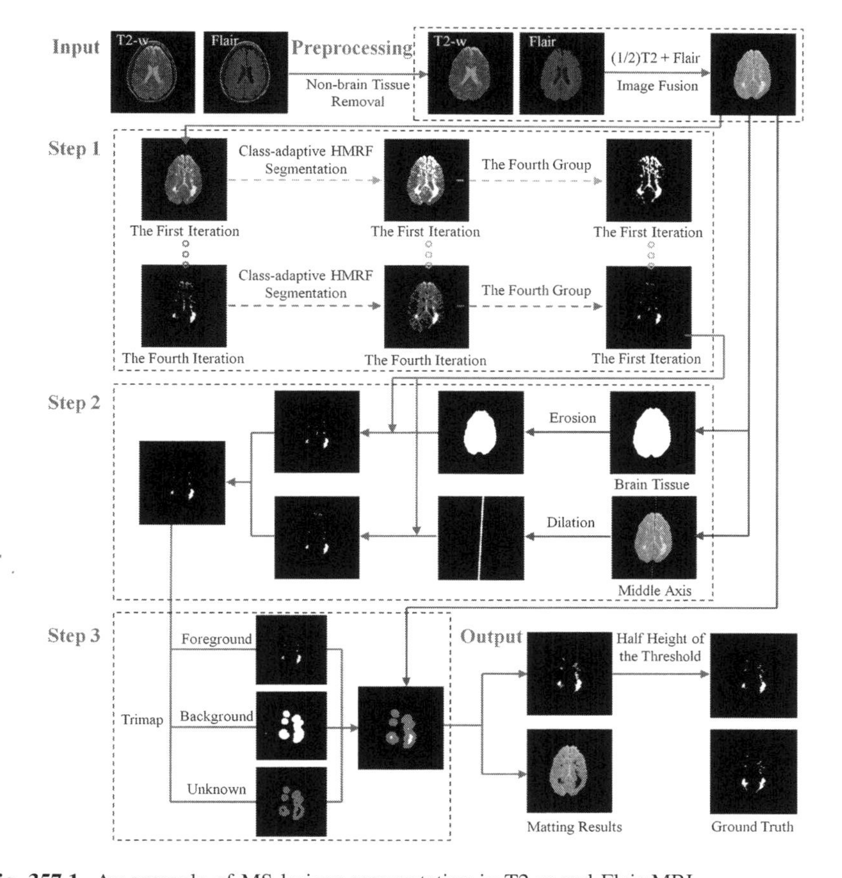

Fig. 357.1 An example of MS lesions segmentation in T2-w and Flair MRI

consider the MS lesions contained in WM in this work. We extract a binary mask of the brain tissue. Then we use the eroded binary region in order to exclude CSF. Subsequently, the generated binary region is utilized to do a logical and with the potential MS lesions in the previous steps. Then the labels which are fully or partially outside of the generated binary region are removed. The second area where false positives commonly occur is in the WM between ventricles. This occurs particularly because this area tends to be enhanced on Flair even if lesions are not present. To address this problem, the symmetry plane [8] is calculated. The generated symmetry axis is dilated. Then it is used to do a logical *and* with the segmentation results in the previous steps and we remove the labels which are connected with the symmetry axis. The processing of this step is shown in Fig. 357.1 Step 2.

357.2.3 Refining the Segmentation Results

Due the results in the previous steps are not accurate enough, an alpha matting is used to refine the segmentation results in this step. To use alpha matting, a trimap has to be generated at first, which separates the image into three regions: definite foreground F, definite background *B*, and the unknown region *U*, as shown in Fig. 357.1 Step 3. Our system automatically generates this trimap. Specifically, we use the morphology method to erode the previous segmentation result with a circular structuring element as the foreground *F* (show in white), then the background *B* (show in black) can be generated by dilating the binary segmentation. The unknown area *U* (show in grey) can be generated by using the fusion image. For the foreground region, we label the binary region and calculate the pixel number for each label. If the number is below nine, the current label will be directly used as the foreground without erosion.

To solve the alpha matting problem, the approach proposed by Levin et al. [9] is used. Using this approach each fusion slice is modeled as $I_i = \alpha_i F_w + (1 - \alpha_i) B_w$, where I is the observed image, F_w and B_w are foreground and background in a small window w, and α is the transparency parameter. This can be rewritten as $\alpha_i = a_w I_i + b_w$ where $a_w = 1/(F_w - B_w)$ and $b_w = -B_w/(F_w - B_w)$. Then the problem is converted into finding a, a and b to minimize the cost function $J(\alpha) = \min_{a,b} J(\alpha, a, b)$. The details of the energy minimization process can be found in [9]. Solving the matting problem leads to a soft segmentation of MS lesions in the fusion MR image.

357.3 Evaluation and Discussion

We evaluated the developed method on some selected images with MS lesions from CHB and UNC datasets [10]. For each case, two MR modalities are made available (T2-w and Flair volumes) which are co-registered.

Table 357.1 TPR, PPV and Dice index for MS lesions segmentation on MR images

Patient cases	Ch. winnner [3]			Context-rich RF [11]			Our method		
	TPR	PPV	DSC	TPR	PPV	DSC	TPR	PPV	DSC
Images1	0.42	0.57	0.48	0.63	0.64	0.63	0.68	0.72	0.70
Images2	0.43	0.52	0.47	0.59	0.59	0.61	0.64	0.53	0.58
Images3	0.46	0.41	0.43	0.58	0.57	0.57	0.56	0.62	0.59
Images4	0.38	0.43	0.40	0.41	0.78	0.54	0.48	0.68	0.56
Images5	0.54	0.48	0.51	0.62	0.52	0.57	0.68	0.51	0.58
Avg	0.45	0.48	0.46	0.57	0.62	0.58	0.61	0.61	0.60
Sd	0.06	0.07	0.04	0.09	0.10	0.04	0.08	0.09	0.05

We take slice 271 in case 01 as an example. The whole segmentation processing on the two modalities is shown in Fig. 357.1. In the first step, the skull in MRI T2-w and Flair are removed by using the BET toolkit [5]. Then we fusion the two different modalities. Subsequently, the generated image is normalized from 0 to 255. In the second step, the fusion image is segmented by using class- adaptive Gaussian Markov modeling [6]. The segmentation group centers of WM and GM are used to estimate the threshold T which is calculated as 0.8 in this first iteration. As the number of iteration increasing, we calculate the mutual information of the enhanced slices in the successive iterations, and the threshold value $S = 0.9$ is used as the stopping criterion. In the third step, the middle axis and the eroded brain mask are used to remove the false positive regions. In the fourth step, the trimap is automatic generated and the alpha matting method is used to refine the previous segmentation results. To compare against the ground truth which are binary image, we threshold the soft segmentation generated by matting at half the maximum value for this image, which leads to the final binary segmentation result. By contrasting with the ground truth, we can see that the potential MS lesions can be successfully detected. To evaluate the accuracy of the proposed segmentation method, we randomly selected a few images with noise and density inhomogenity, and use three measures (true positive rate (TPR), positive predictive value (PPV) and Dice similarity coefficient (DSC)) to evaluate the spatial accuracy of the segmentation results. Table 357.1 shows the segmentation accuracy on each image as well as the overall mean (Avg) and standard deviation (Sd) for all the cases. Comparing with state-of-the-art segmentation method [3, 11], our results show improvements with the overall mean except the mean value in PPV.

357.4 Conclusion

This paper presents a novel segmentation scheme based on the image enhancement and alpha mating techniques. The proposed method can deal well with image noise and density inhomogeneous. In addition, it is a fully automatic and unsupervised segmentation method for MS lesions. In the future, we will evaluate this method on a larger clinical database. Also, the results of the proposed method will be compared with more state-of-the-art methods by using improved evaluation methods.

References

1. Dugas-Phocion G, Gonzalez MA, Lebrun C, Chanalet S, Bensa C, Ma- landain G, Ayache N (2004) Hierarchical segmentation of multiple sclerosis lesions in multi-sequence MRI. In: Biomedical imaging: nano to macro
2. Zeng Z, Zwiggelaar R (2011) Joint histogram modelling for segmentation multiple sclerosis lesions. LNCS 6930:133–144
3. Souplet JC, Lebrun C, Ayache N, Malandain G (2008) An automatic segmentation of T2-FLAIR multiple sclerosis lessions. In: The MIDAS journal—MS lesion segmentation (MICCAI 2008 workshop), pp 1–5
4. Collignon A, Vandermeulen D, Marchal G, Suetens P (1997) Multimodality image registration by maximization of mutual information. IEEE Trans Med Imaging 16(2): 187C198
5. Stephen MS (2002) Fast robust automated brain extraction. Hum Brain Mapp 17(3):143–155
6. Wang W, Feng Q, Liu L, Chen W (2008) Segmentation of brain MR images through class-adaptive Gauss-Markov random field model and the EM algorithm. J Image Graph 13(3): 488–493
7. Grosman RI, Mcgowan JC (1998) Perspectives on multiple sclerosis. AJNR 19:176–186
8. Prima S, Ourselin S, Ayache N (2002) Computation of the mid-sagittal plane in 3-D brain images. IEEE Trans Med Imaging 21(2):122–138
9. Levin A, Lischinski D, Weiss Y (2008) A closed form solution to natural image matting. IEEE Trans Pattern Anal Mach Intell 30(2):228–242
10. Styner M, Lee J, Chin B, Chin MS, Commowick O, Tran HH, Jewells V, Warfield S (2008) 3D segmentation in the clinic: a grand challenge II: MS lesion segmentation. MIDAS J 1–5
11. Geremia E, Menze BH, Clatz O, Konukoglu E, Criminisi A, Ayache N (2010) Spatial decision forests for MS lesion segmentation in multi-channel MR images. LNCS 6361:111–118

Chapter 358
On Aims and Contents of Intercultural Communicative English Teaching

Diao Lijing and Wang Huanyun

Abstract: In the context of globalization, people of different cultural backgrounds need to have effective communication. However, the status quo of China's college English teaching is that the students have very strong linguistic competence and practical skills, but lack social cultural competence and intercultural competence. Language knowledge and skills are emphasized while cultural factors are neglected. Therefore, this paper will analyze College English Teaching aims and contents based on intercultural communication to give some hints to the college English teaching.

Keywords: Intercultural communication · English teaching · Aim · Content

358.1 Introduction

Nowadays, with the rapid development of the globalization, being an organization of cultivating talents, universities must pay attention to equip students with international horizon, master English as a tool and the international communication principle, and understand cultures of different countries and peoples so that they can shoulder the responsibility to achieve communication between cultures. College English is an important tool for cross-culture, where culture teaching should be strengthened to enable students to achieve cross-cultural communication.

D. Lijing (✉)
Department of English, Cangzhou Normal University, Hebei 061001, China
e-mail: dljwhwb@163.com

W. Huanyun
Department of Mechanical Engineering, Cangzhou Normal University, Hebei 061001, China
e-mail: whypwb@126.com

S. Li et al. (eds.), *Frontier and Future Development of Information Technology in Medicine and Education*, Lecture Notes in Electrical Engineering 269,
DOI: 10.1007/978-94-007-7618-0_358,

358.2 College English Teaching Aims

In the light of the principle of intercultural communication, the ideal objective of college English teaching is to help students use English to communicate in the context of the target culture [1], that is, cultivate the students' intercultural communicative competence. Aims of intercultural communication college English teaching can be subdivided into the following aspects:

358.2.1 To Cultivate Students' Comprehensive Practical Ability

As far as English language teaching is concerned, we should cultivate students in terms of language competence, language skills and language use. In six aspects such as listening, speaking, reading, writing, translation and vocabulary, teaching contents, strategies and methods should be determined to offer corresponding courses and improve students' comprehensive practical ability.

358.2.2 To Cultivate Students' Intercultural Communication Cognitive Ability

The ultimate goal of college English teaching is to develop students' intercultural communicative competence, which is necessary for successful cross-cultural communication. Intercultural communication cognition refers to the process in which a person handles and processes language and culture information in a particular communicative environment. Intercultural cognitive ability is the basis to obtain cross-cultural knowledge and communication rules and improve cross-cultural awareness. In college English teaching based on intercultural communication, we should give priority to develop students' cross-cultural cognitive abilities.

358.2.3 To Cultivate Students' Intercultural Emotional Competence

Dictionary of Psychology defines emotion as people's attitude when experiencing whether objective things meet their own needs. In the process of communication, cultural and emotional ability mainly refers to the capacity for empathy communication and self psychological adjustment ability.

358.2.3.1 Empathy Ability

Cultivating empathy ability refers to the cultivation of students' ability to overcome ethnocentrism, empathy and the ability to form appropriate communication motivation. As a member of cultural groups, communicative individuals are ethnocentric and harbour cultural thinking stereotype, prejudice and resentment towards other cultures. The curriculum system based on cultivation of intercultural communication competence can increase the students' understanding of other cultures, improve intercultural communicative awareness and overcome the negative impact of ethnocentrism.

358.2.3.2 Self Psychological Adjustment Ability

In the context of intercultural communication, communicative subjects will have psychological anxiety or feel psychological pressure because of cultural differences such as culture shock. Therefore, to cultivate students' self psychological adjustment ability to accept the uncertain factors in the culture of the target language and maintain self-confidence and tolerance is the important goal of culture teaching.

358.2.4 To Cultivate Students' Intercultural Behavior Ability

Intercultural behaviour ability refers to the various kinds of abilities people use to make effective and appropriate intercultural communication such as the ability to use language appropriately, the ability to exchange information by nonverbal means, the ability to use communication strategies flexibly, the ability to build relationships with each other, and the ability to control the conversation, way and process. Comprehensive language application ability is an important target of cross-cultural teaching, which can be achieved through cross-cultural communication course system.

358.3 Culture Teaching Contents

Cultural contents are complicated, so teachers need to make the appropriate adjustments and classification to the cultural contents and combine with language teaching and science in teaching practice. In English classroom teaching, culture teaching content can be summarized into five aspects:

358.3.1 English Words and Their Cultural Connotations

Words carry a large amount of information on cultures, which is a clue for foreigners to understand national cultures. The cultural connotation of words in English includes the reference category, emotional and associative meaning of English words and the figurative meaning and extended meaning of idioms, proverbs allusions and idioms. The cultural differences between Chinese and English words are one of the main obstacles in English learning.

358.3.2 British and American Cultural Background Knowledge

Background knowledge is an important part of English culture. In the process of reading comprehension, the key is to activate the readers' knowledge schemata, which allows students to use their background knowledge correctly to fill some discontinuous implementation gaps so that other information in the article can become a unified body [2].

358.3.3 English Syntax, Discourse Structure and Thinking Way of British and American People

An English sentence is normally longer than a Chinese one, with verbs as the core and having clear tree structure. It focuses on analysis while a Chinese sentence has no strict linguistic constraints and emphasizes parataxis. English discourse structure is generally straight while Chinese discourse structure is spiral or curved. The theme of an English article is clear and logical while a Chinese article is euphemistic. In the process of language acquisition British and American people form a habit of logical thinking while Chinese form a habit of prominent image thinking.

358.3.4 English Communication and Behavior Style

Communication style differences can be summarized as difference between direct and indirect, difference between linear and circular type, difference between confidence and humility, difference between being scanty of words and speaking with fervor and assurance, difference between being detailed and compact. Only the two sides are aware of the differences in advance and consciously make adjustment can they communicate smoothly. Moreover, teachers should guide students to understand the performance of British and American people in the aspects of verbal behavior performance and nonverbal behavior performance.

358.3.5 British and American Values

Values related to intercultural communication mainly include the relationship between man and nature, interpersonal relationship, attitude to "change", dynamic or static, being or doing and time orientation. In British and American cultural context, people advocate individualism including personal struggle, independence, privacy protection, the pursuit of freedom and difference nonverbal behavior performances.

358.4 Conclusion

All in all, relationship between the language and the culture being the source, linguistic theory and constructivism the base, the author builds the thought of intercultural teaching and discusses in details the aims and contents of college English teaching to provide some references for English teaching reform.

Acknowledgments This work is financially supported by the Social Science Development Research Subject of Cangzhou, Hebei Province, China (201379).

References

1. Nunan D (1991) A communicative tasks and the language curriculum. J TESOL Q 2:25–28
2. Kramsch C (2000) Langauge and culture. Shanghai foreign language education Press, China

Chapter 359
Research on the Cultivation of Applied Innovative Mechanical Talents in Cangzhou

Wang Huanyun

Abstract Based on the analysis of the demands for applied innovative talents in mechanics in Cangzhou, the author puts forward a scientific, advanced, practical and innovative mode to train mechanical talents and makes bold reforms and innovation in terms of theory teaching system, practice teaching system, teaching method and evaluation system. The new attempt and practice in the teaching reform have promoted the construction and development of the discipline construction in mechanics and provided a strong guarantee for the cultivation of applied innovative mechanical talents, and have the promotion value and reference to the talent cultivations in other local colleges.

Keywords Applied talents · Training mode · Teaching reform

359.1 Introduction

At present the phenomenon of college students' difficult employment and the establishment' labor shortage are coexisting, the contradiction between supply and demand is becoming increasingly acute, the knowledge studied in school is seriously incompatible with the engineering practice needed by the establishments and cannot be applied practically, while the majority of private enterprises are unwilling to bear the social responsibility of pre-job training of college students and hope to get technical personnel who can work immediately. In order to meet the needs of the society, applied talents emerge. In order to promote the development of the economy in Cangzhou and enhance the mechanical graduates the overall application abilities such as adaptability to posts and competitiveness.

W. Huanyun (✉)
Department of Mechanical Engineering, Cangzhou Normal University,
Hebei 061001, China
e-mail: whypwb@126.com

S. Li et al. (eds.), *Frontier and Future Development of Information Technology in Medicine and Education*, Lecture Notes in Electrical Engineering 269,
DOI: 10.1007/978-94-007-7618-0_359,

We have researched and practiced the new applied Innovative talent training mode, carried out the reform on the training mode in terms of training target, teaching system, teaching content, practice teaching system and evaluation mechanism to promote the school to meet the needs of economic construction and social development in Cangzhou and solve the problem of students' difficult employment so as to improve the resource allocation efficiency in the society.

359.2 Draft Training Objectives

Our objective is to train applied innovative senior engineering talents, who can adapt to the economic development and the progress of science and technology in Cangzhou, do well in morality, intelligence and physique, have solid basic knowledge of mechanics, materials molding for mechanical engineering, electrical engineering and automation, systematically master the professional knowledge of machinery design, machinery manufacturing, mechanical and electrical observation and control, have higher comprehensive qualities, stronger practical ability and creative and cooperative spirit, have the ability to solve practical engineering problems, and can be engaged in the design and manufacture of electromechanical products, technology application and reconstruction, operation management and sales in the forefront of production in the field of mechanical engineering such as the mechanical equipment and pattern mold.

359.3 Construction and Measures of Talents Cultivation Scheme

Change traditional mode of talent training scheme to construct teaching syllabus aimed at knowledge into carefully designing a training scheme including both knowledge training and quality training with knowledge as carrier around the future engineer vocational quality, social consciousness and the innovative spirit [1].

359.3.1 Optimize Curriculum System and Integrate Teaching Content

To guarantee the smooth realization of the training objectives, it is necessary to establish a reasonable application theory teaching system in which to cope with the relationship between theory and practice, knowledge and quality, and classroom teaching and extracurricular guidance aimed at the actual demands of economic development for applied creative mechanical talents in CangZhou. In the light of talents cultivation, the course design should break the professional disciplinary boundaries, integrate the related subjects, pay attention to of mutual fusion of the contents and cohesion of different courses and construct course system and teaching content for professional ability training, including five major courses such as basic courses, machinery base, machinery manufacturing and processing, electronic technology and control and digital manufacturing technology. On the one hand, make scientific integration among mechanical, electrical and computer courses, on the other hand, put the content of digital design technology into such courses as engineering drawing, mechanical engineering and mechanical design, digital manufacturing technology into such courses as numerical control technology and programming, and CAD/CAM technology, and professional certification and vocational standard into teaching content, lay stress on the fusion with other majors such as other mechanical electricity and computer to highlight the professional characteristics of strong application of digital manufacturing technology. Integrate the traditional mechanical knowledge with modern design methods, modern manufacturing methods, modern measurement and control means, new technology, new technology and new materials to adapt to the development of new mechanical disciplines, develop reasonable curriculum structure and enhance social adaptability of students.

359.3.2 Construct Practice Teaching System and Strengthen the Training of Engineering Practical Ability and Innovative Ability

The teaching contents of Mechanical engineering practice should realize the integration of design and manufacturing, machinery and electronics, basic theory and engineering application, classical content and high technology, unit technology and system thinking, engineering technology and management science, and practical ability and innovative quality and construct engineering practice teaching system in order to improve the students' comprehensive abilities to apply knowledge to solve design problems from the perspective of engineering. Practice teaching system mainly includes the following five modules.

(1) Basic skills module which includes engineering surveying and mapping, engineering dynamics experiment, technology measurement experiment, Metalworking practice, computer application and foreign language application in order to cultivate the basic science literacy of students.
(2) The professional skill module which includes mechanical design, curriculum design, machinery manufacturing base, electrical and electronic curriculum design, and electro-hydraulic control curriculum design to train students' basic skills.

(3) The engineering practice module which comprises the numerical control technology, CAD/CAM/CAE, advanced manufacturing technology and other engineering training to foster students to have a stronger engineering practical ability.
(4) Innovative design module which includes science and technology innovation activities, mechanical design competition and graduation design to foster engineering innovative thinking and technology innovative ability of the students.
(5) Vocational qualification certification training module According to the talent shortage in our country carry out vocational qualification certification training in numerical control technology, PRO/E, UG, Solid-works and CATIA to improve student's vocational skills in digital design and manufacturing.

359.3.3 Reform Teaching Methods, Optimize Teaching Approaches and Improve Assessment Methods

Teaching is the central work in colleges and universities and selecting the flexible and multiply teaching methods and approaches is an important guarantee to achieve educational goals and ensure the teaching effect [2]. Based on the characteristics of mechanical professional courses, innovate and adopt flexible and multiple teaching methods, approaches and assessment methods.

359.3.4 Strengthen School-Enterprise Cooperation to Realize Depth Connection Between Schools and Enterprises, and Form Good Innovation Education Ecology

Explore the running mechanism of school-enterprise cooperation, innovate study-enterprise-research cooperation model and maintain close contact with enterprises to form good engineering and innovation education ecology through deep connection between schools and enterprises [3]. The thinking sources of innovation are all directly driven by the industrial urgent needs, so it is more conducive to improve engineering ability and creative ability of the teachers and students in colleges to solve the engineering practical problems of the enterprises with the industrial personnel.

359.3.5 Strengthen the Innovation Ability and Vocational Training Practice to Realize the Full Employment of the Graduates

Organize students to participate in science and technology activities such as undergraduate mechanical design-innovation competition, mathematical modeling, electronic competition and provide the innovative platforms for students to train students' engineering innovation thinking and technology innovation ability.

Establish the training system in the light of employment need of enterprises, carry out multi-channel vocational skill training, and make efforts to improve the talent-training modes and systems laying equal emphasis on both degree certificates and a variety of occupation qualification certificates to achieve full employment of the graduates.

359.4 Conclusion

Through the practice in training innovative applied mechanical talents we can draw the conclusion:

Adapt to the needs of modernization economic construction and better serve the economic construction and the social developments in Cangzhou, we must strengthen students' moral education, adapt to the requirements of the national economic and social development for the mechanical engineering subjects, lay emphasis on the basic engineering quality required for mechanical engineers, especially the training of the innovation consciousness and practical ability, construct distinctive talent training mode, adhere to combine theory teaching with skill training, cultivate students' engineering application and innovation practical ability to analyze and solve problems, and improve teaching qualities and the talent training level constantly.

Acknowledgments This work is financially supported by the Social Science Development Research Subject of Cangzhou, Hebei Province, China (201335).

References

1. Zhiwei H, Yunfeng B (2011) Professional talents training program exploration in mechanical design manufacturing and automation. J China Adult Educ (20):157–158
2. Zhong L, Shi J, Zhang W (2011) The Exploration of the "3 + 1"applied talents' cultivation in mechanical major under the background of excellent engineers training. J Sci Technol Manage Res 16:158–165
3. Li P (2008) Constructing the system of the cultivation of innovative talents. J Chin high educ 5:20–21

Chapter 360
On Feasibility of Experiential English Teaching in Higher Vocational Institutes

Diao Lijing

Abstract Higher vocational institutes train applied talents who are required to be able to speak and write in English while experiential teaching of English combines language teaching, communication tasks with social activities, which enable students to complete communication goals in the real social interaction. Therefore, this paper probes into the feasibility of experiential teaching of English in higher vocational institutes in terms of the implementation conditions and applicableness in order to provide some references for the English teaching reform.

Keywords Feasibility · Experiential english teaching · Higher vocational institutes · Applicableness

360.1 Introduction

In vocational English teaching, vocabulary and theoretical knowledge should be combined with practice to achieve the basic application level. However, students in vocational colleges possess the relatively poor foundation in English, together with the disadvantage of traditional English teaching mode, which brings great difficulties to vocational English teaching. To meet the needs of national economic construction, reform of higher vocational English teaching has become more and more urgent. Experiential teaching of English requires students to learn in practice, which, to a large extent, improves the English learning method and enables students to combine English learning and practicing. Through practical experience, students' own feelings in learning English are enhanced and their learning interest is cultivated, which helps improve their practical ability. Therefore, the implementation of experimental English teaching in higher vocational institutes should be a beneficial exploration [1].

D. Lijing (✉)
Department of English, Cangzhou Normal University, Hebei 061001, China
e-mail: dljwhwb@163.com

S. Li et al. (eds.), *Frontier and Future Development of Information Technology in Medicine and Education*, Lecture Notes in Electrical Engineering 269,
DOI: 10.1007/978-94-007-7618-0_360,

360.2 Feasibility of Experimental English Teaching

In the recent years, vocational education has undergone considerable development; the relevant policies and regulations put forward by the government guide promote as well as guard the healthy development of higher vocational education. Not only hardware facilities, but also software conditions provide the implementation of higher vocational experiential teaching of English with basic protection [2].

360.2.1 Application of Hardware Facilities

At present, vocational colleges actively introduce and make use of such modern teaching methods as computer multimedia, network technology. Generally speaking, the higher colleges own one or more mufti-media classrooms, which greatly improve English teaching conditions and provide the implementation of experiential teaching and of experiential activities with a hardware support. In addition, Some advanced teaching methods, such as virtual stimulation and stimulation training, are widely used to support teaching, which provides "teaching, learning and practicing" as a unity with strong support. Moreover, such course resources as teaching and training packages are introduced and special web pages are set up in campus network, all of which facilitate students' online learning. Modern educational technology and teaching methods are widely used, which promotes effectively the construction and sharing of excellent college teaching resources and greatly improves students' quality and ability with remarkable results.

360.2.2 Application of Software Conditions

Under the supporting of our country's policy to develop vocational education vigorously, the groups of teacher are continuously optimizing, and the National Ministry of Education has published and distributed the series of Practical English, which provide a favorable blueprint for the implementation of experiential vocational English teaching. Moreover, with the development of economy, and then effective popularization and application of education and teaching research results, all of which provide a powerful safeguard to impel higher English teaching reforms [3].

360.2.2.1 Materials Exclusively for Vocational English Courses

The series of Practical English are materials for vocational English courses planned by Ministry of Education. The material assimilates some arguments suitable for our English teaching reality in modern foreign teaching theory and adopts the reasonable parts in traditional foreign language teaching theory based upon the effective theories, methods and practical reality in the foreign language teaching. It strives to well handle the relationship between language foundation and application, and combined with students' needs for English after graduation, highlights practical English ability and practical application and focuses on the reading and translation of practical style, the training of practical spoken English and simulation writing in practical issues, all of which provide a favorable blue-print for the implementation of experiential vocational English teaching.

360.2.2.2 Talent Training Consistent with the Local Economic Development

The running orientation of vocational colleges is training practical, advanced and technical talents in production, construction, management and services. At present, vocational colleges are devoting to deepening the teaching reforms, intensifying education of English characteristics and developing students' creative spirit and practical ability according to the need of the local economic development.

360.2.2.3 Effective Popularization and Application of Education and Teaching Research Results

In order to develop students' practical English language knowledge and skills and intensify the practical English language ability, many a teacher has done much relevant research related to the subject, all of which provides experiential vocational teaching research with a large amount of research statistics and practical experience.

360.2.2.4 Continuous Optimization of Teaching Staff

The objective of English talent training in vocational college is positioned on developing students' English language knowledge and excellent English listening, speaking, writing as well as translating skills, training advanced and practical talents in reading, translation relevant English materials, which decides that English teachers should not only possess solid English theory and rich teaching experience, but also boast the excellent ability in professional practical work.

360.3 Applicableness of Experimental Teaching

The implementation of experiential vocational English teaching consists of two main evaluation points, one of which gears to students actual situations, namely, their English level and professional practice; the other one of which is to take on course basic requirements, namely, focusing on students' actual using language skills and their English language practice abilities. The very author will analyze the teaching implementation in Practical English Integrated Course (third edition) in the following part.

360.3.1 Combining Emotion with knowledge

Combining emotion with knowledge is to combining "cognitive factors and affective factors in a dialectical unity". Students will be placed in teaching related situations to stimulate their interest and make them experience personally and reflect constantly as well as conclude the knowledge they have learned.

360.3.2 Designing Practical Experiential Activities

Vocational education is to train advanced applied talents, vocational English teaching is mainly to train students' actual English communication ability. Therefore, teachers should design practical experiential activities directed by professional activities to make students to make full use of what they have learned and promote their positive thinking as well as effective expressions, ultimately to enhance students' actual language communication abilities.

Through practical experiential activities, the students will have a better understanding of the learned knowledge and will reflect what they should do better in their later interviews, then apply it in the future professional activities to better their inner knowledge structure and practical abilities.

360.3.3 Constructing Experiential Classes

In the experiential teaching, based on and motivated by new projects and tasks of teaching content, students' emotion experience gets richer, moved by the integration of situations and contents, so the students gain new feelings as well as information and have the desire of creation to achieve the purpose of self-creation based on the association of life experience and emotion experience, through role experience, situation experience, emotion experience and practical activities'.

After finishing the teaching of Surveys, Surveys and More Surveys, teachers draw up a social survey theme and ask students to design questionnaires. Through opinion rolls, discussions, visits and telephone interviews, etc., they collect information as well as data and conduct a series of data analysis and report writing. Motivated by these, students' creation desire is stimulated so that their learned knowledge can be practiced.

360.4 Conclusion

Through the analysis of hardware and software conditions as well as its applicableness, it is quite clear that it is completely feasible to implement the experiential teaching in higher vocational English teaching. Moreover, in the whole teaching process, the teacher, based on students' practical situations, directed by professional activities and motivated by projects and tasks, make his students combine their emotion with knowledge, and make them realize and internalize experiences, which is identical with the aims of higher vocational English teaching, and is also an urgent necessity to reform higher vocational English teaching.

Acknowledgments This work is financially supported by the Social Science Development Research Subject of Cangzhou, Hebei Province, China (201379).

References

1. Lu Z (2008) On application of experimental teaching in oxford higher vocational english teaching. J Shanghai Norm Univ (2):43
2. Huang Z (2008) A probe on experimental english teaching. High Educ Forum 6:100–101
3. Niemi H (2002) Active learning-a cultural change needed in teacher education and schools. Teach Teach Educ 18:763–765

Chapter 361
Vi-RTM: Visualization of Wireless Sensor Networks for Remote Telemedicine Monitoring System

Dianjie Lu, Guijuan Zhang, Yanwei Guo and Jue Hong

Abstract Remote Telemedicine Monitoring Systems (RTMS) based on wireless sensor network give patients more freedom of movement. However, in these systems, numerous biosensors are located on various body parts. Thus, how to manage these sensors to work cooperatively is a challenging problem. Visualization of wireless sensor network for RTMS is a useful tool to solve this problem. This paper presents a framework for visualizing the wireless sensor networks for remote telemedicine monitoring system called Vi-RTM. Our goal is to manage the sensors in a highly convenient form by employing effective visualization algorithms.

Keywords Visualization · Remote telemedicine monitoring system · Wireless sensor networks

361.1 Introduction

RTMS based on wireless sensor network is a kind of modern remote telemedicine monitoring system [1]. It uses the medical sensor as the physiological information acquisition interface, and transmits the collected messages to agent nodes by using the wireless communications technology. The data will be processed by agent node and be switched to remote monitor center. The remote monitor center can analyze and diagnose the physiological data, so as to realize remote monitoring and remote telemedicine treatment. RTMS based on wireless sensor network is a future development trend of the medical field.

D. Lu (✉) · G. Zhang
School of Information Science and Engineering, Shandong Normal University, Jinan, China
e-mail: ludianjie@sina.com

Y. Guo · J. Hong
Shenzhen Institutes of Advanced Technology, Chinese Academy of Sciences, Shenzhen, China

S. Li et al. (eds.), *Frontier and Future Development of Information Technology in Medicine and Education*, Lecture Notes in Electrical Engineering 269,
DOI: 10.1007/978-94-007-7618-0_361,

Despite the exciting possibilities of the remote telemedicine system based on WSNs, there are also some strong challenges and requirements that have to be satisfied such as the sensor management [2]. Visualization of wireless sensor network for RTMS is a useful tool to solve this problem.

There are many research groups developing telemedicine system. CodeBlue [3] telemedicine system is developed by Harvard University to monitor patients' vital information. Researchers at the MIT Media Lab have developed the MIThril, a wearable computing platform compatible with both custom and off-the-shelf sensors [4]. The University of Virginia proposed a prototype of the wireless sensor network called ALARM-NET (Assisted-Living and Residential Monitoring Network). UCLA developed an open and extensible architecture MEDIC (Medical Embedded Device for Individualized Care) [5].

In most of these systems, numerous biosensors are located on various body parts. The system may also include different contextual sensors located in a patient's closer environment. Thus, how to manage these sensors to work cooperatively is a challenging problem. In the following part, we will give a framework of visualized remote telemedicine monitoring system.

Therefore, we formulate a framework to directly address issues with visualizing large sets of physiological data generated by BSNs. We design Vi-RTM to simplify the management and visualization of BSNs, from the perspective of the end user.

361.2 System Structure

As shown in Fig. 361.1, we construct a visualized remote telemedicine monitoring system (Vi-RTM) with three parts: body sensor networks (BSNs), agent and visualized monitor center (VMC). Body sensor network is a wireless network constituted of the micro-nodes, which is responsible for sensor and gather patient's physiological parameters. Agent is responsible for protocol conversion and information transfer. The visualized monitor center includes visualization of real-time information, visualization of history information and visualization of sensor nodes. In this paper, we focus on the visualization of sensor nodes in order to manage them conveniently.

361.2.1 Body Sensor Networks

The main task of BSNs is data collection. It is necessary to define the data format before data acquisition. This framework uses the data frame format based on IEEE802.15.4 protocol. As shown in Fig. 361.2, the collected data are encapsulated into the BSN_Msg format which includes node ID, destination address, group ID, data information etc.

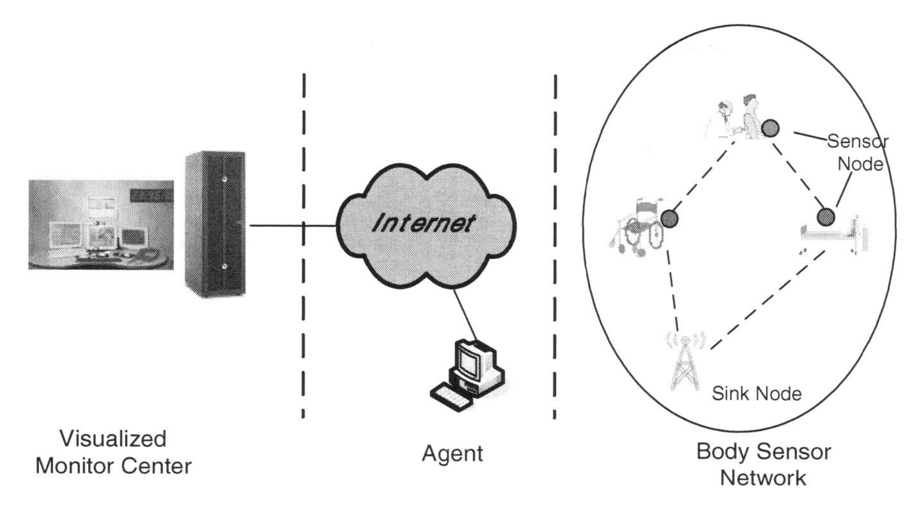

Fig. 361.1 Vi-RTM Framework

Fig. 361.2 BSN_Msg format

Node ID	Dest Addr	Group ID	Data	CRC

Each node has some metadata message such as: ID, energy and transmission radius. The collected data can be routed through a path, and finally reach the sink node. The routing information can be stored in the packet.

361.2.2 Agent

The agent is the intermediate interface between BSNs and VMC. It involves two aspects of communication: The communication with BSNs and the communication with VMC. The agents receive the data transmitted from sensor nodes firstly, and then forward them to the monitor center.

361.2.3 Visualized Monitor Center

VMC can simultaneously monitor multiple patient physiological signs. The monitoring center is responsible for the real-time storage, processing, statistics and display basic information of monitoring patient. It can also provide the basis for the treatment and nursing care of doctors. In addition, VMC can help the doctor on duty to provide remote guidance in emergency.

361.3 Visualization Algorithm

In this section, we investigate the visualization algorithm of BSNs in RTMS. We divide this section into three parts: the topology visualization, energy visualization and routing visualization.

361.3.1 Topology Visualization

The topological structure of BSN can be represented as an undirected graph $G(V, E)$, which records the connections between nodes. The undirected graph is composed of two elements, one is the node position, and another one is the connection between nodes. We assume that the reachability between two nodes depends on the distance between them. A node can communicate with all the nodes covered by its transmission radius. So, $G(V, E)$ can be expressed as an adjacent matrix.

361.3.2 Energy Visualization

Energy of nodes in wireless sensor networks is an important index to evaluate the performance of network. We denote e as the total energy of each node and e_i as the instant energy of node v_i. Thus, the ratio of available energy can be calculated by e_i/e, where $0 \leq e_i/e \leq 1$.

The energy of nodes can be visualized by RGB color. When a node has the maximum energy, it should be colored green ($R = 0, G = 1, B = 0$); When a node has exhausted its energy, it should be colored red ($R = 1, G = 0, B = 0$). The node's color can be obtained by the equation $R = 1 - e_i/e, G = e_i/e, B = 0$. Therefore, the nodes can be mapped into different color through calculating its energy ratio.

361.3.3 Routing Visualization

We use arrowed lines to visualize the routing path. The arrow show the direction of the path and different colors distinguish the different routing packet. For each packet, we connect the traversed node with arrowed line in a random generated color in according to the acquired routing information. Finally, we can get the visualization of all packets' routing.

361.4 Conclusion

The remote telemedicine monitoring system based on wireless networks is becoming a significant enabling technology for a wide variety of wearable applications. In this paper, we present Vi-RTM which can visualize the wireless sensor networks for remote telemedicine monitoring system. By using the effective visualization algorithms, the wireless sensor nodes can be managed conveniently.

Acknowledgments This work is supported by National Natural Science Foundation of P. R. China under Grant Nos. 61202225, 61272094, 61202417, Project of Shandong Province Higher Educational Science and Technology Program under Grant No. J13LN13, and Shenzhen Basic Research Foundation under Grant No. JC201105190934A.

References

1. Yun D, Kang J, Kim J, Kim D (2007) A body sensor network platform with two-level communications. In: Proceedings of the ISCE 2007, June 2007
2. Lorincz K, Malan DJ et al (2004) Sensor networks for emergency response: challenges and opportunities. IEEE Pervasive Comput 4:16–23
3. Shnayder V, Chen BR et al (2005) Sensor networks for medical care. In: Proceedings of the 3rd international conference on em-bedded networked sensor systems
4. DeVaul R, Thril M (2003) Application and architecture. In: Proceedings 7th international symposium on wearable computers, IEEE Press, pp 4–11
5. Wu W, Bui A et al (2008) MEDIC: medical embedded device for individualized care. Artif Intell Med 42:137–152

Chapter 362
The Effect of T-2 Toxin on the Apoptosis of Ameloblasts in Rat's Incisor

Sha-fei Zhai, Zhu Yong, Ma Zheng and Yaochao Zhang

Abstract Trichothecene mycotoxin T-2 toxin is a common contaminant of food and feed and is also present in processed cereal derived products. Cytotoxic effects of T-2 toxin have been already well described with apoptosis being a major action mechanism. It has been reported that T-2 toxin induced the appearance changes in tooth organ. However, effects on the ameloblasts were until now only reported rarely. 60 SD rats were randomly divided into three groups and received gavages containing T-2 toxin in a dosage of 0, 100, and 200 ng/g b.w., respectively. After 4 weeks treatment, the TdT-mediated dUTP nick end labeling (TUNEL) assays were used to investigate the effect of T-2 toxin on the apoptosis of ameloblasts. The imagination analysis of TUNEL showed that there were significantly more apoptotic ameloblasts in the experiment groups than the control group ($P < 0.01$). This effect was more obvious in high-dose T-2 toxin administrated group. Thus, T-2 toxin can accelerate apoptosis of ameloblasts in rat's incisor. This model might provide a potential research tool for studying the influence of T-2 toxin on tooth, and further reveal apoptotic disorders in the tooth development deformity.

Keywords T-2 toxin · Rat ameloblast · Apoptosis

S. Zhai (✉) · Z. Yong
Department of Oral Medicine, Xi'an Medical University, Xinwang Road, Shaanxi 710021, China

M. Zheng · Y. Zhang
Department of Public Health, Xi'an Medical University, Xinwang Road, Shaanxi 710021, China

S. Li et al. (eds.), *Frontier and Future Development of Information Technology in Medicine and Education*, Lecture Notes in Electrical Engineering 269,
DOI: 10.1007/978-94-007-7618-0_362,

362.1 Introduction

The trichothecene mycotoxin T-2 toxin, which is produced by fungi of the Fusarium species, is a worldwide occurring contaminant of cereal based food and feed. The Food and Agricultural Organization (FAO) estimates that mycotoxins contaminate almost 25 % of the world's agricultural commodities [1]. The consumption of food and feed contaminated by mycotoxins is a potential health risk for both humans and animals. Among the trichothecenes, T-2 toxin are the most toxic, because it has radiomimetic effect and is an inhibitor of the synthesis of DNA, RNA and protein. The cytotoxic response of T-2 toxin are already well described with apoptosis being a major mechanism of action in various cell lines of many tissues [2]. It could affect the cell cycle, thus induce apoptosis in vivo and in vitro in the liver, placenta and fetal liver in pregnant rats [3]. Enamel belongs to mineralized tissue. The development processes of tooth enamel include the formation of enamel matrix and mineralization, which are both regulated by the ameloblast [4]. Apoptotic genetic disorders is one of the reasons for tooth development deformity. But the influence of T-2 toxin on the apoptosis of ameloblasts has not been reported.

In the present study, poisoning rat model with T-2 toxin was used to investigate the effect of T-2 toxin on the apoptosis of ameloblasts.

362.2 Experiment

362.2.1 Sample Preparation

Thirty newly born weaning male Sprague-Dawley (60–80 g) rats were purchased from animal center in fourth military medical university (Xian, China) and were subjected to experiment until they were acclimatized for 4 weeks. They were kept under controlled conditions (temperature, 23 ± 2 °C; relative humidity, 55 ± 10 %) using an isolator caging system and fed at libitum.

362.2.2 Chemicals

T-2 toxin was dissolved in 20 % ethanol in 0.01 M phosphate-buffered saline.

362.2.3 Experiment Design

Thirty rats were equally divided into 3 groups. After overnight fasting, 2 groups were intragastric administrated with T-2 toxin at the dose levels of 100 ng/g b. w.

(low T-2 toxin group) and 200 ng/g b. w. (high T-2 toxin group), respectively. The inoculation volume was adjusted to 10 ml/kg b. w. using 0.01 M PB. The control group was given 20 % ethanol in 0.01 M PB in the same way. After 4 weeks gavage, the mice were all killed by heart puncture under ether anesthesia.

362.2.4 Histology and TUNEL Staining

Mandibles including incisors obtained from rat were fixed into 4 % neutral buffered formalin for 24 h, and then they were thoroughly decalcified in EDTA. After water deprivation and paraffin embedding, make 4 μm continued section and HE staining to confirm ameloblasts. After slicing was dewaxed and hydrated, each slicing was incubated with 100 μl TdT enzyme contained reaction liquid at room temperature for 1 h. After rinsed with PBS several times, 100 μl HRP Diluent (1: 500 diluted with PBS) was added and incubated at room temperature for 30 min, then rinse again. Terminated the reaction after DAB color reaction. Nuclei were stained with haematoxylin for 10 s. After deionized water rinsing, the slides were mounted under coverslips. The number of presecretory-stage ameloblast, secretory-stage ameloblast, transition-stage ameloblast and maturation-stage ameloblast in each slide was counted in 5 random high-power fields (×400). Apoptosis rate = Apoptotic cell number/total counting cell number. The experiments were performed in triplicate and repeated twice independently.

362.2.5 Statistical Analysis

The data are expressed as the mean ± standard error of the mean (SEM). The statistical significance of the differences between the groups was analyzed using a two-tailed Student's t test. A P-value of less than 0.05 was considered statistically significant ($P < 0.05$).

362.3 Results

The color of nuclei was dark golden yellow in the TUNEL positive reaction, while the negative nuclei is without staining. In the control group, there is no TUNEL positive reaction in the presecretory-stage and secretory-stage ameloblast, but in the transition-stage and maturation-stage, the TUNEL positive reaction existed not only in the ameloblasts, but also in the neighboring intermedium stratum cells and the stellate reticulum cells, as shown in Figs. 362.1 and 362.2.

In both the high dose and the low dose T-2 toxin poisoning group, TUNEL positive reaction widely distributed not only in the transition-stage and maturation-stage ameloblasts, but also even in the presecretory-stage and secretory-stage ameloblasts, and the neighbouring intermedium stratum cells and the stellate reticulum cells also have positive staining (Figs. 362.3 and 362.4).

Statistical analysis results of showed that there are significant differences in the apoptosis rate between the three experimental groups ($F = 205.883$, $P < 0.01$; $F = 43.397$, $P < 0.01$; $F = 12.095$, $P < 0.01$), as shown in Table 362.1. Thus, apoptosis rate in the two T-2 toxin poisoning groups were higher than the control group and the apoptosis rate in high T-2 toxin group were higher than the low T-2 toxin group.

362.4 Discussion

Both the domestic and foreign research shows that T-2 toxin could induce pathological damage to the body through a variety of ways, of which apoptosis was considered to be a major mechanism of action in various cell lines. Bax and Bcl-2 had inhibitory and promotive effects on T-2 toxin-induced apoptosis of human chondrocytes. However, the specific regulation mechanism of apoptosis is unclear. Our former research showed that T-2 toxin affects the cell morphology of ameloblasts and induces the appearance changes in tooth organ. In the present study, we used T-2 toxin poisoning rat model to investigate the effect of T-2 toxin on the apoptosis of ameloblasts, further revealing the reason for the morphologic changes in ameloblasts.

Enamel development include two process: the formation of enamel matrix and then mineralization of enamel matrix. The two main stages recognized in the formation of enamel are the secretory and maturation stages, both regulated by the ameloblast. Secretory ameloblasts are tall, polarized cells that often reach up to 60–100 μm in length while maintaining a relatively narrow 5–8 μm diameter. Secretory-stage ameloblasts secrete enamel matrix and provide an organic template form for the enamel crystals to grow [4]. The full volume of enamel tissue is built in this stage. Maturation-stage ameloblasts change morphology to become shorter and somewhat more “squat” cells [4]. Maturation-stage ameloblasts remove the water and organic content and finally create the enamel organ containing 95 % mineral by weight. The apoptosis of amelablasts is an important shaping mechanism in tooth development. Our result showed that in the control group there is rarely TUNEL positive in the secretory-stage ameloblast, especially the presecretory-stage ameloblast. Cell proliferation of the presecretory-stage ameloblast is active and secretory-stage ameloblasts begin to divide, thus rarely apoptosis in this two stage is accord with the need for matrix synthesis by a certain amount of secretory-stage ameloblasts [5].

TUNEL positive the presecretory-stage ameloblasts occured in the T-2 toxin poisoning groups, implying that T-2 toxin could induce the normal highly proliferative presecretory-stage ameloblasts to go into premature apoptosis in advance. Apoptosis rate of the transition-stage and maturation-stage ameloblasts in

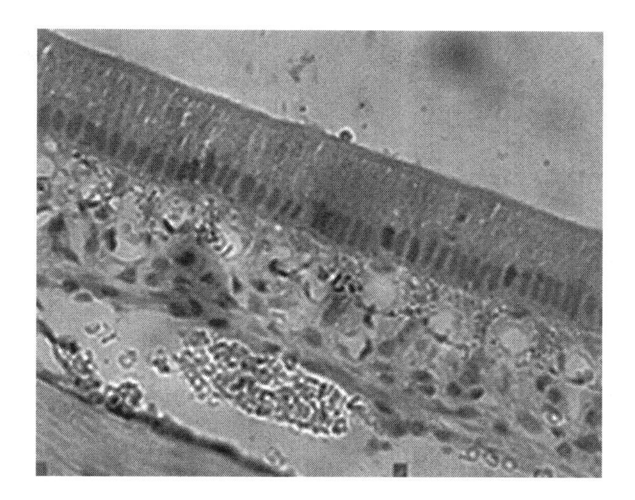

Fig. 362.1 Secretory-stage ameloblast in control group (×400)

the two T-2 toxin poisoning groups were higher than the control group ($P < 0.01$). This indicate that T-2 toxin could further induce the apoptosis in the transition-stage and maturation-stage ameloblasts. This might be related with the morphologic change of transition-stage ameloblasts. In this stage, Tomes's processes of ameloblasts disappear and striated border forms, which is critical for the functional shift of ameloblasts from secreting matrix to synthesizing proteolytic enzymes to promote enamel matrix mineralization. Maturation-stage ameloblasts could secrete many proteolytic enzymes which have effect on the degradation of enamel matrix proteins, regulation of calcium ions deposited into the enamel matrix, keep of the local buffering capacity and promotion of the growth of crystals, thus play an important role in the late stage of enamel development [6]. Increase of apoptotic

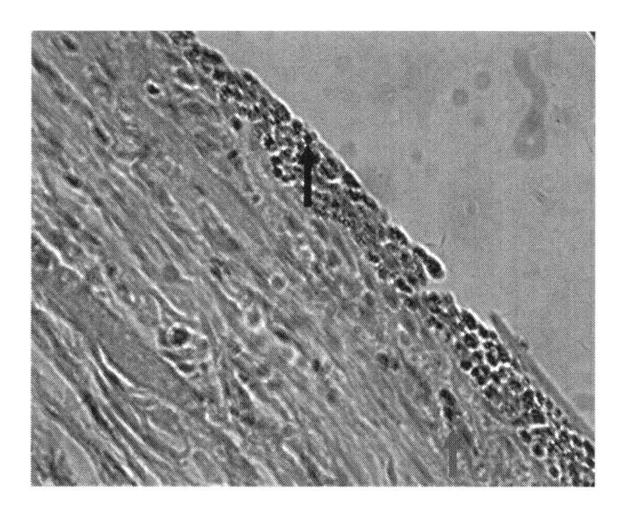

Fig. 362.2 Maturation -stage ameloblast in control group (×400). The *green arrow* represents apoptotic intermedium stratum cells and the stellate reticulum cells

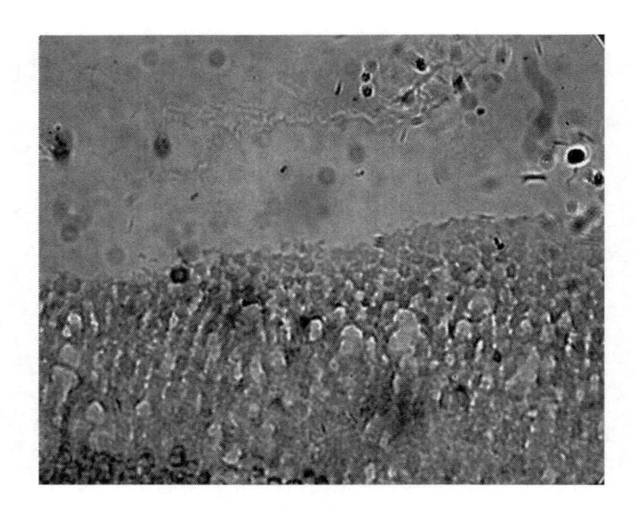

Fig. 362.3 Presecretory-stage ameloblast in high T-2 toxin group (×1000).

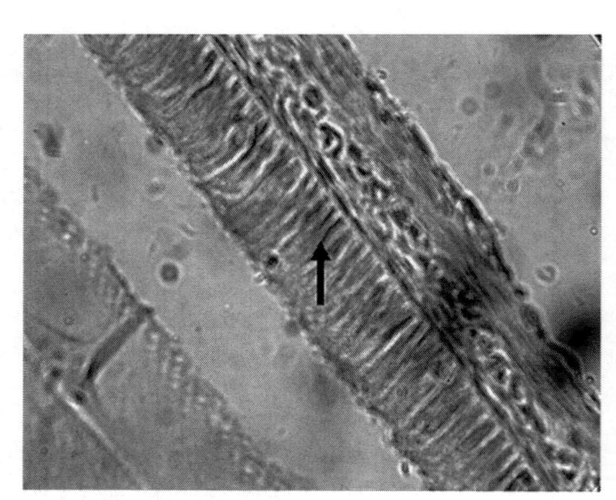

Fig. 362.4 Transition-stage ameloblast in the low T-2 toxin group (×400). The *black arrow* represents apoptotic ameloblast

Table 362.1 Apoptosis rate of ameloblast treated by T-2 toxin in different dose (n = 10, $\bar{X} \pm S$)

Group	Presecretory-stage ameloblast	Secretory-stage ameloblast	Transition-stage ameloblast	Maturation-stage ameloblast
Control group	/	0.014 ± 0.007	0.290 ± 0.012	0.483 ± 0.031
Low T-2 toxin group	0.016 ± 0.007	$0.112 \pm 0.009^{*}$	$0.349 \pm 0.025^{*}$	$0.559 \pm 0.018^{*}$
High T-2 toxin group	0.040 ± 0.006	$0.208 \pm 0.065^{**}$	$0.421 \pm 0.047^{**}$	$0.570 \pm 0.065^{*}$

* Significantly different from control ($p < 0.01$)

** Significantly different from low T-2 toxin group ($p < 0.01$)

cells in the maturation-stage ameloblasts might reduce the amount of proteolytic enzymes, lead retention of enamel protein and water, interfere with the growth of enamel rod and crystals, and thus influence enamel development.

362.5 Conclusion

T-2 toxin can accelerate apoptosis of ameloblasts in rat's incisor. With the increase of T-2 toxin intake dose, the apoptosis rate of ameloblasts increases.

Acknowledgments This research was supported through funding from Scientific Research Program funded by Shaanxi Provincial Education Department (Program No. 12JK0763).

References

1. Seeboth J et al (2012) The fungal T-2 toxin alters the activation of primary macrophages induced by TLR-agonists resulting in a decrease of the inflammatory response in the pig. Vet Res 43(1):35
2. Weidner M et al (2013) Neurotoxic potential and cellular uptake of T-2 toxin in human astrocytes in primary culture. Chem Res Toxicol 26(3):347–355
3. Wu J et al (2011) T-2 toxin induces apoptosis in ovarian granulosa cells of rats through reactive oxygen species-mediated mitochondrial pathway. Toxicol Lett 202(3):168–177
4. Lacruz RS et al (2013) New paradigms on the transport functions of maturation-stage ameloblasts. J Dent Res 92(2):122–129
5. Bronckers AL et al (1996) Nuclear DNA fragmentation during postnatal tooth development of mouse and hamster and during dentin repair in the rat. Eur J Oral Sci 104(2 (Pt 1)):102–111
6. Smith CE (1998) Cellular and chemical events during enamel maturation. Crit Rev Oral Biolo Med Offi Publ Am Assoc Oral Biol 9(2):128–161

Chapter 363
A Preliminary Study of the Influence of T-2 Toxin on the Expressions of Bcl-2 and Bax of Ameloblasts in Rat's Incisor

Sha-fei Zhai, Zhu Yong, Ma Zheng and Yaochao Zhang

Abstract To investigate the effects of T-2 toxin on the protein expression of Bcl-2/Bax of ameloblast in rat's incisor. 30 Wistar rats were divided randomly into 3 groups: control, low dose and high dose T-2 toxin poisoning group. After 4 weeks treatment, immunohisto-chemistry was used to observe the relative intensity of Bax and Bcl-2 expression in the ameloblasts. Quantitative analysis of the expression of Bax and Bcl-2 was performed with a computer image analysis system. Quantitative analysis showed the Bax protein expression was up-regulated, the Bcl-2 protein expression was down-regulated, and the Bax/Bcl-2 expression ratio was up-regulated in the secretory-stage ameloblasts treated with T-2 toxin, and this was significant between three groups ($P < 0.05$). Thus, T-2 toxin can decrease the expression of Bcl-2 and increase the expression of Bax in the secretory-stage ameloblasts of rat's incisor. With the increase of T-2 toxin exposure dose, this effect is much marked.

Keywords T-2 toxin · Rat · Ameloblast

363.1 Introduction

The cytotoxic response of T-2 toxin are already well described with apoptosis being a major mechanism of action in many tissues [1]. It has been reported to affect the cell cycle, thus induce apoptosis in vivo and in vitro in the liver, placenta and fetal liver in pregnant rats [2]. Apoptotic genetic disorders is one of the

S. Zhai (✉) · Z. Yong
Department of Oral Medicine, Xi'an Medical University, Xinwang Road, Xi'an 710021 Shaanxi, China

M. Zheng · Y. Zhang
Department of Public Health, Xi'an medical university, Xinwang Road, Xi'an 710021 Shaanxi, China

S. Li et al. (eds.), *Frontier and Future Development of Information Technology in Medicine and Education*, Lecture Notes in Electrical Engineering 269,
DOI: 10.1007/978-94-007-7618-0_363,

reasons for tooth development deformity. Ameloblasts are the key cells in the enamal formation. They play important role in the formation of enamel matrix and the mineralization of enamel matrix in the enamel development. Our former research showed that T-2 toxin induced the apoptosis of ameloblasts. In the present study, poisoning rat model with T-2 toxin was used to investigate the mechanism of T-2 toxin induced apoptosis of ameloblasts.

363.2 Experiment

363.2.1 Experiment Design

Thirty rats were equally divided into 3 groups. 2 groups were intragastric administrated with T-2 toxin at the dose levels of 100 ng/g b. w. (low T-2 toxin group) and 200 ng/g b. w. (high T-2 toxin group), respectively. After 4 weeks gavage, the mice were all killed by heart puncture under ether anesthesia to obtain the mandibles including incisors.

363.2.2 Immunohistochemical Staining

Using 4 μm continued section and HE staining to confirm ameloblasts. After dewaxed and hydrated, each slicing was incubated with 30 ml/L hydrogen peroxide for 30 min, then microwavely heated in 0.01 mol/L citrate buffer. After rinsed with PBS several times, blocking solution was added for 40 min at room temperature, then primary antibodies diluents (1:1000) at 4 °C overnight. Second antibody was added at 37 °C for 1 h, SABC was added at 37 °C for 40 min. After DAB color reaction, nuclei were stained for 10 s. After rinsing, the slides were mounted. The experiments were repeated twice independently.

363.2.3 Image Analysis and Statistical Analysis

Gray value was analyzed with Image-Pro Plus 5.1 analysis system. Integrated optical density. The average gray value of positive staining ameloblast in each slide was measured in 5 random high-power fields (×400). The integrated optical density (IOD) value was used to detect semi-quantitatively the expression of Bcl-2 and Bax. Optical density value and image grey value is inversely proportional to the quantity of the positive antigen. Thus, high integral optical density value represented low protein expression level. The data are expressed as the mean ± standard error of the mean (SEM). A *P*-value of less than 0.05 was considered statistically significant ($P < 0.05$).

363.3 Results

363.3.1 The Expression of Bcl-2 in Ameloblasts

In the control group, the positive expression of Bcl-2 was pale brown mainly located in cytoplasm. The positive expression of Bcl-2 began in presecretory-stage ameloblasts, and continued to express in secretory-stage, transition-stage and maturation-stage ameloblasts, in which the positive brown staining was deeper in presecretory-stage and secretory-stage ameloblasts (Fig. 363.1a). In the low dose T-2 toxin poisoning group, the positive expression of Bcl-2 could be found in every stage ameloblasts, but the degree of positive staining in presecretory-stage and secretory-stage ameloblasts was weaker than the control group (Fig. 363.1b). In the high dose T-2 toxin poisoning group, the degree of positive staining in every stage ameloblasts was weaker than both the control group and the low dose T-2 toxin poisoning group (Fig. 363.1c). Statistical analysis results of showed that there were significant differences in the IOD of Bcl-2 between the secretory-stage ameloblasts in three experimental groups ($P < 0.05$), as shown in Table 363.1.

363.3.2 The Expression of Bax in Ameloblasts

In the control group, the positive expression of Bax was pale brown. The positive expression of Bax began in secretory-stage ameloblasts, and continued to express in secretory-stage, transition-stage and maturation-stage ameloblasts, in which the

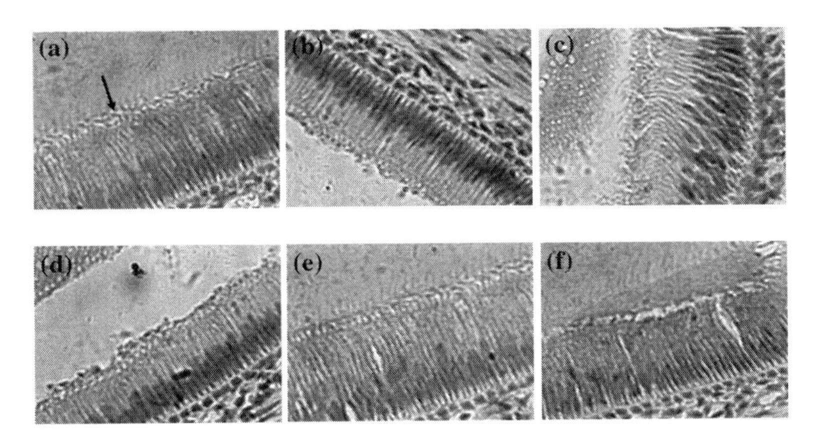

Fig. 363.1 Immunohisto-chemistry staining of ameloblast (×400) (**a**–**c**) are the staining of Bcl-2. (**d**–**f**) are the staining of Bax. (**a**) and (**d**) represent the control group. (**b**) and E represent the low dose T-2 toxin poisoning group. (**c**) and (**f**) represent the high dose T-2 toxin poisoning group. The arrow represents ameloblast.)

Table 363.1 Integrated optical density (IOD) of Bcl-2 (n = 10, $\bar{X} \pm S$)

Group	Presecretory-stage ameloblast	Secretory-stage ameloblast	Transition-stage ameloblast
Control group	116.24 ± 13.79	125.12 ± 14.02	140.79 ± 13.18
Low T-2 toxin group	133.27 ± 17.02[a]	143.83 ± 15.46[a]	145.81 ± 16.43
High T-2 toxin group	155.14 ± 22.04[b]	167.67 ± 24.17[b]	165.70 ± 23.97[b]

[a] Significantly different from control ($p < 0.05$)
[b] Significantly different from low T-2 toxin group ($p < 0.05$)

positive brown staining was deeper in transition-stage ameloblasts (Fig. 363.1d). In the low dose T-2 toxin poisoning group, the positive expression of Bax could be found in every stage ameloblasts as the control group, but the degree of positive staining in secretory-stage ameloblasts was deeper than the control group. The degree of positive staining in transition-stage ameloblasts was almost the same as the control group (Fig. 363.1e). In the high dose T-2 toxin poisoning group, the degree of positive staining in secretory-stage ameloblasts was deeper than the low dose T-2 toxin poisoning group. The degree of positive staining in transition-stage ameloblasts was almost the same as the control group and the low dose T-2 toxin poisoning group (Fig. 363.1f). Statistical analysis results showed that there were significant differences in the IOD of Bax between the secretory-stage ameloblasts in three experimental groups ($P < 0.05$), and there were no significant differences in the IOD of Bax between the transition-stage ameloblasts in three experimental groups ($P < 0.05$), as shown in Table 363.2.

363.3.3 The Expression of Bax/Bcl-2 Ratio in Ameloblasts

Table 363.3 showed that the IOD of Bax/Bcl-2 ratio in the secretory-stage a-meloblasts was maximum in the control group, and the ratio was minimum in the high dose T-2 toxin poisoning group. There were significant differences in three experimental groups ($P < 0.05$).

Table 363.2 Integrated optical density (IOD) of Bax (n = 10, $\bar{X} \pm S$)

Group	Presecretory-stage ameloblast	Secretory-stage ameloblast	Transition-stage ameloblast
Control group	/	178.66 ± 18.73	136.28 ± 15.67
Low T-2 toxin group	/	158.43 ± 11.56[a]	136.52 ± 11.42
High T-2 toxin group	/	130.13 ± 15.58[b]	130.43 ± 12.36

[a] Significantly different from control ($p < 0.05$)
[b] Significantly different from low T-2 toxin group ($p < 0.05$)

Table 363.3 Integrated optical density (IOD) of Bax/Bcl-2 (n = 10, $\bar{X} \pm S$)

Group	Presecretory-stage ameloblast	Secretory-stage ameloblast	Transition-stage ameloblast
Control group	/	1.45 ± 0.22	0.98 ± 0.14
Low T-2 toxin group	/	1.11 ± 0.13[a]	0.95 ± 0.13
High T-2 toxin group	/	0.79 ± 0.12[b]	0.80 ± 0.12[b]

[a] Significantly different from control ($p < 0.05$)
[b] Significantly different from low T-2 toxin group ($p < 0.05$)

363.4 Discussion

Tooth development is a complicated process. The cell growth, proliferation, differentiation and apoptosis in tooth were induced by extracellular signaling molecules and modulated by multiple genes. Bax and Bcl-2 involved in controlling development of teeth through apoptosis by regulation of cell proliferation, differentiation and maturation process. Apoptosis is an important shaping mechanism in the tooth development [3].

Ameloblasts are the key cells in the enamel formation. They play important role in the formation of enamel matrix and the mineralization of enamel matrix in the enamel development [4, 5]. It has been reported that Bax and Bcl-2 have respectively inhibitory and promotive effects on T-2 toxin-induced apoptosis of human chondrocytes. However, the specific regulation mechanism of apoptosis is unclear. In the present study, we used T-2 toxin poisoning rat model to investigate the effect of T-2 toxin on the apoptosis of ameloblasts, further revealing the mechanism for the apoptosis of ameloblasts.

Our present study found positive Bcl-2 expression with no positive Bax expression in the presecretory-stage ameloblasts of each group, and the Bcl-2 expression was reduced in the T-2 toxin poisoning group, and this change was more evident in the high T-2 toxin poisoning group. The Bcl-2 belongs to the genes that could suppress apoptosis, while the Bax belongs to the genes that could promote apoptosis. The reduction of Bcl-2 expression in the T-2 toxin poisoning group imply cell proliferation activity of presecretory-stage ameloblasts was influenced, which could illustrate T-2 toxin induced the apoptosis of ameloblasts in our former research. Secretory-stage ameloblasts exist for a long time in the enamel development. In this stage, ameloblasts were easily interfered by external factors. Statistical analysis of secretory-stage ameloblasts image showed that the Bcl-2 expressions were reduced, the Bax expressions were increased, and ratio of Bax/Bcl-2 was increased in the T-2 toxin poisoning groups as compared with the control group ($P < 0.05$). We speculated that T-2 toxin induced the apoptosis of ameloblasts might be related with the increased Bax expressions. Increased Bax expressions might promote Bax-Bax homodimers formation, which competes the apoptotic suppression effect of Bcl-2, and induce the increase expression of Bax/Bcl-2 ratio.

363.5 Conclusion

T-2 toxin could decrease the expression of Bcl-2 and increase the expression of Bax in the secretory-stage ameloblasts of rat's incisor.

Acknowledgments This research was supported through funding from Scientific Research Program funded by Shaanxi Provincial Education Department (Program No. 12JK0763).

References

1. Weidner M et al (2013) Neurotoxic potential and cellular uptake of T-2 toxin in human astrocytes in primary culture. Chem Res Toxicol 26(3):347–355
2. Wu J et al (2011) T-2 toxin induces apoptosis in ovarian granulosa cells of rats through reactive oxygen species-mediated mitochondrial pathway. Toxicol Lett 202(3):168–177
3. Matalova E, Svandova E, Tucker AS (2012) Apoptotic signaling in mouse odontogenesis. Omics J Integr Biol 16(1–2):60–70
4. Lacruz RS et al (2013) New paradigms on the transport functions of maturation-stage ameloblasts. J Dent Res 92(2):122–129
5. Bronckers AL, Lyaruu DM, DenBesten PK (2009) The impact of fluoride on ameloblasts and the mechanisms of enamel fluorosis. J Dent Res 88(10):877–893

Chapter 364
PET Image Processing in the Early Diagnosis of PD

Kai Ma, Zhi-an Liu, Ya-ping Nie and Dian-shuai Gao

Abstract *Objective* To clear which degree of damage of mice dopamine could change the brain glucose metabolic activity and whether the change can be detected with positron emission tomography imaging processing and to find a positron emission tomography data processing method effectively. *Methods* Using Positron Emission Tomography imaging technology to image 1-methyl-4-phenyl-1,2,3,6-tetrahydropyridine model mice, data analysis after imaging. *Results* The study of Parkinson's disease glucose metabolism found that mice with bilateral striatal glucose metabolism reduced after 2 weeks 1-methyl-4-phenyl -1,2,3,6-tetrahydropyridine administration. And the data processing method of Positron Emission Tomography imaging techniques is discussed in detail, Specific typical statistical parameter mapping processing of positron emission tomography data processing steps and the experimental results are given. *Conclusions* Positron emission tomography imaging can detect early diagnosis of Parkinson's disease and Statistical pixel processing positron emission tomography data image processing method is an effective data image processing methods.

Keywords Parkinson's disease · Positron emission tomography · Dopamine transporter · Glucose metabolism

K. Ma · Y. Nie
Institute of Medical Information Science, Xuzhou Medical College, Xuzhou 221004 Jiangsu, China

Z. Liu · D. Gao (✉)
Department of Basic Medical, Xuzhou Medical College, Xuzhou 221004 Jiangsu, China
e-mail: cumtbmakai@126.com

S. Li et al. (eds.), *Frontier and Future Development of Information Technology in Medicine and Education*, Lecture Notes in Electrical Engineering 269,
DOI: 10.1007/978-94-007-7618-0_364,

364.1 Introduction

Parkinson's disease (PD) is a serious central nervous system degenerative diseases of elderly. The main pathological change is dopamine neuron degeneration and death in the substantia nigra pars compacta, so that the decrease in striatal dopamine (DA) content. Currently, the treatment of PD always supplement the DA and strengthen the DA role of the alternative method, but the long-term effect is not ideal. If early diagnosis of PD could be made before the death of DA neurons degeneration and give neuroprotective treatment rather than an alternative therapy [1]. It is possible to significantly delay the course of the disease and improve the patient's quality of life [2–5].

Positron Emission Tomography (PET) is able to obtain some physiological or biochemical information of the human or animal organs or lesions, is an advanced nuclear medical imaging technique.

This article study the changes in brain glucose metabolism in mice from MPTP injury DA neuron until mice appear symptoms of PD by using PET imaging technology, the main purpose is to clear which degree of damage of mice DA neuron could change the brain glucose metabolic activity and whether the change can be detected with PET imaging processing. To provide a non-invasive means of detection for the early diagnosis of PD by analyzing the signal strength of the PET imaging, and use this case to describe the PET imaging SPM data processing method in detail [6, 7].

364.2 Materials and Methods

364.2.1 Materials

Laboratory reagents 18F-FDG, provided by People's Liberation Army General Hospital, Department of Nuclear Medicine; Experimental animals, C57BL/6 mice, male, weighted 22–25 g, 8–8.5 weeks, provided by experimental animal Centre of Xuzhou medical college.

364.2.2 Methods

Animal grouping, C57BL/6 mice, male, weighted 22–25 g, 8–8.5 weeks, amount is 140. In the position of 24 ± 2 °C room temperature and 12 h/12 h day and night rhythm, intake the water and food freely. All animals begin the experiment after adapting the environment for 2 days. Mice were divided into experimental and control groups, $N = 70$ for each group. Animals in each group have 10 dedicated to FDG-PET imaging, the left 60 were divided into five groups according to five different time points(the first day of the first week after the second time of administration, the second day of the first week after the second time of administration, the third day of the first week after the second time of administration, the forth day of the first week after the second time of administration, the fifth day of the first week after the second time of administration), 12 in each group, take the corresponding group at each time point, to do the behavioral test first, then executed to get the brain for cerebral biological detection. Medication, 1-methyl-4-phenyl-1,2,3,6-tetrahydropyridine model (MPTP) was dissolved in 0.9 % NaCl solution to a concentration of 10 mg/ml. Reference to Lan, Experimental group mice, intraperitoneal injection MPTP 25 mg/kg, twice a week, administration on Monday afternoon and Friday morning, in order to ensure the same time interval, administered for five consecutive weeks for 10 times, give Control group intraperitoneal injection of the same dose of saline at the same time.

PET imaging, The PET apparatus is E-Plus PET. Pixel size: [0.5 0.5 1]; Axial resolution: CFOV 1.67 mm, FOV 1.9 mm; depth of stratum is 2 mm; Meet the window width: 12.5 ns, tracer agent is 18F-FDG. Mice fast for 12 h before detecting. Put the mice in the scan room in the morning for more than 30 min to adapt the environment. Mice tail vein injection 18F-FDG 0.5 mCi, 1 % isoflurane inhalation anesthesia after 35 min, 5 min after anesthesia, begin the PET scanning when mice breathing steadily, end scanning When the total number reaches 30 million. The results are analyzed by SPM software. Imaging time: the first day of the first week after the second time of administration, the second day of the first week after the second time of administration.

Data processing and analysis, the results of mice FDG-PET are proceeded by statistical parametric mapping (SPM2).

364.3 Results

To clear in mice brain of MPTP damage DA neurons model mice whether the glucose metabolism changed from DA neuron degeneration and loss until the onset of PD symptoms, we do a FDG-PET imaging 24 h after the second administration every week. A large number of previously studies about PD brain glucose metabolism show cortex and striatum of PD appears abnormal metabolism, and the damaged DA neuron of PD are most located in the substantia nigra compacta, so we focus on observation the metabolism of nigra, striatum and cortex. Results are shown in Fig. 364.1, 2 weeks after MPTP administration. Bilateral striatum of mice appeared reduced glucose metabolism ($p < 0.001$), the substantia nigra and the cerebral cortex did not show metabolic changes.

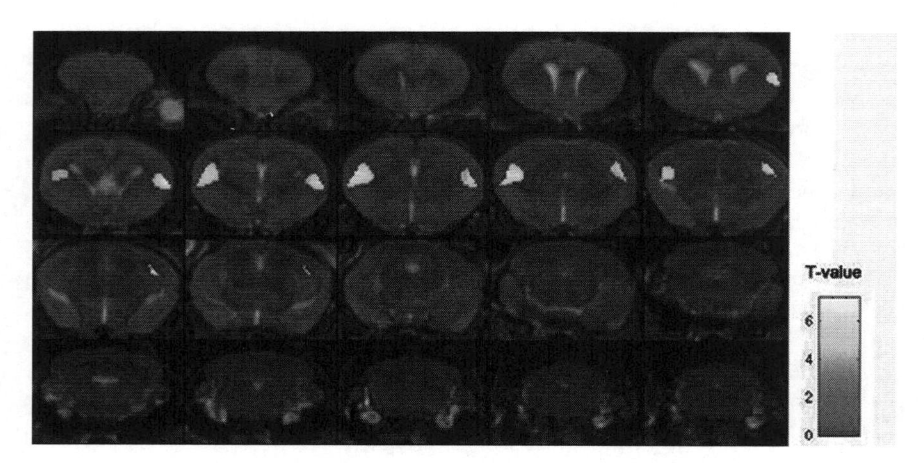

Fig. 364.1 The change of cerebral glucose metabolism in mice treated with MPTP. The PET imaging were performed at the next 24 h after the second-injection of MPTP or saline weekly. The cluster shown encloses some regions of the striatum. Values given at pheight < 0.001, compared to the control group, $n = 10$

364.4 Discussion

As a major molecular imaging technology, the advantages of PET are the radionuclide labeled ligand as inherent mark, not affect the pharmacokinetics of ligand can effectively correct tissue attenuation, preventing radiation diffusion, and has a high sensitivity, benefit for quantitative analysis. 18F-FDG is widely used positron-emitting radiopharmaceuticals and has been widely used imaging of living tissue glucose metabolism. 18F-FDG is glucose isomer, arriving within the organization after inputting and phosphorylated by Hexokinase, but due to the different molecular structure, can not proceed to the next step metabolism immediately, therefore remain in the tissue cells. 18F can release positron, positron annihilation radiation produces γ-ray which is opposite direction and energy equal and can be received by paired detectors in vitro. FDG metabolism in the body distribution can be reconstructed by computer processing. FDG uptake rate can sensitively reflect the glucose metabolism level of body organs and can be applied to PET imaging of the heart, brain and tumor. 30 min after the injection of 18F–FDG, declinding of radioactivity in plasma and various organs become slowly,so 18F–FDG-PET imaging requirements at least 30 min after administration. This article do PET imaging of the brain of mice after 40 min at the administration of 18F-FDG,the FDG uptake in the imaging portion is high, imaging results are reliable.

In the clear early pathological changes in PD, the change of DAT in striatum is One of the most sensitive indicators of early diagnosis of PD, it will be helpful for early diagnosis of PD if more accurate quantitative analysis of striatal DAT can be made. The existing DAT quantitative analysis method, such as the morphometry observation immune -specific staining light combined with electron microscope, immunoblotting gray combined with computer analysis technique, are all biological methods, need the corresponding parts of the organization as experimental specimens for measuring, this is clearly inappropriate for the clinical diagnosis of PD. DAT quantitative measurement method using molecular imaging techniques is using DAT specific ligands labeled with radioactive isotopes (11C, 18F) as a tracer to proceed the DAT - PET imaging and get the quantitative information of DAT content by proceeding the image. So far, there are two quantitative analysis method after DAT-PET imaging: The first is the relative uptake value method, this method first outlined regions of interest then calculate the ratio of the average

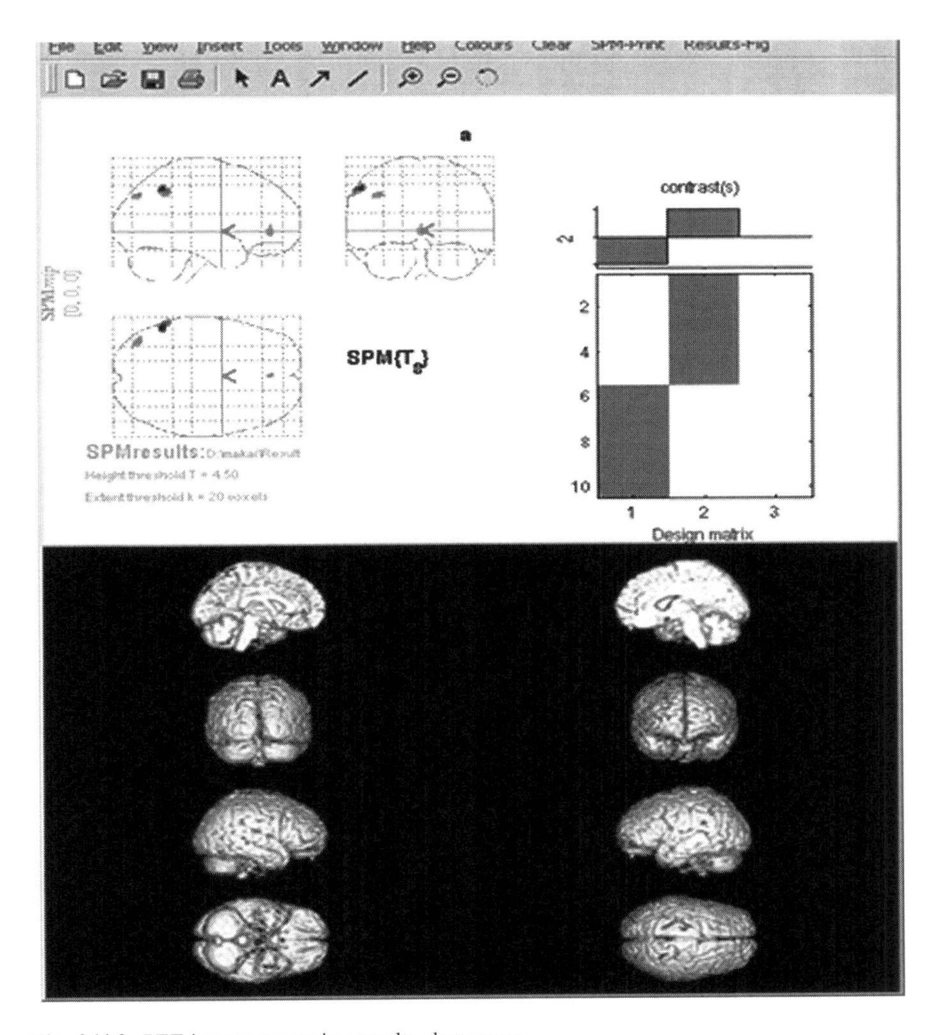

Fig. 364.2 PET image processing results show map

radioactivity count and reference areas. The second is standardized uptake value method, this method take the ratio of average radioactive counts and the radiopharmaceutical injection volume of the unit body weight in the regions of interest as SUV value, it provides a numerical reference for the quantitative analysis of PET imaging, effectively improve the readability of PET imaging and the reliability of results. Both of these methods belong to the semi-quantitative ROI-based analysis and they are all hot topics in the field of imaging diagnosis. But, their reliability are also being questioned. The main influencing factors include: setting of regions of interest, partial volume effect and attenuation correction, plasma level/concentration, the time from injection to imaging, filter function and the cut-off frequency, count of the PET system noise and image reconstruction algorithm and so on.

PET imaging data pretreatment contents: Realign, Co-register of images between the different imaging methods, normalization of images between different subjects and space smooth. The first three are called the image space transformation, common practice is take one of them or a normalizated template image as the base, convert other images (also called object image) to this standard brain. The pretreatment is aimed to fusion the plurality of experimental data of the test object so as to process and analyze together.

Multiple subjects and multiple measurements on the standardization of the resulting image to a standard brain by the pretreatment, improve the signal-to-noise ratio of the data and eliminate the slight brain structure differences between different test objects. Image sequence to the first image as a standard alignment (realign), standardized and Gaussian smoothing.

Estimation process followed the end of the pretreatment of PET, SPM's statistical analysis using two-sample *t* test. The results reconstruct 3D brain activation map and can show as Pseudo-color map as axial, sagittal, coronal projection map. As shown in Fig. 364.2, the upper part of figure is the left side of the bottom to activate the pixel based on the selected value, shows the brain PET activation in Fig. 364.2.

References

1. Shih MC, Hoexter MQ, Andrade LA, Bressan RA et al (2006) Parkinson's disease and dopamine transporter neuroimaging: a critical review. Sao Paulo Med J 124(3):168–175
2. Chitneni SK, Garreau L, Cleynhens B, Evens N, Bex M, Vermaelen P, Chalon S, Busson R, Guilloteau D, Van Laere K, Verbruggen A, Bormans G (2008) Improved synthesis and metabolic stability analysis of the dopamine transporter ligand [$^{(18)}$F]FECT. Nucl Med Biol 35(1):75–82
3. Wuest F, Berndt M, Strobel K et al (2007) Synthesis and radiopharmacological characterization of 2beta-carbo-2'-[^{18}F] fluoroethoxy-3beta-(4-bromo-phenyl) –tropane([18F]MCL-322)as a PET radiotracer for imaging the dopamine transporter (DAT). Bioorg Med Chem 15(13):4511–4519

4. Saba W, Valette H, Schöllhorn-Peyronneau MA et al (2007) [^{11}C]LBT-999: a suitable radioligand for investigation of extra-striatal dopamine transporter with PET. Synapse 61(1):17–23
5. Wang J, Zuo CT, Jiang YP et al (2007) ^{18}F-FP-CIT PET imaging and SPM analysis of dopamine transporters in Parkinson's disease in various Hoehn&Yahr stages. J Neurol 254(2):185–190
6. Shi J, Zhao LY, Copersino ML et al (2008) PET imaging of dopamine transporter and drug craving during methadone maintenance treatment and after prolonged abstinence in heroin users. Eur J Pharmacol 579(1–3):160–166
7. Sekine Y, Minabe Y, Ouchi Y et al (2003) Association of dopamine transporter loss in the orbitofrontal and dorsolateral prefrontal cortices with methamphetamine-related psychiatric symptoms. Am J Psychiatry 160:1699–1701

Chapter 365
"4 Steps" in Problem Based Teaching in the Medical Internship: Experiences from China

Huasheng Liu, Mei Zhang, Richard Bae, Muxing Li, Xiaoping Xi, Qin Gao, Yan Li, Di Wu and Bingyin Shi

Abstract *Background* The clinical internship represents a crucial time in medical education. Our study looks at the effects of our problem-based teaching "4 steps" method in the training of the interns in our center. *Methods* 35 final-year medical students were enrolled in our study. We investigated the main problems they encountered as well as their suggested resolutions to these problems using personal interviews and e-mail. We guided every medical student through our problem-based teaching "4 steps" method. The supervision of the interns was adjusted according to the feedback from the survey. We later rated the effects of the changes by soliciting their feedback. *Results* All the students received training in critical thinking and practice which helped them better make the transition from being a medical student to a junior medical doctor. Most of the 35 students received an offer from our hospital, which is one of the best hospitals according to the Ministry of Public Health. *Conclusion* Our problem-based teaching "4 steps" strategy was shown to improve the quality of our medical internship.

Keywords Problem based teaching · 4 steps method · Reflective practice · Medical internship

---

H. Liu · M. Zhang · M. Li · X. Xi · D. Wu
Department of Hematology, First Affiliated Hospital of Xi'an Jiaotong University School of Medicine, NO. 277, Yanta West Road, Xi'an 710061, People's Republic of China
e-mail: lhs681995@126.com

R. Bae · Q. Gao · Y. Li · B. Shi
Department of Medical Education, First Affiliated Hospital of Xi'an Jiaotong University School of Medicine, NO. 277, Yanta West Road, Xi'an 710061, People's Republic of China

B. Shi (✉)
Department of Endocrinology, First Affiliated Hospital of Xi'an Jiaotong University School of Medicine, NO. 277, Yanta West Road, Xi'an 710061, People's Republic of China
e-mail: shibingy@126.com

S. Li et al. (eds.), *Frontier and Future Development of Information Technology in Medicine and Education*, Lecture Notes in Electrical Engineering 269,
DOI: 10.1007/978-94-007-7618-0_365,

365.1 Background

Internship is a significant part of medical education as it bridges the gap between being a medical student and becoming a doctor. Undergoing a valuable internship is the prelude to becoming an outstanding doctor. As the competition among the students increases, all medical students, during their internship year, hope to improve the 3 pillars of being a doctor—theory, skill, and communication. However, many reports show that the educational quality of the internship is not as highly regarded by the students and society as we expected. On one hand, insufficient supervision, instruction, and guidance does not remove the blame for inferior quality. On the other hand, students may not be diligent or motivated enough to perform well in their rotation. Under the condition of escalating workloads and scientific research requirements, residents may find themselves being not able to afford enough time and effort to teach their followers. A heavy workload was associated with disorganized surface-learning for residents and clerks [1]. Students may not get in-depth clinical practice or understanding of the internship, and thus residents should reform their strategy towards their interns in their teaching programs. In addition, the residents may not be experienced enough to perform their didactic duties for the medical students. Therefore, emphasis should be exerted on an effective teaching approach.

Reflection may be most useful when viewed as a learning strategy [2]. A clear understanding of deep and surface learning related to reflective and non-reflective thinking has yet to be developed [3]. We examined 35 medical students' reflective thinking using a structured activity called the "4-step method". Most students who completed the exercise demonstrated reflection at deeper, as well as more descriptive, levels.

The aim of our study is to determine the students' difficulties in their final year clinical internship through their written reports, and then raise strategies targeting the main problems. Finally, we assess the outcomes by looking at variables such as the students' future publications and jobs and investigate the effects of our Problem-based Teaching "4-step method" in the clinical internship.

365.2 Materials and Methods

365.2.1 Internship

In our department the final year medical student is trained by the residents. Every student is required to attend an 18 week internship in Internal Medicine, Surgery, Gynecology, Obstetrics, and Pediatrics, rotating in each department for 3 weeks, respectively.

365.2.2 Methods

The largest issue for interns is assuming and coping with the increasing responsibilities of patient care. They are often confused during the internship because they suddenly find themselves facing many problems at the same time. Every case is so different. How should they deal with clinical problems and find a suitable way that leads to the desired endpoint? This is not an easy task, especially because there is only 1 year for medical students in China to practice before they graduate and get a job.

In our clinical teaching practice, we tried to find an easy method to help the medical students' thinking and practice. It is called the four steps problem-based teaching method for assisting the medical intern transition to being a full doctor.

The first step, identify all the problems encountered in the interns' clinical practice.

The second step, divide all the problems into multiple aspects.

The third step, reorder the problems according to personal need.

The fourth step, try to answer every question.

The methods have been performed with the approval of The Medical Ethics Committee of The First Affiliated Hospital of Xi'an Jiaotong University School of Medicine. The written informed consent for participation in the study were obtained from participants. More details can be found in the attachment below.

365.2.3 The Survey

From November 2010 to May 2012,a total of 35 students were surveyed during their clinical rotation in the Department of Hematology, the 1st Affiliated Hospital, School of Medicine, Xi'an Jiaotong University. Of the 35 students, 19 were in the Seven-Year Program, 6 were in the Five-Year Program, and 5 were in the Eight-Year Program. In addition, there were also 5 foreign students in our survey pool. At the end of their 1st week of their rotation in our department, the students were required to submit a report of the main problems they encountered along with suggestions on how to improve the experience of their clinical internship. We developed a rating system for the survey (Table 365.1). We later subdivided the surveyed students into 4 levels according to their scores. At 14.3, 28.6, 37.1, and 20.0 %, the surveys were respectively in levels A, B, C and D (Table 365.2). Furthermore, the students from the 8-Year Program received higher scores than students from the 7-Year Program, and the students from 7-Year Program received higher scores than students from the 5-Year Program and the Foreign Students (Table 365.3).

Table 365.1 The rating system of the survey

Criteria	Score
Whether they raised problems?	50
Whether they divided their problems into different groups?	20
Whether they listed the problems as a priority?	10
Whether they proposed their view on the resolution of the problems?	20
Total	100

Table 365.2 The distribution of the scores of the survey

Level	Score	Number of Students
A	>85	5/35 (14.3 %)
B	70–85	10/35 (28.6 %)
C	50–70	13/35 (37.1 %)
D	<50	7/35 (20.0 %)

Table 365.3 The score of the students from different programs

Student group by program	Score
8-Year program (5/35)	80 ± 1.02
7-Year program (19/35)	78 ± 9.81
5-Year program (6/35)	70 ± 5.23
Foreign students (5/35)	72 ± 6.97

The students from 8-Year Program and 7-Year Program received higher scores than students from 5-Year Program and the Foreign Students

365.2.4 The Main Problems (in Descending Order) and Our Strategy Targeting the Problems

Our survey of the final-year clinical students in their internship program consistently showed several problems. The top 5 problems they faced were: "how to consolidate medical theories throughout the internship" (35/35, 100 %), "how to get more 'physical contact' with the residents' work" (31/35, 88.5 %), "how to practice basic clinical skills" (26/35, 74.3 %), "How to communicate with patients and their relatives? How to answer the questions of patients and their relatives?" (22/35, 62.8 %) and "How to deal with the unconventional work assigned by the residents and maximize efficiency?" (18/35, 51.4 %).

1. How to consolidate medical theories throughout the internship?
   After finishing a rotation in a department, many students will find that even though they were busy every day, they did not learn much specialized knowledge in the specific department.
   Someone once said there are three prerequisites to be an excellent surgeon—an eagle's eyes, a lion's mind, and a woman's hands. In our view, the three factors

are not only advisable for the surgeon but also worthwhile for all doctors.
Our strategy

a. Be patient with the students.
b. Ask the students to prepare the tools for internship: pocketsize reference manual, notebook, medical apps in their smartphone (if available), and stethoscope.
c. Most students report that they value the ward rounds as the main platform for them to enhance their understanding of medical knowledge. We perform ward rounds every morning. Time permitting,we conduct detailed explanations of the related theories, especially the practical experience that goes beyond the medical textbook. When conducting ward rounds, we are mindful to show the students the significant pathology of the patients and review the related knowledge with them. Reviewing differential diagnoses is a good way to practice clinical thinking. We should ask the students' opinions first and then correct their mistakes.
d. If the students come up with questions, especially contradictory questions, we can guide the students to search for the answer from reference books, data in the internet, or the experience of a teacher. And later we may have a meeting with the students to discuss the crux of the issue at hand.

2. How to get more "physical contact" with the resident's work?
The medical students are eager to receive hands-on experience the resident's work during their internship. However, in some cases, they are not fortunate enough to involve themselves in the resident's life. Some residents hold the idea that teaching interns is a waste of time. They are prone not to assign work to the intern because they may have to do it a second time if the intern fails to accomplish it well.
Our strategy

a. Build friendship and trust with the students.
b. Prolong the internship time so that they have enough time to adapt to the situation.
c. Evaluate the capability of the student first. If they are capable enough to perform some of the resident's duty, allow them to have a try under supervision.

3. How to practice basic clinical skills?
Our strategy

a. Encourage the students to perform clinical skills, such as bone marrow puncture, lumbar puncture, and so on. Of course, they should be carefully supervised and their mistakes quickly corrected. Also provide them more chances.
b. Before they conduct the skills, ask them to learn the guidelines and watch the videos. Additionally, ask them to observe our practice when we are performing the skills for the patients. Field teaching is indeed important.

4. How to communicate with patients and their relatives? How to answer the questions from patients and their relatives?
   Our strategy
   a. Love the patients. Thank them for providing the chances for the students to learn during the internship. Our attitude towards the patients will greatly influence our students' attitude.
   b. When talking with the patients or their relatives, bring the students along to listen to the conversation. Be aware of the risk factors for possible medical disputes and tell them to the students. Sum up communication skills to instruct them.
5. How to deal with the unconventional work assigned by the residents and maximize efficiency?
   Many final-year medical students complain about the lack of time the ward doctors have available for supervision and even about being exploited for non-medical activities (activities that could be delegated to nurses or non-medical staff) in order to help doctors cope with an increasing workload in patient care [4].
   Our strategy
   a. Do not ask the students just to do the odd jobs and never teach them clinical knowledge. They come to the hospital for learning, not only to do odd jobs that can be delegated to nurses or non-medical staff. We can teach them how to obtain knowledge from the odd jobs.
   b. Faced with many non-medical activities, the students can discuss and share them with the staff together.

365.2.5 The Outcome

All the students were followed up on their short-period internship performance and their subsequent career achievements in order to evaluate the effects of the Problem-based teaching "4 steps method". All the students received a novel and deep experience in thinking and practicing, which helped them transition from being a medical student to becoming a medical doctor. Most of the 35 students received job offers from our hospital, which is one of the best hospitals according to the Ministry of Public Health.

365.3 Discussion

Learning by rote memorization has been widely accepted and practiced for hundreds of years in China, fueled by the exam-oriented mindset that has historically flourished in China [5]. In light of that, medical internship, as a practical and hands-on educational process, is an indispensable part of the development of future doctors. Medical education reform is taking place in China now. In China, medical education reform lags behind its economic reform in depth and in scope. To cope with increasing societal needs, the innovation of medical education in China has become an urgent and important issue [6, 7]. Our institution has already been devoted to the reforming of the medical internship for a long time.

How can we help the medical students assume more responsibility as they transition to becoming full medical doctors? It is a big problem for the interns. Other longstanding problems in the medical internship include: ① reduced communication between the teachers and students; ② brief evaluations of the internship by the students themselves.

The "4 steps methods" not only prompts the students to think over their internship by themselves, but also provides the teachers a simple but effective way to reform their teaching methods. Thus, it is a mutually beneficial strategy for conducting medical education. We examined 35 medical students' reflective thinking using a structured activity called the "4-steps method". All the students received a novel and deep experience in thinking and practicing, which helped them transition from being a medical student to a medical doctor. This may be particularly beneficial in the clinical learning environment, where many aspects of the professional role are learned through experience. It appears that it fulfills several functions, including helping to make meaning of complex situations and enabling learning from experience [2].

365.4 Summary

Judging from the students' short period performance and their subsequent career achievements, the "4 steps methods" approach, a kind of reflective practice as well as a problem based teaching strategy, is indeed an effective strategy in reforming the internship education.

Acknowledgments Many thanks to the surveyed students and all the staff in the Department of Hematology, the 1st Affiliated Hospital, School of Medicine, Xi'an Jiaotong University.

Funding/Support:

2011 Shaanxi ordinary undergraduate universities teaching reform research project named "Construction and application of eight-year problem-based learning (PBL) integrated course's teaching mode and evaluation system for clinical medical specialty in Xi'an Jiaotong University"

Other disclosures:

None

Ethical approval:

The methods of this project have been performed with the approval of The Medical Ethics Committee of The First Affiliated Hospital of Xi'an Jiaotong University School of Medicine and the written informed consent for participation in the study were obtained from participants. The more detail can be check in the attachment.

Previous presentations:

None

References

1. Delva MD, Kirby J, Schultz K, Godwin M (2004) Assessing the relationship of learning approaches to workplace climate in clerkship and residency. Acad Med 79(11):1120–1126
2. Mann K, Gordon J, MacLeod A (2009) Reflection and reflective practice in health professions education: a systematic review. Adv Health Sci Educ Theory Pract 14(4):595–621
3. Leung D, Kember D (2003) The relationship between approaches to learning and reflection upon practice. Educ Psychol 23:61–71
4. Ramani S, Leinster S (2008) AMEE Guide no. 34: teaching in the clinical environment. Med Teach 30(4):347–364
5. Lam TP, Wan XH, Ip MS (2006) Current perspectives on medical education in China. Med Educ 40(10):940–949
6. Howley LD, Wilson WG (2004) Direct observation of students during clerkship rotations a multiyear descriptive study. Acad Med 79(3):276–280
7. Remmen R, Derese A, Scherpbier A, Denekens J, Hermann I, van der Vleuten C, Van Royen P, Bossaert L(1999).Can medical schools rely on clerkships to train students in basic clinical skills. Med Educ 33(8):600–605

Chapter 366
Applications of Pitch Pattern in Chinese Tone Learning System

Song Liu and Peng Liu

Abstract Mandarin Chinese is a tonal language and it is a big barrier for foreign learners in the understanding of the features of the tones when studying Chinese. In order to give them a more direct understanding of the Chinese tones, this paper presents a visualized pitch pattern of the tones and gives effective guidance derived from the analysis of tone discrimination error corpus. The system is mainly designed for elementary level students. Precise acoustic data of the Chinese tones have been utilized for designing the system. Characteristics of the errors found in the examination have been analyzed, and these characteristics have been carefully considered while constructing the system.

Keywords Pitch pattern · Tone discrimination · Speech analysis · Learning system · Learner corpus

366.1 Introduction

Mandarin Chinese is a tonal language and it is a big barrier for foreign learners in the understanding of the features of the tones when studying Chinese. Tonal language has been defined as a kind of language that even the same phonemes consisted in one syllable; the dictionary meaning will be different because of the existing of high/low pitch, or relative rise/fall of pitch in this syllable [1]. Chinese is tone language but not the only one. Some languages of Southeast Asia such as Vietnamese language, Burmese, Thai; Parts of Africa such as Western Ethiopia, Southern Sahara; and those of Latin American Indians are also tone languages. Because Japanese is not tone language, when Japanese students study Chinese

S. Liu (✉) · P. Liu
School of Electrical and Electronic Engineering, North China Electric Power University, No.2 Beinong Road, Beijing 102206, China
e-mail: liusongjp@gmail.com

S. Li et al. (eds.), *Frontier and Future Development of Information Technology in Medicine and Education*, Lecture Notes in Electrical Engineering 269,
DOI: 10.1007/978-94-007-7618-0_366, © Springer Science+Business Media Dordrecht 2014

language, especially in the early stage, it is very difficult to discriminate the difference among tones. The purpose of this study is to design and construct a learning system for discriminating Chinese four tones and provided through the Internet to Japanese college students in beginner's course of Chinese language. In this paper, the issues about applications of pitch pattern considered in system construction are described.

366.2 Standard Pitch Pattern of Chinese Tones

The visualization characteristic of acoustic analysis has recently spread into general education of foreign language [2]. In Chinese language education, the visual presentation using voice pitch pattern has also been tried [3, 4]. However, in the education and training of discriminating tones, there is still no effective tool using voice pitch pattern designed based on the analysis of learners' characteristics. In this system, visualized pitch pattern of tones plays very important role, and should be expressed as easy as possible to learners. For this purpose, from the precise acoustic analysis results, standard pitch pattern images of mono-syllabic word and bi-syllabic word have been derived and based on these standard visualized pitch patterns, guidance manual for tones discrimination has also been made.

Standard pitch pattern of mono-syllabic Chinese word is shown in the figure below. Solid straight line is the fundamental part and dotted curve line is part of accompanying change. Six diatonic (whole tone) has been used in the notation [5–7]. The change in fundamental part of pitch pattern shows the features of each kind of tone. Tone-1 is flat pattern in mid-high level. Tone-2 is rising pattern from mid-low to mid-high. Tone-3 is long pattern with low flat beginning and rising end. Tone-4 is short falling pattern from high to low (Fig. 366.1).

Japanese also has the feature of pitch accent. It also uses phonemic tone, but only one or two syllables in a word can be phonemically marked for tone, and many words are not marked for tone at all. Because of the difference between Japanese and Chinese, in the elementary stage of studying, Japanese learners will

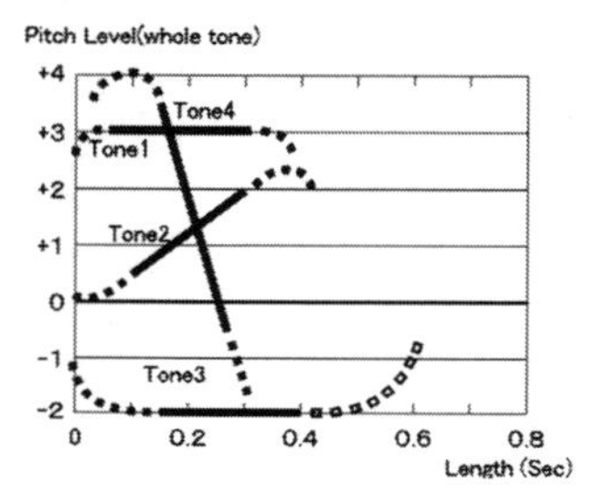

Fig. 366.1 Standard pitch pattern of Chinese mono-syllabic word

encounter many difficulties in discriminating of Chinese tones. In this background, this CAI system has been designed for Japanese students for self-teaching of discriminating Chinese four tones outside classroom.

366.3 Construction of Pitch Pattern

Through the display of visualized pitch pattern, the utilization of visual images to reinforce the auditory discrimination is a significant feature of this system. Therefore, the accuracy in constructing of visualized pitch pattern is very important. This process consists of the following steps.

(1) To Get Pitch Contour with WaveSurfer

In order to get visualized pitch pattern of each word, free software named WaveSurfer have been used [8], which is an open source tool for sound processing and visualization. As the figure below shows, the panels from top to bottom are respectively waveform, spectrogram, pitch contour and time axis. By setting up parameters of pitch tracking algorithm according to speaker's sound characteristics, the pitch contour will be analyzed and constructed (Fig. 366.2).

(2) To Get Data of Pitch Contour

With WaveSurfer, the fundamental frequency (F0) of pitch contour can be saved as a group of data in text file. Each point of data represents frequency (Hz) of sound in a moment, where the time difference between adjacent two points is to 10 ms of time units.

(3) To Process Raw Data

Because people's hearing sense to sound is proportional to the logarithm of fundamental frequency, macro program in excel has been written to calculate the logarithm of F0.

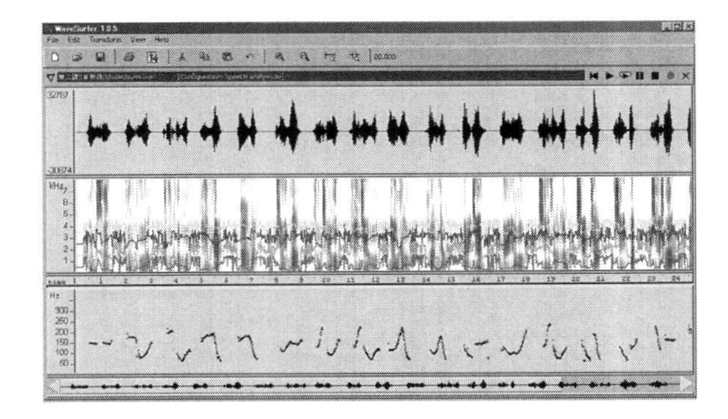

Fig. 366.2 Construction of pitch pattern with WaveSurfer

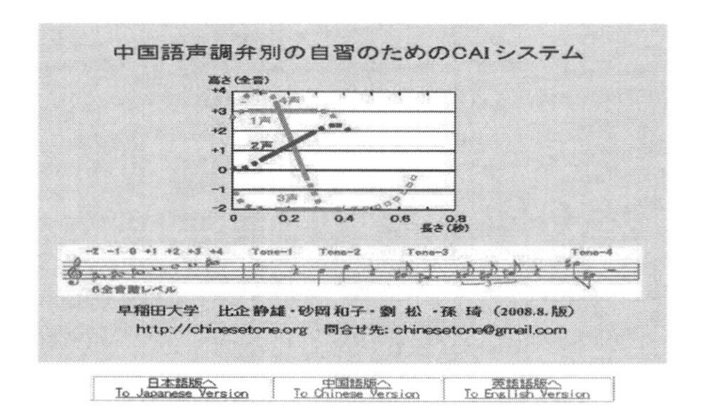

Fig. 366.3 Login interface of system

366.4 Implementation of System

This system has been carried out through Internet [9, 10], so learners can make use of system to practice their discrimination ability in anytime and anywhere. In order to record learners' studying history, it is necessary for users to input their ID when login the system (Fig. 366.3).

There are two kinds of course carried out in the system: standard course and intensive course. The main difference between two courses is that, in standard course, the sequence of presented word tables is step by step based on level of difficulty. While in intensive course, the sequence of presented word tables is according to the students' learning result and appropriate word table will be presented to them based on their practice result. Therefore, it will not waste learners' time to practice tables too easy or too difficult for them. Of course, even in intensive course, learners can also choose word table they want to practice freely, apart from the intensive sequence (Fig. 366.4).

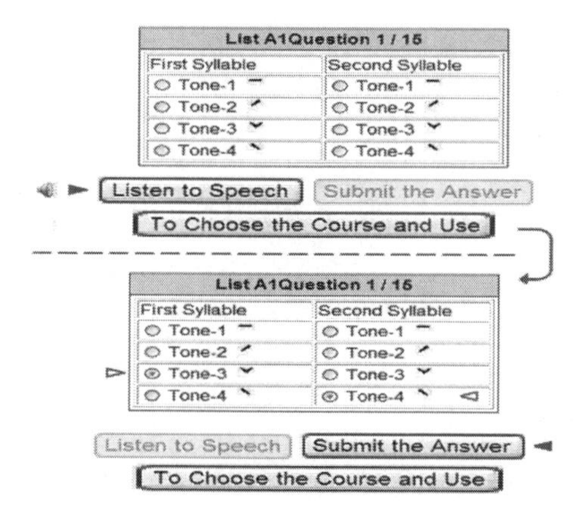

Fig. 366.4 Interface of practice

366.5 Conclusion

Tone is a great difficulty for Japanese students to study Chinese. How to guide students to master the discriminating skill of tones is one of key points of Chinese language education. In this research, we have constructed a learning system discriminating Chinese four tones. Precise acoustical data of Chinese tones have been utilized for designing the system. This system provides students more direct perception of Chinese tones through presenting images of different tones' pitch patterns and gives an effective guidance for tone discrimination. There still remain many topics for further research. For example, the selection of a word corpus is mainly based on teachers' experience. In order to further leverage this system, it is necessary to automate the word corpus selection process. Rules that predict the difficulty of discriminating Chinese words have already been examined [11]. In the next step, our objective is to make use of these rules to achieve the function of automatically selecting appropriate words for students.

Acknowledgments This work is supported by "the Fundamental Research Funds for the Central Universities". We greatly appreciate the aid of Professor Shizuo Hiki, Mrs. Qi Sun, Professor Kazuko Sunaoka and Professor Yoshiyori Urano.

References

1. Chuang CK, Hiki S, Sone T, Nimura T (1975) Acoustical features of the four tones in monosyllabic utterances of standard chinese. Acoust Soc Jpn 31(6):369–380
2. Sakamoto T (2003) Studies on the use of advanced multi-media contribute to the reform of higher education. Research report for scientific research grant in aid for scientific research on priority area
3. Takagi T, Hattori A, Momiya M, Imai A, Kishi K, Ito T (2005) A Chinese language learning system with visualization and speech correction for prosody. IEICE Trans 88-D1:478–487
4. Anhui USTC iFLYTEC. http://www.iflytek.com/Html/cpfw/newyuyin/kypc/pthmn. Accessed on 15 April 2012
5. Hiki S, Sunaoka K, Yang LM, Tokuhiro Y (2004) Occurrence frequency and transition probability of the Chinese tones. Proceedings of international symposium on tonal aspects of languages: emphasis on tone languages, Beijing, pp 73–76, March 2004
6. Hiki S, Imaizumi K, Sunaoka K (2005) A CAI system for self-teaching Chinese tones based on their acoustical properties. IEICE technical report, SP, 105(198):37–42
7. Kakita Y, Hiki S (1976) Investigation of laryngeal control in speech by use of thyrometer. J Acoust Soc Am 59(3):669–674
8. http://www.speech.kth.se/wavesurfer. Accessed on 15 April 2012
9. A computer-assisted instruction system for self-teaching of discriminating Chinese four tones. http://chinesetone.org. Accessed on 15 April 2012
10. Liu S, Urano Y, Hiki S (2010) A computer-assisted instruction system for self-teaching of discriminating Chinese four tones. Educ Technol Res, Jpn Soc Educ Technol 34(3):223–233
11. Liu S, Hiki S (2009) Predicting rules of difficulty in discriminating bi-syllabic Chinese tones for compiling word lists in a CAI self-teaching system. IEICE technical report, ET, 109(268):57–62

Chapter 367
Detection of Onset and Offset of QRS Complex Based a Modified Triangle Morphology

Xiao Hu, Jingjing Liu, Jiaqing Wang and Zhong Xiao

Abstract It was important to detect onset and offset of QRS complex from ECG signal in order to accurately and effectively obtain some clinic parameters about ECG signal. Based on a conventional triangle morphology method, this paper introduced a modified triangle morphology algorithm (MTM). In the algorithm, a triangle shape was firstly built from the ECG signal processed by local normalization, and then the vertex angle of the formed triangle shape was calculated for each sample point. At last, the sample points, whose angles satisfied with some preset conditions, were regarded as onset or offset of QRS complex. Seven 12-lead ECG records obtained from the public standard database MIT-BIH twadb were employed to evaluate the proposed method. The results showed that MTM method could accurately detect onset and offset of QRS complex even though ECG signal was contaminated by baseline wander (BW), and these onset and offset of QRS complex identified by the proposed method were more reasonable than those by other methods.

Keywords ECG signal · QRS complex · Morphology · Characteristic point

367.1 Introduction

ECG signal, which was suggested by Einthoven, was an oldest and most commonly used cardiology method [1]. Among all feature segments (e.g. ST and PR), intervals (e.g. RR) or waves (e.g. T wave) of ECG signal, QRS complex might be the most significant and important, because QRS complex could not only provides rich clinic information, but also was a reference point through which one measured

X. Hu (✉) · J. Liu · J. Wang · Z. Xiao
Department of Electronic Information Engineering, School of Mechanical and Electrical Engineering, Guangzhou University, Guangzhou 510006, China
e-mail: huxiao@gzhu.edu.cn

S. Li et al. (eds.), *Frontier and Future Development of Information Technology in Medicine and Education*, Lecture Notes in Electrical Engineering 269,
DOI: 10.1007/978-94-007-7618-0_367,

or detected other physical features. So it was important to detect QRS complex from ECG signal. On the other hand, onset (marked as $\boldsymbol{\mu}$ in this paper) and the offset (marked as $\boldsymbol{J}$) of QRS complex common need be detected before one measured accurately other characteristic waves, segments and intervals [2]. For example, $\boldsymbol{\mu}$ point and $\boldsymbol{J}$ point was respectively one end of PR segment and ST segment. However, so far $\boldsymbol{\mu}$ and $\boldsymbol{J}$ used by most investigators have depended on visual assessment given by specialist observers. Recently, computer-based algorithms for ECG signal have been a significant research topic more than ever. For these above reasons, it became more important and necessary to automatically detect $\boldsymbol{\mu}$ point and $\boldsymbol{J}$ point than ever.

So far many algorithms have been proposed to locate QRS complex. Due to their sharper slope information than other waves, QRS complexes were usually detected by differentiation methods such as PT algorithm [2] and first-order derivatives [3]. Because of the impulse-like morphology of QRS complex, template matching method [4] was used to identify QRS complex as well. In the last decade, QRS complex were recognized by searching for simultaneous modulus maxima in the relevant scales of the wavelet coefficients [5]. In addition, empirical mode decomposition [6] and phasor transform [7] were proposed to detect QRS complex. However, most detection algorithms of QRS complex were common designed to locate QRS complex's position other than exact positions of R peak, Q peak and S peak. As a result, the calculated RR interval calculated from QRS complex's positions was not the exact RR interval measured by cardiovascular specialists. It was therefore important and necessary to exploit a new algorithm to locate the exact position of R peak and $\boldsymbol{\mu}$ and $\boldsymbol{J}$ points. In Daskalov and Christov's (DC) algorithm [8], PR segment and ST segment were firstly searched, and then $\boldsymbol{\mu}$ and $\boldsymbol{J}$ points were respectively decided from these segments. However, if PR/ST segment changed or were not isoelectric, they would not be found accurately according to DC algorithm. If firstly to detect $\boldsymbol{\mu}/\boldsymbol{J}$ point and then to look for PR/ST segment, the algorithm would perform better. For this reason, it was also important and necessary to explore an algorithm independent of PR/ST segment to locate $\boldsymbol{\mu}/\boldsymbol{J}$ point. Recently, an algorithm based on triangle was proposed to detect $\boldsymbol{\mu}$ and $\boldsymbol{J}$ points [9]. In the triangle method, three samples $ecg(\mathrm{n}-2)$, $ecg(\mathrm{n})$ and $ecg(\mathrm{n}+2)$ were used to form a triangle shape ABC. The vertex angle of vertex A and the vertical distance between the vertex A and the base BC were used as the features to recognize QRS complex and its onset and offset. Although this algorithm could detect QRS complex, $\boldsymbol{\mu}$ and $\boldsymbol{J}$ points, the algorithm need two features: angle and height. The later feature measuring the amplitude of peak, which was applied to distinguish peaks from noise, was easy interrupted by noise.

Hence, in this paper a modified triangle method without height feature was introduced to detect QRS complex's characteristic points.

367.2 Modified Triangle Morphology Method

The modified triangle morphology included three steps: local normalization, formation of triangle shape and calculation of the vertex angle.

367.2.1 Local Normalization

Obviously, θ at Δ ABC at Fig. 367.1 was related with amplitude of sample point and sampling cycle by which ECG signal was acquired. During ECG signal was recorded, ECG-acquired machine's gain might change because of the change of environmental temperature and contact resistance of electrode. The phenomenon inevitably leads to the fluctuation of signal's amplitude. It was possible that the angle values of characteristic points belonging to the same class distribute too dispersedly to be distinguished with other points. Hence, in this proposed method local normalization was applied to adjust the same class of peaks with different amplitudes into peaks with similar equal amplitude, so that the angles of peaks belonging to the same category became equal or similar equal.

For each ECG sample ecg(n), a moving window consisted of 2m + 1 sample points [ecg(n − m),..., ecg(n − 1), ecg(n), ecg(n + 1),..., ecg(n + m)], every ecg(k) was normalized as

$$x(k) = \frac{ecg(k)}{Max} \%\% \quad \%\%\% \quad \%\%\% \quad k = n - m, \ldots, n - 1, n, n + 1, \ldots, n + m\%\% \tag{367.1}$$

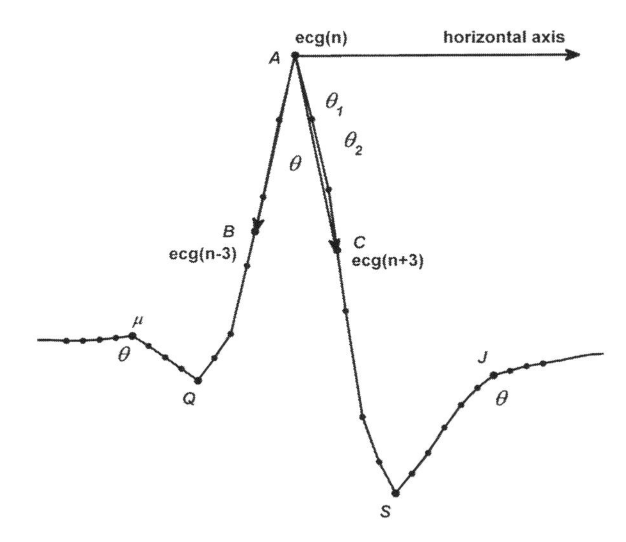

Fig. 367.1 Construction of triangle shape

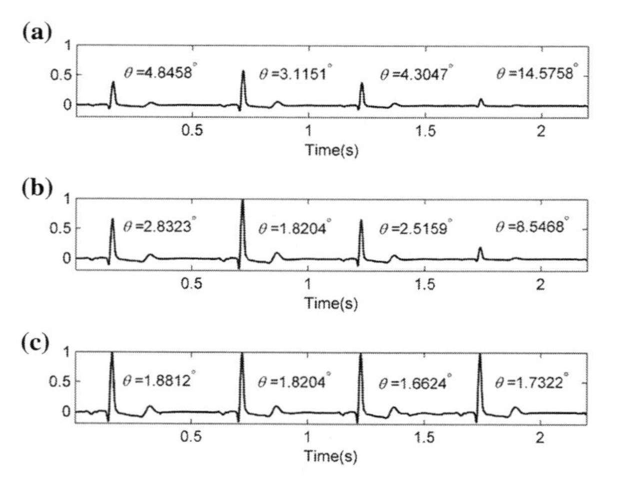

Fig. 367.2 Normalization's Results. **a** Raw ECG signal; **b** ECG signal after overall normalization; **c** ECG after local normalization. Θ were angle of R peaks at corresponding positions

Here, *Max* is the maximum of absolute value of the ECG signal series within the moving window. 2m + 1 should last for about one cardiac cycle.

Figure 367.2 illustrated the different results between overall normalization and local normalization. There were four QRS complexes with unequal amplitude on the original signal with sampling frequency $f_s = 500$ Hz in Fig. 367.2. From left to right, amplitude of the second QRS complex was the highest and that of the fourth QRS complex was the lowest. Although the ECG signal in Fig. 367.2b had been globally normalized, the four QRS complexes still kept the same size ratio as QRS complexes of raw ECG signal on Fig. 367.2a. These angles θ in Fig. 367.2 were of R peaks at corresponding positions. Though angles of R peaks on ECG signal after globally normalized were changed, their zoom ratio was near equal (2.8323/4.8458 $\approx$ 1.8204/3.1151 $\approx$ 8.5468/14.5758). Obviously R peak with the highest amplitude held the smallest angle and the R peak with lowest amplitude held the biggest angle. Fortunately after local normalization was applied to ECG signal, four R peaks' amplitude became one. The angle of the R peak with the highest amplitude in Fig. 367.2a decreased in the smallest ratio (3.1151/1.8204 $\approx$ 1.72), and the angle of R peak with the lowest amplitude in Fig. 367.2a did in the biggest ratio (14.5758/1.732 $\approx$ 8.42). Figure 367.2c distinctly showed that four R peaks' angles were almost equal after ECG signal was locally normalized. Obviously the clustering of θ favored the recognition of characteristic points.

367.2.2 Formation of Triangle Shape

In previous triangle morphology algorithm [9], three vertex of $\triangle ABC$ were $ecg(\mathrm{n}-2)$, $ecg(\mathrm{n})$ and $ecg(\mathrm{n}+2)$. The side *AB* or *AC* spanned only three samples and lasted for two sample points. The height, the distance from vertex *A* to the opposite side BC, might usually be smaller than noise's amplitude. On the other hand, the span of side AB or AC should not beyond the span covered by one peak's slope. Among these ECG signal used in this paper, there were a part of small peaks (such as r, q and s) whose slope covered only about 10 sample points and even fewer. After some experiments about the span, four sample points (lasted for three sample cycles) were more appropriate than other number. So in the modified triangle morphology, for every $ecg(\mathrm{n})$, three samples $ecg(\mathrm{n}-3)$, $ecg(\mathrm{n})$ and $ecg(\mathrm{n}+3)$ were chosen to construct $\triangle ABC$.

367.2.3 Calculation of the Vertex Angle

From Fig. 367.1, the interior angle corresponding to the vertex A of $\triangle ABC$ was the difference of the primary phases of vectors $\overrightarrow{AB}$ and $\overrightarrow{AC}$. Thus, θ could be calculated by

$$\theta = |\theta_1 - \theta_2| \tag{367.2}$$

Here, θ_1 and θ_2 were the primary phases of vectors $\overrightarrow{AB}$ and $\overrightarrow{AC}$ respectively.

For different class of characteristic points, their morphology was different. R peak, S peak and Q peak appeared one kind of morphology while $\boldsymbol{\mu}$, $\boldsymbol{J}$ and T wave did more than one. Their angles (θ, θ_1 and θ_2) were consequently not uniform in polarity and magnitude. Table 367.1 listed the polarity about these angles of different peaks, $\boldsymbol{\mu}$, $\boldsymbol{J}$ or T wave.

367.3 Detection Tactic

Commonly, R peak was firstly detected, and then served as a reference to detect other characteristic points if they exist.

367.3.1 To Detect R Peak

The detection of R peak was the first step to recognize other characteristic points of ECG signal. Table 367.1 showed that all R peaks and some T peaks were rounded up and other fiducial points were rounded down. Both θ_1 and θ_2 of the rounded up peak were negative and below -90 and above -90 respectively. On the contrary, both θ_1 and θ_2 of the rounded down peak were positive and more than 90 and less than 90 respectively. Thus, all R peaks and some T waves could easily be distinguished from other characteristic points according to the polarity of θ_1 and θ_2. However, another difficulty to recognize R peak from ECG signal was how to

Table 367.1 Comparison of angles about different characteristic points

	Morphology	θ_1	θ_2	θ
μ point		$90 < \theta_1 \leq 180$	$-90 < \theta_2 < 0$	Bigger
		$-180 < \theta_1 < -90$	$-90 < \theta_2 < 0$	Bigger
		$\theta_1 \approx 180$	$0 < \theta_2 < 90$	Bigger
Q peak		$90 < \theta_1 < 180$	$0 < \theta_2 < 90$	Smaller
R peak		$-180 < \theta_1 < 90$	$-90 < \theta_2 < 0$	Smaller
S peak		$90 < \theta_1 < 180$	$0 < \theta_2 < 90$	Smaller
J point		$-180 < \theta_1 < -90$	$0 \leq \theta_2 < 90$	Bigger
		$-180 < \theta_1 < -90$	$-90 < \theta_2 < 0$	Bigger
		$90 < \theta_1 < 180$	≈ 0	Bigger
T peak		$-180 < \theta_1 < 90$	$-90 < \theta_2 < 0$	Bigger
		$90 < \theta_1 < 180$	$0 < \theta_2 < 90$	Bigger

distinguish R peaks from T waves and P waves. Because both slopes of R peak were sharper than these slopes of T wave and P wave, θ of R peak was smaller than that of T wave and P wave. Hence R peaks could be selected from P waves and T waves by θ with rounding up peak.

Both Q peak and S peak were rounded down. If R peak, Q peak and S peak existed within one QRS complex, Q peak and S peak stand before and behind R peak respectively. So in the proposed method, Q peak was researched within a seek window preceding R peak, and S peak was researched within another seek window following R peak. These samples, whose θ_1 were between 90 and 180° and whose θ_2 were between 0 and 90°, were taken as candidates of Q peak or S peak. Then from Q peak candidates, the sample with minimal θ was taken as Q peak, and from S peak candidates, the sample with minimal θ was taken as S peak.

367.3.2 To Detect μ Point and *J* Point

In this paper, μ point was researched from a seek window before Q peak or R peak without Q peak, and *J* point was researched from another seek window after S peak or R peak without S peak. If there was Q peak in one QRS complex, these samples with $\theta_1 \approx 180^o$ and $0 < \theta_2 < 90^o$ were classified as candidates of $\boldsymbol{\mu}$ point. The candidate with minimal θ was regarded as $\boldsymbol{\mu}$ point. If there was not Q peak in one QRS complex, these samples with $-90^o < \theta_2 < 0$ and $90 < \theta_1 \leq 180$ or $-180 < \theta_1 < -90$ were candidates of $\boldsymbol{\mu}$ point, then the candidate with minimal θ was regarded as $\boldsymbol{\mu}$ point. If there was S peak in one QRS complex, these samples with $90 < \theta_1 < 180$ and $\theta_2 \approx 0^\circ$ were classified as candidates of $\boldsymbol{J}$ point. The candidate with minimal θ was thought as J point. If there was not Q peak in one QRS complex, these samples with $-180 < \theta_1 < -90$ and $0 \leq \theta_2 < 90$ or $-90 < \theta_2 < 0$ were candidates of $\boldsymbol{J}$ point, then the candidate with minimal θ was thought as $\boldsymbol{J}$ point.

367.4 Experiments and Results

In this paper, the public standard database MIT-BIH twadb [10] was used to test the proposed method. The database contained 100 multichannel ECG records sampled at sampling frequency 500 Hz with 16 bit resolution over a ±32 mV range. From the ECG database, seven records with 12 lead-ECG signal were chosen to evaluate the performance of the proposed method.

367.4.1 Result of μ and J point

Figure 367.3 displayed one example of onsets and offset of QRS complexes detected by four methods. A cardiologist's annotations were marked with a vertical slash. If the difference between the position by the cardiologist and the position by one algorithm was below five samples (0.001 s), the located position was thought to be right. Hence, all onsets and offsets had been accurately detected by MTM. While some of these $\boldsymbol{\mu}$ and J estimated by the other three algorithms were far away the cardiologist's annotations.

367.4.2 Robust on Baseline Wander

Figure 367.4 depicted robust to BW with low frequency. TM algorithm did not detect $\boldsymbol{J}$ point on the third QRS complex of ECG signal with BW, and DC algorithm only detected $\boldsymbol{\mu}$ and J on the second QRS complex of ECG signal with BW because of the change of PR segment and ST segment. Both MTM algorithm and PT algorithm estimated all $\boldsymbol{\mu}$ and J points on ECG signal with BW, and their estimated positions remained unchanged as on original ECG signal without BW.

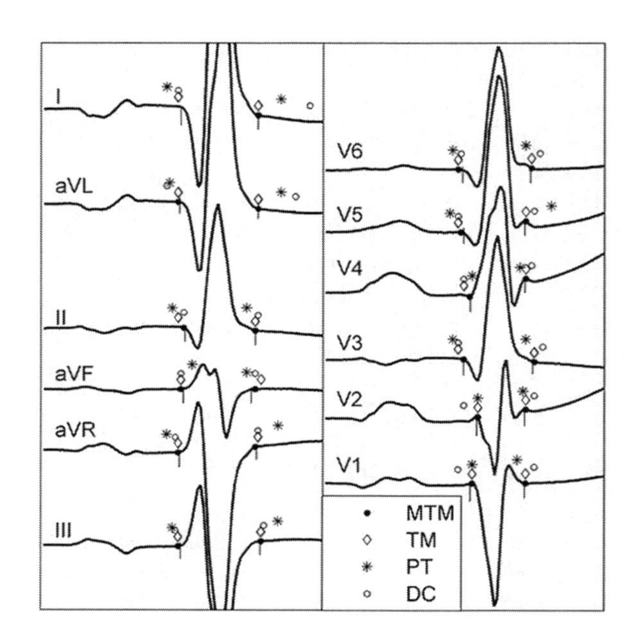

Fig. 367.3 One example of onsets and offset of QRS complexes detected by the four methods: MTM (*filled dots marked*), MT algorithm (*rhombus* '◇' *marked*), PT algorithm (*star* '*' *marked*), and DC algorithm (*hollow dots marked*). These vertical slashes were cardiologist's annotations. The ECG signals on the figure were from 12-lead ECG signals of twa21. Because of overlapping, these curves were shifted vertically

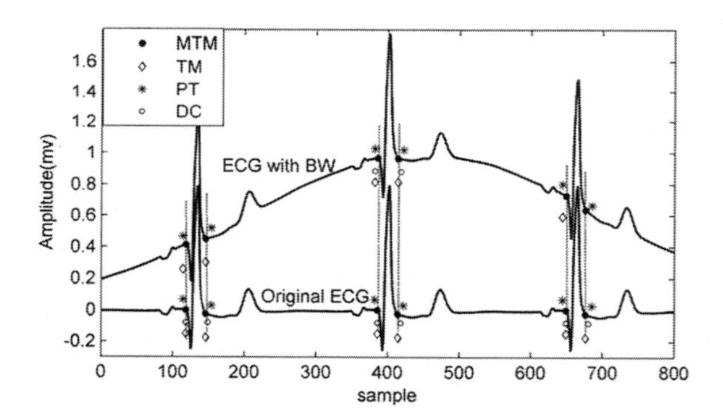

Fig. 367.4 Boundaries detection immunity to baseline shift. MTM (*filled dots marked*), MT algorithm (*rhombus* '◇' *marked*), PT algorithm (*star* '*' *marked*), and DC algorithm (*hollow dots marked*)

367.5 Conclusion

Characteristic points could be accurately detected by the modified triangle morphology algorithm even though the ECG signal was interrupted by baseline wander. Furthermore during detecting R peak, onset and offset of QRS complex, the proposed method achieved to 100 % accurate detection rate. Compared with traditional methods, the modified triangle morphology could achieve more reasonable onset and offset of QRS complex. Therefore, the detection algorithm based on the modified triangle shape was an effective and reliable means to detect characteristic point from ECG signal.

Acknowledgments This work was supported the National Natural Science Foundation of China (No. 61100150 and No.51207027).

References

1. Hu X, Xiao Z, Zhang N (2011) Removal of baseline wander from ECG signal based on a statistical weighted moving average filter. J Zhejiang Univ Sci C (Comput Electron) 12(5):397–403
2. Jiapu P, Willis JT (1985) A real-time QRS detection algorithm. IEEE Trans Biomed Eng 32(3):230–236
3. Arzeno NM, Deng ZD, Poon CS (2008) Analysis of first-derivative based QRS detection algorithms. IEEE Trans Biomed Eng 55:478–484
4. Suarez KV, Silva JC, Berthoumieu Y, Gomis P, Najim M (2007) ECG beat detection using a geometrical matching approach. IEEE Trans Biomed Eng 54(4):641–650
5. Ghaffari A, Golbayani H, Ghasemi M (2008) A new mathematical based QRS detector using continuous wavelet transform. Comput Electr Eng 34:81–91
6. Hadj Slimane Z-E, Naït Ali A (2010) QRS complex detection using empirical mode decomposition. Dig Sig Proc 20:1221–1228
7. Martínez A, Alcaraz R, Rieta JJ (2011) Application of the phasor transform for automatic delineation of single-lead ECG characteristics points. Physiol Meas 31:1467–1485
8. Daskalov IK, Christov II (1999) Electrocardiogram signal preprocessing for automatic detection of QRS boundaries. Med Eng Phys 22:37–44
9. Hu X, Wang JQ, Zhang N (2011) Detecting onset and offset of QRS complex based on measurement of a triangle. J Appl Sci 29(3):289–293
10. PhysioNet Resource. National Institutes of Health. http://physionet.org/pn3/twadb/

Chapter 368
Ecological Characters of Truffles

Hai-feng Wang, Yan-ling Zhao and Yong-jun Fan

Abstract We undertook an overview of the physical and chemical quality of soil characteristics, features of morphology, distribution and mycorrhizal relationships of Tuberaceae in China. The topsoil is found to be limestone region, abundant organic matter and the soil type is determined to be sand-clay-slimy. Various characteristics are recorded including ascocarp features (hypogenous, like tubers) and color (peridium, glebe red tones, brown), time of appearance (October to April), host (*Pinus, Rhododendron polifolium, Eragrostis piosa*), habitat (basic soil, sand-clay-slimy, and semi-arid zone), fresh weight (8–150 g) and ascospore morphology (3–5warty spherics, medium size). The relationship between truffle growth and weather, soil, vegetation are particularly elaborated. A general overview of the characteristic of many ecosystem factors of region is described, especially where truffles grow. In conclusion, the habitats of tuberaceae should be protected by turning those fields into natural protected areas.

Keywords Truffles · Ecological · Review · Characters

368.1 Introduction

Truffles are true tuber if it belongs to the section of Ascomycotina, and it is a type of ectomycorrhizal fungus of symbiosis relation with trees such as Pinaceae and Fagaceae etc. [22, 27]. Ascocarp living underground can be eaten so be called

---

H. Wang
Department of Biology Engineering, Baotou Light Industry
Vocational Technical College, Baotou, China

Y. Zhao · Y. Fan (✉)
Department of Biology Science and Technology,
Baotou Teacher's College, Baotou, China
e-mail: fanyj1975@163.com

S. Li et al. (eds.), *Frontier and Future Development of Information Technology in Medicine and Education*, Lecture Notes in Electrical Engineering 269,
DOI: 10.1007/978-94-007-7618-0_368,

"Truffle". Some truffles are highly prized as edible fungi [2]. Because of rare product area, scarce yield, vagary scent and expensive delicacy, they are the rarest edible fungi. Meanwhile, truffle mycorrhizal fungi have been recognized as providing "keystone" ecosystem functions, because of their direct access to plant carbon that drives below-ground microbial communities. Truffles as one of mycorrhizas, they assist plants in obtaining water and nutrients, protect plant roots from pathogens, and form below-ground networks that link above-ground plant communities [1, 21, 10, 18]. For the sake of better the development and make use of this rare resources, we carried on initial summary of the physiology ecology characteristic of truffle, be reported as follows:

368.2 Morphological Feature and Emergence Period of Sporocarp

Ascocarp of truffle is subglobose, semi-sphericity, tuber and irregular tuber. Diameter 1.5–12 cm, Fresh weight ranges between 8 and 150 g per ascocarp with the color being brown to dark brown, blackish brown or especially glebe red tones. When dry dust-color. Its surface have different small wart, which are made up of 3–5 pyramids [20, 23]. If carved, there are uncounted rein like marble in ascocarp, when rape from hoar to taupe, vein of truffle are very small and have many branches which arrive epidermis, hypha in vein are distinct with others, they no color, array sparseness [2, 12, 14]. Peridium of ascocarp is more sturdily, so they are not easy to be putrefied. The growth of them experience several months. If the conditions are suitable, we can collect them from midmonth of October to April of second year. If collected earlier, ascocarp is small, few and has bad quality [16]. Ascus is sphericity, semi-sphericity or pyriform, no suspensor, including 1–4 ascospores in each [8, 20]. These data are similar to the data in our work. It is the first time that members of our team find truffles lay in Helan Mountain.

368.3 Ecological Factors

368.3.1 Climatic Factors

Truffles and hosts need light, caloric, water etc. All of them rest on its distribution region. So distribution of them has connected with Climatic factors. Truffles live in southwest, northwest of China, and mainly distribute the broad-leaved wood of the elevation between 1600 and 2400 m and dark coniferous forest of the elevation 2600 m in the mountain [4, 20]. Huidong Country is one of the most outputs of truffles in Sichuan province. It lays low degree of latitude area, elevation 1500–2500 m. Shining ample, the calories abundant, the year average temperature is 16.1 °C, the month average temperature changes small. Cumulative temperature for $\geq$10 °C is up to 5117 °C, sunshine of year counts to 2322.8 h, frost-free season for 279 days, rainfall is plentiful, the dry and damp seasons are obvious, the year average rainfall 1056 mm, rain day of whole year 123 days, appearing from June to October. The mountainous country weather shows perpendicular difference [12, 20] following the altitude rising, air temperature and ground temperature falls. On the contrary, air humidity, rainfall and rain day increase. This environmental is suit to propagate for truffle. Another typical area of truffle growth pigeons is Panzhihua city. Altitude 1100–2600 m, sunshine of year count 1900-2700 h, rainfall of year 700–1700 mm, day average temperature is 3.5–11.4 °C. Many research showed that truffle has different temperature in different stage of growth, for example hyphae can grow under 10–35 °C [9], if over 25 °C, grow rapidly. Rapid growth period is summer, soil temperature is 25–30 °C, truffles will ripe in autumn, so the weather would be nice and cool, and not below 0 °C in winter. Other reports consider that the truffles need water differently in different phase of vegetate. Rainfall of spring influences remarkably on producing and yield. If it is dry or little rain in spring and summer, the ascocarp can not form or grow slowly, so yield and quality would be decrease. It is wet in autumn, but not over, thus will benefit on develop of truffles.

368.3.2 Soil Characteristics

Soil is the base material where truffles lies and its host lived. The growths of truffles were closely related with soil type, structure, fertility, degree of consolidation and pH. Some studies consider that soil that produces truffles generally takes place at the limestone region. It implies not only abundant calcium quality, but also magnesium, phosphorus and other various minerals. Including dinas, weathering rock fragment or thick bone scraps. The colour of soil is various, such as: red, purple, yellow–red, brownish red etc. pH is between subacidity and a tiny alkalescence [7, 5]. Mehmet akyüz [16] pointed the topsoil of the fields are found to be 54.73 % sand, 21.97 % clay, 23.30 % dust, 45.27 % dust-clay, 0.126 % nitrogen, 1.848 % organic matter, 3.78 % total lime, 40.92 ppm P_2O_5, 613.0 ppm K_2O, 28.82 ppm Na, 0.164 mmhos/cm salt, 7.12 pH, and a sand-clay-slimy soil type. Studies [4] indicate that those soils contained mental ion and red limestone soil that are in favour of the development of truffles. The truffles are not suitable to develop in viscosity soil. And study indicate that they like living where are many dry branches and fallen leaves, preferable soil fertility, better aerating, higher contain of organic matter. Wang Yue-hua [28] discovers the growth of truffles includes certain directions orientation. They lived the colder northwest slope avoiding the influence of dry wind from south. On the other hand, the degree of slope would influence the yield and quality of truffles, and it is below 32 degree, because it can hold back the phenomenon of soil run off [7].

368.3.3 Host and Vegetation Factors

The truffle is one of the main symbiosis fungi of ectotrophic mycorrhiza. The fact is that ectomycorrhizal roots gain much more mineral substance with the help of hyphae. Plant roots help ectomycorrhizal fungi to overcome carbohydrate limitation and increase their competitive ability in soil. Both the fungi and the plant can profit from the interaction and absorbe major nutrients (nitrogen, phosphate) fixed in the organic layer [24].

Different truffle formed different mutualistic symbios with advanced plants. The survey from Huidong country indicated that the truffles occurred in the region of mixed coniferous broad leaved forest. The ectomycorrhizal associations are long considered to be rare in the tropics, but much knowledge suggests that all tropical regions support at least five lineages of host plants [15, 25]. It has mycorrhizal associations with the roots of *pinus yunnanensis, Keteleeria evelyniana, pinus armandii*. [16, 29]. Other authers point that thier host are *Quercus, Corylus, Ostrya, Carpinus, Tilid, Populus, Salix, Alnus, Fagus, Castaned, Pinus, Cedrus, Abies, Juglans, Helianthemum* etc. by cultivating [7, 16, 29]. Our team found that the truffles become symbiosis with the root of *Picea crassifolia.* There are about 202 families and 1554 species, the forest fraction of coverage leads to 30.02 % in Huidong country. Research of Panzhihua city showed that the frequentness of producing truffles in theropencedrymion is more than other forest. Vegetation cover degree attains 77 %. The truffle secrete the substance which are harmful to ruderal, so there are little weed in the region of them, weed springs up out of the region.

368.3.4 Wild ANIMAL of the Truffles Region

Fungi are indispensable components of the biota of any region. Their presence and distribution are of paramount importance to flora and fauna, and their ecological function may be responsible for the presence or absence of many other species, particularly animals [19]. The wildlife category of the truffle habitat is a lot. However rodents associate closely with the growth of truffles. The investigation indicated there are 6 families and 34 species in the region of the district where truffles grew in Huidong country. Major in *Petaurista clarkei, Petaurista alborufus, Drmorays pernyipernyi, Callosciurus evythracus, Apodemus sylvaticus, Apodemus chevrieri* [3, 4]. They liked to eat truffles depending on their sharp olfaction, thus spores are spread in anywhere by them [7].

368.4 Appropriate Habitats of Truffles

Truffles are nutritive symbiosis of ectotrophic mycorrhiza fungus. Their development has closely associate with Climatic factors, Soil characteristics, earth slope features, host, vegetation factors and wild animal of producing truffles area etc. [3, 17, 26]. Appropriate the ground temperature and rainfall are two most important climate factors for truffle to develop. The soil is found to be limestone region, abundant organic matter, the soil type is determined to be sand-clay-slimy. The hosts of truffles are *pinus, Quercus fabri, Rhododendron polifolium, eragrostis piosa* et al. Animals became the best medium for truffles multiply in the nature. They can spread spores through eating ascocarp and expelling dejecta.

Although we summarize all of those, some fundamental aspects concerning truffles have not yet to be fully elucidated. All of us will keep trying to protect, exploit and study truffles. As a beginner of studying truffle, the author strongly recommended that the habitats of the species should be protected by turning those fields into natural protected areas.

References

1. Solti A, Tamaskó G, Lenk S et al (2011) Detection of the vitalization effect of tuber mycorrhiza on sessile oak by the recently-innovated FMM chlorophyll fluorometer. Acta Biologica Szegediensis 55(1):147–149
2. Pavić A, Stanković S, Marjanović Ž (2011) Biochemical characterization of a sphingomonad isolate from the ascocarp of white truffle (tuber magnatum pico). Arch Biol Sci 63(3):697–704
3. Cheng H-q, Liu H-y, Li Z (1995) A primary study on ecological property of truffle. Acta Edulis Fungi 5(1):39–44
4. Chen H-q, Liu H-y, Yang Y-m et al (1999) Studied on the ecological and physiology property of truffle. Resour Dev Mark 15(1):11–15
5. Chen J, Deng X-j, Chen J-y et al (2011) A checklist of the genustuber(pezizales, ascomycota) in china. J Fungal Res 9(4):244–254
6. Chen J, Liu P-g (2007)Tuber *latisporumsp.* nov. and related taxa, based on morphology and DNA sequence data. Mycologia 99(3):475–481
7. Chen Y-l (2000) Ecological studies on truffles (tuber spp.). Edible Fungi China 20(5):28–30
8. Hu R-f, Zang C-r, Huang J-c (2003) Research progress in the ecology, physiology and artificial cultivation of truffles. Fujian J Agric Sci 18(2):112–115
9. Nascimento JS, da Eira AF (2007) Isolation and mycelial growth of diehliomyces microsporus: effect of culture medium and incubation temperature. Brazilian Arch Biol Technol 50(4):587–595
10. Kong Q-l, Tai L-m, Liu B, Fan J, Zhao T-r (2012) Research of chemical properties bioactivity and preservation on the genus tuber. Edible Fungi China 31(6):1–4
11. Li J-z (2008) Study on wild edible fungi species diversity from human. Life Sci Res 12(4):314–321
12. Long Y-j, Li R-c (2009) Ecological investigation of Tuber indicum around Dianchi Lake in Kunming of Yunnan Province. J Fujian Agric For Univ (Natural Science Edition). 38(2):192–197

13. Long Y-j, Li R-c (2009) Research on anatomical structure of tuber indicum ascocarps of Kunming, Yunnan Province. Acta Bot Boreal-Occident Sin 29(2):0269–0274
14. Long Y-j, Chen y-p, Li R-c (2011) Anatomical structure of tuber indicum ascocarps with scanning electron microscope. Acta Bot Boreal-Occident Sin 31(11):2222–2225
15. Tedersoo L, Sadam A, Zambrano M et al (2010) Low diversity and high host preference of ectomycorrhizal fungi in Western Amazonia, a neotropical biodiversity hotspot. Int Soc Microb Ecol J 4:465–471
16. Akyüz M, Kirbağ S, kurşat M (2012) Ecological aspects of the arid and semi-arid truffle in Turkey: evaluation of soil characteristics, morphology, distribution, and mycorrhizal relationships. Turk J Bot 36:386–391
17. Outerbridge RA, Trofymow JA (2009) Forest management and maintenance of ectomycorrhizae: a case study of green tree retention in south-coastal British Columbia. BC J Ecosyst Manag 10(2):59–80
18. Shi Z-y, Zhang X-f, Wang F-y (2010) Ecology and environmental sciences influence of mycorrhizal fungi on soil respiration. Ecol Environ Sci 19(1):233–238
19. Helfer S (2008) Mycota of south-west Asia. Turk J Bot 32:481–484
20. Tang P, Lan H, Lei C-h et al (2005) A study of truffle resources and optimal niches in panzhihua region. J Sichuan For Sci Technol 26(2):71–75
21. McLenon-Porter TM (2008) Above and below ground fungal diversity in a hemlock-dominated forest plot in southern ontario and the phylogenetic placement of a new ascomycota subphylum. Ecol Evolut Biol Univ Toronto 3–4
22. Tang C, Chen Y-L, Liu R-J (2011) Advances in studies of edible mycorrhizal fungi. Mycosystema 30(3):367–378
23. Lebel T, Castellano MA (2002) Type studies of sequestrate Russulales II. Australian and New Zealand species related to Russula. Mycologia 94(2):327–354
24. Nehls U (2008) Mastering ectomycorrhizal symbiosis: the impact of carbohydrates. J Exp Bot 59(5):1097–1108
25. Kagan-Zur V, Roth-Bejerano N (2008) Unresolved problems in the life cycle of truffles. The Open Mycology J 2:86–88
26. Wang X-e, Yao F-j, Li Y (2005) Research advancement of truffles. Edible Fungi China 24(5):6–9
27. Wang Y, Liu P-g (2011) Verification of Chinese names of truffles and their conservation in natural habitats. Plant Diversity Resour 33(6):625–642
28. Wang Y-h, Ren J-m, Lin Y-f (2001) Research advances on the ecology of tuber melanosporum. J Foshan Univ (Natural Science Edition) 19(4):66–68
29. Zhong K, Liu H-x (2008) The new characters and application of mycorrhizal studies. Ecol Sci 27(3):169–178

Chapter 369
A Study on Mobile Phone-Based Practice Teaching System

Tiejun Zhang

Abstract Students mainly adopt independent, extracurricular and spaced learning for distance open education. In order to allow students to practice in a mobile manner, this study adopts B/S structure and MVC framework mode to build an overall structure of the practice teaching system; design MIDlets of mobile phones with Java ME; and design Web Servlets with Java EE. Students can conveniently select practice items, check practice steps and submit practice assignments with mobile phones.

Keywords Mobile phones · Practice teaching · Java ME · Java EE

369.1 Introduction

Practice teaching of distance open education means the learning practice completed by students including everyday exercise [1], and field trip under the instruction of the education and learning practice is an important process for cultivating applied talent [2]. Adopting advanced technologies like Java ME and Java EE, this study is intended to design and development the mobile phone practice teaching system to allow students to conveniently obtain practice content, steps and requirements in a mobile manner so as to independently and flexibly arrange the time, place and progress of practice and reflect the practice conditions and submit assignments in time; allow teachers to publish practice teaching information in time, instruct the practice of students, know about the conditions of the students' practice and carry out scientific management and assessment, which will play a positive role in expanding the improvement of practice teaching.

T. Zhang (✉)
Department of Computer and IT Engineering, Dezhou Vocational Technical College,
Dezhou 253034, China
e-mail: zzttjj24@126.com

S. Li et al. (eds.), *Frontier and Future Development of Information Technology in Medicine and Education*, Lecture Notes in Electrical Engineering 269,
DOI: 10.1007/978-94-007-7618-0_369,

369.2 Analysis on Mobile Learning

369.2.1 Development Status

Mobile phone is a common terminal device of mobile learning. Compared with other terminal devices of mobile learning, such as PDAs, e-dictionaries and learning aids, it is advantageous in portability, easy access to network and declining rates, and furthermore, with the continuous consummation of mobile phone functions and mobile communication technologies, mobile phones are often preferred tools of the masses for mobile learning. Mobile learning with mobile phone is highly regarded by relevant institutions and enterprises, and research programs and applications like EU's "M-Learning", "Mobile Education" of the Ministry of Education of China and Nokia's "Mobiledu" have exercised broad influence [3, 4]. However, in general, mobile learning with mobile phone is still in the stage of simple applications and needs more powerful technical support [5].

At present, practice teaching of distance open education is relatively backward, so it is required to make full use of IT means to facilitate the practice of students [2, 6]. So designing and developing practice teaching systems for mobile phones to achieve practice teaching with mobile phones have become an option for aiding learning.

369.2.2 Case Analysis

Besides radio and TV university education, Dezhou Vocational Technical College also undertakes training programs for corporate employees, migrant workers, community residents and veterans, etc., and such education modes and training programs, mainly in the form of open education and targeting the cultivation of applied talent, urgently need consummated supporting services for practice teaching to effectively assist and manage routine practice of students.

Let's take the program "Chinese cooking" as an example. Students need a lot of practice to master the processes and essentials of Chinese cuisines. However, existing teaching methods cannot fully satisfy the demand of students for daily practice. Firstly, because the students mainly adopt independent, extracurricular and spaced learning, they are restrained from long-term centralized practice training. Secondly, during independent practice, because students need to complete operation steps like material purchase, material forming and cooking, etc., it is hard for them to obtain help information about the operations in time and conveniently while moving, and it is also difficult for teachers to grasp the actual operations of students. Thirdly, many migrant workers, community residents and older students, etc. lack fundamental knowledge about computer or the conditions for online learning with computers., and besides, desktop computers or laptop computers are not easily movable.

In 2012, the colleague launched the study on "Work Management on the Basis of Network Environment", which has been confirmed and initiated by Dezhou City as a development plan for science and technology; one of its purpose is to solve issues like checking practice teaching information and submitting practice assignments, etc. of students while moving and to provide the practice teaching of open education with technical support by virtue of mobile phones.

369.2.3 Demand Analysis

To achieve practice teaching of "Chinese cooking" with mobile phones, it is required to satisfy users' demands, teaching functionality and data storage according to the actual situation of the program.

Students need to obtain practice teaching information with mobile phone to select practice items, follow the stimulated steps and requirements, and submit the process and results of practice, the practice assignments. The teachers need to release practice teaching information and instruct and manage the practice of students by viewing practice assignments of students. If the demands above can be satisfied, the integration of "teaching, learning and practicing" can be achieved. Administrators need to set user privilege, manage web resources and maintain routine operation of websites.

The first function is login verification, namely, correctly recognizing and validating various users to ensure normal operation of the system. The second function is releasing practice information, namely, editing the items, steps, content and requirements of practice. The third is submitting practice assignments, namely, selecting practice items, checking practice steps, contents and requirements. It allows submission of practice assignments along with time of submission to relevant teachers with mobile phone. The fourth is Q&A, which allows bilateral communication between students and teachers via questions and answers. The fifth is management of practice assignments, which allows sorting, checking, review, approval and deletion of assignments as required. And the sixth is background management, which allows the users to add, delete, edit or modify data of the website.

The background database should be capable of ensuring storage of practice information and facilitating data operation and management. It is required to build databases for publishing practice information, submitting practice assignment information, Q&A and user information, etc.

369.2.4 Technical Analysis

The development of mobile phone, computer and mobile communication network has provided mobile phone-based practice teaching with technical support. It is required to focus on critical technical factors like overall structure, language platform and organization code during the design and development of software systems.

The three-layer structure of B/S (Browser/Server) consists of the Presentation Layer, the Business Logic Layer and the Data Access Layer. Compared with the 2-layer structure of traditional C/S (Client/Server), B/S structure's main service logic is achieved on the server side, and thus the installation of client applications and the development and maintenance of the system are simplified. B/S structure is a nice choice for reducing client load of mobile phones and offering PC browser services.

Java language targets objects of multiple platforms and is widely used. Java ME, Java SE and Java EE are important members of Sun's Java platforms. Where, Java ME, the major platform for the development of mobile phone applications at present, adopts the B/S structure. Mobile phone MIDlets (Mobile Information Devices applet) developed with Java ME are easy to use; Java ME offers support for multiple protocols including HTTP (Hypertext transfer protocol) and solves the limit of WML (Wireless Markup Language) that requires mobile phones to access the Internet via WAP (Wireless Application Protocol). Java SE is applicable to fundamental applications of desktop computers, while the advantage of Java EE lies in the application of the B/S structure on the server side. The relations between the three are shown in Fig. 369.1.

MVC (Model View Controller) separates service logic from data display relatively. Core components of MVC are Model, View and Controller, each of which is responsible for its respective tasks to provide the system with good serviceability and reproducibility, and facilitate expansion of functions [7]. It is a typical framing model of MVC to combine JSP (Java Server Pages), Servlet and JavaBean.

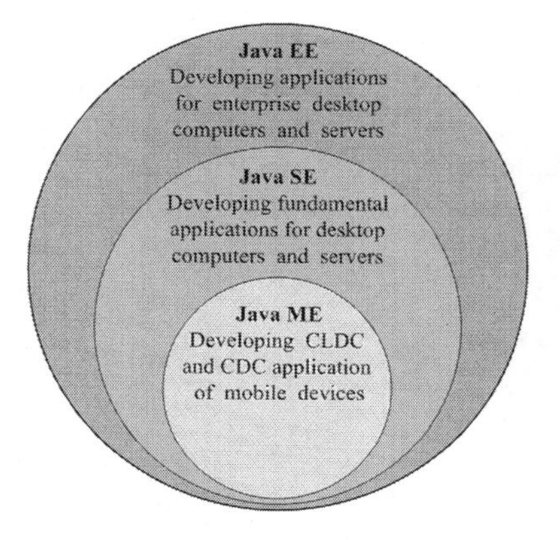

Fig. 369.1 Relations of Java ME, Java SE and Java EE

369.3 Design of the Practice Teaching System

369.3.1 Design Objective and Ideas

The objective is to build a practice teaching system of "Chinese cooking" for mobile phones. Students can access internal Web server of the college to obtain relevant practice information and submit practice assignments via mobile learning with mobile phones; teachers and administrators can effectively manage practice information, practice assignments and the website.

Since mobile phones are not as powerful as PCs in terms of internal memory, input, output and network transmission, it is required to provide mobile phone users with concise and user-friendly interfaces, maximally reduce the data handling load of mobile phones, reduce the fees for internet surfing via mobile phones, improve the universality of mobile phones and users, and meet the daily demands for practice teaching.

It is decided to design MIDlets of mobile phones with Java ME, design Web Servlets with Java EE and adopt MVC framing model based on the B/S structure to achieve efficient, rapid and flexible design and development.

369.3.2 Overall Structure of the System Design

The overall structure of the system is shown in Fig. 369.2.

The three layers of the structure and their functions are as follows:

The Presentation Layer is located on the client. Mobile phone users design MIDlets with Java ME and establish connection between the MIDlets and Java EE server through protocols like HTTP, HTTPS (Hypertext Transfer Protocol over Secure Socket Layer) or XML to send HttpRequests. Furthermore, users are also provided with PC browser service.

The Service Logic Layer is located on the server side. It runs Servlets designed with Java EE, which receives HttpRequests from MIDlets of mobile phone users. The service logic processing program processes requests of mobile phone users, or connect with the database with JDBC, the database system processes the data and

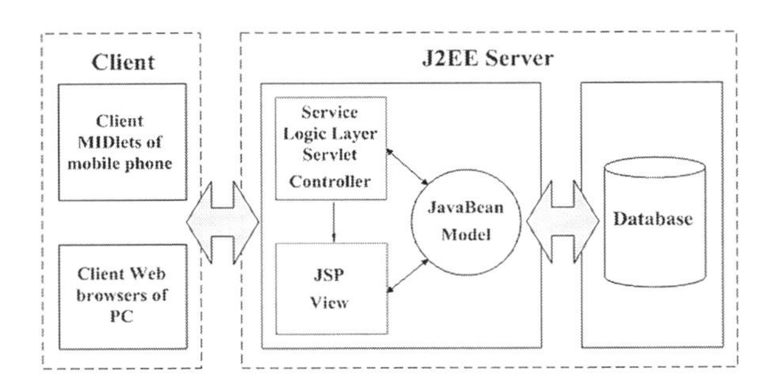

Fig. 369.2 Overall structure of the practice teaching system

send the results back to the Service Logic Layer, where the service logic processing program receives data processing results. Servlet returns Response information to mobile phone clients.

The Data Access Layer is also located on the server side. It serves to store data required for the system or results processed in the SQL session, and send the results back to the mobile phone clients through the Service Logic Layer.

In term of MVC, Servlet acts as the Controller for receiving user's requests and invoke relevant Model, which returns data and invoke View, through which the response information is returned to the user. JavaBean acts as the Model responsible for data processing and returning results of data processing. And JSP acts as the View for handling and returning page display.

369.3.3 Design of Mobile Phone Client

Functions of mobile phone client include: mobile phone user login, selecting practice items, checking practice steps and requirements, inputting new practice process information (text, photos), viewing previous practice process information (editing, clearance), asking questions and submitting practice process information. The operation flow of mobile phone client is shown in Fig. 369.3.

The mobile phone user will firstly enter the login menu for user verification. After the verification, the user will enter the practice item menu for selecting practice items. After selecting a practice item, the user can check the steps and requirements of practice and carry out the practice activities according to the practice steps and requirements. After completing each step, the user can input and then submit the practice information of corresponding step. The mobile phone can also check, edit and clear submitted practice process information and resubmit the practice process information.

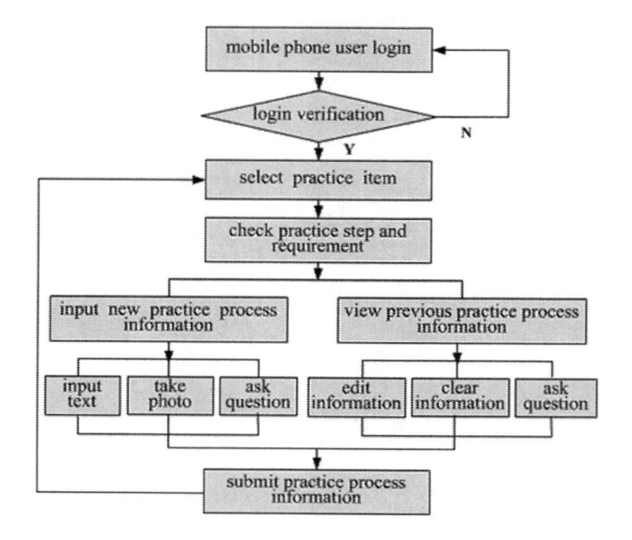

Fig. 369.3 Operation flow of the mobile phone client

369.4 Realization of Functions of Mobile Phone Clients

369.4.1 Development Environment

Hardware environment:PC. OS:Windows XP. Software environment:jdk1.5.0, WTK2.5.2, MyEclipse6.5, SQL Server.

369.4.2 Programming

"Select practice item", "Check practice steps and requirements" and "Submit practice process information" are important functions of the system and the key to realize learning practice with mobile phone. The main programming method is as follows:

Select practice item. When there are many practice items, it is required to set up multiple item options. IMPLICIT in List class can be used for realizing multiple choices of mobile phone users.

Check practice steps and requirements. Text information can be displayed with Label or TextBox, and if Form is used, both text and images can be displayed.

Input and submit practice process information. Public TextBox (String title, String text, int maxSize, int constraints) is used to create TextBox [8]. Text data is sent via HTTP protocol in the form of POST, and it is required to generate HttpConnection object and invoke setRequestMethod in the configuration mode of POST. It is also required to set the HTTP header and check whether the data is sent successfully.

Take phone and submit image information. Both deprive class of Cavans or classes like Form may be used to launch the camera shooting program. After taking a phone with the mobile phone, the mobile phone user will be asked to input the local directory of images, and send the image data to the server side with byte stream. Because POST also support sending binary data without limitation of the data size, the image data are still sent by means of POST.

Besides, to label the time of submission, the user can adopt currentTimeMillis in System class, Date in Date class or getInstance in Calendar class, but they need to be converted into routine format.

369.4.3 Running Results

The running results are shown in Figs. 369.4, 369.5 and 369.6.

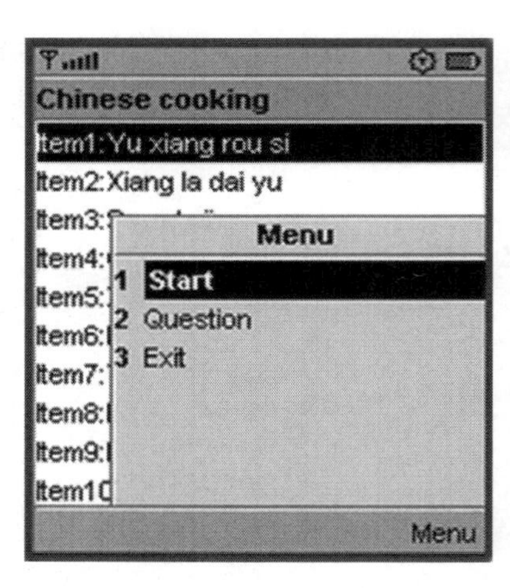

Fig. 369.4 Selecting practice items

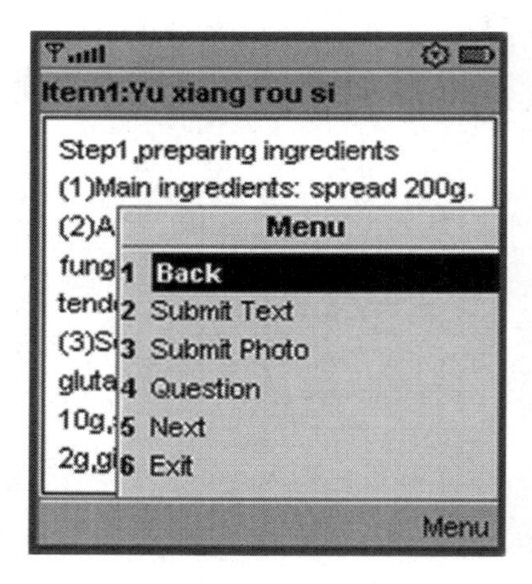

Fig. 369.5 Viewing practice steps and requirements

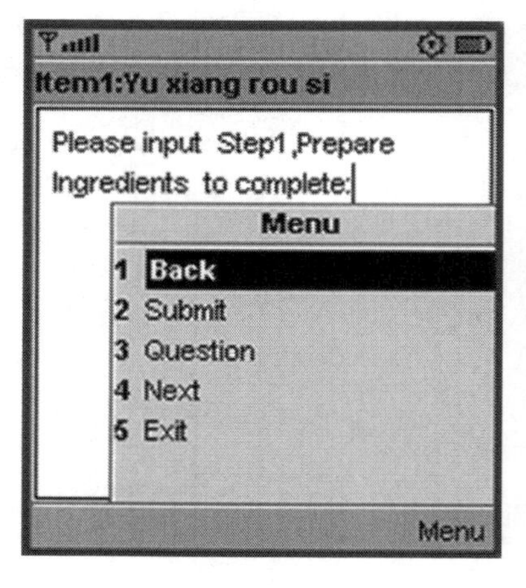

Fig. 369.6 Inputting new practice process information

369.5 Conclusion

Practice teaching with mobile phones can be achieved according to actual situation of distance open education. B/S structure and MVC framing model are adopted to build the overall structure of the practice teaching system; Java ME and Java EE are used for detailed design of mobile phone clients and servers. Having passed the commissioning test, the system allows students can obtain practice teaching information and submit practice assignments anywhere at any time, and compared with the practice teaching merely with PC browsers or paper materials, this more convenient and efficient method can stimulate the communication between teaching and learning, help enhancing the efficiency of practice teaching and reinforce the management of the students' practice. In addition, the students are provided with PC browser services, which further enhanced the universality and practicality of the practice teaching system.

References

1. Zhang S, Huang Y, Xue F (2013) Conceptual categories of modern distance open education [EB/OL]. 2013-3-12. http://www.crtvu.edu.cn/ddsx/file.php?id=788
2. Ren W (2012) Practice teaching is a systematic project [J]. Distance Educ China 4:15–16
3. Guo S, Huang J, Yuan Q (2011) A summary of overseas application and development of mobile learning. E Educ Res 5:105–107
4. Fang H, Wang H, Huang R (2011) Route chart of systematic environment for mobile learning. Mod Educ Technol 21(1):14
5. Gao M (2013) Research and realization of key technologies for mobile phone-based mobile learning system [EB/OL]. 2013-3-12. http://www.pep.com.cn/rjwk/zjyj/2012/201202_1/zjgl/201209/t20120914_1138367.htm
6. Yin K, Yao F, Wan L et al (2010) A discussion on existing problems and countermeasures of practice teaching of distance open education. Adult Educ 8:27
7. Sun W. Mastering struts: MVC-based java web design and development [M]. Publishing House of Electronics Industry, 2004: 9-11
8. Lu J, Yue X, Zhou H (2011) Programming of J2ME mobile learning software. China WaterPower Press, p 54

Chapter 370
Study on Application of Online Education Based on Interactive Platform

Li Fengyun

Abstract Although the network platform as an assistant teaching system has been used in most colleges and universities, the whole teaching effect has not been to the satisfactory results. This thesis put forward the solution of the interactive teaching platform, and has made some applied research regarding the new teaching mode based on the interactive platform. The purpose of this teaching mode is to extend the class teaching from in-class to both pre-class and after-class, and the three parts must been treated as equal importance so they could form a whole teaching process. The platform not only provides the documents for learning but also becomes an online communication platform between teachers and students outside class. It was proved an effective teaching mode based on the interactive online platform through the trial use last year.

Keywords Teaching mode · Teaching platform · Online education · Interactive

370.1 The Background to Improve Teaching Platform and Teaching Mode

As we know, the traditional teaching mode has been changed lots with the application of computer network technology in the past ten years. The whole teaching effect also has been improved. For example, the network teaching platform and excellent course website have been used in almost universities, distance education platform has been used in continual education and vocational education, multimedia teaching system has been used in most of classroom. However, we has

L. Fengyun (✉)
School of Information Science and Electronic Engineering,
Shandong Jiaotong University, Jinan, China
e-mail: 1982600936@qq.com

S. Li et al. (eds.), *Frontier and Future Development of Information Technology in Medicine and Education*, Lecture Notes in Electrical Engineering 269,
DOI: 10.1007/978-94-007-7618-0_370,

found that the whole teaching effect is not ideal and there are many aspects to improve based on our investigation and analysis to these systems function and application methods.

370.1.1 Improve the Teaching Mode

Why should we improve the teaching mode to further engage students spending more time on their leaning task?

At the present, most of teachers and education administration departments in universities and colleges focus on the in-class and don't pay attention to the preview and review. They have researched the teaching methods in-class, designed the PPT and assignment but they haven't checked the preview results and controlled the students to finish all the assignment according to the desire. On the one hand, some of teachers could remind the students to preview but not give them the detailed foundational knowledge and the appropriate basic exercises for testing the preview effect. So most of students always attend the class without previewing and the teachers must insure the foundational knowledge rather than some in-depth knowledge. On the other hand, the teachers often give some written assignments related to the class contents for review but less some questions to guiding the students to learning in-depth. Although the teachers have a fixed Q & A time per week but it isn't convenient for students to ask the questions in office. At the same time, most of students always take less time after class so they often are in a state of passive learning especially in the ordinary universities and colleges because of lacking the guiding and checking for preview and review [1]. As a result, the teaching mode must be reformed so as to achieve an ideal teaching effect.

370.1.2 Improve the Current Teaching Platform

Another important factor to affect the teaching effect is the limited functions of the network platform and it hasn't been used well with the class teaching. Now most network teaching platform can provide the course documents such as course syllabus, PPT, handouts, unit quizzes, document links and message board etc. But they seldom provide online teaching like face to face in-class to answer the students' questions to guide them to review and in-depth learn. At the same time, they have not provided the function for teachers to guide the students to preview. The students could view and download the course documents but don't get the guide for learning method because of the documents organized by their categories but not around the knowledge point. So the platform needs to be improved with the new teaching model.

370.2 Overall Solution

The overall design goal is to improve the teaching effect by changing the teaching mode and to support the teaching mode by using the new teaching platform. In other words, the teaching process for each chapter/topic includes three parts which are preview, lecture and review and they have equal importance. At the same time, the teacher must divide the contents around the chapter/topic into three parts to respectively fit the preview, lecture and review. So the teaching in-class will be combined with both pre-class and after-class learning which guide the students' active learning by specific learning tasks and thinking problems. As a result, it has extended the teaching in-class to outside class with the interactive online education and changed the knowledge-based learning into the ability-based learning.

370.2.1 New Teaching Mode

Each teaching contents for a chapter/topic will be divided into three equally important components: the pre-class contents and the related exercises, lectures in-class, review questions and assignments for in-depth leaning. The teacher must check most students' performance at each stage, adjust the class session, grade students' assignment and provide online teaching. Of course, the teacher must carefully design the three parts for each knowledge point to guide the students to spend more time on learning and researching both in-class and outside-class. That will guide and engage the students to learn actively in a measurable way.

370.2.2 New Platform

Unlike the current network teaching platform, the organizational structure of the new teaching platform has been re-built according to the new teaching mode. On the one hand, some new functions have been added based on the original network teaching platform, such as interactive online teaching, preview guide and evaluation, review guide and thinking problems, time record of students' learning online, and so on. So the teachers can control the three teaching stages with the platform and realize the face-to-face teaching at anytime and anywhere. On the other hand, the documents for each chapter/topic must be re-organized around the topic and formed a learning guide.

370.3 Implement

The new teaching mode changes the teaching organization method and its performance depends on the new platform. So there are two important aspects which must be done well during the implement of this teaching mode: the re-designed teaching process and the re-built platform.

370.3.1 Determining the Content of the Leaning Guide

How to design the course content for each chapter/topic and how to arrange the content into a learning guide are the two keys during the implement. A design team included some teachers who are all familiar to this course must be formed because of the heavy workload. At the beginning of design, the team must review and identify the course's goals and objectives, then further break them down into specific learning outcomes for each topic/chapter of content, and at last all of the small learning outcomes would cover the entire course. Then they could begin to arrange all the detailed contents according to the requirements of the following three stages.

The first is to design the pre-class study guides that would lead students with a series of key points, activities, and graded assignments which can motivate them to use the resource. But the content must focus on the foundational knowledge, it can be shown on the website or indicate the places on the textbook or other links. Foundational knowledge is always specific, and the questions asked by the teachers are well-defined and have correct answers. All the students can check the correct answers after they have submitted their answers.

Unlike previous lectures, which offered a long and static learning model, the teachers could break the preview content into segments as short as 10–15 min and offers quick online quizzes as a part of each segment. A short time studying can often be acceptable and be successful for the learner than a long time.

The second is to design the lecture in-class based on the result of preview and the difficult content of each chapter/topic. Moving foundational knowledge to the platform will give the teachers more in-class time available to teach in-depth knowledge face-to-face [2].

On the one hand, the contents in-class must contain the review of the pre-class and the analysis to some problems which concluded from all the students' preview situation. So the teachers must check all the students' answer and the grade to find their common problems. On the other hand, the highlights critical information in each chapter/topic must be as well as a variety of supplementary materials to help students decipher difficult concepts in the textbook. These include key points, brief notes, summaries, examples, and identification of important materials. Of course, the study guide in-class must integrate the students' response into the course content. In order to enhance the efficiency and flexible of the class teaching, each knowledge point will be introduced into the class by some related questions. If the students could answer the questions easily, so the teacher could skip this content and move to the next new topic. This way allows the teachers to tailor the class session based on students needs.

The content in-class is also be released to the teaching platform as the pre-view contents and review contents so it can also be accessed easily and conveniently outside of the classroom both before and after class on this platform.

The third is to design the content after-class to guide the student review and learn in-depth. The review questions must be designed for students to check their study by themselves through answer each question. Then some more difficult questions or assignments must be provided to guide the students leaning more related knowledge which always belongs to the non-foundational content. The non-foundational knowledge is often less specific, and the questions created by teachers might have more than one correct answer. These questions focus on the application of knowledge such as thinking problems, comprehensive training problems and even small thesis.

370.3.2 Constructing the Platform

The structure of the new platform system has been designed according to the requirements of the above teaching mode. It has three main features except the similar functions with the current network teaching platform. In other words, the platform can also provide the regular functions such as view and update the course documents, answer question and submit the assignment online, multimedia resources and links etc. It has some special functions as below.

The first feature is that the platform has re-adjusted the documents organization structure. Unlike most of the current network teaching platform which organized the documents according to the content classification, the new platform system has organized the documents around the chapter/topic. It means that all documents which include goal, preview content, test exercises, lecture, review questions and thesis are organized as a whole—online study guide. It likes an instructor to lead the student to lean the course for each chapter/topic at anytime.

In order to facilitate the students to use the study guide, the documents will be arranged both in liner and nonlinear. So the linear structure enables the teacher to guide students based on the class guide content. However, the nonlinear structure allows the students to quickly jump to a specific section of content for view.

The second feature is the platform could provide the students' learning evaluation online which includes the learning time record and statistical analysis, the evaluation of objective exercises [3]. It allows the teacher to adjust the content in-class and the review contents according to these. At the same time, the teacher can control the whole teaching process with the platform.

The third feature is interactive and online. It is different from the current network teaching platform that the newer platform provides the online interactive teaching and discuss. Specifically, the teacher can provide a face-to-face teaching on this platform, and the students can ask the questions or attend the discussion group after class [4]. But as you know, the teacher couldn't have enough time online. There are at least two solutions. On the one hand, the course team can arrange the in-turn tutoring plan and announce it on the website. On the other hand, the teachers could rely on the elder students who has learned this course or who is learning better to attend the tutoring online, in effect turning them into teaching assistants.

370.4 Application and Development Trend

370.4.1 Application

We have a difficult problem in course *C Language Programming*. It means that there are more than 15 % and sometime more than 20 % students are failed in the course examination in recent years. And we find there are more and more students would not be interested in this course from the start of the semester to the end. And this problem looks more serious because it would affect the students to continue learning the next related courses. So we selected this course which has a low retention and success to reform the teaching mode and built the new platform as a trial last year.

Another reason for us to choice this course is that the test paper always be extracted randomly from a general exam-paper database. It is convenient for us to identify the difference of using this teaching mode with the previous.

About the students, we selected two specialties which are C*omputer Science* and *Information Management* in our school. There are 6 classes and nearly 600 students, so we could avoid the accidental caused by lacking of enough samples.

About the teacher, we arranged two teachers to take 3 classes task for each one. So we can study the effect to the teaching result from the teacher.

During the phases of development and the trial, the teacher team and the development team brainstormed and paid a great of effort.

There are some experiences to show as bellow.

- All the students must complete the assignment in the pre-class study guide prior to each class. The teachers can view the website and check who has spending time on the preview and remind those who hasn't completed in timely.
- The teachers must view the students' preview results so as to adjust the class contents.
- The teachers could verify how much time each student has spent on a specific task and intervene where necessary.
- In order to make the study guide student-centered and provide an activity-based learning environment, each study guide includes both textbook chapter practice

exercises and some pre-class assignment created by teachers, and even the questions for review focus on the program training.
- The use method of review is similar to preview.
- The teachers must conclude the number of students online in different time so adjust the schedule for Q & A.

During the course term, most students followed the study guide to finish each chapter more easily so they had more interesting than the previous students. A relaxed and happy learning atmosphere has been made slowly so it could allow the students to study to his full potential.

At the end of last semester, we made a statistics about the students' grade of this course, the attendance rate, the average number of exercises finished by the students for each chapter/topic, the total time spent by the students online, etc. As the result, more than 64 % students spent at least twice times as much as the previous students who never used this platform and this teaching method. At the same time, the number of exercises done by the students out-class time is almost the 1.5 times as much as before.. The retention and success rate were all be increased in the last semester. There were only 7 % students failed.

In addition, there is another important factor which will determine the effect of using this platform. It is the control ability of the teacher. It means that, the teacher should know about the situation of pre-view for each student and then arrange each lecture, even to remind a few students who haven't finished the pre-view or the review task in time.

370.4.2 Trend of Development

This teaching mode and the platform not only can be used in the programming course but also any courses. The key factor lies in the teacher how to prepare his course contents for each chapter/topic and how control the process of teaching during using the platform successfully. But it is suitable better for universities or colleges because it demands the students have the better self-learning ability in some degree and have more time outside class [5].

The platform might offer an online student community in a university or the global world. So there are more and more students who can help the learner answer the questions in timely.

Although the platform and the teaching mode are not perfect, we still hope the online platform could replace the classroom in the future in universities. And even it can open to all learners in the world. So a teacher could teach more and more students than in classroom. It will reduce the education cost and enhance the teaching effect.

370.5 Conclusion

This is a typical case to use information technology to improve the teaching mode. It changes the current education model from the knowledge education to the ability education. It is in favor of training the students' self-learning ability, extending the teaching from classroom to the outside class, providing a interactive online communication, engaging the students' active learning and increase the student success.

References

1. Randy Garrison D, Vaughan ND (2008) Blended leaning in higher education: framework, principles and guidelines, Jossey-Bass, San Francisco
2. Means B, Toyama Y, Murphy R, Bakia M, Jones K (2009) Evaluation of evidence-based practices online learning: a meta-analysis and review of online learning studies, U.S. Department of Education, Washington, D. C
3. Bruffee KA (1999) Collaborative learning: higher education, interdependence and the authority of knowledge, 2nd edn. John Hopkins University Press, Baltimere
4. Tan L, Chen Y (2007) The construction of online teaching platform based on campus network. Educ Info Technol (11):31–33
5. Li F, Cao M (2009) Building the online project training base based on the campus network. ITME 2009, Jinan

Chapter 371
Analysis on Curative Effect of Exercise Therapy Combined with Joint Mobilization in the Treatment of Knee Osteoarthritis

Wang Hongliang

Abstract *Objective* compare and analyze the curative effect of exercise therapy combined with joint mobilization in the treatment of knee osteoarthritis. *Methods* This paper studies the cases dated from March 2011 to March 2012, including 28 cases of knee osteoarthritis patients who are randomly divided into observation group and control group, and each group contains 14 cases. Both groups of patients are taking joint mobilization to alleviate symptoms but only the observation group is supplemented with exercise therapy, then researcher compares and analyzes the curative effect of the two therapies. After treatment, both groups' scores of JOA are improved ($P < 0.05$). The efficiency of observation group is higher than the control group ($\chi2 = 9.001$, $P < 0.05$) and the JOA scores of observation group improves more significantly than that of the control group ($t = -2.114$, $P < 0.05$). *Conclusion* the exercise therapy combined with joint mobilization has an obvious curative effect on the treatment of knee osteoarthritis and provides a practical value in the clinical application.

Keywords Exercise therapy · Joint mobilization · Knee osteoarthritis

With the increasing world population, aging problem has attracted global attention. Meanwhile, cardiovascular disease, tumour, obesity, diabetes and other serious diseases endangering human health has been paid great attention by the whole society. Many specialized institutions have been established all over the world to study these diseases, and public awareness towards the prevention and harm degree of these diseases has also been greatly improved. But the importance of osteoarthritis was so neglected that most patients think that the disease is not a threat to life. If patients do not pay enough attention to the early disease which

W. Hongliang (✉)
Qinhuangda, P R China
e-mail: hongliangwang2013@163.com

S. Li et al. (eds.), *Frontier and Future Development of Information Technology in Medicine and Education*, Lecture Notes in Electrical Engineering 269,
DOI: 10.1007/978-94-007-7618-0_371,

may causes treatment delay or inappropriate and unsystematic treatment, these diseases will bring pain, limb dysfunction, deformity and expensive medical expenses to them when these diseases came into the advanced stage. This has become a medically social problem that cannot be ignored.

Although there have been many researches about the knee osteoarthritis treatment, less patients receive formal treatment. For doctor, the understanding from non-specialized doctors on the disease is quite superficial, resulting treatment still in informal stage, i.e. mainly depends on pure analgesic drug treatment, but lack of individualized treatment and systematic and comprehensive treatment. The comforting thing is that, in recent years, with the rapid development of medicine, clinical diagnosis technology appeared qualitative leap, and there has emerged many pragmatic methods concerning the treatment of knee osteoarthritis. For patients with early stage joint diseases, they can take positive and targeted drug therapy, physical therapy, functional training as well as joint protection measures [1]; patients in the early and middle stages can take internal medicine treatment supplemented with minimally invasive surgical arthroscopic knee treatment;— patients in the middle and advanced stages may take the osteochondral grafting, joint orthopedic surgery, arthrodesis, artificial joint replacement and arthroplasty, etc. Clinical application of these methods can save the joint function of the patients to a large extent and greatly improve the quality of patients' life, which may relieve the burden of their family and society. This paper focuses on the curative effect of exercise therapy combined with joint mobilization in the treatment of knee osteoarthritis. The report is as follows.

371.1 Data and Methods

371.1.1 General Data

We studied the cases from March 2011 to March 2012, including 28 cases of knee osteoarthritis patients who were randomly divided into two groups, i.e. observation group and control group, each group 14 cases. The observation group included 8 male cases and 6 female cases aging between 41 and 68 years old, which make their average age 53.16 ± 10.04 years old and their average duration of 5.39 ± 1.33 months; The control group included nine male cases, five female cases aging between 40–67 years old which make their average age 51.99 ± 12.18 years old and their average duration of 5.47 ± 1.41 months. Both groups of patients showed no significant statistical difference in general data and are comparable ($P > 0.05$).

371.1.2 Methods

Both groups of patients were taking joint mobilization to alleviate their symptoms. The specific method is:

(1) Patient position: comfortable, relaxed and painless position;
(2) Treatment position: treatment should be close to the joint that need to be treated, then one hand fix one end of the joint and the other hand start to loosen the other end;
(3) Evaluation before treatment: identify the existing problem (e.g. pain, stiffness and its degree);
(4) Methods of application: (1) the direction of manipulated movement: can be vertical or parallel to the treatment plane. The plane of treatment defines a plane perpendicular to the rotation axis of the articular surface of the midpoint. Separation is perpendicular to the plane of the treatment; sliding and long axis traction are parallel to the plane of treatment; (2) the degree of manipulation, should reach the limit of joint activities. Pain—no more than the pain point. Stiff—more than stiff point. Balanced movement with rhythm lasts 30 s–1 min. If the pain is not relieved and even getting worse after 24 h, it indicates that the treatment intensity or duration is so long that we must reduce the intensity of treatment or shorten the treatment time.

The observation group was taking joint mobilization and supplemented with exercise therapy, including the following contents:

(1) Warm up: refers to the preparation that must be done before exercise, for example, muscles and joints relaxation;
(2) Isometric exercise: one maximum contraction every 5 s, and a total of 2 h, 3–4 times per day;
(3) Isotonic contraction exercise: refers to the movement under constant resistance load, which need rehabilitation therapist put certain resistance during patients' muscle contraction;
(4) Continuous Passive Motion (CPM): if patients use CPM exercise, it is necessary to follow the principle of using early, improving gradually and individual dose;
(5) Proprioception training: utilizing simple instrument such as a seesaw, a trampoline or a hanging rack, and adjustable platform is also usable. By standing on an unstable device, patients try to find balance, firstly through their visual and vestibular sense, and finally find their own body positions by proprioceptive sense;
(6) Functional exercise: lower limb joint walking needs gradual training. Start with one leg walk aided by two crutches, after patients regain their confidence, begin to walk with two leg aided by two crutches. Then, gradually get rid of the crutches and begin postural stability and coordination training with rehabilitation therapist's help until they can walk freely.

371.1.3 The Criteria for JOA Patients with Knee Joint Osteoarthritis

Table 371.1.

371.1.4 Curative Effect Criterion

Cure: the disappearance of joint pain and the function of knee joint resume normal. Availability: the disappearance of joint pain and the function of knee joint resume normal almost resume normal. Mend: the alleviation of joint pain and the function of knee joint a bit improve. Invalidation: no alleviation of joint pain and the

Table 371.1 Knee osteoarthritis curative effect criteria

Index	Grade point (Full mark is 100)	
	Right	Left
1. Pain but able to walk		
(1) Walking more than 1000 m, usually without pain. Occasional pain during activity	30	30
(2) Walking more than 1000 m, but feel painful	25	25
(3) Walking more than 500 m and less than 1000 m, but feel painful	20	20
(4) Walking more than 100 m and less than 500 m, but feel painful	15	15
(5) Indoor walking or walking less than 100 m, but feel painful	10	10
(6) Unable to walk	5	5
(7) Unable to stand	0	0
2. Pain but able to go up and down stairs		
(1) Able to go up and down stairs without pain.	25	25
(2) Able to go up and down stairs but feel painful, while no pain using handrail	20	20
(3) Painful with handrail, while no pain if walking step by step	15	15
(4) With or without handrail, no pain if walking step by step	10	10
(5) With handrail, painful if walking step by step	5	5
(6) Unable to walk	0	0
3. Flexion angle, ankylosis and highly contracture		
(1) Able to reach normal sitting posture	35	35
(2) Able to sit sideways and cross-legged	30	30
(3) Flexion angle more than 110°	25	25
(4) Flexion angle more than 75°	20	20
(5) Flexion angle more than 35°	10	10
(6) Flexion angle less than 35°, ankylosis and highly contracture	0	0
4. Swelling		
(1) Neither edema nor swelling	10	10
(2) Sometimes need to puncture	5	5
(3) Often need to puncture	0	0

function of knee joint don not improve. The total efficient ratio = the Cure ratio + the Availability ratio + the Mend ratio.

371.1.5 Statistical Analysis

Data were analyzed through SPSS19.0 statistical software. Measurement data were compared by t test while count data were compared using $\chi 2$ test. $P < 0.05$ had statistical significance.

371.2 Results

371.2.1 Compare the JOA Scores of Two Groups

After treatment, both groups' scores of JOA were improved ($P < 0.05$), but the JOA scores of observation group improved more significantly than that of the control group ($t = -2.114$, $P < 0.05$). Table 371.2 shows the JOA scores comparison of the two groups.

Note: compared with the control group, *$P < 0.05$.

371.2.2 Compare the Curative Effects of Two Groups

Table 371.3 shows the curative effects comparison of the two groups. The total efficient ratio of observation group improved more significantly than that of the control group ($\chi 2 = 9.001$, $P < 0.05$).

371.3 Discussion

In the treatment of knee osteoarthritis, physical therapy, to some extent, could relieve local pain and muscle spasm. As one of these methods, joint mobilization is

Table 371.2 Compare the curative effects of the two groups [$\bar{r} \pm S$]

Group category	Amount of cases	Before treatment	After treatment
Observation group	14	38.65 ± 14.11	87.99 ± 10.32
Control group	14	39.77 ± 13.54	62.45 ± 11.88
t		1.305	−2.114
P		>0.05	<0.05

Table 371.3 Compare curative effects of the two groups (case %)

Group category	Amount of cases	Cure	Availability	Mend	Invalidation	The total efficient ratio
Observation group	14	6(42.9)	4(28.6)	3(21.4)	1(7.1)	13(92.9)
Control group	14	0(0)	2(14.3)	5(35.7)	7(50)	7(50)
$\chi 2$						9.001
P						<0.05

the manipulation technique treatment for joint activities within the scope permitted, belonging to the category of passive movement. The basic principle of joint mobilization is to use joint physiological movement and affiliated exercise as a therapy technique. The physiological movement refers to the joint motion completed in the physiological range, such as flexion and extension, adduction, abduction and rotation, etc. Physiological exercise could not only be completed by patients themselves, but can also be accomplished by therapists. The affiliated exercise refers to the joint movement completed within the permissible range of motion in itself and its surrounding tissue. It is a kind of indispensable movement to maintain normal joint activities. And generally, it cannot be completed by patients themselves but needs to be done with others' assistance. The therapeutic effects of joint mobilization techniques are mainly embodied in the following aspects:

(1) Pain relief: when the joint swelling and patients cannot do full range of activities, joint mobilization can promote joint fluid flow, increase the nutrition of the avascular zone in the articular cartilage and cartilage disc and finally relieve pain; Meanwhile, prevent joint degeneration caused by activity number reduction. This is the mechanical effect of joint mobilization.
(2) Improving the range of joint motion: regarding clinical findings, joint immobilization may cause tissue fibrosis hyperplasia, joint adhesion and contracture of tendon, ligament and joint capsule.

As directly pulling tissues around joint, joint mobilization techniques, therefore, can maintain or increase its extension and improve the range of joint motion. However, these methods only serve the purpose for relieving symptoms, still they has no effect on the disease process.

In recent years, knee rehabilitation exercise gains more and more widespread attention [2]. It is an essential link for knee osteoarthritis patients in the whole process of the treatment and prevention of diseases. WHO define rehabilitation as: for the people who suffer from body, mind or spirit obstacle threats, and can neither rely on themselves to eliminate the obstacles nor help other people eliminate consequences caused by the obstacles, rehabilitation measures can explore patients' abilities and promote its function so that the patients can soon recover their daily life and restart work.

Therefore, whether adopt operation treatment or the non-operation therapy, rehabilitation exercise as an adjunctive therapy is indispensible. If lack of correct rehabilitation exercise or proper functional guidance, it will not achieve the desired treatment effect. In particular, due to joint pain, the majority of osteoarthritis patients reduce the volume of activities, resulting in the thigh muscle begins atrophy and weakness. And as a result of long disuse of knee joint, the joint gradually appears deformity. Hence, for those osteoarthritis patients, exercise can not only increase the flexibility of the joints, also due to enhanced muscle strength, the joint stability has been well protected, easing the symptom to a certain extent [3]. But on the other hand, strenuous activities, such as running, jumping and climbing, etc. should be avoided, because instead of protecting joints, these activities will further aggravate the burden of joint and make the joint disease worse.

In other words, the motion of knee joint should be mainly active with no weight-bearing activities, such as isometric muscle contraction, relaxation, no weight-bearing joint flexion activities, walking, cycling and swimming, etc. Through these exercises, patients can prevent muscle contraction, enhance the muscle strength and increase the range of joint motion. Based on the above contents, this study designs one treatment group using exercise therapy and supplemented with joint mobilization, and one simple group only using joint mobilization in the treatment to discuss therapeutic effect on knee osteoarthritis. Assisted exercises that have been taken in this study includes warm-up, isometric exercise, isotonic contraction exercise, CPM, proprioceptive training and functional exercise. The warm-up movement is of great importance to all exercises, because it can prevent muscle and soft tissue injury in sports. It is the start overture for all training; Isometric contraction plays a significant role in the early postoperative period, for its capability to prevent muscle contraction, restore force and ensure the wound healing; Isotonic contraction emphasizes low repeatability, high resistance to achieve the maximum strength; CPM has become a vital content in the rehabilitation of joint surgery and increasingly accepted by the orthopedics doctors. It depends on the joint activities stimulation to synovial, simulate microenvironment of normal articular, increase nutrition and metabolism of articular cartilage and promote the transformation from the repair of articular cartilage to normal articular cartilage, preventing degeneration of articular cartilage and tissue adhesion caused due to braking, and promoting the recovery of joint function; Many patients with knee osteoarthritis suffer from proprioceptive disorder and they need other normal feelings such as visual and vestibular sense to help recover training. Proprioceptive training and functional exercise should be carried out at the same time and run through the whole process of rehabilitation to improve the reaction time and coordination of lower limb muscle. This kind of comprehensive exercise therapy used in this study has achieved excellent results, i.e. the JOA score of the observation group was 38.65 ± 14.11 before treatment, while after treatment JOA score increased to 87.99 ± 10.32 ($P < 0.05$); Before treatment, the JOA score of the control group was 39.77 ± 13.54, while the JOA score increased to 62.45 ± 11.88 after treatment ($P < 0.05$). Statistical analysis indicates that before treatment there is no obvious difference between the two groups($P < 0.05$), but differences became more significant after treatment($t = -2.114$, $P < 0.05$). And the total efficient ratio is 92.8 % in the observation group, which is much higher than 50 % in control group ($\chi2 = 9.001$, $P < 0.05$). The JOA score of observation group improved owing to the comparison with the control group. Furthermore, with the proprioceptive and balance training, it will finally reach a certain level of joint function. The result of this study provides an outstanding guidance for the rehabilitation treatment of knee osteoarthritis and is of great significance for the clinical diagnosis and treatment.

371.4 Conclusion

Combination of exercise therapy and joint mobilization provides obvious curative effect in the treatment of knee osteoarthritis, and worthy of clinical application.

References

1. Jin J, Yao B, Zhai W (2006) Massage combined with strength training in the treatment of knee osteoarthritis. Chin J Rehabilit 21(1):42–43
2. Pan H (2006) Exercise therapy combined with block therapy for knee osteoarthritis. Chin J Rehabilit 21(6):384–385
3. Lin H, He C (2008) Foreign research progress of clinical study of exercise therapy on the treatment of knee osteoarthritis. China Reconstr Surg 22(11):1389–1342

Chapter 372
Predictions with Intuitionistic Fuzzy Soft Sets

Sylvia Encheva

Abstract This paper is applying methods from soft sets theory for timely identification of students who are in danger to fail their exam in a particular subject. The work exploits the advantages of soft sets compare to fuzzy logics and statistical methods. While most statistical methods require large data sets and perform well in stochastically stable environments, the ones we have been addressing in this paper can give results within a very small data sets and can accommodate additional information derived from later experiments.

Keywords Soft sets · Uncertainties · Decision making

372.1 Introduction

Molodtsov introduced the theory of soft sets [8], which can be seen as a new mathematical approach to vagueness, [1]. Soft set theory is very useful in the presence of uncertainties since it does not require special functions like in fuzzy set theory. The choice of convenient parametrization strategies such as real numbers, functions, and mappings makes soft-set theory very convenient and practicable for decision making applications, [9].

Correlations between midterm tests outcomes and exam results derived from available data can be summarized and applied on new cases. As pointed in [11] similar inductions can be found in statistical reasoning and are more or less unavoidable if a model is to be applied in real life situations. Therefore, all conclusions derived from sample data are true only with respect to that set of data,

S. Encheva (✉)
Stord/Haugesund University College, Bjørnsong. 45 5528 Haugesund, Norway
e-mail: sbe@hsh.no

S. Li et al. (eds.), *Frontier and Future Development of Information Technology in Medicine and Education*, Lecture Notes in Electrical Engineering 269,
DOI: 10.1007/978-94-007-7618-0_372,

and, they should be treated as uncertain hypotheses about properties of a large universe, [11].

In our case preliminary data on students taking intermediate tests and final exams is extracted from already completed courses. New students who experience problems with these topics (i.e. failed on the corresponding intermediate tests) are to receive special attention. They are offered extra tutorials in digital form or face to face tutoring when ever needed. Contents providers can use tests outcomes for further adjustment of the related teaching materials.

372.2 Preliminaries

In the soft set theory, the initial description of the object has an approximate nature, [9]. Notions regarding soft sets follow [1]. Let U be an initial universe set and E_U be the set of all possible parameters under consideration with respect to U. The power set of U (i.e., the set of all subsets of U) is denoted by $P(U)$ and $A \subseteq E$. Intuitionistic fuzzy sets were introduced in [3] and further developed by many authors, see f. ex. [2, 5, 6, 10].

A pair (F,A) is called a soft set over U, where F is a mapping given by $F : A \rightarrow P(U)$. A soft set over U is a parametrized family of subsets of the universe U. For $\varepsilon \in A, F(\varepsilon)$ may be considered as the set of ε-approximate elements of the soft set (F,A).

An intuitionistic fuzzy set (IFS) A in a nonempty set U a universe of discourse is an object having the form $A = \{\langle x, \mu_A(x), \upsilon_A(x)\rangle : x \in U\}$, where the functions $\mu_A(x) : U \rightarrow [0, 1], \upsilon_A(x) : U \rightarrow [0, 1]$, denotes the degree of membership and degree of nonmembership of each element $x \in U$ to the set A, respectively, and $0 \leq \mu_A(x) + \upsilon_A(x) \leq 1$ for all $x \in U$.

372.3 Tests and Exam Results

Initially we prepare information table with students and their results on intermediate tests (Test 1, Test 2, Test 3) and final exam (Exam), Table 372.1. The soft set (F,A) shows students who failed some or all of the intermediate tests (F), just managed to pass some or all of the intermediate tests (J), and passed the intermediate tests (P). Different topics under tests (Test 1, Test 2, Test 3) are denoted by $x_i, y_j z_k$ for simplicity, empty cells under tests indicate that a student has not answered that question.

The soft set (G,B) shows students who failed the final exam, just managed to pass the final exam, and passed the final exam.

We then use a soft function $f(F(a)) = G(b)$ that identifies students who failed some or all of the intermediate tests, just managed to pass some or all of the

Table 372.1 Students and their results on intermediate tests and final exam

	Test 1			Test 2			Test 3			Exam		
	F	J	P	F	J	P	F	J	P	F	J	P
*St*1	x1	x3	x1	y2	y1		z2	z1			×	
*St*2	x2	x3		y3	y1	y2	z2		z3		×	
*St*3		x3	x1		y1			z1				×
*St*4	x3			y3	y2		z3			×		
*St*5			x2			y1	z3		z1			×
*St*6	x1		x2	y3		y1			z2			×
*St*7		x1		y1				z2			×	
*St*8	x1		x3		y2			z3			×	
*St*9		x1				y2	z1			×		
*St*10	x2		x1	y3				z1	z3	×		

intermediate tests, and failed the final exam, or just managed to pass the final exam, respectively. Once these students are identified we go back to the information table and extract the specific topics from the tests on which they failed.

If necessary it is possible to insert weights reflecting the significance of different topics and or the level of difficulties of concepts and problems included in tests. Another important variable related to tests is the number of students who fail or just managed to pass.

Suppose new groups of students are added to the database. The value of the attribute A for a student is then calculated according to the function

$$A = \frac{\Sigma If(C_i) \cdot \alpha_{C_i} \cdot w_{n,If}}{l}$$

where $w_{n,if}$ is the weight obtained after the nth interaction for the attribute A.

The weights $\frac{w_{n1}}{w_{n-1,1}}$ are determined via normalization of the number of elements in the two iterations: $n-1$th iteration—ϕ elements, nth iteration—ψ elements

$$w_{n-1,1} = \frac{\phi}{\phi + \psi}, w_{n,1} = \frac{\psi}{\phi + \psi}$$

Another interesting question is related to the significance of each of tests students are suggested to take. Obviously if they cannot pass a particular test they have to work further in order to obtain the required knowledge and skills. The not so obvious part is which of these tests or which combination of these tests results gives better indication about possible exam failure. To the rest of this subsection we follow an approach in [5].

In our example the universe consists of ten elements $St1, St2, \ldots, St10$ corresponding to the ten students, and three parameters $T1, T2, T3$ corresponding to the three tests, see Table 372.1.

Applying function $F_p(e) = (F(e)(x), p(e)(x))$ as defined earlier we conclude that students $St2, St4, St9, St10$ are likely to fail their exam. These students do not receive satisfactory tests results. They are offered additional help and asked to repeat those tests. As in Definition 2 we calculate

$H_\lambda(e_1, e_1), H_\lambda(e_1, e_2), H_\lambda(e_1, e_3), H_\lambda(e_2, e_2), \ldots, H_\lambda(e_2, e_3)$, where $H_\lambda(e_i, e_j) = (H(e_i, e_j)(St_k), \wedge(e_i, e_j)(St_k)), \ \ i,j = 1,2,3, \ \ k = 1, \ldots, 10.$

Then we proceed with calculations of the difference between the membership and non-membership values and note the maximal numerical grade $M_{ij}, i,j = 1,2,3$, $Score(St_k) = \sum_{i,j=1,2,3} M_{ij}(e_i, e_j) \times \lambda_i$.

After calculating scores for students and tests we conclude that results from Test 1 and Test 2 are sufficient to predict possible exam failure.

In a future work we would like to explore the idea of following tests outcomes with respect single topics. Experienced lectures know very well that certain topics and concepts appear to be difficult for the majority of the students but it still not quite clear to which topics in particular and to which degree these topics happen to cause exam failure or even drop outs.

372.4 Conclusion

The main idea in this paper is to work out an approach for identifying students who might be in danger of exam failure. A soft set function is applied to point which tests' results indicate exam failure in a course completed by a group of students. New students with similar tests results are considered to be in danger to fail their exam as well. Thus identified students receive additional help. At the same time contents of topics included in such tests have to be reworked by the corresponding content developer.

References

1. Ali MI, Feng F, Liu X, Min WK, Shabir M (2009) On some new operations in soft set theory. Comput Math Appl 57:1547–1553
2. Alhazaymeh K, Halim SA, Salleh AR, Hassan N (2012) Soft Intuitionistic Fuzzy Sets. Appl Math Sci 6(54):2669–2680
3. Atanassov KT (1986) Intuitionistic fuzzy sets. Fuzzy Sets Syst 20(1):87–96
4. Babitha KV, Sunil JJ (2010) Soft set relations and functions. Comput Math Appl 60:1840–1849
5. Bashir M, Salleh AR, Alkhazaleh S (2012) Possibility Intuitionistic fuzzy soft set. Adv Decis Sci 2012:1–24
6. Dinda B, Bera T, Samanta TK (2012) Generalised intuitionistic fuzzy soft sets and its application in decision making. Ann Fuzzy Math Inform 4(2):207–215
7. Maji PK, Biswas R, Roy AR (2003) Soft set theory. Comput Math Appl 45(4–5):555–562
8. Molodtsov D (1999) Soft set theory's first results. Comput Math Appl 37(4–5):19–31
9. Mushrif MM, Sengupta S, Ray AK (2006) Texture classification using a novel, soft-set theory based classification algorithm, ACCV 2006, LNCS 3851, Springer, Berlin, pp 246–254
10. Roy AR, Maji PK (2007) A fuzzy soft set theoretic approach to decision making problems. J Comput Appl Math 203(2):412–418
11. Ziarko M (1993) Variable precision rough set model. J Comput Syst Sci 46:39–59

Chapter 373
Eliciting the Most Desirable Information with Residuated Lattices

Sylvia Encheva

Abstract Current technologies for collecting and storing data allow users to gather it without been too much concern about devices' capacities. At the same time a very serious question on how to extract significant knowledge from available datasets remains quite open. One non trivial attempt to provide an adequate answer involves residuated lattices.

Keywords Residuated lattices · Concept lattices · Evaluation

373.1 Introduction

Studying and learning seems to be of ever growing interest to researches from various fields. New types of learning materials and evaluation tools are introduced in all educational levels and their usefulness has to be considered. The right amount of information should be presented to the right person while person to person teaching is very rear. In this work we looking at another way of filtering the most desirable information.

Current technologies for collecting and storing data allow users to gather it without been too much concern about devices' capacities. At the same time a very serious question on how to extract significant knowledge from available datasets remains quite open. One non trivial attempt to provide an adequate answer involves residuated lattices, [1].

S. Encheva (✉)
Stord/Haugesund University College, Bjørnsong. 45, 5528 Haugesund, Norway
e-mail: sbe@hsh.no

S. Li et al. (eds.), *Frontier and Future Development of Information Technology in Medicine and Education*, Lecture Notes in Electrical Engineering 269,
DOI: 10.1007/978-94-007-7618-0_373,

373.2 Preliminaries

A lattice is a partially ordered set, closed under least upper and greatest lower bounds. The least upper bound of x and y is called the join of x and y, and is sometimes written as $x + y$; the greatest lower bound is called the meet and is sometimes written as $x\dot{y}$, [2–4].

A complete residuated lattice is a structure $L = \langle L, \wedge, \vee, \otimes, \Rightarrow, 0, 1\rangle$ such that

(i) $\langle L, \wedge, \vee, 0, 1\rangle$ is a complete lattice, i.e., a partially ordered set in which arbitrary infima and suprema exist;
(ii) $\langle L, \otimes, 1\rangle$ is a commutative monoid, i.e., $\otimes$ is a binary operation which is commutative, associative, and $a \otimes 1 = a$ for each $a \in L$;
(iii) $\otimes$ and $\Rightarrow$ satisfy adjointness, i.e., $a \otimes bc$ if $a \leq b \Rightarrow c$.
0 and 1 denote the least and greatest elements. The partial order of L is denoted by $\leq$. To the rest of this article, L is to be understood as an arbitrary complete residuated lattice.
Elements of L are called truth degrees while $\otimes$ and $\Rightarrow$ are 'fuzzy conjunction' and 'fuzzy implication', respectively.
Lukasiewicz pairs of adjoint operations on the unit interval are

$$a \otimes b = \max(a + b - 1, 0)$$

$$a \Rightarrow b = \min(1 - a + b, 1).$$

An L-set (or fuzzy set) A in a universe set X is a mapping assigning to each $x \in X$ some truth degree $A(x) \in L$ where L is the support of a complete residuated lattice. The set of all L-sets in a universe X is denoted L^X.

Binary L-relations (binary fuzzy relations) between X and Y can be thought of as L-sets in the universe $X \times Y$. That is, a binary L-relation $I \in L^{X \times Y}$ between a set X and a set Y is a mapping assigning to each $x \in X$ and each $y \in Y$ a truth degree $I(x, y) \in L$ (a degree to which x and y are related by I). For an L-set $A \in L^X$ and $a \in L$, the a-cut of A is a crisp subset ${}^aA \subseteq X$ such that $x \in^a A$ if $a \leq A(x)$. This definition applies also to binary L-relations, whose a-cuts are interpreted as classical (crisp) binary relations.

For universe X we define L-relation graded subsethood $L^X \times L^X \Rightarrow L$ by: $S(A, B) = \bigwedge_{x \in X} A(x) \Rightarrow B(x)$. $S(A, B)$ represents a degree to which A is a subset of B. The value $A \approx^X B = S(A, B) \wedge S(B, A)$ is interpreted as the degree to which the sets A and B are similar.

A binary L-relation R on a set X is called an *L-tolerance*, if it is reflexive and symmetric, *L-equivalence* if it is reflexive, symmetric and transitive, [5]. Another approach is presented in [6].

Table 373.1

	G1	G2	G3	G4	G5	G6	G7	G8
Theory		0.6		0.8	0.8	1		0.6
Applications	0.6	0.6	0.8		1	0.8		1
Exercises	1	0.8	0.8	1	0.6		0.6	
Visualization	0.8		1	1	0.8	0.6		0.6
Self evaluation tests		1	0.6		1	0.8	0.6	
Help functions	0.8		0.6		1			0.8

373.3 Size of a Concept Lattice

Concept lattices are very useful for unveiling dependences among objects and attributes. A node of a concept lattice is a pair of elements representing objects and attributes. A node in a concept lattice is a formal concept containing the extension and the intension of the concept.

Their readability is considerably decreased with a larger number of objects and attributes. We use the techniques presented in Sect. 373.2 for reducing the size of a concept lattice by applying a-cut.

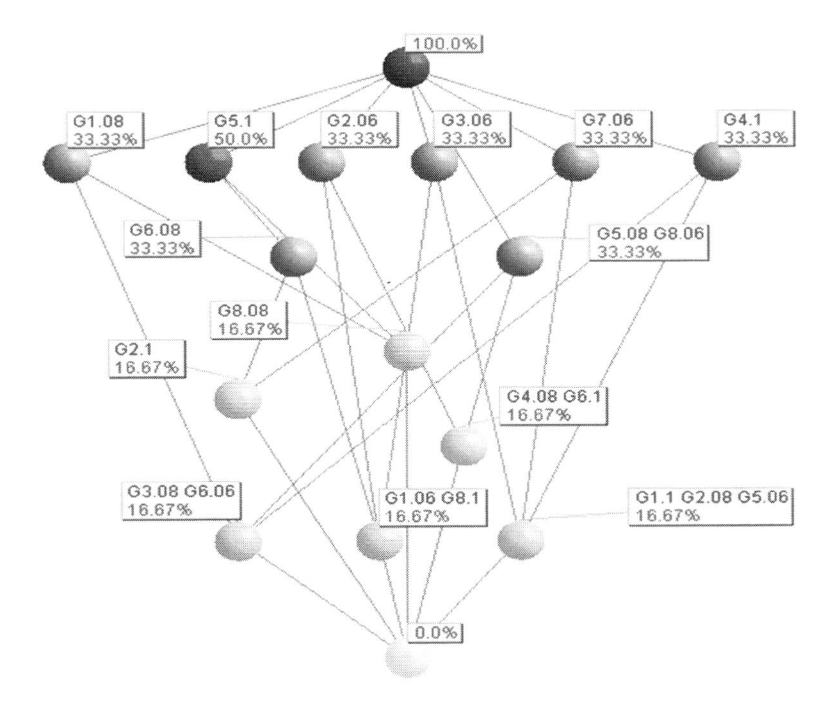

Fig. 373.1 Hasse diagram corresponding to information from Table 373.1

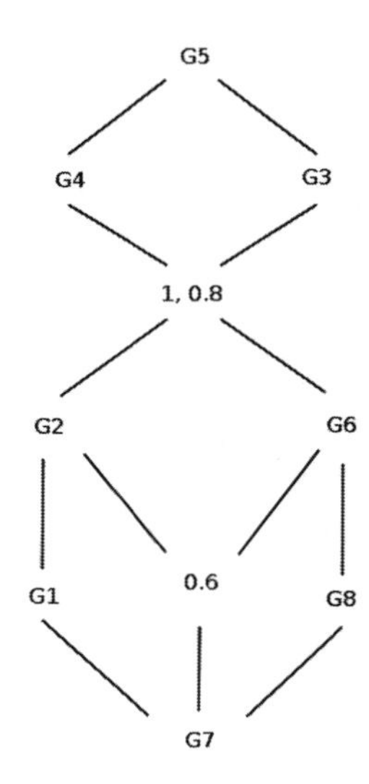

Fig. 373.2 Simplified Hasse diagram corresponding to information from Table 373.1

In particular we are investigating responses of students to questions regarding usefulness of learning materials and applications. Students are grouped according to gender and results obtained from a preliminary test. Students opinions are summarized in Table 373.1.

By 'Applications' (A) we mean illustrative examples where students can see how the presented theory is used in real life situations. 'Exercises' (E) refer to examples which students can try to solve. 'Visualizations' (V) are actually interactive Java applets showing how changing values of some elements is effecting the final outcome. 'Help functions' (H) are understood to be the automated messages assisting students in solving problems without the presence of a human tutor.

Evaluations are based on 10 points scale and responses below 0.6 are not shown to avoid difficulties in reading the corresponding lattice in Fig. 373.1. The result after a-cut of 0.7 is presented in Fig. 373.2. This way the number of nodes in the simplified Hasse diagram is reduced by about 50 %.

373.4 Conclusion

The a-cut approach is certainly useful for reducing the size of a concept lattice but it is too laborious. While the techniques to realize an a-cut are known it is still unclear how to determine a proper size for an a-cut. Balancing between readability and not loosing important information is an interesting question for future work.

References

1. Wille R (1985) Complete tolerance relations of concept lattices. In: Eigenthaler G et al (eds) Contributions to general algebra, vol 3, pp 397–415
2. Carpineto C, Romano G (2004) Concept data analysis: theory and applications. Wiley, Chichester
3. Davey BA, Priestley HA (2005) Introduction to lattices and order. Cambridge University Press, Cambridge
4. Ganter B, Wille R (1999) Formal concept analysis—mathematical foundations. Springer, Berlin
5. Czedli G (1982) Factor lattices by tolerances. Acta Sci Math 44:35–42
6. Meschke C (2010) Approximations in concept lattices. In: Kwuida L, Sertkaya B (eds) Formal concept analysis, Lecture notes in computer science, vol 5986. Springer, Berlin, pp 104–123
7. Ward M, Dilworth RP (1939) Residuated lattices. Trans Am Math Soc 45:335–354

Chapter 374
Research on Data Exchange Platform Based on IPSec and XML

Li Bo

Abstract Collaborative management and administrative examination and approval requires a large amount of data exchange across different management systems. In order to solve the problem of data format between different management systems and ensure the security and integrity of data exchange, using the data exchange sub-platform in walling management platform of Jinan city as an example, a new scheme of data exchange platform based on IPSec and XML is presented. This scheme use XML to realize the standardization of data and achieve reliable transmission of data using IPSec.

Keywords Data exchange · IPSec · XML

374.1 Introduction

E-government construction of China has a rapid development, but it also brought the problems of data sharing across different platforms: various government departments and various social units constructed their information systems independently with different standards and different platforms, formed numerous of isolated islands of information. Data exchange between different management systems is needed for the collaborative management and administrative examination and approval. How to realize the secure, convenient data exchange between government departments, enterprises, banks and other units is one of the technical problems need to be solved in the current construction of e-government.

This paper designs a secure data exchange platform model based on IPSec and XML technology to provide a reliable, safe, correct data exchange service for all

L. Bo (✉)
Shandong Polytechnic, No.23000 East Jingshi Road, Jinan, Shandong, China
e-mail: 24874890@qq.com

S. Li et al. (eds.), *Frontier and Future Development of Information Technology in Medicine and Education*, Lecture Notes in Electrical Engineering 269,
DOI: 10.1007/978-94-007-7618-0_374,

types of cross-sectors, cross-platform isomeric application systems. It will greatly improve the work efficiency and information security of the government administrative examination and approval.

374.2 Requirements of the Data Exchange Platform

Data exchange platform is one of the core contents of the e-government constructions, is the key of success or failure of e-government system construction. The e-government data exchange platform must meet the following requirements [1]: unified data standard, stronger safety, good data format, immediate data integration and other requirements. In addition, the data exchange platform should own the characteristics of loosely-coupled, flexibility, scalability, availability.

374.3 Structural Framework of the Data Exchange Platform

This paper adopts star topology using the data exchange platform as the central node, all data exchange between application nodes through the central node, so if any communication node changes, other nodes basically do not need to be modified.

An end-to-end secure connection to ensure the data security between management systems and data exchange platform can be realized by the use of IPSec [2]. XML is used by each system to format and transform the heterogeneous data for sharing [3]. The overall designed framework is shown in Fig. 374.1, mainly composed of the data conversion module, IPSec driver module, security policy module and IKE service module [4].

374.4 Module Function Design of the Data Exchange Platform

374.4.1 Data Conversion Module

Data conversion module works on the application layer, locates in the interface of each management systems. It mainly includes two functions: first is the conversion of outgoing data, forming the standard data marked by XML; second is converts the received standard data to specific data that could be recognized and used by local management system. Middleware technology can be used for data conversion of those databases which cannot support XML. Data exchange model based on

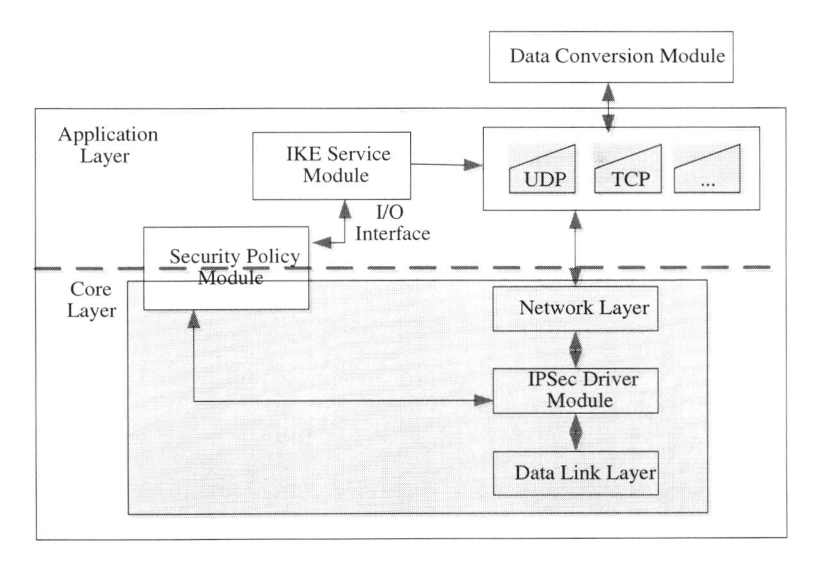

Fig. 374.1 System structure framework

XML is shown in Fig. 374.2. We can use the XML parser Xerces for mapping data to XML documents and use DOM (Document Object Model) for mapping XML files to local database. IPSec is used to encrypt data between source and destination to ensure the information security.

374.4.2 IPSec Driver Module

This is the core module to ensure the data security of the data exchange platform, responsible for processing IPSec security protocol, executing the authentication algorithm and encryption algorithm. It is divided into 3 sub-modules as shown in Fig. 374.3 [5].

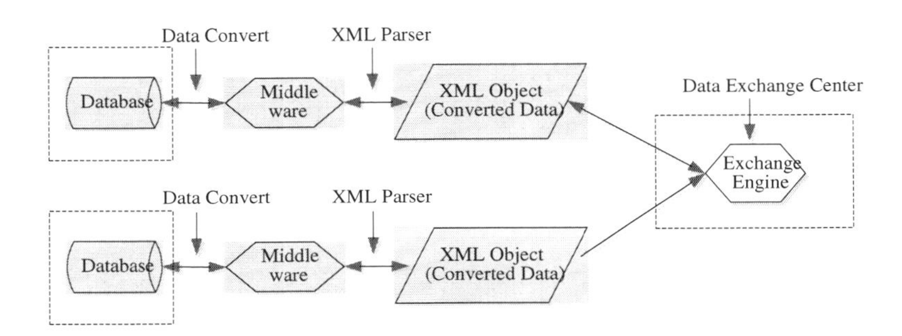

Fig. 374.2 Data exchange model of the data conversion module

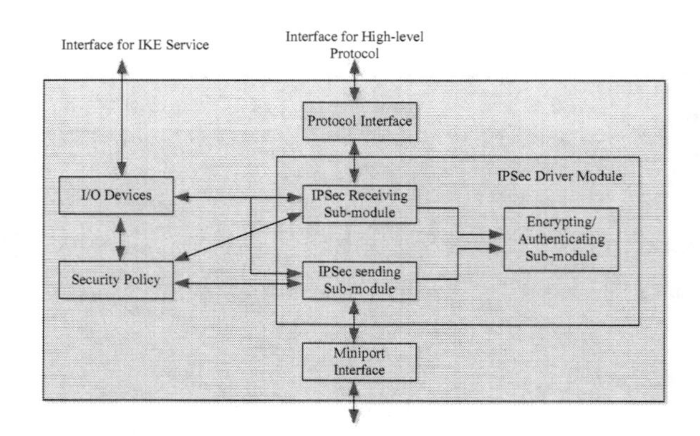

Fig. 374.3 IPSec drive module structure

(1) IPSec receiving sub-module. Mainly used to receive the data frames, execute AH and ESP deblocking, dispose the received data frames with IPSec and then send to the high-level TCP/IP protocol.

(2) IPSec sending sub-module. Mainly used to complete the ESP package, AH package and IPSec transmission, process the data frames sent by high-level protocol and then send them to the NIC driver. The data frames will be sent to the data exchange platform by the physical network card.

(3) Encrypting/authenticating sub-module. Mainly used to implements DES-CBC or 3DES-CBC encryption algorithms in accordance with the IPSec protocol and provide the API call interface [6].

374.4.3 IPSec Security Policy Module

Security policy module runs on the application layer and in the system's kernel, composed of policy server, policy client and policy database. Policy server provides an interactive operating interface for adding, deleting and modifying the policy configurations. Policy client exists in the operating systems in the form of services, sends policy requirements to policy server and monitors policy changes at the same time. Policy database module is implemented in the kernel, mainly used to preserve policy information.

374.4.4 IKE Service Module

The Internet Key Exchange (IKE) service module executes IKE protocol, is responsible for the identity authentication and policy negotiation between two communicators, and establishes Security Association (SA), dynamically manages and updates the SA, deletes expired SA. In addition, also need to be responsible for handling users' configuration commands, processing of IKE data packet, verification and encryption of IKE load.

374.5 Summaries and Acknowledgments

This paper carries on the detailed function design of the e-government data exchange platform based on XML and IPsec. Practice found that encryption, authentication and encapsulation of data using IPSec will reduce the efficiency of the system in a certain extent. In the following work, further study and research is needed to carry on the more efficient data exchange platform.

This research was supported by the Project of Shandong Province Higher Educational Science and Technology Program under Grant No.J12LN61. It was also supported by the Project of Shandong Province Higher Educational Science and Technology Program under Grant No.J13LN64. In addition, the author would like to thank the reviewers for their valuable comments and suggestions.

References

1. Post G, Ahmadi S, Daskalaki S, Kingston JH, Kyngas J, Nurmi C, Ranson D (2012) An XML format for benchmarks in High School Timetabling. Ann Oper Res 194(1):385–397. doi:10.1007/s10479-010-0699-9
2. Wang A-m, Li X, Song Q (2012) Key technologies research of transfer rate test in electronic information exchange platform. Advances in mechanical and electronic engineering, Lecture notes in electrical engineering, vol 177, pp 627–631. DOI: 10.1007/978-3-642-31516-9_101
3. Migault D (2012) E2E: an optimized IPsec architecture for secure and fast offload., 2012 Seventh international conference on availability, reliability and security (ARES). 20–24 Aug 2012, pp 365–374. doi: 10.1109/ARES.2012.80
4. Luniya R, Agarwal A, Bhatnagar M, Rathod V, Unwalla D (2012) SmartX–advanced network security for windows operating system. Third international conference on intelligent systems, modelling and simulation (ISMS), 2012, pp 680–683. doi: 10.1109/ISMS.2012.43
5. Zhang Y, Zhang Y (2012) Cloud computing and cloud security challenges. Proceedings of 2012 international symposium on ITME, 2012, issue no I, pp 1084–1088
6. Tan W, Xie Y, Li D, Liu M (2011) A modified securities model based on public key infrastructure. Commun Comput Info Sci 226:252–259

Chapter 375
Integration and Utilization of Digital Learning Resources in Community Education

Liangtao Yang

Abstract Community education is an important part to advance the construction of learning society. In the process of the development of community education, digital learning resources will greatly improve the learning effectiveness and quality; effectively expand the public space for learning and it can create new options and opportunities for learners. Based on analyzing the advantages of digital learning resources, this paper shows the strategy of integration and utilization of digital learning resources in community education.

Keywords Community education · Digital learning resources · Integration sharing

375.1 Introduction

With the application of multimedia technology and network technology in education and teaching, a new learning mode—digital learning came into being. Digital learning resources are the multimedia material which has been digitized and can be run in a multimedia computer or network environment. It can stimulate the students through independent, cooperative, creative way to find and process information, so that the digital learning becomes possible. Digital learning resources include digital video, digital audio, multimedia software, learning sites, online learning management system, computer simulation, online discussions and databases. Digital learning resources are the foundation for E-learning and its construction and application will directly impact on the level of the digital learning

---

L. Yang (✉)
Shanghai Second Polytechnic University, Shanghai, China
e-mail: ltyang@sspu.cn

S. Li et al. (eds.), *Frontier and Future Development of Information Technology in Medicine and Education*, Lecture Notes in Electrical Engineering 269,
DOI: 10.1007/978-94-007-7618-0_375,

effect. It is foreseeable that in the upcoming learning society, learning will rely more on digital learning resources [1].

Community education is self-generated by the community residents in a certain geographical area to improve the overall quality of the community. It is public education activities promoted by the government joint efforts with local grassroots organizations to promote regional economic construction and social development. The development of community education is an important way to create a learning society and harmonious society. Digital learning resources should be rich, sharing, personalization, dynamic update, which coincides with the characteristics of the community education. It is very important to make full use of digital learning resources for community education. This paper focuses on how to integrate and use digital learning resources for community education.

375.2 The Advantages of Digital Learning Resources in Community Education

As a product of the progress and development of information technology, digital learning resources have some features such as development, openness, comprehensiveness and diversity, which are closely related to the characteristics of the community education. Because of the many advantages of digital learning resources, it has a very important practical significance to explore the integration and application of digital learning resources for the construction of a learning society [2].

375.2.1 The Expansibility of Digital Learning Resources According with the Lifetime of Community Education

Compared with other learning media, digital learning resources has the incomparable advantage and has become the people's most convenient learning resources. Most of the traditional learning resources are made on paper as a carrier and its presentation form is single. In addition to text and image, digital learning resources can present the information by others ways as well as audio, video, animation and other forms of multimedia information. It can mobilize people's senses receive information from visual, hearing, etc., can be fully, accurately and efficiently present information, people use it to learn to be able to master knowledge and skills better and faster. As digital technology continues to improve, digital learning resources will be more advanced and convenient form of expression. At the same time, the expansion and the reproducibility of digital learning resources can integrate and expand the knowledge to meet the learning needs of different learners and the same learning needs of learners in different periods. Digital learning resources can provide the residents with education platform and the development of digital learning resources make community education become a good relying on the resources.

375.2.2 The Openness of Digital Learning Resources According with the Popularity of Community Education

The openness of digital learning resources refers to the resource for all sectors of industry, the comprehensive public service. At present, the main way by which presents digital learning resources includes network, TV, digital library, mobile communication network. The network is the main way of presenting digital learning resources. Various educational resources including government departments and educational institutions construction, relying on the advantages of the network and the auxiliary and the other way, will make digital learning resources everywhere. Thus it can be seen that digital learning resources are available to all learning resources, is conducive to learning effective carrier of society, so that each person has an equal rights to get free, public resources. The spread of digital learning resources to learners is not affected by time, region and the location. Coverage of digital learning resources make all kinds of people carry out learning exchanges in different regions, different time and learning methods. Therefore, as long as the digital learning resources can be reasonable uses by the whole society, the goal of community education will certainly be achieved.

375.2.3 The Comprehensiveness of Digital Learning Resources According with the Universality of Community Education

The comprehensiveness of digital learning resources refers that in a small physical space, information unlimited, covering all kinds of people with different learning content. Resources can stored various achievements of human civilization and different cultures, ideas and concepts for people to understand from a different perspective, absorption. Resources contain all kinds of skills, knowledge and common sense on work, entertainment, family and social life, which is beneficial to human and life improvement. Resources can contain at all times and in all countries the wealth of knowledge, let people learn and appreciate from all sides. Community education is a breakthrough to the school education in the knowledge and skills, comprehensive digital learning resources can meet the different needs of various groups, let the young students to acquire knowledge, let the occupation of people skills, let the laid-off workers obtain employment, let the elderly residents get happiness...... This is the pursuit of the value of the learning type society.

375.2.4 The Diversity of Digital Learning Resources According with the Flexibility of Community Education

The diversity of digital learning resources refers that resources have different manifestations, transmission carrier, form of access, communication methods by the technical support. On the one hand, the digital learning content can be presented by the form of hypertext structure, multimedia integration manifested; on the other hand, network transmission and remote sharing, reading, watching, download free become quick and easy. At the same time, the digital learning resources are convenient and effective between the learner and the learner to achieve the two-way transfer between the learner and the learning content and feedback function. Digital learning resources can make learners choose a different form of resources, to achieve the best learning effect according to their own needs. Digital learning resources can be no time limit open, provides flexible learning time for learning, people can independently determine the learning objectives, plan the learning process and achieve the aims of learning. Community education is the learner's self-directed learning, and digital learning resources are conducive to flexible learning, which reflects the learner-centered ideology in community education.

375.3 The Integration of Digital Learning Resources in Community Education

375.3.1 To Strengthen the Overall Leadership of the Government

With a deeper understanding of role and function of Community Education in the Learning Society and harmonious society, our government and the relevant departments at all levels start to lead, manage and supervise the community education. On the one hand, extensive service object in community education demands that the construction of educational resources must be multiple and rich; On the other hand, the awareness and the concept that community resources should be integrated and shared needs to be strengthened. The advantage of power and the ability of government in social resources planning directly affect the degree of integration of education resources and the development of community education [3]. Therefore, the integration of digital education resources demands our government lead, organize, coordinate and mobilize the aspects of community education to form a stable relationship.

In the process of integration of educational resources, there is arbitrariness and instability. Therefore, the government must formulate relevant policies and regulations to safeguard the stability. Perfect regulation policy can overcome arbitrariness and guarantee the healthy, stable development of community education. The government should use policy means to show the importance of resources integration, to show the responsibilities and obligations which the government departments should take. Only in this way, we can ensure the long-term and stable community education resource integration.

375.3.2 To Realize the Sharing of Digital Learning Resources

Resource sharing is to uniformly plan and commonly use the resources which belong to different organizations through a variety of methods, techniques and strategies. From a technical point of view, it is to achieve a variety of types of distribution of resources to watch and download in support of the relevant technical standards. From the operational point of view, it is to establish learning resource nodes throughout the whole of society to form the open learning resource service network to provide the whole society.

Abundant digital learning resources provide the powerful support for the people's learning. Resource construction is a huge engineering which cost a lot of human, material and financial resources. If digital learning resources are self-occupied, its efficiency is extremely low. To achieve the greatest degree of sharing is the fundamental way for the construction of digital learning resources. First of all, the integration of resources through the network can realize retrieval and hyperlinks. Secondly, the integration of resources can realize common construction and common use.

375.3.3 To Strengthen the Integration of Digital Learning Resources

At present, all levels of the community college is committed to creating community digital learning platform, the platform construction are mostly single centralized resource storage model based on their own, and community education massive resource demand and fast access to, any single community college to all tasks, so common problems we encounter is: multiple learning needs and single supply of resources. To resolve this contradiction, the key is to change the single point mode of resources supply and try to establish a multi-node distributed storage. At the same time we must set up a special community education institution to coordinate resources integration and sharing.

375.4 The Effective Use of Digital Learning Resources

375.4.1 Establishing Measures to Generalize Digital Learning Resources

The focus is to improve the degree of awareness, recognition and participation of digital learning resources to promote digital learning resources. We should use the network, newspapers, radio, television and other ways to promote digital learning resources and public resources information. We should form a communication mechanism led by the government, civil society organizations actively involved in, the social parties responded positively. We should improve the people's information literacy, and foster the people's attitude and ability about information integration and utilization. We should mobilize all digital learning enthusiasm and improve the participation of citizens by creating the environment, theme activities, achievements and example encouragement [4].

375.4.2 Improving the Service System of Digital Learning Resources

The service system of digital learning resources includes platform support services and technical support services. The so-called platform support service is the basis of digital learning. The learner can carry out all kinds of learning, completion of the learning task through a variety of platforms. These platforms are: network platform support services, learning platform and management platform [5]. The so-called technical support services, is an important part of the technical problems to solve learners, designed to help learners to overcome the digital learning disorder, make full use of good digitization facilities, so that the digital learning to maximize the benefits. They are: technical guidance services, technical maintenance services, software development and technical training support services.

375.4.3 Generalizing Learning Methods in Digital Learning Environment

Learning methods mean that learners carry out a variety of learning activities in the digital learning environment by using digital learning resources, which reflects the learner' basic characteristics such as autonomy, explore and collaborative. In digital learning, learning methods are not only to optimize the learning process but also are to play an orientation, stimulation and polymerization role. So-called orientation is a certain way by which we can learn in accordance with the process of the right. The so-called excitation is to use a scientific method to mobilize everyone's enthusiasm for learning, and lead to a wider range of learning. The so-called polymerization is a specific learning by which we will gather together to learn together.

375.4.4 Improving the Training System

The construction of teachers is an important part of effective application of digital learning resources. However, the majority of teachers who are lack of information literacy are not able to meet the needs of the development of the digital age. Because of lack of effective guidance, students cannot efficiently and quickly get the information in the digital learning environment. Especially in the digital library, network environment, a virtual community learning, our students will become lost easily. Thus it is an urgent need to carry out comprehensive and systematic training for teachers and students.

375.5 Conclusion

In short, the digital learning resources is an important material resources to carry out community education, is an important part to create a learning society. Digital learning resources is an integral part in future society, is an important social resource to guide the new trend of development and application of learning resources. With the deepening of construction of learning social and the growing dependence on digital learning resources, the integration of digital learning resources and integration strategy will be our exhaustive research topics.

References

1. He KK (2009) Present situation and countermeasures of digital learning resources construction in China. China Audiovisual Educ 11:5–9
2. Wang J, Yang G, Kong L (2011) Research on the development strategy of domestic digital learning resources. J Distance Educ 5:41–44
3. Song Y (2011) Analysis of integration strategy of digital learning resources from the perspective of learning society. China Adult Educ 2011(3):46–49
4. Hao M, Zhang W (2010) On the resource development of universities in community education. Adult Educ 8:23–24
5. Li X, Han J (2012) The integration of community education resources under the framework of learning society. Educ Vocat 2012(11):167–168

Chapter 376
Correlation of Aberrant Methylation of APC Gene to MTHFR C677T Genetic Polymorphisms in Hepatic Carcinoma

Lian-Hua Cui, Meng Liu, Hong-Zong Si, Min-Ho Shin, Hee Nam Kim and Jin-Su Choi

Abstract *Object* To investigate the relationship between aberrant hypermethylation of APC gene and methylenetetrahydrofolate reductase (MTHFR) C677T genetic polymorphisms in Hepatic Carcinoma. *Method* Hepatic Carcinoma cancer tissues and para-cancerous normal tissues were collected. CpG island methylation status of APC gene and MTHFR gene polymorphisms were analyzed by Real-time quantitative polymerase chain reaction (Real-time PCR). The associations between methylation status of APC gene and clinical characteristics, as well as the relationship between *APC* methylation and MTHFR C677T polymorphisms, were evaluated. *Results* Among 86 HCC patients, the aberrant hypermethylation rate of APC gene in tumorous tissues (77.9 %) was significantly higher than that in para-cancerous normal tissues (46.5 %). No relationship was found between APC gene methylation and selected factors including sex, age, tumor size, TNM stage, HBsAg and AFP. After adjustment for potential confounders, individuals carrying MTHFR 677 T allele gene have higher frequency of hypermethylation in APC gene in cancer tissues, with odds ratio of 3.64(95 % CI: 1.13–11.79). Our results suggested that MTHFR 677 T allele might be associated with aberrant methylation of APC gene.

Keywords APC methylation · MTHFR gene polymorphism · Hepatic carcinoma

---

L.-H. Cui (✉) · M. Liu
Department of Public Health, Qingdao University, Qingdao, China
e-mail: qdlhcui@163.com

H.-Z. Si
Institute for Computational Science and Engineering, the Growing Base for State Key Laboratory, Qingdao University, Qingdao, China

M.-H. Shin · J.-S. Choi
Department of Preventive Medicine, Chonnam National University Medical School, Gwangju, South Korea

H. N. Kim
Genome Research Center for Hematopoietic Diseases, Chonnam National University Hwasun Hospital, Hwasun, Jeollanam-do, South Korea

S. Li et al. (eds.), *Frontier and Future Development of Information Technology in Medicine and Education*, Lecture Notes in Electrical Engineering 269,
DOI: 10.1007/978-94-007-7618-0_376,

376.1 Introduction

DNA methylation, an epigenetic modification, is the process by which DNA methyltransferase (DNMTs) catalyzes a methyl group from S-adenosylmethionine (SAM) and attaches it to the 5′carbon of a cytosine pyrimidine ring, resulting in 5-methylcytosine. DNA methylation is common on endogenous genes in eukaryotic cells. It plays an important role in gene mutation, genetic imprinting, the regulation of gene expression, and cell proliferation, differentiation, and development [1]. DNA methylation usually occurs in CpG islands, which are CG-rich regions upstream of the promoter region. Methylation of CpG islands rarely occurs in normal cells but frequently occurs in tumor cells, where it causes the silencing of tumor suppressor genes [2, 3]. The methyl group required for DNA methylation is provided by the folate metabolic pathway. In this way, DNA methylation is closely correlated with folate metabolism. Folic acid is an essential nutrient in the body, and its main biological function is to donate a methyl group for cellular DNA methylation and synthesis.

Recently, some studies showed that genetic polymorphisms in MTHFR might be associated with aberrant methylation in tumor-related genes in gastric cancer and esophageal cancer [4, 5]. However, to our knowledge, there is no study on the association between aberrant DNA methylation in tumor-related genes and polymorphisms in genes involved in folate metabolism in liver cancer patients. Therefore, we evaluated APC gene promoter methylation in 86 liver tumors and corresponding adjacent tissues and performed an association analysis with the polymorphism of the MTHFR C677T gene.

376.2 Materials and Methods

376.2.1 Subjects Selection

The tumor tissues of HCC and corresponding adjacent nontumorous liver tissue were obtained from 86 patients who underwent radical surgical resection for hepatocellular carcinoma between 2008 and 2009 at affiliated Hospital of Medical College Qingdao University in Qingdao, China. Patients undergoing any therapeutic intervention were excluded. Fresh samples from tumor and corresponding adjacent nontumorous liver tissue (2–5 cm from the tumor) were frozen at −80 °C immediately after resection. Informed consent was obtained from all patients. This study was approved by the Institutional Review Board of the Affiliated Hospital of Medical College Qingdao University, China.

376.2.2 Outcome Collection

Data were collected from the questionnaire survey on the content includes general case such as age, gender, and clinical characteristics following with HBsAg, tumor size, tumor stage and AFP. Stage was in the light of the TNM staging standards for primary hepatic carcinoma, formulated by Union for International Cancer Control (UICC). Collection was performed by laboratory personnel undergone normal training.

376.2.3 DNA Extraction

DNA was extracted from fresh frozen tumor tissues using Animal DNAout kit (TianDZ, Beijing, China), following the manufacturer's recommendations. The indicators A260‘ A280 and A260/A280 need to be measured and counted to meet the quality and purity. Finally, available DNA was stored at −80 °C until used.

376.2.4 Methylation Analysis of the APC Gene Promoter

Real-time quantitative polymerase chain reaction (Real-time PCR) was used to detect the CpG island methylation status of the APC gene. PCR amplification and HRM analysis were performed on the Rotor-Gene 6000TM (Corbett Research, Mortlake, Australia).The sequences of the primers used were as follows: APC forward primer, GAACCAAAACGCTCCCCAT, APC reverse primer, TTATA TGTCGGTTACGTGCGTTTATAT. PCR was carried out in 10 μl total volume containing: 2× Epitech HRM Master Mix (containg HotStarTaq® Plus DNA Polymerase, EpiTect HRM PCR Buffer, EvaGreen® dye and dNTP mix), 200 nmol/l of each primer, 25 ng of bisulphite-modified template. The following PCR conditions were performed: 20 s of initial denaturation at 95 °C; 30 s of anneal at the appropriate temperature (63 °C) followed by 45 cycles of 72 °C for 30 s, 95 °C for 1 min; HRM was performed from 55 to 90 °C, with a temperature increase at the rate of 0.2 °C/s for all assays. The annealing temperature was experimentally determined for each assay to ensure that only methylated templates were amplified. The control of fully methylated and fully unmethylated, as well as no template control were also included in every run.

376.2.5 Genotyping

Genotyping for the detection of the MTHFR C677T polymorphism was performed by real-time polymerase chain reaction (PCR), using dual-labeled probes containing locked nucleic acids (LNA), in a real-time PCR assay [6]. PCR primers and LNA probes were designed and synthesized by Intergrated DNA Technologies (IDT, Coralville, IA, USA).

376.2.6 Statistical Analyses

All analyses were performed using the Statistical Package for the Social Sciences software (ver. 13.0; SPSS, Chicago, IL, USA). Pearson's Chi square tests and Fisher's Exact tests were used in univariate analyses. A logistic regression analysis was used to analyze the correlation between APC methylation and the polymorphism of MTHFR.

376.3 Results

376.3.1 Patient Characteristics

The 86 Patients with HCC consisted of 69 (80.2 %) men and 17 (19.8 %) women; 57 (66.3 %) samples aged 60 and below, and 29 (33.7 %) cases more than 60 - years of age; 71 HBsAg positive (82.6 %) and 15 HBsAg negative (17.4 %).

376.3.2 Methylation Analysis of APC Gene Promoter

Genotype frequencies of APC gene promoter is as follows: for methylated cancer tissue 77.9 % (67) and for methylated paracancerous normal tissues 46.5 % (40). The results showed that compared with the corresponding adjacent nontumorous liver tissue, the frequency of methylation in APC gene promoter area of cancer tissue was significantly higher ($p < 0.05$).

376.3.3 Association between APC Methylation and Clinical Characteristics in the HCC Patients Tissue

Table 376.1 showed association between APC gene Methylation and Clinical Characteristics in the HCC. The aberrant methylation status in the promoter region of APC gene in tumor tissues were not correlated with age, sex, tumor stage, tumor size, HBsAg and the level of AFP ($p > 0.05$).

376.3.4 Association between APC Gene Methylation and MTHFR Genetic Polymorphisms in Liver Cancer Patients

Association between APC gene methylation and MTHFR C677T genetic polymorphisms in liver cancer patients was present in Table 376.2. After adjusting other potential confounders such as age and gender, we found that the APC gene methylation frequency in the hepatic carcinoma cancer tissue from carriers of MTHFR677 TT genotypes was significantly increased, compared with MTHFR 677 CC genotype, with the OR of 3.91(95 % CI: 0.98–15.59).

376.4 Discussion

DNA methylation has been found to be a common epigenetic modification. It plays an important role in the regulation of gene expression and the maintenance of normal cell differentiation. Changes in the levels and patterns of genomic

Table 376.1 Association between APC methylation and clinical characteristics in the HCC

Clinical characteristics		Number	HCC cancer tissue	
			Methylated N (%)	P Value
Sex	Male	69	53 (76.8)	
	Female	17	14(82.4)	0.662
Age (years)	<60	57	45(78.9)	
	≥60	29	22(75.9)	0.744
HBsAg	Negative	15	10(66.7)	
	Positive	71	57(80.3)	0.248
TNM stage	I + II	53	42(72.9)	
	III + IV	33	25(75.8)	0.705
Tumor size(cm)	<5	46	37(80.4)	
	≥5	40	30(70.5)	0.545
AFP (μg/l)	≤7.02	24	18(75.0)	
	>7.02	62	49(79.0)	0.686

Compared with Paracancerous normal tissues, $p < 0.05$

Table 376.2 Association between methylation of APC gene and MTHFR C677T polymorphism in HCC

MTHFR C677T	Cancer tissue		
Genotype	Methylated (N %)	OR[a] (95 %CI)	P Value
CC	9(13.4)	1	
CT	32(47.8)	3.45(0.95–12.53)	0.060
TT	26(38.8)	3.91(0.98–15.59)	0.053
CT + TT	58(86.6)	3.64(1.13–11.79)	0.031

OR[a] , adjusted by sex and age

methylation may result in gene silencing and deficits in corresponding proteins. These are the early events in HCC [7].

The adenomatous polyposis col (APC) gene is located in 5q21-q22 and encodes varieties of tumor suppressor proteins connected with the Wnt signaling pathway. In the pathway, the APC protein forms a complex with actin, causingβ-catenin degradation by the proteasome. Allelic loss, mutation, or hypermethylation may lead to the lack of APC protein expression, which preventingβ-catenin degradation, thus stimulating the abnormal transcription of several oncogenes [8].

APC gene is frequently inactivated by DNA mutations, but also an epigenetic mechanism that involves aberrant DNA methylation of promoters which is a form of non-gene mutations in tumor formation [9]. During carcinogenesis, DNA hypermethylation-induced silencing of tumor suppressor is a frequent phenomenon. Guoren et al. [9] reported that the methylation of CpG island in APC promoter silenced gene expression by changing the chromatin conformation and interfering with the binding of transcription factor CCAAT binding factor, aberrant promoter methylation may suppress the expression of adenomatous polyposis col. In addition, several studies demonstrate that APC methylation is associated with some cancers, for instance, human prostate cancer, breast cancer,lung cancer and colorectal cancer, also including HCC [10–14]. Dong et al. [15]. and Priyanka et al. [16] showed that the frequency of APC gene promoter methylation in cancer tissue of HCC was significantly higher than those of surrounding nontumorous tissues and the control group ($p < 0.05$).Also, Feng et al. [14] investigated APC methylation levels are significantly higher in hepatocellular carcinoma tissues compare to adjacent tissues and liver cirrhosis. Similarly, our results showed the frequency of APC gene promoter methylation in HCC (77.9 %) to be significantly higher than in adjacent tissues (46.5 %).However, in another study, APC methylation was not detectable in HCC, adjacent tissues, or normal liver tissue; the researchers performing that study speculated that APC gene methylation might not play a role in the development of liver cancer and that there might not be any functional genetic or epigenetic loss [17]. These inconsistent results may be due to patient sample size and different methods of methylation detection. Dong et al. [15] and Priyanka et al. [16] have investigated that APC hypermethylation is not association with age or gender, TNM stage, tumor size, HBV infection, smoking, drinking, and serum AFP levels in HCC patients tissues. Concordantly, we did not observe a significant relationship between APC methylation and clinical characteristics.

MTHFR is the key enzymes in folate metabolism. Mutations in the MTHFR gene may reduce the thermal stability and activity of the resulting enzymes, thereby affecting normal folate metabolism and the supply of methyl groups in vivo, affecting the normal intracellular DNA methylation and promoting tumor development. With the development of molecular biology, the association between polymorphisms in MTHFR and cancer-related gene methylation has seen increasing study. Currently, some studies showed that polymorphisms in *MTHFR* was connected with several cancers, such as gastric, esophageal, and prostate cancer,in which tumor–related genes are aberrant methylation [18, 19]. However, few study demonstrated the association between MTHFR C677T gene polymorphism and aberrant APC methylation in HCC patients.

Our study reported that the frequencies of APC gene promoter methylation was significantly increased in carriers of the MTHFR C677T mutation relative to individuals with the wild type MTHFR 677CC genotype. The frequencies of APC gene promoter methylation significantly increased up to 3.64-fold, in carriers of the MTHFR C677T mutation versus those with the wild type MTHFR 677CC genotype. Our results suggested that MTHFR 677 C > T SNP might be a risk factor for APC gene promoter methylation. MTHFR C677T polymorphism increased the frequencies of APC gene promoter methylation in liver cancer, which may promote tumor development.

Acknowledgments This work was supported, in part, by the National Natural Science Foundation of China (Contract No. 30872169) and the Natural Science Foundation of China (Contract No. ZR2011HM031).

References

1. Laird PW, Jaenisch R (1996) The role of DNA methylation in cancer genetic and epigenetics. Annu Rev Genet 30:441–464
2. Baylin SB (2005) DNA methylation and gene silencing in cancer. Nat Clin Pract Oncol 2(Suppl 1):S4–11
3. Baoxing FKZ, Dechang W (2002) DNA methylation and tumor. Foreign Med Mole Biol 24(3):139–143
4. Graziano F, Kawakami K, Ruzzo A et al (2006) Methylenetetrahydrofolate reductase 677C/T gene polymorphism, gastric cancer susceptibility and genomic DNA hypomethylation in an at-risk Italian population. Int J Cancer J Int Du Cancer 118(3):628–632
5. Wang J, Sasco AJ, Fu C et al (2008) Aberrant DNA methylation of P16, MGMT, and hMLH1 genes in combination with MTHFR C677T genetic polymorphism in esophageal squamous cell carcinoma. Cancer Epidemiol Biomark Prev 17(1):118–125
6. Kim HN, Lee IK, Kim YK et al (2008) Association between folate-metabolizing pathway polymorphism and non-Hodgkin lymphoma. Br J Haematol 140(3):287–294
7. Bárbara do Nascimento Borges RMRB MLH (2013) Analysis of the methylation patterns of the p16INK4A, p15INK4B, and APC genes in gastric adenocarcinoma patients from a Brazilian population. Tumor Biol doi: 101007/s13277-013-0742-y

8. Kondo Y, Kanai Y, Sakamoto M et al (2000) Genetic instability and aberrant DNA methylation in chronic hepatitis and cirrhosis–A comprehensive study of loss of heterozygosity and microsatellite instability at 39 loci and DNA hypermethylation on 8 CpG islands in microdissected specimens from patients with hepatocellular carcinoma. Hepatology 32(5):970–979
9. Deng G, Song GA, Pong E et al (2004) Promoter methylation inhibits APC gene expression by causing changes in chromatin conformation and interfering with the binding of transcription factor CCAAT-binding factor. Cancer Res 64(8):2692–2698
10. Yoon HY, Kim YW, Kang HW et al (2013) Pyrosequencing analysis of APC methylation level in human prostate tissues: a molecular marker for prostate cancer. Korean J Urol 54(3):194–198
11. Tserga AMN, Levidou G, Korkolopoulou P et al (2012) Association of aberrant DNA methylation with clinicopathological features in breast cancer. Oncol Reports 27(5):1630–1638
12. Begum S, Brait M, Dasgupta S et al (2011) An epigenetic marker panel for detection of lung cancer using cell-free serum DNA. Clin Cancer Res 17(13):4494–4503
13. Kang HJ, Kim EJ, Kim BG et al (2012) Quantitative analysis of cancer-associated gene methylation connected to risk factors in Korean colorectal cancer patients. J Prev Med Public Health 45:251–258
14. Feng Q, Stern JE, Hawes SE et al (2010) DNA methylation changes in normal liver tissues and hepatocellular carcinoma with different viral infection. Exp Mol Pathol 88(2):287–292
15. Hua D, Hu Y, Wu YY et al (2011) Quantitative methylation analysis of multiple genes using methylation-sensitive restriction enzyme-based quantitative PCR for the detection of hepatocellular carcinoma. Exp Mol Pathol 91:455–460
16. Iyer P, Zekri AR, Hung CW et al (2010) Concordance of DNA methylation pattern in plasma and tumor DNA of Egyptian hepatocellular carcinoma patients. Exp Mol Pathol 88(1):107–111
17. Yu J, Ni M, Xu J et al (2002) Methylation Profiling of twenty Promoter CpG islands of genes which may contribute to hepatocellular carcinogenesis. BMC Cancer 29(2):1–14
18. Gao S, Ding LH, Wang JW et al (2013) Diet folate, DNA methylation and polymorphisms in Methylenetetrahydrofolate reductase in association with the susceptibility to gastric cancer. Asian Pacific J Cancer Prev 14(1):299–302
19. Zhao P, Lin F, Li Z et al (2011) Folate Intake, Methylenetetrahydrofolate Reductase Polymorphisms, and Risk of Esophageal Cancer. Asian Pac J Cancer Prev 12:2019–2023

Chapter 377
The Application of Humane Care in Clinical Medical Treatment

Chunhua Su

Abstract Humane care is a new more recognized medical model of care, the rehabilitation of the main purpose of the application is to make the patient's medical care environment warm and comfortable satisfaction, so that patients maintain a pleasant mood, is conducive to the patient's condition. Humane care and use of a creative, personalized, holistic, effective care model, its purpose is to create a comfortable environment for patients, so that patients in the whole process of medical treatment convenience, comfort and satisfaction kinds of care, so that patients in the physical, psychological, social and spiritual in a healthy and comfortable state, to avoid the occurrence of discomfort.

Keywords Humane care · Care · Application

377.1 Introduction

With the development of socio-economic and medical model change, the requirements for medical services, and are constantly improving. Medical services, nursing services were the main face of a services, humane nursing care model gradually people identify with, humane care is people-oriented, to the fundamental interests of the patient as a starting point, with full respect of some of the patient's own select to better provide clinical care for patients, to promote the rehabilitation of patients faster.

Social development continue to pursue human services, personalized service throughout the process to do to adapt to the personal habits, and with full respect of clients and meet their needs, thereby enabling clients to have a good moodstate

C. Su (✉)
University Hospital, Beihua University, Jilin 132013, China
e-mail: suchunhua@126.com

S. Li et al. (eds.), *Frontier and Future Development of Information Technology in Medicine and Education*, Lecture Notes in Electrical Engineering 269,
DOI: 10.1007/978-94-007-7618-0_377, © Springer Science+Business Media Dordrecht 2014

hospital humane care with emphasis on human culture based on patient-centred care, the purpose is to make the patient in a natural and comfortable in the physical, mental and spiritual state, promote physical rehabilitation. In the care of people text, let the patients or their families to fully understand their illness and treatment process, and the main contents of the care and some of the results may occur. Encounter patients with psychological mood swings, must promptly give communication to eliminate negative emotions, as far as possible to meet the needs of patients are conducive to disease treatment.

377.2 Enhance the Awareness of Humane Care Services

Gradually increase the requirements for humane care patients in nursing, nurses the patients health protection and supervisors as medical services to fully establish the concept of human services to people-oriented comprehensive services for patients. Care workers to fully enhance the awareness of humane care, you need to have a sense of communication, have some flexible communication skills. While strengthening some of its own to enhance the quality, keep the foundation of professional knowledge, expand horizons, do patient-cantered, all for the patient multi-level awareness of humane care. Hospitals throughout the specification should also establish a sense of humane care.

377.3 Section Heading

When the patient entered the hospital, psychological health from a familiar environment into the strange medical environment, there is anxiety and negative emotions. Workers in every aspect of the medical services need to be fully prepared human services, the gradual elimination of all the confusion of the patient. Nurse workers to be patient to communicate, try to meet some of the requirements of the patients, and effectively create a good user-friendly environment.

377.3.1 Active Humane Care Services Training

Through a series of humane care training, nurses aware of the requirements of all aspects of human services. The language and the overall image of the nurse constantly upgrading the formation of a good image of the nursing, dedication, more personalized service philosophy applied to the work. The training is not only a moment of proposed evaluation system to form an effective humane care, real people work carried out, so that patients get more benefits. Complete training and evaluation system of human services, regular training evaluation, self-evaluation checks in a timely manner.

377.3.2 Full Respect for the Patient, Indeed, for Patients

Human services patients, as a part of the social role, care workers, respect for the patient's personality and some privacy for patients and set up a good fight against the disease state of mind. Patients in either the heart or emotionally very sensitive fragile and in need of care workers to give more humane care. Respect for the patient, can be conversational questionnaire to understand the needs of patients and the work of some of the opinions and suggestions, according to some reasonable suggestions in the nursing work correct. Care workers should strengthen exchanges, some of the problems encountered in the implementation of humane care and ways to resolve through discussions and exchange of state-of-the-art found to identify deficiencies and enhance awareness of personal care human services, awareness of human services for the entire care team also improved. Each care workers in the exchanges and discussions to further enhance awareness of humane care, full respect for patients, improve the quality of care.

377.3.3 Good at Applied Affinity Language

Humane care services emphasis on human factors, not only the medical care of the mechanical work, the work should be adept at some affinity language skills, closer relationships between patients. Especially for patients just admitted to hospital, and my impatience, more patient, and careful use of the humane language skills, communication affinity language, to eliminate the tension of patients, so that patients fully appreciate the words and deeds of the nursing work human services. Application of affinity language communication, enhance the sense of the relatives of patients, so that patients feel sincerely and genuinely care nurses.

377.3.4 Elegant Humane Care Environment

Different conditions for different patients, individualized assessment. Depending on the results of the assessment, the specific implementation of the application of humane care of an important aspect is the health education publicity. Through the preaching of patients with disease-related knowledge, so that patients' awareness of the disease have a certain understanding, and then the patient care workers fully understand the important role in the implementation of humane care services, and actively cooperate to promote physical rehabilitation. Patient care workers are also more of a understanding and support.

For the environment in which the reaction is relatively straightforward, especially in the mood, a good environment will make the patients feel more comfortable, feel more pleasure, this is also an important humane care services.

For the layout of the ward to comfortable, clean, practical, reasonable criteria. Indoor environment is bright, pastel shades, ground clean items neatly. And according to the needs of the patient in the case does not affect the care and treatment, can be appropriate for some other arrangement. Is also conducive to the humane care work carried out by the layout of the ward to meet the wishes of the families of patients.

377.4 Surgical System of Humane Care Services

Surgical ward received most patients need surgery, some elective some deadline surgery, emergency surgery. Matter what type of surgery, there will be a certain degree of trauma and risk. Patients this will produce different degrees of negative psychological, can not adapt to sudden changing roles, the heart will produce some of the psychological fear and resistance. No matter in the preoperative or post-operative treatment of diseases and rehabilitation of the body are very unfavorable. Positive patients with human services, to create a comfortable medical environment for the patient, the patient's fear gradual elimination of the psychological fear, establish the faith to overcome the disease, more recognition and support of humane care.

Care workers in the preoperative humane care education to patients to explain some of the disease-related knowledge, so that the patient's afraid to worry about the gradual elimination of gradually accept the current treatment options, especially the need for surgery. You can put some easy songs into the operating room to make patients feel relaxed; care workers actively with patients communicate mitigation preoperative anxiety. Postoperative patients must also be humane care health education, to enable patients to understand after some considerations, humane mode for some care operations should also be fully applied. Some adverse reactions after surgery, to be patient with the patient communication, to enable patients to avoidance of doubt, in need of care treatment should be promptly humane care treatment. Enhanced surgical system humane care of all aspects of the service system.

The humane care of the surgical system due to the services of different objects, especially talked about the need for surgery, the heart is full of all kinds of fear and disgust. The nurses and doctors to cooperate fully with the good patients the humane care services to promote the patient's body to a speedy recovery.

377.5 Some of the Issues of Humane Care

Care in the patient's medical treatment is an important job. Humanistic nursing services is necessary. However, in the specific implementation, there are some problems. For example, the lack of human and financial capital. A question of money through increased investment. But for the introduction of talent. Human services staff with the same need to strengthen the present situation, the use of medical resources is not very high. Need positive psychological problems of some specific initiatives for service survey. In short, the humane care system is applied to all aspects of patient care. From patients admitted to hospital someone answered, check care procedures was guiding handled in a timely manner for someone to go home to visit, so that patients everywhere can enjoy someone to love, someone to help. Humane care is strictly regulated services, standardized operation, standardized management for patients at ease, Heart, a comfortable medical care; through the whole care, general care, comprehensive care, close nurse-patient relationship, reduce nurse-patient disputes improve quality of care, enhance the overall image of the hospital.

References

1. Gu ZY (2005) Present situation and enlightenment of the Japanese hospitals humane care. J Nursing Zhi 40(7):550–552
2. Wang Y, Zhang L, Liu C (2009) Nurse to carry out the effect of humane care training intervention. Chongqing Med 38(6):685–685, 687
3. Huang L, Yao YW, Hubin C et al (2005) Humane care for nurses cognition investigation and analysis. Chinese Hospital Manag 25(5):45–47
4. INVENTORY AND. Humane care in elderly hypertensive patients with blood pressure control effect. Chinese J Pract Nurs 27(15):4–6
5. Li J (2012) The application of the results of humane care in emergency patient care evaluation. Chinese J Pract Nurs 28(12):28–29
6. Yu Z (2011) The humane care anorectal surgery patients. Chin J Pract Nurs 27(18):21–22
7. Fan L (2011) Specification humane care of the surgical patient satisfaction. Chin J Pract Nurs 27(6):63–64
8. Son Y (2011) The humane care cardiac medical care. Chin J Pract Nurs 27(29):11–12

Chapter 378
Chinese EFL Learners' Metacognitive Knowledge in Listening: A Survey Study

Zeng Yajun and Zeng Yi

Abstract This study investigated Chinese EFL learners' ($N = 1{,}044$) current level of metacognitive knowledge in listening. Results show that Chinese undergraduates have a fairly high degree of metacognitive awareness of listening learning in aspects like person knowledge, planning, and problem solving but not in strategies like directed attention, online-appraisal and mental translation. The finding lends further evidence to what was reported by other scholars. Finally, the pedagogical implications of findings from this study are discussed.

Keywords Metacognitive knowledge · MALQ · L2 listening

378.1 Introduction

The role of metacognition in second language learning has gained recognition in the last few decades. However, the significance and contribution of metacognitive awareness to learner listening has yet to be discussed extensively, and more importantly, supported by empirical evidence.

This study investigated Chinese EFL learners' ($N = 1{,}044$) current level of metacognitive knowledge in listening. An analysis of metacognitive awareness listening questionnaire (MALQ in [1]) demonstrates that Chinese undergraduates have a fairly high degree of metacognitive awareness of listening learning in aspects like person knowledge, planning, and problem solving. Students are, however, still limited in their use of strategies like directed attention and online-appraisal. Furthermore, most participants are found to have a misconception of the

Z. Yajun (✉) · Z. Yi
Yangtze University, Jingzhou 434023, People's Republic of China
e-mail: zyajun@gmail.com

S. Li et al. (eds.), *Frontier and Future Development of Information Technology in Medicine and Education*, Lecture Notes in Electrical Engineering 269,
DOI: 10.1007/978-94-007-7618-0_378, © Springer Science+Business Media Dordrecht 2014

mental translation strategy, a debilitating strategy according to the MALQ. The finding lends further evidence to what was reported by other scholars.

Finally, the pedagogical implications of findings from this study are discussed. We argue that future studies direct more attention to examining the connection and interactions between EFL learners' metacognitive awareness and their strategy use as dynamic systems [2] in relation to L2 listening achievement.

378.2 Literature Review

Listening plays a critical role in second language curriculum in China, where English is learned as the foreign language (EFL). Apart from being an important component in the current curriculum of college english and an essential and compulsory module for all non-English major undergraduates, listening is also an essential language communication skill in the current educational and economic landscape in the country. Furthermore, listening assumes greater importance by its growing weightage in large-scale high-stake language tests like the college english test (CET) and public english test (PET) in China. However, listening is the least understood and least researched skill in China, although L2 listening experts have long stressed its central role in language learning [3, 4]. Listening classes in Chinese universities are still dominated by the product-based approach, where learners are asked to listen to given oral texts and complete the comprehension questions.

Metacognitive knowledge is believed to be important for language learning. However, contrary to the emerging interest of metacognition in reading and writing research, empirical study on eliciting and raising L2 listeners' awareness of the listening process itself is a more recent development [4] despite the fact that listening experts have advocated to raise learners' metacognitive knowledge about listening for some time now [5, 6]. We adopted MALQ in the present study as the main instrument to measure the level of metacognitive awareness of Chinese EFL learners in English listening.

378.3 Methodology

The informants of the survey study ($n = 1{,}044$) were all native speakers of Chinese learning english as a foreign language for academic purposes in a Chinese provincial university. Randomly chosen out of a cohort of over 8,000 freshmen students, they belonged to different disciplines of study, such as sciences, medicine, engineering, agriculture, and economics.

This study used MALQ as a key instrument to assess Chinese EFL learners' metacognitive awareness and perceived use of strategies while listening to oral texts. For the survey, 1,044 copies of MALQ were distributed and completed by

Chinese EFL undergraduates after the listening task so that learners could capitalize on the MALQ by reflecting on their listening process and comprehension. Data collected were expected to address one main research question. SPSS16 was used to analyse the survey data, with frequencies and percentages calculated to examine certain central tendency of five major metacognitive factors in the MALQ framework.

1. "What are Chinese EFL learners' level of metacognitive knowledge in listening?"

378.4 Results and Discussions

Table 378.1 provides the descriptive statistics of level of Chinese undergraduates' metacognitive knowledge in listening based on MALQ. As can be seen from the table, the comparatively high mean scores of two metacognitive factors: directed attention (M = 4.55, SD = 0.783) and problem-solving (M = 4.44, SD = 0.756) suggest that the participants have reported using these two groups of strategies quite frequently to help them comprehend while listening. Meanwhile, the participants also reported frequent use of another set of strategies: planning and evaluation (M = 3.94, SD = 0.856), although participants were less inclined to reflect on their listening and evaluated the effectiveness of their strategy use in L2 listening.

In contrast, participants scored quite high on the person knowledge factor (M = 3.96, SD = 1.295), indicating a high level of anxiety and a lack of confidence in listening. Furthermore, most participants reported to have relied on the mental translation strategy (M = 3.55, SD = 1.020) to achieve better understanding of the oral texts. Around 60 % of them believed translating help ensure their understanding and they would translate whatever they hear, key words in particular to help them comprehend.

With respect to the research question, the survey study found that Chinese undergraduates have a fairly high degree of metacognitive awareness of listening learning about directed attention (M = 4.55, SD = 0.783), problem-solving (M = 4.44, SD = 0.756), and planning and evaluation (M = 3.94, SD = 0.856), suggesting learners' frequent use of such effective strategies in listening activities. However, the comparatively high mean score on the person knowledge factor

Table 378.1 Descriptive statistics of level of Chinese undergraduates' metacognitive knowledge in listening based on MALQ (N = 1044)

Metacognitive factor	MALQ item	Mean	S D
Directed attention	2, 6,12, 16	4.55	0.783
Problem-solving	5, 7, 9, 13, 17, 19	4.44	0.756
Planning/evaluation	1, 10, 14, 20, 21	3.94	0.856
Person knowledge	3, 8, 15	3.96	1.295
Mental translation	4, 11, 18	3.55	1.020

(M = 3.96, SD = 1.295) indicates a high level of anxiety and a lack of confidence, which might negatively influence participants' listening comprehension abilities. Meanwhile, most participants were found to rely heavily on the mental translation strategy (M = 3.55, SD = 1.020), a debilitating strategy according to [1] and should, therefore, be overcome if learners are to become skilled L2 listeners.

To sum up, the above analysis could shed light on some important aspects concerning Chinese non-english major undergraduates' varied perception in five distinct factors related to learners' metacognitive awareness and regulation of listening comprehension strategies: directed attention, problem-solving, planning and evaluation, person knowledge, and mental translation. More than two-thirds of the participants focused harder when they had difficulty understanding and even higher percentage of participants were able to recover their concentration and get back on track when their minds wandered or when concentration drifted or was lost while listening. However, it was also found that over a quarter of the 1,044 participants experienced anxiety and opted for giving up when they had difficulties understanding in L2 listening. Second, as many as four-fifths of the participants were aware of problem-solving strategies and employed them frequently when needed to enhance their comprehension. Third, most of the participants had a plan in their heads for how they were going to listen before they started to listen. And over two-thirds of the participants tried to recall their past listening experience and prior knowledge to help them comprehend and more percentage of participants had a goal in mind for what they were going to listen. Fourth, about two-fifths of the participants regarded listening in English a real challenge and around one-third of the participants felt that listening is more difficult than other three macro-skills of english. This might indicate learners' lack of confidence or high levels of anxiety, both of which can negatively influence listening success. However, most of the participants did not feel nervous when they listened to english. Finally, most participants in the survey were found to rely heavily on the mental translation strategy, a debilitating strategy, according to [1]. While an ability to identify key words may be useful, Chinese EFL learners should be cautioned that conscious translation would hinder the speed and efficiency of processing, and is thus detrimental to listening success.

378.5 Implications

Besides heightening the importance of metacognition in L2 listening, the study also made important contributions to listening pedagogy in China. First, the metacognitive knowledge profile reported in the study enriched our understanding of Chinese EFL learners' knowledge base and strategy preference in L2 listening. Second, the study confirmed that the MALQ could provide a relatively reliable and valid means of tapping into learners' metacognitive knowledge and perceived strategy use in listening and could therefore be applied into L2 listening teaching and learning. Furthermore, listening teachers can use the MALQ as a diagnostic or consciousness-raising tool. When particular strategies or set of strategies are found to be underused, instruction can be adjusted to place greater emphasis on those strategies in listening classes.

References

1. Vandergrift L, Goh C, Mareschal C, Tafaghodtari M (2006) The metacognitive awareness listening questionnaire: development and validation. Lang Learn 56:431–462
2. Zhang LJ (2010) A dynamic metacognitive systems account of Chinese university students' knowledge about EFL reading. TESOL Quarterly 44:320–353
3. Nunan D (1997) Approaches to teaching listening in the language classroom. Paper presented at the 1997 national Korea TESOL conference, Taejon
4. Vandergrift L (2007) Recent developments in second and foreign language listening comprehension research. Lang Teach 40:191–210
5. Mendelsohn D (2006) Learning how to listen using learning strategies. In: Juan E, Martínez-Flor A (eds) Current trends in the development and teaching of the four language skills. Mouton De Gruyter, New York, pp 75–89
6. Morley J (2001) Aural comprehension instruction: principles and practices. In: Celce-Murcia M (ed) Teaching english as a second or foreign language. Heinle & Heinle, Boston, pp 69–85
7. Goh C (2008) Metacognitive instruction for second language listening development: theory, practice and research implications. RELC 39:188–213
8. Nation ISP, Newton J (2008) Teaching ESL/EFL listening and speaking. Routledge, New York

Chapter 379
Research on Mobile Learning Games in Engineering Graphics Education

Huang Chen, Liang Chen, Jinchang Chen and Jin Xu

Abstract With the rapid development of smart mobile terminals, mobile learning games have shown great potential in future engineering graphics education. In this research, mobile learning games in engineering graphics curriculums are introduced, and the 4 Layers Design Method for game design with the Memory Forgotten Law was put forward. By applying mobile learning games to the engineering drawing lessons, students' self-learning ability and spatial imagination ability are enhanced obviously.

Keywords Mobile learning games · Self-learning · Engineering graphics

---

*This research is supported by the education information technology program of the Guangdong Education Science 12th Five-Year Plan (11JXN027).

H. Chen · L. Chen · J. Chen
School of Design, South China University of Technology, Guangzhou 510006, People's Republic of China
e-mail: 490922513@163.com

L. Chen
e-mail: earchen@scut.edu.cn

J. Chen
e-mail: jcchen@scut.edu.cn

J. Xu (✉)
Department of Computer Science and Engineering, Guangdong Peizheng College, Guangzhou 510830, People's Republic of China
e-mail: jinerxu@163.com

S. Li et al. (eds.), *Frontier and Future Development of Information Technology in Medicine and Education*, Lecture Notes in Electrical Engineering 269,
DOI: 10.1007/978-94-007-7618-0_379,

379.1 Introduction

With the development of the wireless communication technology and smart mobile terminals, such as smart phones, iPads, PDAs, laptops and so on, mobile learning (m-learning) is becoming more and more popular [1]. M-learning is a new learning way that can take place at anytime and anywhere with the help of smart mobile terminals. Modern smart mobile terminals can provide the bidirectional communication for teachers and learners [2]. The strong interest of self-learning for students is the primary driving force of m-learning. In some countries, educators have been studying on issues of combining smart mobile terminals with education. One of the typical applications is the applying of iPads in the primary and secondary schools of the United States. In addition, the portability of smart mobile terminals can facilitate teachers and students to communicate and interact with each other more conveniently. However, the research of m-learning is insufficiently in generally. So far, most m-learning resources are focused on early childhood education, and few of professional courses at university are combined with m-learning.

In addition, according to our research in South China University of Technology, 90 % of undergraduates have smart phones. However, these smart mobile terminals are rarely used in learning. Most of them are used for enjoying entertainment and playing games. It proves that m-learning games based on smart mobile terminals have the great potential in the education field. It can better arouse students' interest to learn the knowledge in the m-learning field. The strong learning interest can drive students to learn the knowledge well and quickly by themselves without teachers' help. What's more, the teaching features of engineering graphics curriculums require students to have the strong self-learning ability in fact. In order to gradually cultivate the interest of learning knowledge by their own, it is helpful and meaningful for such students to play funny m-learning games. Therefore, we choose the engineering drawing curriculums as the object of m-learning games.

379.2 Advantages of M-Learning Games in Graphics Education

For students in China, the traditional learning mode is passively listening to the teacher in class. There is less communication or interaction between teachers and students. Combining engineering graphics study with m-learning games is a new learning mode. In this mode, students can understand knowledge easily and insensibly through playing the funny m-learning games which are designed specially for the engineering drawing curriculums. It enriches learning resources and forms of engineering graphics education. It is useful for students to deeply thinking and improves their self-learning ability. The new education way of introducing m-learning games into the engineering drawing curriculums owns the follow four advantages.

(1) Pleasure: Studying by m-learning games is an enjoyable learning experience. Students can master the knowledge of engineering graphics easily and insensibly through playing the funny m-learning games designed for the engineering drawing curriculums.
(2) Self-learning: When playing the m-learning games in their free time, students may meet unknowing problems or new knowledge which they will study in class of engineering drawing in the future. Obviously, it can help them solve these problems or learn the new knowledge of the engineering drawing curriculums by themselves.
(3) Portability: Because of the portability of smart mobile terminals, students do not need to sit in a fixed place anymore. They can play m-learning games in the smart mobile terminals at anytime and anywhere, such as waiting for bus, beginning to sleep, relaxing after dinner and so on. Their boring time can be reasonably used for learning knowledge by playing the m-learning game.
(4) Interactivity: Students can rotate the virtual objects, such as basic geometrical shapes, combined solids, the strange solids, as the way they like in the funny m-learning games. These will help them to better understand the three-dimensional spatial features of objects, just like touching the real objects.

379.3 Design of M-learning Games

379.3.1 Choice and Arrangement of Knowledge

German psychologist Hermann Ebbinghaus found people's Memory Forgotten Law (MFL) by doing a lot of experiments [3]. But it is emotional, and it is difficult to measure data of the MFL. In order to quantitatively study the MFL, we improve the law as shown in Fig. 379.1. Students can obtain the short-term memory (SM) after the initial learning for new knowledge (NK). These short-term memory will become their long-term memory (LM) after reviewing, which will form their retention of memorization (RM) at last. But if you never review those knowledge, the short-term memory will be forgotten (FK) slowly. We establish the quantitative mathematical model of the modified MFL.

The SM, LM and RM can be calculated by

$$SM = NK - FK \tag{379.1}$$

$$LM = f(f(SM)) \tag{379.2}$$

$$RM = (LM/NK) * 100\% \tag{379.3}$$

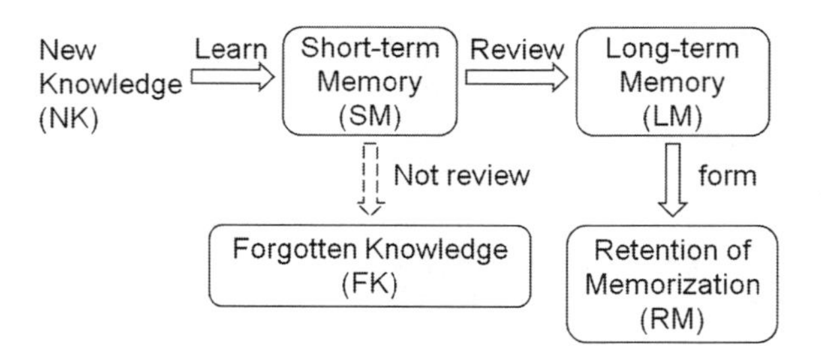

Fig. 379.1 The improvement of MFL

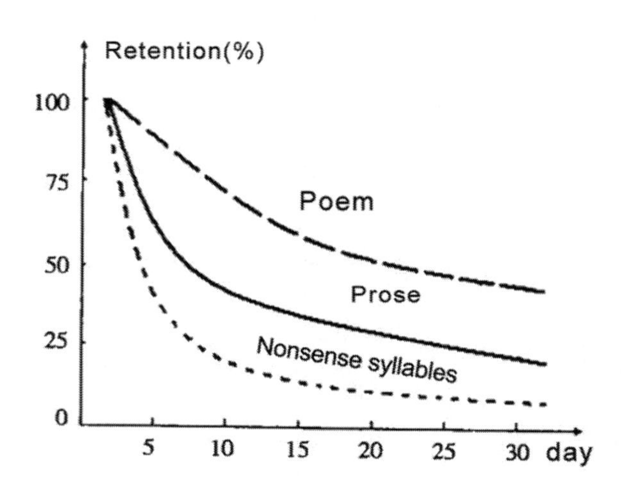

Fig. 379.2 The MFL for different knowledge

The MFL reveals the learning method and the learning law. The knowledge which is easy to be understood and regular will be easier to be remembered, such as poem, prose and so on, as shown in Fig. 379.2. The m-learning game with interesting story backgrounds or funny experiences can make students learn and remember the knowledge easily. In order to design the excellent game levels of the m-learning game for the engineering drawing curriculums, we choose the basic project theory, simple solid projection and the composite solid projection as the game story and the stage. We design complex combined solids which consist of basic geometrical shapes through Boolean operation, including intersection, union and subtraction.

379.3.2 The Design Method of M-Learning Games

By analyzing the surveys, researching the popular mobile games and studying the cognitive psychology, we find that intellectual micro-tasks and funny emotion-motivation are two key factors in designing m-learning games [4]. Further, we put forward the 4 Layers Design Method (4LDM).

(1) The theme layer: M-learning games need to establish the story background about the knowledge of the engineering drawing curriculums [5]. It can increase the interest of the m-learning game to students.
(2) The knowledge layer: The design of game levels must combine the chosen knowledge of the engineering drawing curriculums with the content of micro-tasks in game levels reasonably. It enables students to learn the knowledge easily and insensibly when playing the funny m-learning game.
(3) The goal layer: The goal of the m-learning game is keeping the high user participation in the game. Only by this way, students can be gradually cultivating their learning interest in engineering drawing lesson, improving their self-learning ability and mastering the learning method.
(4) The extending layer: The learning method by playing m-learning games of the engineering drawing curriculums can be extended to other knowledge.

379.3.3 The Example of the M-Learning Game

Repair UFO is the m-learning game that we designed for learning the engineering drawing lessons. The interface and knowledge are shown in Fig. 379.3. The story background is that Frankenstein, controlled by the player, identifies the parts and repairs the UFO seized from the alien. The player must find the right parts from their projection. The game levels are divided into the single-plane projection of basic geometrical shapes, single-plane projection of combined solids, double-plane projection of combined solids and three-plane projection of combined solids.

The game has been tested by undergraduates in their engineering drawing lessons in South China University of Technology. When students test the game, they need to rotate the object to get through the hole on the wall. After they pass a game stage, the picture of victory will display their score and three-plane projection of the part they have repaired. Therefore, they can better master the learning method, three-dimensional spatial imagination and three-plane projection drawing easily and insensibly by overcoming the interesting problems in the game

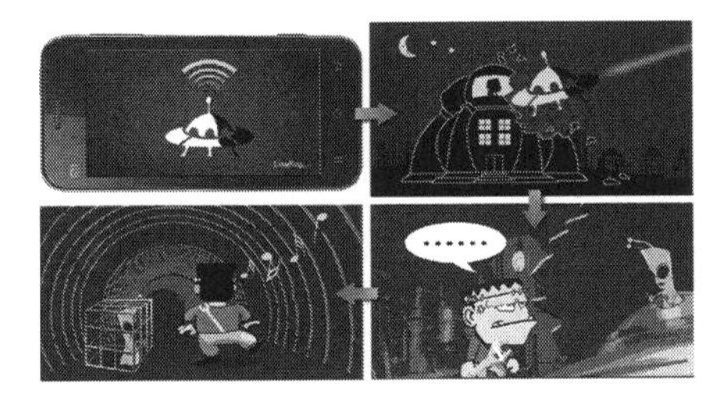

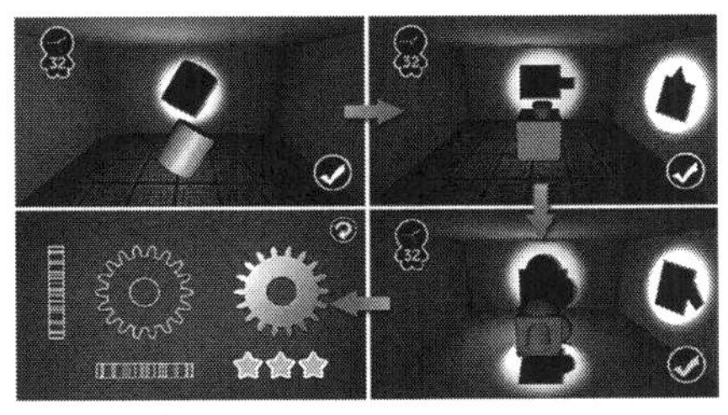

Fig. 379.3 The interface and knowledge of the m-learning game

levels of the m-learning game without teachers' help. Since the m-learning game of the engineering drawing curriculums is so interesting and funny, students are willing to take their initiative to learn the knowledge which is related to the engineering graphic for expanding extra-curricular knowledge and supplementing classroom learning. They can play the m-learning game at anytime and anywhere, such as waiting for a bus, relaxing after dinner, before sleeping and so on.

379.4 Conclusions

Through studying the advantages of m-learning games in engineering graphics education, we combine the m-learning game with the engineering drawing curriculums. Under the guidance of the Memory Forgotten Law, we put forward the 4LDM for how to design a good m-learning game of the engineering drawing curriculums. Eventually, we develop the m-learning game named Repair UFO. Through applying this game in the engineering drawing curriculums, students' interest of self-learning, ability of spatial thinking and ability of reading engineering drawing have been greatly improved.

References

1. Ling-mei K (2012)The development of mobile learning system based on the android platform. In: Proceedings of the 2012 international conference of modern computer science and applications advances in intelligent systems and computing. 191: 701–706
2. Aleksander D Mobile education—a glance at the future. http://www.nettskolen.com/forskning/mobile_education.pdf. 2001-10-04
3. Guo-an Y. Professor of psychology on memory magic—ebbinghaus forgetting curve. http://www.sina.com.cn. Sina Education, 2002-11-21
4. Lynch T, Gregor S (2004) User participation in decision support systems development: Influencing system outcomes. Eur J Inf Sys 13:286–301
5. Gómez-Martín MA, Gómez-Martín PP, González-Calero PA (2004) Game-driven intelligent tutoring systems. Lect Notes Comput Sci 3166:108–113

Chapter 380
Design and Implementation of a New Generation of Service-Oriented Graduate Enrollment System

Shao Zhenglong, Li Yanxia and Zhong Wenfeng

Abstract Based on the "enrollment is service, management is service" working concept, the new generation of service-oriented graduate enrollment system was optimized and improved on information organization mode, design of the registration process, communication with the examinee communication, service providing way, information push service and data interoperability. It fully reflects the idea of service examinees. This system was constructed and used in Tsinghua University. It plays an important role in the selection of high-quality talents.

Keywords Graduate enrollment system · Service-oriented · Websites group · Mobile application · Video service

380.1 Introduction

Postgraduate education is the highest level of education in the education structure. It takes up the heavy responsibility for cultivating high-quality innovative talents. Admission of postgraduates is an indispensable part of the education of graduate work. It has a crucial impact on the quality of postgraduate education [1]. Since China resumed the graduate enrollment, after 30 years of reform and development, the graduate enrollment scale increasing rapidly. Postgraduate entrance examination system was established and gradually formed the current exam and selection system. With the demand for the development of graduate education and the social and economic development, the number of graduate applicants rose year after year. According to the statistics of Ministry of education, the number of the

S. Zhenglong (✉) · L. Yanxia · Z. Wenfeng
Information Technology Center, Tsinghua University, Beijing, China
e-mail: szl@cic.tsinghua.edu.cn

S. Li et al. (eds.), *Frontier and Future Development of Information Technology in Medicine and Education*, Lecture Notes in Electrical Engineering 269,
DOI: 10.1007/978-94-007-7618-0_380,

national graduate entrance examination candidates in 2010 to reach 1,400,000 people, an increase of 13 % over the previous year [2].

In 2005, the Ministry of education opened the graduate entrance examination online registration system. The system greatly eased the information management work pressure of the registration points [2]. Many colleges and universities have opened the graduate enrollment information system. These systems provide stable support for Master enrollment, Doctor enrollment and recommended exemption of enrollment, improve the management standard and efficiency and provide accurate, high-quality information service for colleges, teachers and students.

Along with the reform of postgraduate training mechanism unceasingly thorough, the graduate enrollment is more and more outstanding top-notch innovative talents selection. It makes emphasis on building the fair admissions environment. It needs to achieve precision management of examinee information and targeted enrollment information. The working concept of admission of postgraduates also changes from mainly in the recruitment process management to serving the examinees to choose suitable schools and professional. The original system for registration, examination, admission and enrollment process management has deficiencies in many aspects, as design of enrollment process, interaction with candidates, personalized information service for the candidates and diversity of the way for enrollment information service. A new generation of service-oriented graduate enrollment system is needed.

380.2 The Service-Oriented Design

380.2.1 Optimization of Information Organization, Rich the Forms of Propaganda for Enrollment

The main service object of graduate admissions web site is the candidates. It is the professional site for communication enrollment information and publicity enrollment policy [3]. In addition to providing enrollment system outside the entrance, it is mainly used for various information publish as enrollment directory, recruit students general rules and dynamic news related to the graduate admissions. In the website design of the new generation of postgraduate enrollment system, the information is not organized by its attribute (as notice, news, enrollment directory), but is organized by its publicity objects (as master's degree candidates, Ph.D. candidates, school recommendation of candidates). This organization can better embody the people-oriented and service candidate concept. At the same time, the introduction of school life is added making the candidates know school environment in advance. In the form of publicity in addition to traditional text, pictures, video service is used to add videos in the site.

380.2.2 Application Materials Submitted by No-Paper Way, Reducing the Examinee Registration Cost

In the old admissions process, the examinee should register and provide personal information on the website; they also need to submit photos, certificates and other materials by post. When the submitted materials have problems, they must communicate with enrollment management department and resubmit modified materials. Sometimes they need to mail several times before successful submit the material. In the functional design of the new generation of postgraduate enrollment system, through the optimization of enrollment management process, function of photo and application materials submission and review is added. Application materials submitted by no-paper way is implemented, it reduces the examinee registration cost, improves the efficiency of the material review and realizes the information management of application materials.

380.2.3 Collecting the Views of Candidates by Multi-channel, Strengthen the Communication with Candidates

Before, candidates as applicants are mainly passive acceptance of the postgraduate enrollment management arrangements. There is no way for candidates to express opinions and suggestions about propaganda of enrollment and enrollment process. A survey module is added in the new generation of postgraduate enrollment system. It embodies the concept of service candidates. This online survey module realizes reusable, customizable questionnaire. And it can be used for statistical analysis of survey results.

380.2.4 Using Mobile Internet Technology, Providing more Convenient Information Service

Mobile Internet technology is used to construct mobile edition enrollment information network. It allows candidates to query about admissions policies and notice through the mobile terminal whenever and wherever. The mobile version of personal examination query system is integrated with the mobile version of graduate enrollment information network. It allows candidates to query material examination, interview, results and other information through the mobile phone.

380.2.5 Using Email, Text Messages and Information Push Service, Achieving Accurate Delivery of Personal Information

Graduate admissions process includes registration, material review, interview and admitted. Each step has relevant information needed to inform to the examinee. The enrollment system in the past requires candidates to login the system with their own account repeatedly to query. Email, text messages and information push service is used in the new generation of service-oriented graduate enrollment system. Personal related information can be accurate delivery to the candidates. At the same time, mobile phone client software message pushing mechanism can further realize the information push.

380.2.6 Sharing the Enrollment Data, to Strengthen Inter-Agency Coordination

After the new graduate students are admitted, they will face the following steps such as register, studying. They need to be associated with the other information systems of the university. Such as they need to create one's status as a student in the educational administration system, need to allocate the beds in the property management system, need to get campus card from campus card management system. The data sharing between graduate enrollment system and the other systems in digital campus is fully considered, to provide data basis for interagency work. This makes the admitted students participating in advance to the campus life.

380.3 Implementation of the System

The new generation of postgraduate enrollment system's architecture is shown in Fig. 380.1. This system is divided into publicity platform, operation system, basic services and enrollment database. Publicity platform contains the WEB website and mobile App. This platform implements information publicity for all kinds of recruitment. Operation system contains all kinds of enrollment management and the questionnaire for students. This system implements information management for enrollment. Basic services provide basic services for advertising platform and operation system, such as identity authentication service, authority management service, video service, message service and email service. Graduate enrollment database stores data related to the graduate admissions and provides data sharing.

The key technology of the new generation of postgraduate enrollment system as follows:

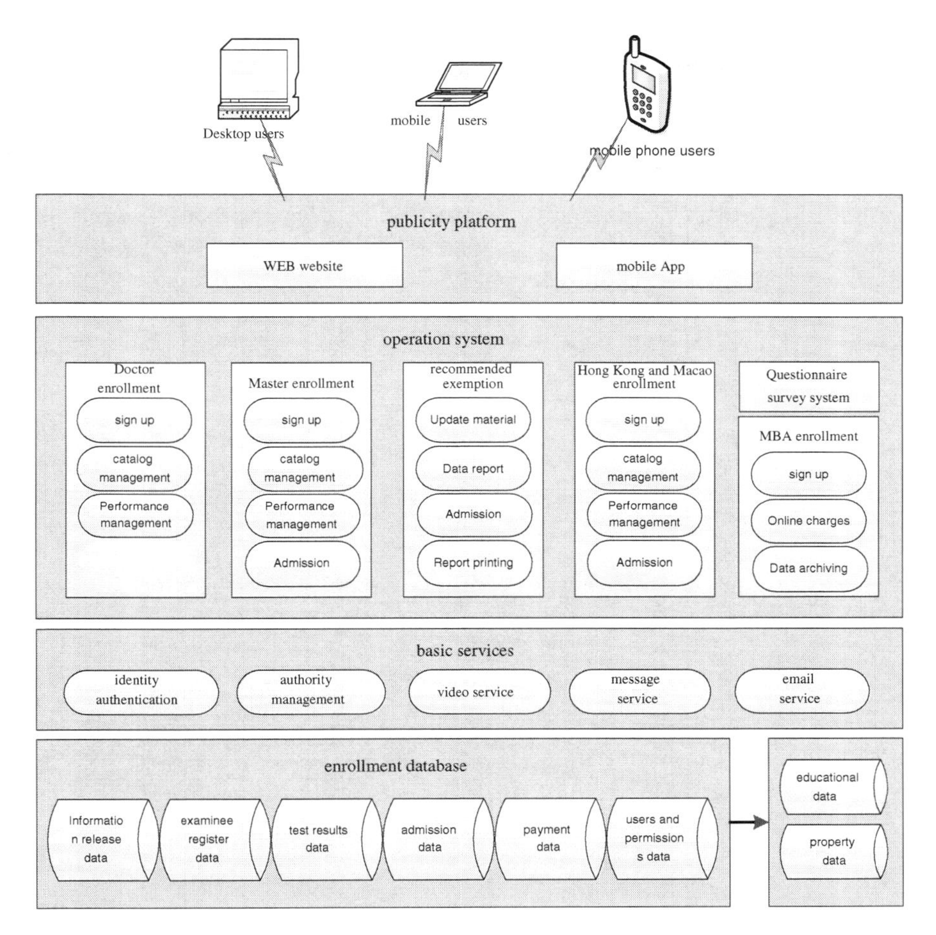

Fig. 380.1 Structure of the new generation of service-oriented graduate enrollment system

380.3.1 Websites Group and Content Management Technology

Publicity platform is constructed based on websites group and content management technology. Website group is a sites collection. The sites are unified planned and constructed. They are organized together according to some membership. They not only can be unified managed and can also be an independent management system formation. Content management system is a software system located between the Web front-end and back-end business application systems, office systems or processes. It focuses on the acquisition, management, utilization, transmission and value-added of digital resources of different unstructured or semi-structured [4]. At the same time, static technology is used to ensure the site safety, efficient access.

380.3.2 Mobile Information Push Technology

In the age of Internet, due to the complexity of the structure characteristics, distribution of the scattered, dynamic changes and the irregular change of the massive information, information overload and information puzzle becomes the main reason to hinder the efficiency problem of Internet [5]. The traditional information search is not enough to solve these problems. Information push technology can solve these problems as an information service technology obtaining the required information from massive information and transmitting the information to the user. It can provide efficient information services.

380.3.3 Video Service Technology

With the development of information technology, the video service has become one of the basic services of campus network [6]. The graduate enrollment system integrates a multifunctional video service system, which has on demand, rebroadcast and broadcast functions. The system adopts the technology of streaming media. Graduate enrollment system focuses on the application of VOD function. Transcoding Center does video transcoding and sends the video to the VOD server. The transcoding center also provides interactive API with application systems. It also provides FTP service for video uploading and stores the video in a distributed file system.

380.4 Conclusions

The design of new generation of service-oriented graduate enrollment system was based on the "enrollment is service, management is service" working concept. Relying on advanced information technology, it achieves a comprehensive, harmonious, stable and sustainable development of the enrollment work .

References

1. Jing G, Zhaozhao Z (2007) Discuss on strengthening and improvement of graduate enrollment management. Educ Sci Culture Mag 102–103
2. Gang H (2011) Research and practice of postgraduate admission information management system. Heilongjiang Res High Educ 205:124–126
3. Guodong Z (2003) Discussion on the function of graduate school admissions Website. Acad Degrees Grad Edu 8:27–29

4. Jing H, Kejun D, Fudong L (2011) The application of CMS in construction of Website group in colleges and universities. Exp Technol Manag 28(4):220–222
5. Yuetian Z, Zhongshan X (2009) Discussion on the information push technology in the internet. Shanxi Libr J 112:18–22
6. Qun C (2009) Realization of multifunctional video service system based on campus network. China Edu Info 43–45

Chapter 381
Research on the Quality of Life of Cancer Patients Based on Music Therapy

He Wei

Abstract The impact of music therapy on the quality of life of cancer patients has been explored. The 38 cases of cancer patients receiving radiotherapy or chemotherapy during treatment with the music, a measured assessment of the quality of life of the indicators of quality of life questionnaire (QLQ-C30) before and after the intervention. Insomnia score was statistically significant ($P < 0.05$) before and after the intervention. Application of music therapy can improve sleep, improve patients' quality of life.

Keywords Music therapy · Cancer · Quality of life

381.1 Introduction

Music therapy as a method of psychological intervention clinical application in various fields will help ease the patient tense psychological pressure, lower blood pressure. Studies have shown that music therapy on patients rebuild the emotional activities, motivate thinking, increased interest in the surrounding, to motivate behaviours, improve retreat tend to have a positive effect. Especially in the field of cancer treatment, because cancer patient anxiety, depressive disorder incidence of up to 48, 45 %. Cancer is a treatment and recovery a long illness, it will make the patient is subjected to the pain of the different stages of treatment and quality of life have also been varying degrees of impact. In recent years, the quality of life of cancer patients there is a growing trend, on this basis; we explore the application of music therapy on the quality of life of cancer patients.

H. Wei (✉)
Affiliated Hospital, Beihua University, Jilin 132013, China
e-mail: hewei@126.com

S. Li et al. (eds.), *Frontier and Future Development of Information Technology in Medicine and Education*, Lecture Notes in Electrical Engineering 269,
DOI: 10.1007/978-94-007-7618-0_381,

381.2 Materials and Methods

Clinical data 2004 January 2007–April sick patients, diagnosed with cancer, and more than a primary school education, no previous history of mental illness and disturbance of consciousness, Karnofsky Functioning Scale (Karnof-sky performance status, KPS) score\ 60. Into the group of patients with a total of 38 cases, of which 15 cases of nasopharyngeal carcinoma, lung cancer in 11 cases, six cases of breast cancer after six cases of liver cancer; youngest 19 years old, maximum 76 years, an average of 45.56 years.

381.2.1 Rating Scale

Cancer patients quality of life scale (Quality of Life Questionnaire-Core 30 QLQ-C30), a total of 30 projects, functional subscale physical functioning (PF), role function (RF), cognitive function (CF), emotional function (EF), social function (SF), three symptom subscales (fatigue, pain, nausea, vomiting), an overall health subscale (GH) and a single measurement projects (difficulty breathing constitute, insomnia, lack of appetite, constipation, diarrheal, financial difficulties). The Functioning Scale the PF, RF and GH higher the score, the better quality of life; CF, EF, SF and symptom scale and individual measurements project the higher the score, the worse the quality of life. The questionnaire was comparable with that in different countries and regions, its reliability and validity and sensitivity has been validated in a number of countries, successfully used in the clinical studies of cancer patients. Questionnaire by the researchers under the unified guidance language.

381.2.2 Cartesian Functioning Scale

KPS into 10 grades, according to the assessment of the functional status of patients given the range of 0–100 points, the higher the score, the better physical function. Up to 100 points, followed by 90, 80, 70 points, which means that researchers different assessment of the patient's physical condition from high to low. 100 indicating normal, with 10 indicating critically ill dying, with 0 representing death. Space environment to a certain extent affect the patient's therapeutic effect, and should therefore be avoided noisy interference environment. We choose a single area of 26 m^2, and from the wards, offices at some distance from a dedicated treatment room; built-in with living flowers and murals with health education, information, and as warm as possible, so that the patient is relaxed, natural and comfortable environment.

381.2.3 Music Selection

The principles of the "symptomatic soundtrack", based on the patient's level of cultural enrichment, music appreciation and hobby selections. Nervousness, irritability patients election relaxation, quiet music, such as the "Palace Moon" "cold duck swimming" mysterious circle ; "dizziness, weakness, fatigue, physical decline the patients selected cheerful kind of music, such as" Clouds Chasing the Moon "Red Beans Love" Minuet ; "upset, palpitations, chest tightness patients choose the soft, beautiful, lyrical music, such as" Spring Song "Gorillas in the Mist"; "the depression patients election cheerful kind of music, such as" step by step "radiant", "Swan Lake Waltz". Based on content classification in compiling the music CD, each music CD playback time of 30 min Table 381.1.

381.2.4 Interfere with the Preparation and Methods

Before the intervention, the patient emptying urine, lying in bed, eyes closed, in a natural state of relaxation. Music player, stereo space surround playback, and in order to avoid the interference of others, each time only one person, per day, each time 30 min, five times a week for 4 weeks for an intervention treatment. All patients studied before and after the intervention test of the quality of life; 1st measurement time after the patient is admitted to the acoustic space around the player, in order to avoid the interference of others, each time only one person, once a day, each time for 30 min per week 5 for 4 weeks for an intervention treatment. All the patients studied in the test of the quality of life before and after the intervention; 1st measurement time of patients admitted to hospital after receiving radiation therapy and chemotherapy before intervention. 2nd measurement time 2 days after the end of the intervention applied again QLQ-C30 quality of life assessment situation Table 381.2.

381.3 Statistical Results

SPSS 10.0 statistical package for statistical analysis using the t test was used to compare the before and after intervention quality of life.

Shown in the table, after the intervention the insomnia score is lower than before the intervention ($P < 0.05$), other quality of life and overall health evaluation before the intervention were not statistically significant ($P > 0.05$) Table 381.3.

Table 381.1 The intervention QLQ-C30 in function subscale scores

Time	Number of cases	Physical function	Role and function	Cognitive function	Emotional function	Social function
Before intervention	38	7.84 ± 1.44	3.65 ± 0.73	3.52 ± 1.63	7.76 ± 2.47	5.24 ± 2.15
After intervention	38	7.77 ± 1.45	3.64 ± 0.62	3.54 ± 1.29	7.80 ± 2.22	5.25 ± 1.86
t		0.175	0.465	−0.865	−1.499	−0.634
P		0.862	0.645	0.394	0.144	0.531

Table 381.2 QLQ-C30 score of six individual measurement items

Time	Number of cases	Difficulty breathing	Insomnia	Lack of appetite	Constipation	Diarrhea	Economic difficulties
Before intervention	38	1.65 ± 0.86	2.11 ± 0.98	1.67 ± 1.02	1.87 ± 1.03	1.11 ± 0.30	3.02 ± 1.15
After intervention	38	1.63 ± 0.79	1.51 ± 0.62	1.70 ± 1.06	2.21 ± 0.76	1.21 ± 0.42	3.05 ± 1.12
t		1.099	2.516	−0.229	−1.871	−1.680	−1.648
P		0.280	0.017	0.820	0.071	0.103	0.110

Table 381.3 QLQ-C30 symptom subscale and overall health subscale score

Time	Cases	Fatigue	Pain	Nausea of vomiting	Overal health
Before intervention	38	5.05 ± 2.69	3.25 ± 1.93	2.89 ± 1.305	9.21 ± 2.21
After intervention	38	5.06 ± 2.59	3.13 ± 1.86	2.88 ± 0.987	9.23 ± 1.95
t		−0.205	1.928	1.222	−0.316
P		0.839	0.190	0.231	0.754

381.4 Conclusion

According to foreign Derogates (1983) reported that 47 % of cancer patients have significant psychological stress response or psychological disorders. As Hang said, fear of cancer is global, because cancer means extreme suffering and death. Due to the incidence of cancer usually does not cause people's attention, so many patients are diagnosed in the late often accompanied by other symptoms, such as pain, insomnia, indigestion, and most patients; and the long duration of treatment, the patient need to face treatment the emergence of side effects, such as chemotherapy, nausea, vomiting, constipation, fatigue, mouth ulcers, these factors could materially and adversely affect the patient's overall quality of life. This study is based cancer patients psychological and disease characteristics, the implementation of the principle of mainly symptomatic soundtrack. When people get sick, the rhythm of the body is in an abnormal state, choose the appropriate music, harmony through music audio, allows the body to a variety of vibration frequency coordination of activities, to the benefit of the patient back to health. The results of this study show that music therapy has a good effect to improve the quality of sleep in patients with cancer, statistically significant ($P < 0.05$) before and after the intervention. Due to the application of nature music easily beat the promotion of sound waves of sleep, the sleep center of the brain gradually relaxed, and goes to sleep. Johnson and abroad personalized music for insomnia in elderly women (age > 70 years) is similar to the findings, both of which can improve the patient's quality of sleep. On the positive side, the music as a wonderful sound waves, the role of the human brain, people feel the life force from the natural world, in order to stimulate the love of life; the other hand, it can enrich people's imagination, people with good ideas and vision for the future. For cancer patients, to arouse their courageous battle with cancer, recognizing the value of self-existence, face reality, cherish every second of life, actively cooperate with treatment, improve treatment compliance, you can improve the patient's quality of life.

References

1. Min L, Xu H, Xia Y (1999) cancer patients with anxiety and depression survey. Chin Ment Health J 13(3):187
2. Huilan Z, Chen R (2000) Chen Rong Fang tumor, Nursing. Tianjin Science and Technology Press, Tianjin, p 261

3. Wang J, Cuijun N, Chen Z (2000) Cancer patients quality of life and related factors. Chin J Clin Psychol 8(1):23–26
4. Huang YB, Wang KO (2004) Cancer quality of life survey and analysis. J Nurs 19(10):938
5. Olschewski M, Schulgen G, Schumacher M et al (1994) Quality of life assessment in clinical cancer research. Br J Cancer 70(1):1–5
6. Hang X, Butow PN, Mciscr B et al (1999) Attitudes and information needs of Chinese migrant cancer patients and their relatives. Aust NZ J Med 29:207–213

Chapter 382
Design, Synthesis and Biological Evaluation of the Novel Antitumor Agent 2*H*-benzo[b][1, 4]oxazin-3(4*H*)-one and Its Derivatives

Huanhuan Li, Kailin Han, Qiannan Guo, Fengxi Liu, Peng Yu and Yuou Teng

Abstract In order to further explore the potential pharmaceutical application of the benzoxazine type molecules, a series of novel 4 and 6 substituted 2*H*-benzo[b] [1, 4]-oxazin-3(4*H*)-one derivatives were prepared by a convenient Microwave-assistant four-step synthetic approach in 20–30 % overall yield. All the newly synthesized compounds were characterized by ^{1}H NMR and ^{13}C NMR. 7 of the 8 target compounds among them have not been reported yet. The primary antitumor activities of the target compounds and key intermediates against HT-29, K562 and HepG2 cell lines have been evaluated and result of the test shows that 6 benzoxazine derivatives demonstrated certain inhibition against those tumor cells, especially 6-bromo-4-(4-(trifluoromethyl)benzyl)-2*H*-benzo[b][1, 4]oxazin-3(4*H*)-one possessed good antitumor activity against HepG2 cancer cell with an IC_{50} of 6 μM.

Keywords Benzoxazine · Heck reaction · Antitumor activity

382.1 Introduction

WHO survey data shows that cancer is the second leading cause of death after cardiovascular diseases [1]. At present, cancer mortality rate is still on the rise. The existing chemotherapy drugs kill cancer cells mostly by interfering cell division.

H. Li · K. Han · Q. Guo · F. Liu · P. Yu
Key Laboratory of Industrial Microbiology, Ministry of Education,
College of Biotechnology, Tianjin University of Science and Technology, Tianjin 300457, People's Republic of China

Y. Teng (✉)
Tianjin Key Laboratory of Industry Microbiology, College of Biotechnology,
Tianjin University of Science and Technology, 300457 Tianjin, People's Republic of China
e-mail: tyo201485@tust.edu.cn

S. Li et al. (eds.), *Frontier and Future Development of Information Technology in Medicine and Education*, Lecture Notes in Electrical Engineering 269,
DOI: 10.1007/978-94-007-7618-0_382,

As the phenomenon of resistance gradually emerged in clinical practice using anti-cancer drugs, there is an urgent need for more effective anti-cancer drugs.

Benzoxazine-based compounds are a large class of novel heterocyclic compounds and possess a wide range of biological activities, such as antitumor [2], anti-inflammatory [3], antiulcer [4]. *2H*-benzo[b][1, 4]oxazin-3(*4H*)-one derivatives also exhibit other bioactivities, such as antipyretic [5], antihypertensive [6], antifungal [7] and potassium channel modulators [8] and so on [9, 10], which attracts the interest of many research groups.

Previous studies of *2H*-benzo[b][1, 4]oxazin-3(*4H*)-one derivatives were mainly focused on the substitution at 2 and 4 positions, but the substitution at 4 and 6 positions of Benzoxazine was rarely reported. In this paper, we would like to report the design and Microwave-assistant four-step synthesis of novel 4- and 6-substituted *2H*-benzo[b][1, 4]oxazin-3(*4H*)-one analogues as well as the primary evaluation of their antitumor activities against K562, HT-29 and HepG2 cancer cells.

382.2 Materials and Methods

382.2.1 Materials and Measurements

All reagents and solvents used in this paper were of reagent grade. Reaction temperatures were controlled using oil bath temperature modulator. Thin layer chromatography (TLC) was performed using E. Merck silica gel 60 GF254 precoated plates (0.25 mm) and visualized using a combination of UV. Silica gel (particle size 200–400 mesh) was used for flash chromatography. ^{1}H NMR spectra was recorded on Bruker AM-400 NMR spectrometers in deuterated chloroform or deuterated DMSO. The chemical shifts are reported in δ (ppm) relative to tetramethylsilane as internal standard.

382.2.2 Chemistry

The synthetic approaches of target compounds **4a–4d** and **5a–5d** were demonstrated in Fig. 382.1.

2-aminophenol **1** was employed to react with chloroacetyl chloride at 55 °C to provide compound **2** which was then reacted with bromine in acetic acid at 0 °C to afford the key intermediate **3**. Compound **3** was reacted with NaH and all kinds of benzyl chloride at room temperature to provide compound **4** (**4a, 4b, 4c and 4d**) in yield (66 %). A mixture of compound 4, N,N-Dimethylformamide, methyl acrylate, $PdCl_2(PPh_3)_2$ and $K_3PO_4 3H_2O$ were heated to 145 °C for 0.5 h in microwave reactor to afford compound **5** (**5a, 5b, 5c and 5d**).

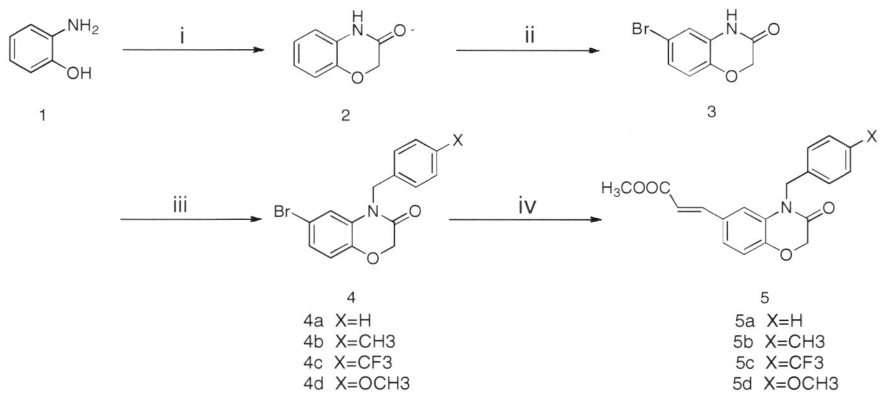

Fig. 382.1 Synthesis of compounds **4a–4d** and **5a−5d**

Reagents and conditions: (i) TEBAC, $NaHCO_3$, chloroform, 55 °C, 16 h, 60 %; (ii) Br_2, CH_3COOH, 0 °C,1 h,46 %; (iii) NaH, DMF, benzyl chloride,rt,10 h,65 %; (iv) methyl acrylate, $PdCl_2(PPh_3)_2$, $K_3PO_4 \cdot 3H_2O$, DMF,145 °C,0.5 h,45 %.

382.2.3 Biological Assay

The antiproliferative effects of the target compounds were determined by using MTT assay [11]. In briefly, K562, HepG2 and HT-29 cells were seeded at a density of 5×10^4 cells/mL in 96-well plate (100 μL/well). After incubating for 24 h, test compounds were added to cells for 48 h incubation. The media were replaced by PBS (-) medium (containing 0.5 mg/mL MTT) and incubated for another 4 h. Then the medium was replaced by 100 μL DMSO and incubated for 10 min to dissolve formazan crystals. The absorbances at 570/630 nm were measured for K562 cells and the absorbances at 490/630 nm were measured for HepG2 and HT-29 cells using Thermo microplate reader. Cell viability was calculated from measurements of OD value according to the corresponding formula and a graph is plotted of Cell viability (y-axis) against drug concentration (x-axis) [12]. OD value of DMSO-treated cells was used as 100 % cell viability. The inhibitory concentrations by 50 % values (IC_{50}) of sample compounds toward test cell proliferation were obtained by nonlinear regression. IC_{50} measurements for each compound were repeated three times.

382.3 Results and Discussion

382.3.1 Experimental Section

382.3.1.1 2*H*-benzo[b][1, 4]oxazin-3(4*H*)-one (2) [13]

To a solution of 2-chloroacetyl chloride (8.14 g, 72.20 mmol) in chloroform (5 mL) was added over 20 min to a suspension of 2-aminophenol (5.45 g, 50.00 mmol), TEBA (11.38 g, 50.00 mmol), and sodium bicarbonate (16.80 g, 200.00 mmol) in chloroform (30 mL) at 0 °C. The reaction mixture was maintained for 1 h and then was heated at 55 °C for 16 h. The reaction mixture was concentrated and was diluted with water. The precipitated solids were collected by filtration, washed with water (2 × 50 mL), and dried under high vacuum. The final product was purified by recrystallization from ethanol to provide 2*H*-benzo[b][1, 4]oxazin-3(4*H*)-one (**2**) in 60 % yield as a white solid.

^{1}H NMR ($CDCl_3$ 400 MHz): δ/ppm 4.55 (s, 2H, CH_2), 6.87-6.96 (m, 4H, Ar–H), 10.68(s, 1H, N–H).

382.3.1.2 6-bromo-2*H*-benzo[b][1, 4]oxazin-3(4*H*)-one (3) [14]

Bromine (1 mL) was slowly added to a solution of (2*H*)-1,4-benzoxazin-3(4*H*)-one **(2)** (1.50 g, 10.06 mmol) in glacial acetic acid (20 mL). The mixture was left to stand in ice for 1 h and then poured into aqueous sodium sulfite. The product was recovered in ethyl acetate. The extract was washed with aqueous sodium hydrogen carbonate, dried and the solvent was evaporated. The residue was chromatographed on silica. Elution with 30 % ethyl acetate: light petroleum gave 6-bromo-(2*H*)-1,4-benzoxazin-3(4*H*)-one **(3)** (1.06 g, 46 %) which crystallized from methanol as white prisms.

^{1}H NMR ($CDCl_3$ 400 MHz): δ/ppm 4.60 (s, 2H, CH_2), 6.90 (d, J = 8.4 Hz, 1H, Ar–H), 7.01 (d, J = 2 Hz, 1H, Ar–H), 7.06 (m, 1H, Ar–H), 10.80 (s, 1H, N–H).

382.3.1.3 4-benzyl-6-bromo-2*H*-benzo[b][1,4]oxazin-3(4*H*)-one(4a)[15]

To a flask (25 mL) which contained the solution of 6-bromo-2*H*-benzo[b][1, 4]oxazin-3(4*H*)-one **(3)** (0.20 g, 0.87 mmol) in dry N,N-Dimethylformamide (1 mL).The reaction temperature was maintained at 0 °C followed by the dropwise addition sodium hydride (0.04 g, 1.75 mmol). Stirring 5 min, was added benzyl chloride (0.13 g, 1.02 mmol) and the mixture allowed warm to room temperature. The reaction mixture was stirred at room temperature for 10 h. The orange solution was poured into water (25 mL) and extracted with dichloromethane (3 × 100 mL). The combined extracts were dried over anhydrous magnesium sulfate, filtered and evaporated.Chromatography (petroleum ether/ethyl acetate 10:1) afforded the title compound **4a** (0.19 g, 66 %).

^{1}H NMR ($CDCl_3$ 400 MHz): δ/ppm 4.71 (s, 2H, CH_2), 5.12 (s, 2H, CH_2), 6.85 (d, J = 8.4 Hz, 1H, Ar–H), 7.01 (s, 1H, Ar–H), 7.05 (d, J = 8 Hz,1H,Ar–H), 7.25–7.23 (m, 3H, Ar–H), 7.34–7.33 (m, 2H, Ar–H).

382.3.1.4 6-bromo-4-(4-methylbenzyl)-2*H*-benzo[b][1, 4]oxazin-3(4*H*)-one (4b)

Starting from compound **3** (0.20 g, 0.87 mmol) and 1-(chloromethyl)-4-methylbenzene (0.15 g, 1.05 mmol), compound **4b** was obtained in 60 % yield.

^{1}H NMR ($CDCl_3$ 400 MHz): δ/ppm 2.32 (s, 3H, CH_3), 4.7 (s, 2H, CH_2), 5.07 (s, 2H, CH_2), 6.84 (d, J = 8.4 Hz, 1H,Ar–H), 7.05–7.03 (m,2H,Ar–H),7.14–7.06 (m,4H,Ar–H).

382.3.1.5 6-bromo-4-(4-(trifluoromethyl)benzyl)-2*H*-benzo[b] [1, 4]oxazin-3(4*H*)-one (4c)

Starting from compound **3** (0.20 g, 0.87 mmol) and 1-(chloromethyl)-4-(trifluoromethyl) benzene (0.20 g, 1.04 mmol), compound **4c** was obtained in 70 % yield.

^{1}H NMR ($CDCl_3$ 400 MHz): δ/ppm 4.72 (s, 2H, CH_2), 5.17 (s, 2H, CH_2), 6.93–6.88 (m, 2H, Ar–H), 7.11–7.08 (m, 1H, Ar–H), 7.35 (d, J = 8 Hz, 2H, Ar–H), 7.60 (d, J = 8.4 Hz, 2H,Ar–H).'

382.3.1.6 6-bromo-4-(4-methoxybenzyl)-2*H*-benzo[b][1, 4]oxazin-3(4*H*)-one (4d)

Starting from compound **3** (0.2 g, 0.87 mmol) and 1-(chloromethyl)-4-methoxybenzene (0.20 g, 1.04 mmol), compound **4d** was obtained in 65 % yield.

^{1}H NMR ($CDCl_3$ 400 MHz): δ/ppm 3.79 (s, 3H, CH_3), 4.69 (s, 2H, CH_2), 5.05 (s, 2H, CH_2), 6.88–6.84 (m, 3H, Ar–H), 7.06–7.05 (m, 2H, Ar–H), 7.17 (d, J = 1.2 Hz, 2H, Ar–H).

382.3.1.7 (E)-methyl 3-(4-benzyl-3-oxo-3,4-dihydro-2*H*-benzo[b] [1, 4]oxazin-6-yl)acrylate (5a)

To a microwave reactor vial (2 mL) which contained the solution of 4-benzyl-6-bromo-2*H*-benzo- 2*H*-benzo[b][1, 4]oxazin-3(4*H*)-one (**4a)** (0.2 g, 0.63 mmol) in DMF (1 mL) were added methyl acrylate (0.08 g, 0.94 mmol) $PdCl_2(PPh_3)_2$ (0.02 g, 0.03 mmol) $K_3PO_4 3H_2O$ (0.22 g, 0.82 mmol) under the atmosphere of Ar. The microwave reactor vial was caped and placed into the microwave cavity.

The reaction mixture was irradiated at high level for 0.5 h at 145 °C. The reaction mixture was cooled down to room temperature and poured onto 20 mL ice-water then extracted with ethyl acetate (3 × 50 mL). The combined organic layers were washed with water (100 mL), brine (100 mL) and dried over anhydrous magnesium sulfate. The solvent was removed under vacuum to afford the crude which was purified by flash column chromatography (silica gel, petroleum ether/ethyl acetate 20:1) to yield the desired compound (E)-methyl3-(4-benzyl-3-oxo-3,4-dihydro-2*H*-benzo[b][1, 4]oxazin-6-yl)acrylate **(5a)** (0.1 g, 50 %)

^{1}H NMR ($CDCl_3$ 400 MHz): δ/ppm 3.77 (d, J = 1.2 Hz, 3H, CH_3), 4.77 (d, J = 1.2 Hz, 2H, CH_2), 5.18 (s, 2H, CH_2), 6.18–6.14 (m, 1H, CH), 7.02–6.98 (m, 2H, Ar–H), 7.15 (d, J = 8 Hz,1H, Ar–H), 7.29–7.26 (m, 3H, Ar–H), 7.35–7.33 (m, 2H, Ar–H), 7.47 (d, J = 1.5 Hz, 1H, CH), ^{13}C NMR (400 MHz $CDCl_3$) : δ 167.29, 164.14, 146.92, 143.84, 135.49, 129.23, 129.06, 129.00, 127.75, 126.62, 123.97, 117.45, 116.83, 115.31, 67.58, 51.72, 44.95.

382.3.1.8 (E)-methyl 3-(4-(4-methylbenzyl)-3-oxo-3,4-dihydro-2*H*-benzo[b][1, 4]oxazin-6-yl)acrylate (5b)

Starting from compound **4b** (0.2 g, 0.60 mmol) and methyl acrylate (0.07 g, 0.90 mmol), compound **5b** was obtained in 45 % yield.

^{1}H NMR ($CDCl_3$ 400 MHz): δ/ppm 2.32 (s, 3H, CH_3), 3.78 (s, 3H, CH_3), 4.75 (s, 2H, CH_2), 5.13 (s, 2H, CH_2), 6.16 (d, J = 1.6 Hz, 1H, CH), 6.97 (d, ;J = 8.4 Hz, 1H, Ar–H), 7.03 (d, J = 2.0 Hz, 1H,Ar–H),7.16–7.15 (m, 5H, Ar–H), 7.48(d, J = 16 Hz, 1H, CH). ^{13}C NMR (400 MHz CDCl3): δ 167.33, 164.10, 146.96, 143.91, 137.44, 132.43, 129.73, 129.20, 129.04, 126.64, 123.89, 117.41, 116.78, 115.39, 67.59, 51.73, 44.74, 21.10.

382.3.1.9 (E)-methyl3-(3-oxo-4-(4-(trifluoromethyl)benzyl)-3,4-dihydro-2*H*-benzo[b][1, 4]oxazin-6-yl)acryl-ate (5c)

Starting from compound **4c** (0.20 g, 0.51 mmol) and methyl acrylate (0.06 g, 0.77 mmol), compound **5c** was obtained in 47 % yield.

^{1}H NMR($CDCl_3$ 400 MHz): δ/ppm 3.78 (s, 3H, CH_3), 4.78 (s, 2H, CH_2), 5.23 (s, 2H, CH_2), 6.16 (d, J = 16 Hz, 1H, CH), 6.92 (d, J = 2 Hz, 1H, Ar–H), 7.01 (d, J = 8.4 Hz, 1H, Ar–H), 7.18 (d, J = 2 Hz, 1H, Ar–H), 7.37 (d, J = 8.4 Hz, 2H, Ar–H), 7.48 (d, J = 16 Hz, 1H, CH), 7.60 (d, J = 8 Hz, 2H, Ar–H). ^{13}C NMR (400 MHz CDCl3); δ 167.19, 164.19, 146.86, 143.57, 139.57, 129.41, 128.73, 126.90, 126.09, 126.05, 124.08, 117.74, 117.11, 114.99, 67.54, 51.75, 44.50.

Table 382.1 Inhibition activity of the compounds **4a–4d** and **5a–5d**

Cells	Compounds ((IC_{50}, μM))							
	4a	**4b**	**4c**	**4d**	**5a**	**5b**	**5c**	**5d**
K562	>50	>50	30	35	>50	45	45	30
HepG2	>50	>50	6	30	>50	>50	>50	>50
HT-29	>50	>50	30	>50	>50	>50	>50	>50

382.3.1.10 (E)-methyl 3-(4-(4-methoxybenzyl)-3-oxo-3,4-dihydro-2*H*-benzo[b][1, 4]oxazin-6-yl)acrylate (5d)

Starting from compound **4d** (0.20 g, 0.57 mmol) and methyl acrylate (0.07 g, 0.86 mmol), compound **5d** was obtained in 40 % yield.

^{1}H NMR ($CDCl_3$ 400 MHz): δ/ppm 3.78 (d,J = 0.8 Hz,6H,CH_3),4.74 (s,2H,CH_2), 5.11 (s, 2H, CH_2), 6.17 (d, J = 15.6 Hz, 1H, CH), 6.88–6.86 (m, 2H, Ar–H), 6.97 (d, J = 8 Hz, 1H, Ar–H), 7.06 (d, J = 2 Hz, 1H, Ar–H), 7.14 (d, J = 2 Hz, 1H, Ar–H), 7.16 (d, J = 1.6 Hz, 1H, Ar–H), 7.20 (d, J = 8.8 Hz, 2H, Ar–H), 7.49 (d, J = 16 Hz, 1H, CH). ^{13}C NMR (400 MHz, CDCl3): δ 167.31, 164.09, 159.09, 146.95, 143.90, 129.18, 128.99, 128.07, 127.50, 123.91, 117.42, 116.79, 115.34, 114.44, 67.58, 55.27, 51.72, 44.41.

382.3.2 Biological Assay

The in vitro antitumor activities of the target compounds **4a–4d** and **5a–5d** against three human tumor cells, K562, HepG2 and HT-29 were evaluated by MTT assay. The inhibitory concentrations by 50 % values (IC_{50}) of sample compounds toward test cell proliferation were presented in Table 382.1. Their biological activity results indicated that 6-bromo-4-(4-trifluoromethyl)benzyl)-2*H*-benzo-[b][1, 4]oxazin-3(4*H*)-one **(4c)** showed good antitumor activity against HepG2 cells with an IC_{50} of 6 μM.

382.4 Conclusions

The design and synthesis of novel benzoxazine derivatives have been reported in this paper. Several steps among this route were optimized, such as cyclization, bromination, N-Alkylation, Microwave-assistant Heck coupling reaction and so on. The Microwave-assistant Heck coupling reaction was the key step. The reactions reported in other articles mainly modified at 4 position of (2H)-1,4-benzoxazin-3(4H)-one (2) by aldol condensation, which result in lower yields (only 10–30 %), and need higher temperature over 110 °C, or it will be difficult to react. In this paper, all the target compounds were synthesized in four steps with the overall yield of 20–30 % at 30–60 °C, respectively. The structures of these novel targets and all of intermediates were confirmed by ^{1}H NMR and ^{13}C NMR. Biological activity test indicated that 6-bromo-4-(4-(trifluoromethyl) benzyl)-2*H*-benzo[b] [1, 4]- oxazin -3(4*H*)-one **(4c)** has good antitumor activity against HepG2 cells. The probably reason for the antitumor activity of 4c better than other derivatives is that the trifluoromethyl shows stronger electrical absorption effect. Moreover, methyl acrylate can increase the liposolubility of 4c and makes it more easily penetrate the cell membrane. In order to improve the antitumor activity, further modification based on compound **(4c)** is ongoing in our lab.

Acknowledgments The authors sincerely thank the financial support from the Tianjin Municipal Science and Technology Commission (11ZCGHHZ00400,10ZCKFSY07700) and National Natural Science Foundation of China (81241104).

References

1. Parkin DM, Bray F, Ferlay J, P et al (2005) Global cancer statistics, 55:74–108 2002
2. Minami Y, Yoshida K, Azuma R et al (1993) Structure of an aromatization product of C-1027 Chromophore. Tetrahedron Lett 34:2633–2636
3. Smid P, Coolen HKAC, Keizer HG et al (2005) Synthesis, Structure–activity relationships, and biological properties of 1-Heteroaryl-4-[ω-(1*H*-indol-3-yl)alkyl] piperazines, Novel potential antipsychotics combining potent dopamine D_2 receptor antagonism with potent serotonin reuptake inhibition. J Med Chem 48:6855–6869
4. Fringuelli R, Pietrella D, Schiaffella F et al (2002) Anti-*candida albicans* properties of novel benzoxazine analogues. Bioorg Med Chem 10:1681–1686
5. Macchiarulo A, Costantino G, Fringuelli D et al (2002) 1,4-Benzothiazine and 1,4-Benzoxazine imidazole derivatives with antifungal activity: A docking study. Bioorg Med Chem 10:3415–3423
6. Lanni T, Greene KL, Kolz CN et al (2007) Design and synthesis of phenethyl benzo[1,4]oxazine-3-ones as potent inhibitors of PI3Kinaseγ. Bioorg Med Chem Lett 17:756–760
7. Huang M-Z, Huang K-L, Ren Y-G et al (2005) Synthesis and herbicidal activity of 2-(7-fluoro-3-oxo-3,4-dihydro-2H- benzo[b][1, 4]oxazin-6-yl)isoindoline- 1,3- diones. Agric Food Chem 53:7908–7914
8. Anderluh M, Cesar J, Stefanic P et al (2005) Design and synthesis of novel platelet fibrinogen receptor antagonists with 2*H*-1,4-benzoxazine-3(4*H*)-one scaffold. A systematic study J Med Chem 40:25–49
9. Scheunemann M, Sorger D, Kouznetsova E et al (2007) Sequential ring-opening of *trans*-1,4-cyclohexadiene dioxide for an expedient modular approach to 6,7-disubstituted ($\pm$)-hexahydro-benzo[1, 4]oxazin-3-ones. Tetrahedron Lett 48:5497–5501
10. Niemeyer H (1988) Hydroxamic acids (4-hydroxy-1,4-benzoxazin-3-ones), defence chemicals in the gramineae M. Phytochemistry 27:3349–3358
11. Mosmann T (1983) Rapid colorimetric assay for cellular growth and survival: application to proliferation and cytotoxicity assays. J Immunol Methods 65:55–63
12. Haudecoeur R, Ahmed-Belkacem A, Yi W et al (2011) Discovery of naturally occurring aurones that are potent allosteric inhibitors of hepatitis C virus RNA-dependent RNA polymerase. J Med Chem 54:5395–5402

13. Robert D, Wenge X, Ashok T et al (2009) Preparation of 3-substituted pyrrolo[3,2-b]pyridin- es having 5-HT6 receptor affinity, WO 2009023844. Feb 19, (A2) English
14. Hanson* JR, Richards L Rozas P et al (2003) The bromination and nitration of some (2H)-1,4-benzoxa- zin-3(4H)-ones.11:681–681
15. Torres JC, Pinto AC, Garden SJ et al (2004) Application of a catalytic palladium biaryl synthesis reaction, via C–H functionalization, to the total synthesis of Amaryllidaceae alkaloids. Tetrahedron 60:9889–9900

Chapter 383
On Structural Model of Knowledge Points in View of Intelligent Teaching

Jun Li

Abstract With the advancement of IT technology, intelligent teaching is increasingly valued stressed. Structural model of knowledge points constitutes the basis and core of computer intelligent teaching. By studying the characteristics of structure of knowledge points and its construction kernels, this thesis has summarized two structural models of knowledge points and put forward suggestions for a complete expression of the structure in tree-like XML, so as to provide a reference for researchers and designers concerned.

Keywords Intelligent teaching · Knowledge points · Structural model

383.1 Introduction

The rapid development of IT technology and the universal application of such learning devices as tablet PCs and smart phones have provided people with more diversified and convenient learning styles, which give learners an intelligent teaching environment that is otherwise inaccessible by traditional classroom and media. Therefore, intelligent teaching means, on the basis of new technology, plays an increasingly important role in modern education. Intelligent teaching, in a attempt to use research achievements of artificial intelligence, cognitive psychology and science of thinking, is designed to improve the adaptability and interaction of CAI to efficiently accomplish the teaching task by flexibly adjusting teaching plans and organizing teaching courses according to the differences in teaching goals and ability of students, forming favorable information communication and exchange mechanism by a timely feedback of teaching situation.

J. Li (✉)
Southwest China University Press, Southwest China University, Chongqing, China
e-mail: 765770633@qq.com

S. Li et al. (eds.), *Frontier and Future Development of Information Technology in Medicine and Education*, Lecture Notes in Electrical Engineering 269,
DOI: 10.1007/978-94-007-7618-0_383,

Composed of intelligent teaching model, intelligent teaching system and knowledge base, the intelligent teaching environment has structural model of knowledge points as its internal kernel connection. Though knowledge points, the basic unit of teaching content, are the indispensable foundation of teaching activities, they are often ignored in design as people have long focused their attention on the design of classroom teaching model, leading to the inadaptation of teaching model and teaching content of original class towards the needs of computer intelligent teaching.

383.2 Key Points in Construction of Structural Model of Knowledge Points

383.2.1 Appropriate Grading of Knowledge Points

In an intelligent teaching environment, it is important to have a dynamic construction of learning content for learners based on their individual needs. Learning content is made up in a particular combined way by countless independent learning units that consist of a number of knowledge points. As a learning object, a knowledge point may appear in different learning content, which makes the selection of its grading size the basic problem in effectively organizing and scheduling resources. The basic principle for selecting grading is to ensure the partial integrity of knowledge content whose size is determined by specific requirements. Research shows that the smaller the object grading is, the more flexible the content organization and reconstruction is, and the more complex the whole process becomes. On the contrary, bigger grading, though explains the teaching content better, will restrict the flexibility and the quality to amend, making it difficult to properly schedule and reconstruct the resources.

383.2.2 Avoiding Overlapping Relation in Knowledge Points

Difference in standards of grading and constructing knowledge points will contribute to different forms of knowledge points and affect their interrelations, which is particularly true to subjects in which the structure of knowledge points is flexible and the classification standards are numerous, and the Chinese subject is good example in case here. This phenomenon will form three types of relations among knowledge points, namely, inclusion, intersection and disjointing. It is normal to have relations of inclusion and disjointing in the structure of knowledge points, while the intersecting implies the partly same semanteme between different knowledge points, leading to chaos in the organization and scheduling of content of knowledge points, which must be avoided.

383.2.3 Expandability of Structure of Knowledge Points

The structure characteristics of knowledge points variation depends on teaching stage and subjects. Comparatively speaking, the structure of knowledge points in basic education is stable, while higher education and professional education has a fast knowledge updating pace for their touch upon a variety of fields. Furthermore, in the same teaching stage, knowledge points of different subjects may differ in their structure, for instance, the structure of knowledge points of math is clearer and more explicit than Chinese. Thus, while ensuring meeting the basic demands of users, the structure of knowledge points must be flexible so that its expansion can be realized, which is especially important to subjects with fast changing quality and flexible structural classifications. The expandability of the structure of knowledge points is the precondition for users to modify based on specific needs and form demanded structure of knowledge points.

383.3 Structural Model of Knowledge Points

The structural model of knowledge points mainly focuses on the interrelationships of individual knowledge point that can be categorized into the following four groups:

1. Parent–child relationship: the "parent knowledge point" is the summary and consists of his "child knowledge point".
2. Sibling relationship: this indicates the intimate relationships of "child knowledge points" under one "parent point".
3. Dependence relationship: dependent knowledge point, seen as the must-have before learning others, is the basis and precondition for new knowledge.
4. Association relationship: this indicates the knowledge points that are similar or relative to others. To be specific, those aforesaid points may have reference values or similarities for learning some knowledge, or often appear in same issue generating a more complex question.

383.3.1 Tree-Relationship Model of Knowledge Points

Parent–child relationship and sibling relationship are of vital importance which constitute the foundation of structural model of knowledge points. Through those two relationships above we are able to see clearly the trunk of knowledge tree-relationship model. Furthermore, organizing and scheduling learning content is mainly dependent on this model (Fig. 383.1).

Through this hierarchy those knowledge can be seen as a knowledge tree featuring: when the level is higher, its integrity will be stronger with more content

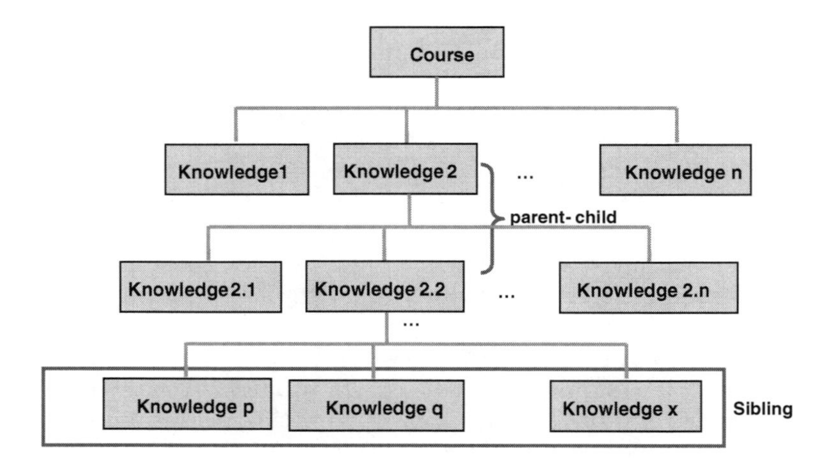

Fig. 383.1 Knowledge tree-relationship model

contained and more abstract issues expressed; when the level is lower, its integrity will be less with more specific object expressed. The knowledge levels in the course shall be arranged from top to bottom, each subordinate level is the development of its upper. When designing teaching content from top level to the lowest, the area concerned in each level becomes narrower and the basic units separated are more specific so that teaching staff are able to comprehend and grasp the course from the whole and develop a teaching design.

383.3.2 Net-Relationship Model of Knowledge Points

Dependence and association relationship supplement the knowledge model and usually determine the intellectuality of intelligent teaching. Dependence influences the content organization of intelligent teaching and secures the acquisition of adequate knowledge for learner; association relationship will benefit the integration of knowledge and the formation of knowledge system. Each knowledge association relationship can be regarded as a model of one-to-many (Fig. 383.2).

383.4 Expression Approaches of Structural Model of Knowledge Points

Graphical knowledge structural model is not suitable to be a general expression approach due to its numerous knowledge points, complex relations and indistinguishableness by computer system. Considering the requirement for standardization

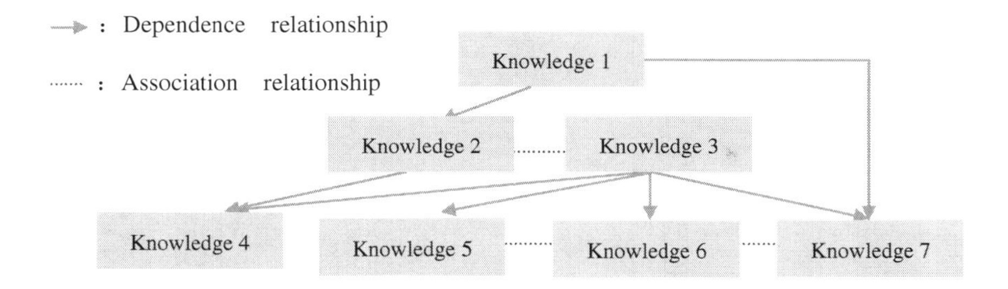

Fig. 383.2 Knowledge net-relationship model

and generality, XML language is a better choice for expressing knowledge structural model with the following advantages:

1. XML can describe the structure, performance and interrelation of knowledge points well.
2. XML is adequate and convenient for describing, organizing, quote and interaction of net resource.
3. XML is a standard formal specification language that is convenient for designing and interaction within intelligent teaching system.
4. XML features flexible expression that is convenient for development of knowledge structure.

XML can express semantic knowledge net-structure model with the tree-like XML by effectively integrating different tree structures and graphic structures. For instance:

```
⟨?xml  version="1.0"  encoding="gb2312" ?⟩
        ⟨knowledge⟩
                ⟨knowledge 1⟩
                        ⟨association relationship⟩
                                ⟨close relation⟩ knowledge n ⟨/ close relation⟩
                         ⟨similarity relation⟩ knowledge m ⟨/ similarity relation⟩
                         ...
⟨/ association relationship⟩
              ⟨/ knowledge 1⟩
        ⟨knowledge 2⟩ ... ⟨/ knowledge 2⟩
...
        ⟨/ knowledge⟩
```

383.5 Conclusion

Based on the analysis of the characteristics of knowledge points structure and its construction features, the thesis has summarized the structural model of knowledge points and put forward suggestions for complete expression of the structure, which laid a foundation for the construction of intelligent teaching environment.

Acknowledgments This work has been supported by the Fundamental Research Funds for National Culture and Science and Technology Innovation Project of National Scinece and Technology Support Plan in the Twelfth Five-year Plan (project No.2012BAH55F02,project No. 2012BAH55F04).

References

1. Kang J, Liu C, Luo N (2009) Research and construction of intelligent tutoring system based on knowledge-point as the center. Comput Program Skills Maint (s1)
2. Jiang Z (2005) The application study of knowledge point relation and its structure diagram and knowledge network. J Anshan Normal Univ 7(5):99–101
3. Teng M, Chen Y (2004) Construction and application of a knowledge structure graph. Modern Educational Technology (05)
4. Lin B (2007) The design for XML-based knowledge node of web courseware. J Shaoxing Univ (Natural Science) (03)

Chapter 384
Evaluation Model of Medical English Teaching Effect Based on Item Response Theory

Lanfen Ji, Dianjun Lu and Dianxiang Lu

Abstract The teaching effect of medical English involves learning competence of students and teaching level of teachers, at medical college its significance has immediate influence on the vocational skills and knowledge absorbing capacity of students. As one of modern psychometric techniques, item response theory provides more insights over and above those gained from classical psychometric techniques. Using item response theory to evaluate medical English teaching effect is a new attempt. This paper presents an introduction to item response theory and demonstrates the evaluation model of the teaching effect of medical English based on item response theory.

Keywords Item response theory · Cumulative IRT models · Psychometric techniques · Medical english

384.1 Introduction

Studies done by many researchers shows that medical English teaching effect has much to do with learning competence of students and teaching level of teachers, at medical college its significance has immediate influence on the vocational skills

L. Ji
Foreign Language Department of Qinghai Normal University,
Xining 810008, People's Republic of China

D. Lu
Department of Mathematics of Qinghai Normal University, Xining 810008,
People's Republic of China

D. Lu (✉)
Research center for high altitude medicine in Qinghai University,
Xining 810001, People's Republic of China
e-mail: ludianxiang@qhu.edu.cn

S. Li et al. (eds.), *Frontier and Future Development of Information Technology in Medicine and Education*, Lecture Notes in Electrical Engineering 269,
DOI: 10.1007/978-94-007-7618-0_384, © Springer Science+Business Media Dordrecht 2014

and knowledge absorbing capacity of students. The content of evaluation is based on medical College English Teaching Programs. Basic teaching goal of medical English is to train students' practical abilities to use the target language. As an important subject in college education, it also has the important task of improving students' autonomy and creativity. Based on the participation of all students, the methods of multivariate evaluation are in accordance with the realization of medical English teaching goals.

The process is often concerned with the measurement of psychological, attitudinal, and cognitive constructs from followers about their teacher and vice versa. Measurement of these constructs can be a very complicated and difficult issue for evaluation of medical English teaching effect. Recently, there has been a marked increase of interest in more detailed treatments of the psychometric properties of the measures used in the evaluation we talk about. Moreover, there are several excellent demonstrations of the consequences that insufficient attention to psychometric properties can have on the nature of the conclusions drawn from evaluation of it. Despite the importance of measurement for evaluation of the teaching effect of medical English, the use of psychometric techniques has not kept pace with the advances in psychometric theory and methods.

The most notable development in techniques for understanding the psychometric properties is item response theory (IRT). IRT is a family of techniques for understanding the psychometric properties of measures and relationships between properties of the measures and the individuals completing those measures [1–4]. These techniques have been used to advance our understanding in a variety of domains of organizational research ranging from multisource performance ratings [5], to cross-cultural differences in employee attitudes.

It is easy to find out that researchers haven't used these techniques to carry out studies on evaluation of medical English teaching effect. This is regrettable as modern psychometric techniques provide additional insights over and above those gained from classical psychometric techniques [6]. As noted above, many of the constructs of interest in evaluation of medical English teaching effect are assessed using self-report or other-report measures and the conceptualization of these constructs is becoming more complex. As such, gaining a better understanding of the measures used to support evaluation of English learning competence theories and constructs is a prudent course for related researchers to take.

In this paper an introduction to item response theory is presented and the application of IRT models in evaluation of medical English teaching effect research is demonstrated. We focus this demonstration on the aspects of IRT that allow for a deeper understanding of the psychometric measures and the application of the recently developed IRT models. In the subsequent sections, we briefly review issues surrounding measurement techniques in the area of medical English teaching and we will further discuss and present the basic principles of IRT.

384.2 Item Response Theory

As we know, researchers use item response theory, which is a model-based (i.e. mathematical) approach, to understand the non-linear relationships between individual characteristics (e.g. ability, traits), item characteristics (e.g. difficulty) and individuals' response patterns [7]. Thus, IRT is concerned with estimating parameters of the items on a measure and parameters of the individuals who complete those measures.

Total scores and correlations are considered to be a basis for the person and item parameters in the course of classical psychometric procedures. IRT, on the other hand, estimates latent parameters for the persons (i.e. the characteristic underlying the total scores) and items using the responses gathered from the sample of data. Moreover, the estimated person and item parameters in IRT are invariant. That is, they are independent of one another. The item parameters do not depend on the distribution of the characteristic in the sample and the person parameters do not depend on particular items on a measure [8]. Therefore, the item parameters are not needed to interpret the person parameters and vice versa.

With classical psychometric techniques, this is not the case, as the person parameters or item parameters cannot be understood out of the context of each other. Moreover, with IRT, the items and persons are on the same metric (i.e. z-scores). Therefore, the level of a characteristic an individual possesses can be compared to the level of the characteristic required by the item. With classical methods, individuals can only be compared to other individuals or an external standard (e.g. a cut score).

A family of different models can be used when we look through IRT. Although there are many differences between the available models (e.g. use of binary vs. polytomous data), one major distinction between IRT models concerns the assumption about the relationship between the selection of a response options and the level of the latent trait. For "cumulative" IRT models the assumption is that there is an increased probability of selecting the correct or higher-ordered response options as the level of the latent trait increases. That is, there is a monotonic relationship between the response choice and the level of the latent trait. Consequently, the individuals with the highest levels of the latent trait will have the highest scores on the items. Another possible assumption is that the relationship is non-monotonic. More specifically, there is an ideal point for each individual on the continuum of a latent trait and the response option nearest the ideal point will be selected. Consequently, the individuals with a level of the latent trait that is closest to the level expressed in the item will have the highest score on the item. This notion is based on Coomb's [9] and Thurstone's [10] research on ideal point response processes. This class of IRT models is referred to as "unfolding" models [11]. These models are relatively new and not widely known outside of the measurement literature.

In the subsequent sections, a cumulative IRT model that is commonly used with graded response data is briefly described.

384.3 Cumulative IRT Models

When we talk about the basis of cumulative IRT models, we surely hold the notion that the relationship between individuals' latent characteristics (i.e. intelligence, exchange quality) and individuals' response selection is a monotonic function. Many of the well-known IRT models (e.g. Rasch models, logistic models, Samejima's (1969) graded response model, Master's (1982) partial credit model) [12] are cumulative models. In this paper, three parameters logistic model is discussed.

On how to evaluate medical English teaching effect, the measures utilize response options that are ordered and the data are used to make conclusions concerning the level of the construct that is assessed by the measure. In these cases, graded response models can be used. In these models, the IRT analysis examines the relationships between item or option parameters, person parameters, and the selection of a particular option. For cumulative graded response models, it is assumed that the value of the latent trait is smaller for individuals who choose the first response option than for individuals who choose the second response option in an ordered response set.

The latent trait of teaching effect is referred to as theta (i.e., θ). The values of theta are expressed as standardized scores (i.e., z-scores). Thus, an individual with $\theta = 1.0$ has a value on the latent trait that is one standard deviation above the mean. Using the first response option as an example, the probability of selecting this option is greatest for individuals with low levels of exchange quality ($\theta < 0.0$) and the probability becomes smaller as the exchange quality increases.

A full understanding of three parameters logistic model, a particular cumulative model, is needed. In three parameters logistic model, three parameters associated with the items are estimated. The first is an option difficulty parameter. The difficulty parameter is referred to as the 'threshold' parameter. This refers to the probability of an individual with a given level of the latent trait selecting a given option or any of the subsequent higher ordered options. Specifically, this parameter is the point on the theta scale where there is a 50 % chance that a given option or a higher ordered option will be selected (i.e. $P(\theta) = 0.5$). In other words, this parameter represents the thresholds between the response options. The second parameter is the discrimination parameter. This parameter represents how well an option discriminates between individuals at different levels of the latent trait. The larger the value, the better the option is at discriminating between individuals at different levels of the latent trait. The third parameter is a parameter of conjecture.

We need to estimate the boundary response functions before we estimate the option characteristic. Boundary response functions are the cumulative probability of selecting a response option equal to or higher than the current response option. Option difficulty parameters are estimated for $m_i - 1$ boundary response functions where mi equals the number of response options. Each boundary response function has a difficulty parameter, but only one discrimination parameter is estimated for each item. The boundary response functions are used to estimate the option characteristic. Mathematically, the boundary response function is expressed as, $P_{i3}(\theta) = {[c_i + \exp(Da_i(\theta - b_i))]}/{[1 + \exp(Da_i(\theta - b_i))]}$, where $P_{i3}(\theta)$ is the probability of a respondent at a particular level of theta responding to option k or any of the other higher ordered options on item i, b_i is the option difficulty parameter, a_i is the discrimination parameter, c_i is the parameter of conjucture, D is a scaling constant equal to 1.702, and exp represents an exponential function. Thus, the probability of selecting option is a function of the level of the latent trait, the difficulty of the option, the discrimination, and the conjucture. In essence, the boundary response functions are estimated by utilizing a three-parameter logistic IRT model on the response option data. From the boundary response functions, the probability of selecting a particular option and the OCCs are estimated.

384.4 Summary

In conclusion, item response theory provides useful models for evaluating medical English learning competence. This paper gives cumulative IRT models that we argue have the potential to contribute to evaluating medical English learning competence and teaching practice. We hope that these techniques will lead to a greater understanding of the nature and measurement of learning competence.

References

1. Ackerman TA (1994) Using multidimensional item response theory to understand what items and tests are measuring. Appl Measur Educ 7:255–278
2. Ackerman TA, Gierl MJ, Walker CM (2003) Using multidimensional item response theory to evaluate educational and psychological tests. Educ Measur Issues Pract 22:37–53
3. Foti RJ, Lord RG (1987) Prototypes and scripts: the effects of alternative methods of processing information on rating accuracy. Organ Behav Hum Decis Process 39:318–341
4. Tejeda MJ, Scandura TA, Pillai R (2001) The MLQ revisited: psychometric properties and recommendations. Leadersh Quart 12:31–52
5. Facteau JD, Craig SB (2001) Are performance appraisal ratings from different rating sources comparable? J Appl Psychol 86:215–227
6. Reise SP, Henson JM (2003) A discussion of modern versus traditional psychometrics as applied to personality assessment scales. J Pers Assess 81:93–103
7. Drasgow F, Hulin CL (1990) Item response theory. In: Dunnette MD and Hough LM (eds) Handbook of industrial and organizational psychology, 2nd ed, vol 1. Consulting Psychologists Press, Palo Alto, pp 577–636
8. Hambleton RK, Swaminathan H, Rogers HJ (1991) Fundamentals of item response theory. Sage, Newbury Park
9. Coombs CH (1950) Psychological scaling without a unit of measurement. Psychol Rev 57:145–158
10. Thurstone LL (1928) Attitudes can be measures. Am J Sociol 33:529–554

11. Roberts JS (1995) Item response theory approaches to attitude measurement. Dissertation Abstracts International, 1995, 56, 7089B, Doctoral Dissertation, University of South Carolina, Columbia
12. Charles, Scherbaum, Finlinson S, Barden K, Tamanini K(2006) Applications of item response theory to measurement issues in leadership research. Leadersh Q 17:366–386

Chapter 385
Discussion on Intervention of Chinese Culture in Chinese College Students' English Writing and Dealing Strategies

Ruxiang Ye

Abstract Owing to the high frequent emergence of errors in Chinese college students' English writing, the paper tries to analyze and discuss the types and reasons of these errors, identifying that most of the mistakes in college students' English writing are caused by the interference of Chinese language, that is, negative transfer of the first language strategy on the second language writing, should not be ignored. Therefore, the author suggests that the development of cultural awareness and reasoning patterns of the target language and trying to reduce the intervention of the first language culture on the second language writing will be the solution.

Keywords Language learning · English writing · Chinese culture · Negative transfer

385.1 Introduction

In recent years, there are growing researches on the correlation between the mother tongue and the L2 writing, which have achieved considerable results. For example, ZHANG Wen-tao believes linguistic errors in China's college students' L2 writing arising from the interference of the structure of mother tongue are relatively conspicuous and its role of negative transfer could not be overlooked [1]. JIANG Pin points out that the negative transfer not only occurs in such aspects as grammar and vocabulary, but in culture and thinking modes [2]. Kaplan thinks our native culture thinking and knowledge will affect the organization in the second language learners' writing [3]. YAN Li-dong thinks that the researchers' interpretation and

R. Ye (✉)
School of Foreign Languages, Anhui University of Science and Technology, Dongshanzhong Road 232001 Huainan, People's Republic of China
e-mail: rxye1975@163.com

S. Li et al. (eds.), *Frontier and Future Development of Information Technology in Medicine and Education*, Lecture Notes in Electrical Engineering 269,
DOI: 10.1007/978-94-007-7618-0_385,

description on the errors not only strengthens the bidirectional study both as a theory and as a method, but also has an important inspiration on second language learning and foreign languages teaching [4]. However, the above researches for mistakes in Chinese students' English writing caused by native culture seem to offer no further presentation, or detailed analyses. This paper will discuss the specific types of mistakes interfered with by Chinese language conventions and the reasons in Chinese students' English writing and suggest appropriate strategies.

385.2 Types of Mistakes

Generally, in English learning there are four basic skills, listening, speaking, reading, and writing. The ability to write, the fourth level of these abilities, is the improvement of the other three abilities and it is understandable that English writing ability has always been the main item in various levels of the examination. For non-English majors in college, through 2 years of English learning, they should be grasping certain level of listening, reading, speaking and writing abilities, meeting the requirements of the college English teaching program. In reality, however, most students, including those who have passed CET-4 or CET-6, there are great disproportions in the development of various English language abilities. For instance, their abilities of reading and listening are usually better, while speaking and writing abilities are relatively weak. I launched a survey on the correction of English compositions of 200 students who come from Grade 2006 and Grade 2008, and found more than 73 % of the mistakes in their compositions are related to the influence of our native culture (the rest mistakes belong to word spelling mistakes). Specifically, these culturally affected mistakes can be divided into several categories.

385.2.1 Poor Diction

This kind of mistakes was made largely because of the fact that English words and Chinese words do not belong to one–one corresponding. Usually a Chinese word can have a few English corresponding words. As an example, "*Kan*" in Chinese, can be translated into several words in English like "see", "look", "watch", "peer" and "glance", etc. When Chinese students write compositions in English, owing to the influence of their mother tongue, they simply want to use the vocabulary of the translation from Chinese into English, not considering the deep semantic meaning of Chinese word and the limitation of English words in use. For example:

(1) Their family can't *give* their education costs.
(2) A part-time job can *contribute to increase* their experience.

385.2.2 Chinese Thinking Pattern

In China, most learners have at least 10 years of Chinese-learning experience before they begin to learn English, and their thought patterns are inevitably influenced by their mother tongue, Chinese. Even learners who perform better in English learning can't avoid making mistakes in writing. After all, the time spent on English can never be parallel to that on Chinese. For students, there are only 4 or 5 h exposed to English learning, which is absolutely insufficient. Therefore, "Chinglish" becomes a common phenomenon in Chinese students' English compositions. For example:

(1) When he smiles, you will see that *his teeth lost many*.
(2) *There are a lot of things changed* in my home town since reforming and opening.

385.2.3 Mixture of Sentence Structure

Strictly, such mistakes should be avoided; they are only grammatical mistakes, represented by double predicates, redundancy of sentence structure and variety of mixed patterns, etc. At first glance, these statements seemed to be understandable, especially for Chinese readers, but foreign readers will feel confused with the exact meaning. For instance:

(1) *There are have* all kinds of sports we can take part in for the well-being of our bodies.
(2) *In spite of sports have* its passive sides, for instance, it can cause injury, it can bring some bad manners, but sports still attract more and more people.

385.2.4 Incoherence in Statement

For an internally coherent sentence, the following information introduced by its connecting part or concessive clue is usually consistent to the direction of the receiver's mental expectations, while coherence of a passage depends more on orderly connection between the sentences with semantic relations. There is numerous occurrence of incoherence with students' English writing. It is not a grammatical mistake, but consistence and combination. Even though there are no obvious mistakes in grammar with some students' English compositions, but they sound influent, incoherent and inconsistent when read, for example:

(1) Nowadays, education is very important to a modern man. In my opinion, the concept of education has been broadened.
(2) In modern time, everyone wants to find a good job, a good job can earn much money, also make people happy.

385.3 Analysis on the Causes of Mistakes

From the above existing problems in Chinese college students' English compositions, the main reason for them lies in the following aspects:

First of all, influence of the mother-tongue culture. A language is the embodiment of the culture it belongs to, and acquisition of a language and understanding its culture are complementary and inseparable with each other. Learning a language equals learning its culture. Writing, as one of the purpose of attaining basic skills of the language output, must reflect the culture it represents. Chinese college students, who are affected deeply by the Chinese language, still cannot avoid the mode of thinking and reasoning process disturbed by Chinese language habits, and write the Chinese-style English compositions that sometimes Chinese can understand while foreigners do not.

Secondly, Chinese college students lack understanding for the features of English writing. It is common for an English writer to put forward the point at the beginning and it is more straightforward and direct. There will be details or facts supporting after presentation of the viewpoint. In contrast, Chinese prefer indirect ways of expressing their ideas in writing. They seldom make the subject clear at the beginning, but reaffirm the viewpoints in many different ways, leaving readers enough room for reflection. In thinking pattern and organization of materials, English writing accents logical reasoning and clear organization and the finished article is always coherent and clear, thus an organic unity. While Chinese way of thinking pays little attention to the logical reasoning. In expression, English writing prefers deduction and places emphasis on originality and personalization. Therefore, the writer is encouraged to use his own words and unique way to present his points after the main idea made clear. Chinese writing tends to generalize and the main idea is often delayed till the end of the article. When writing, Chinese Students don't know how to use English to express and organize their ideas since they do not understand the differences between two languages, only to mechanically turn the Chinese ways of expression into English. No wonder that Chinese students' English writing to some foreign teachers is artificial and unnatural with logical confusion [5].

Finally, students' misconception on English writing, most students hold a wrong idea that learning foreign languages is just learning the grammatical rules, remembering words, phrases and set terms, and writing is not as important as reading. This misconception largely influences students' attitudes towards learning tasks, and further affects the development of students' various abilities in English. Along with the deeply rooted tendency of emphasizing reading and ignoring writing in English teaching approach in China, there is much less time for writing training compared with other language skills, and some teachers even arrange writing activities totally at extracurricular period. Moreover, no enough attention is paid to writing in the college English test at present. Instead, grammar and vocabulary are offered more attention to improve students' reading comprehension. Under this guideline, both teachers and students show no respect for English writing. Even though students are offered time for writing in class, they usually do not take it seriously, so it is difficult to achieve the aim of this activity.

385.4 Suggestions to the Problem

In view of the common occurrence of errors caused by the interference of mother-tongue culture in college students' English composition in China, solutions to cope with the problem lie in the fact that in the teaching of English writing we should urge students to cultivate students' English cultural awareness, sense the differences between English and Chinese, and avoid the interference of Chinese and think in English. Specifically, desirable are the following strategies in college English class.

385.4.1 Pay Attention to the Accumulation of the Cultural Knowledge Related to the Language We Are Learning

As mentioned above, a language is medium of its culture, and learning a language is indispensable to acquiring its culture. Since we are learning English, our English compositions shall be natural and authentic, apprehensible to readers from English-countries. In English class, as teachers, we should guide the students to realize the essential differences between two languages and the differences in thinking patterns between west people and Chinese people, and try to conceive and write in English reasoning. In addition, attention should be paid to cultivation of English language and culture, and students should take notice of the differences between two languages in usage, function and context of vocabulary and phrases; teachers should strengthen students' English way of thinking and approach of expression in explaining grammar and presenting articles.

385.4.2 Make Use of Students' Reading Materials as the Guide to Cultivate Their Ability to Write

Reading course, especially intensive reading, is the most important among the courses offered by Chinese universities. And this course always centers on articles, which is the focus of the college English teaching and learning. There is a need of detailed explanation and solid grasp of these articles with which the students are quite familiar. For example, when we explain these articles to the students, we may require our students to pay special attention to the diction like the word choice, usage of pronouns, adjectives and connectives within these articles, and the logical relations and linguistic ties between sentences, etc. Meanwhile, the articles are usually written by native speakers of English, and they are certainly natural and authentic in usage of language, reflecting the characteristics of contemporary English language. Frequent exposure to such cultivation, students will apply what they have acquired from the articles to his writing and gradually improve their English writing.

385.4.3 Stress Cultivation of Writing Process, Including Collection of Writing Materials, Definition of Genre, Organization of Materials, Development of a Composition and Ultimate Improvement

English writing teaching in China is result-oriented and the teacher assigns a writing task after roughly introducing certain type of writing skills, then compositions students completed independently were handed into teachers. In judging, teachers accent the form of students' writing instead of the content, which is suitable for the education reality in China but has little help for students' writing. Process-oriented Writing can make up for the disadvantages of product-oriented writing. In process writing, students are not alone in a given topic and offer their products for correction, but write the preparation and plan to action steps, for example, discussion, debate, reading, thinking of ideas and listing. Many students work together to plan how to begin and how to organize a writing assignment. They conceive ideas, choose words and make sentences together, then write the first draft to submit to the teacher or the other students for feedback and revision. Accordingly the second draft can be achieved after attentive correction. The process of writing provides students with an opportunity to reflect, innovate, help and learn from each other. Consequently the students improve their English writing ability in practice.

385.5 Conclusion

Above all, it is quite common and severe that there are numerous errors in college students' English compositions in China. Because Chinese college students seldom touch natural and authentic English writing materials and they also have few opportunities to contact the native English speakers. Chinese traditional English teaching methods emphasize grammar, vocabulary and reading skills. Hence, English writing ability has long been ignored and Chinese students' English writing ability is still weak. In their English compositions there are a great amount of mistakes interfered with by Chinese language. We need to take effective teaching methods and ensure that adequate teaching time to improve students' writing ability, but this is not enough. It is more important to help students develop a thorough sense of the nature of writing assignment, raising the awareness of English language and culture, to overcome the negative influence or negative transfer of Chinese language and culture in English writing.

References

1. Zhang WT (2003) Analysis of interlingual and intralingual errors made by college students. Teach Engl China Vol 26:48
2. Jiang P (2001) Negative transfer in the aspects of language, culture and thinking pattern. Teach Engl China 20:36
3. Kaplan RB (1996) Cultural patterns in intercultural education. Lang Learn pp 16
4. Yan LD (2004) Implication for second language pedagogy by analyzing errors in college students writing. Teach Engl China 27:27
5. Houston A (1994) Learning writing through writing: the Chendu approach to teaching written composition. Teach Engl China 26:100–110

Chapter 386
Investigation and Analysis of Undergraduate Students' Critical Thinking Ability in College of Stomatology Lanzhou University

Li ZhiGe, Wang Xuefeng, Zhang Yulin, Weng Wulian, WuFan Bieke, Na Li and Liu Bin

Abstract *Objective* To investigate the status of undergraduates' critical thinking ability and improve medical students thinking ability and comprehensive quality in college of Stomatology Lanzhou University. *Methods* 238 undergraduates of Stomatology Lanzhou University were selected by cluster sampling method of the United States California critical thinking disposition questionnaire (CCTDI). *Results* the average total score of critical thinking ability of undergraduate students of Stomatology Lanzhou University was more than 280 points which showed positive effect on critical thinking ability. Among all the seven critical thinking characteristics, average scores of each item were all positive (>40 points) except that the score of Truth seeking (38.98 ± 5.304) and Systematicity (39.01 ± 4.406) were not meaning.There were statistically significant differences among different grades students loving this profession, strengthening the understanding of critical thinking ability ($P < 0.05$). *Conclusions:* Undergraduates' critical thinking is showed positive effect in college of Stomatology Lanzhou University. However, there still are some shortages. The traditional course system should be continuously reformed; a variety of teaching methods can be implemented to further strengthen the critical thinking ability of medical students.

Keywords: Stomatology · Undergraduate students · Critical thinking ability · Investigation and analysis

L. ZhiGe (✉) · W. Xuefeng · Z. Yulin · W. Wulian · W. Bieke · N. Li · L. Bin
Department of Stomatology, College of Stomatology, Lanzhou University, Lanzhou 730000, People's Republic of China
e-mail: Liubkq@lzu.edu.cn

Z. Yulin
e-mail: siqz@lzu.edu.cn

S. Li et al. (eds.), *Frontier and Future Development of Information Technology in Medicine and Education*, Lecture Notes in Electrical Engineering 269,
DOI: 10.1007/978-94-007-7618-0_386,

386.1 Introduction

Critical thinking was defined as the combination of logical reasoning, problem-solving, and reflection [1]. The investigations in China had showed [2] that the majority of medical graduates in seven areas covered GMER to think the ability to occupy an important position. Little is known about the ability of medical undergraduates' critical thinking ability. So in my paper, the aim is to investigate the status of undergraduates' critical thinking ability and improve medical students thinking ability and comprehensive quality in College of Stomatology Lanzhou University.

386.2 Objects and Methods

386.2.1 Objects

A total of 238 undergraduate students of Stomatology Lanzhou University, 92 boys (38.66 %),146 girls (61.34 %),76 of the grade 2012 students (34.9 %), 62 of the grade 2011(28.4 %), 20 of the grade 2010 students (10 %), 60 of the grade 2009 students (27.6 %), 20 of the grade 2008 students (8.4 %).

386.2.2 Testing Tools

A total of two parts: (1) Basic information of the respondents. (2) characteristics of thinking with Critical thinking tendencies questionnaire (CCTDI) Revision, which is an effective tool to evaluate the critical thinking ability, including Truth-Seeking, Open-Mindedness, Analyticity, SystemAticity. Self-confidence, Inquisitiveness and Maturity. Answer options from full compliance with the completely in line is divided into six negative entry score of 1–6, the positive entries in reverse assignment. Each score is between 10–60 points. The range of total score is 70–420 points. more than 210 points shows negative effect on critical thinking ability. The score between 11 and 279 points is not meaning, more than 280 points demonstrates positive effect on critical thinking ability,more than 350 points shows strong critical thinking. Each dimension is divided into 10–60 points, less than 30 points shows negative effect on critical thinking, the meaning between 31 and 39 points is not clear, more than 40 points illustrates positive effect on critical thinking, more than 50 points is strong tendency.

386.2.3 Survey Methods

Using cluster sampling method. Description of the purpose and significance of the research, to gain understanding and support to the survey, 238 questionnaires are handed out.After filling in the recovery of 238 on the spot, the recovery rate of 100 %,valid questionnaires were 223 copies, Effective rate was 93.7 % 0.76, 62, 20, 60, 20 questionnaires were distributed to Grade 2012, 2011, 2010, 2009, 2008 students,74, 58, 18, 56, 17 valid questionnaires with efficiency of 97.4, 93.5, 90.0, 93.3, 85 %,,respectively.. The internal consistency of the questionnaire CCTDI the coefficient is 0.898, the reliability.

386.2.4 Statistical Treatment

SPSS18.0 statistical software for processing is used to analysis the data. Critical thinking scores using the form, independent samples *t* test, one-way ANOVA and Pearson correlation analysis, and two analyzes were performed using the Bonferroni method to conduct a comparative analysis of the information obtained. $P < 0.05$ indicated that it was a statistically difference.

386.3 Results

The overall situation of critical thinking skills of Stomatology medical undergraduates in Lanzhou University

Overall situation of Lanzhou University School of Stomatology undergraduate critical thinking ability (Table 386.1), 218 total score (292.56 ± 30.726) points (280 points), the overall performance of positive critical thinking skills, and less than 210 points. Among of seven dimensions showed positive traits (>40 points) except that truth capacity, the systematic (<40 points) are not clear.

Lanzhou University School of Stomatology year undergraduate critical thinking ability to analyze the relationship with each factor

The sequence of all grades score is 2012 > 2011 > 2010 > 2009 > 2008 (Table 2), the score of 2008, 2009, and between 2010 and 2011 students have no statistically difference. But compared with the score of grade 2012 students, the rest of the year showed a larger difference with statistically difference,which is considered stronger effect than the grade 2012 students in critical thinking ability, different grade students have statistically differences about loving the professional, strengthening critical thinking skills to understand(*P* value < 0.05). Tables 2–4.

Table 386.1 Analyze the overall situation of critical thinking skills of Stomatology medical undergraduates in Lanzhou University. ($n_1 = 420$, $n_2 = 102$, points)

Dimensions	$\overline{X} \pm S$
Truth-Seeking	38.98 ± 5.304
Open-Mindedness	42.23 ± 5.163
Analyticity	41.73 ± 6.192
Systematicity	39.01 ± 4.406
Self-confidence	43.12 ± 6.086
Inquisitiveness	44.40 ± 5.704
Maturity	43.09 ± 5.964
Total points of CCTDI	292.56 ± 30.726

Table 386.2 Compare the influence of different grades to critical thinking of Stomatology undergraduates in Lanzhou University

Grades	N	Total scores of CCTDI $(\overline{X} \pm S)$
2008	17	275.37 ± 28.242①
2009	56	283.48 ± 30.302②
2010	18	285.06 ± 29.433③
2011	58	291.55 ± 28.336④
2012	74	305.99 ± 26.209
F value		13.537
P value		0.000

386.4 Discussion

It showed positive effects that are similar to the results of Peng Meici [3] about the critical thinking ability of undergraduates. The score of Truth seeking and Systematicity (less than 40 points) were not meaning in the ability of critical thinking ability,whose results also showed agreement with previous results [4, 5]. Some scholars had pointed out that low ability was showed in the searching for Truth [6]. As shown in Table 3: the critical thinking ability about the students liking to learn stomatology was higher than that the specialty "did not feel" undergraduates.Interest is the best teacher, only one person to love what you do can actively and constantly improve their own qualities to try to make things better. As shown in Table 4: Understand the critical thinking ability of critical thinking levels in college of Stomatology Lanzhou University were significantly higher than that of students who do not understand the critical thinking. The results agreement well with previous research by Zhang Tingting [7], who had reported that the ability of clinical nurses who understanded critical thinking were significantly higher than others. Our goal is to improve medical students thinking ability and comprehensive quality.

In the study, Interesting,the score of different grades about critical thinking ability in college of Stomatology Lanzhou University decreased. In 5 years' leaning,this problem that the critical thinking ability did not not only increase but also decrease significantly has to ponder, after interviewing with some teachers and students, we think that students' critical thinking ability have been influenced

Table 386.3 Compare the influence of if like their major to critical thinking of stomatology undergraduates in Lanzhou University

Content	N	Total scores of CCTDI $(\overline{X} \pm S)$
Like	135	297.12 ± 29.655①
No feelings	78	286.16 ± 30.420
dislike	10	280.88 ± 30.423
F value		6.422
P value		0.002

Table 386.4 Compare the influence of the understanding of critical thinking skills to critical thinking of oral medical undergraduates in Lanzhou University

Content	N	Total scores of CCTDI $(\overline{X} \pm S)$
Know	12	309.44 ± 32.788①
Know a little	100	300.16 ± 31.846②
Do not know	111	283.89 ± 28.250
F value		5.073
P value		0.01

by the factors that are as follows : concerning with "traditional teaching to the test–oriented", Furthermore, relating to the influence of Chinese traditional culture. The research shows that the scores of truth seeking and systematicity are low (<40 points), which correspond to the studies in home and abroad [4–8].

In short, it is important for higher medical education to cultivate medical students'critical thinking ability. Education should be comprehensive and systematic to improve the link of teaching and practice, and cultivate medical students to adapt to the development of social economy, thus they can make the wisdom choice in complicated clinical environment. In this study, students' critical thinking ability in college of Lanzhou University are investigated.However,which cannot be broadly representative of other domestic college students'critical thinking in stomatology. Further investigation should also be expanded the depth and breadth to provide the reliable basis for further strengthening the cultivation of critical thinking of students in stomatology.

References

1. ZhiHua S, Peichun H (2011) Investigation and analysis present situation of critical thinking ability of our school students'. J Health Vocat Educ 121–122
2. Rosy clouds, GuQiMei (2004) Investigation and analysis of the attitude of the "Global Minimum basic requirements" of the TCM college students. J Northw Med Educ 12(5):352–354
3. Peng MC, Wang GC, Chen JL et al (2004) The reliability and validity testing of critical thinking skills meter. Chin J Nurs 644–647
4. Guo RH (2007) Status survey and analyse of influencing factors of nursing Undergraduates' Critical thinking attitude tendency. J China Med Univ

5. Zhao M, Wang WL, Zhang XQ (2008) Investigate of Medical Students' critical thinking skills. Chin Doct 2008:269–271
6. Giancarlo CA, Facione PA (2001) A look across four years at the disposition toward critical thinking among undergraduate students. J Gen Educ 50(1):29–55
7. Zhang T, BaoLing, ZhangYaQing (2011) The correlation between clinical nurse critical thinking skills and general self-efficacy. Shanghai Nurs J 11 (6):5–8
8. Yem ML (2002) Assessing the reliability and validity of the Chinese version of the California critical thinking disposition inventory. Int J Nurs Stud 39(2):123–132

Chapter 387
Surgeons' Experience in Reviewing Computer Tomography Influence the Diagnosis Accuracy of Blunt Abdominal Trauma

Sun Libo, Xu Meng, Chen Lin, Su Yanzhuo, Li Chang and Shu Zhenbo

Abstract Computer Tomography (CT) plays an important role in the diagnosis and treatment strategy in blunt abdominal trauma (BAT). The aim of this study was to evaluate the surgeons experience in CT reviewing in the diagnosis accuracy in the early stage of BAT. Altogether 82 patients with BAT were retrospectively reviewed, and the final diagnosis was confirmed according to intra-operative exploration and post-operative pathological examination. Surgeons were classified into senior and junior groups. Double blind method was used to evaluate the accuracy of injury judgement from CT scan. Totally the accuracy in the senior group was significantly higher than the junior group (73.9 vs. 34.1 %, $P < 0.05$). Compared with junior group, senior group showed significant higher diagnosis accuracy both in the hollow and solid organ injuries (90.1 vs. 78.9 %; 88.4 vs. 58.3 %, respectively, $P < 0.05$). It is concluded that surgeon's experience in the reviewing of CT scan significantly influence the diagnosis accuracy of viscera injury in BAT. Senior surgeon's attendance can help the diagnosis of viscera injury in the early stage of BAT.

Keywords Computer tomography · Blunt abdominal trauma · Diagnosis

387.1 Introduction

Abdominal trauma is one of the emergency diseases usually following traffic accident and industrial injuries. Blunt abdominal trauma (BAT) has not superficial wound, so it is difficult to judge the location and extent of injury. Besides clinical findings, image examinations, especially computer tomography (CT), plays an

S. Libo (✉) · X. Meng · C. Lin · S. Yanzhuo · L. Chang · S. Zhenbo
Department of Gastrointestinal Surgery, China-Japan Union Hospital, Jilin University, Changchun 130033, China
e-mail: sunlibo0431@sina.com

S. Li et al. (eds.), *Frontier and Future Development of Information Technology in Medicine and Education*, Lecture Notes in Electrical Engineering 269,
DOI: 10.1007/978-94-007-7618-0_387,

important role in the diagnosis and treatment strategy [1–3]. In emergency case, the report of CT examination was usually delayed compared with CT films. In order to get the injury information in the early stage of BAT, it is necessary for surgeons to have the ability in reviewing CT films. The aim of this study was to evaluate the surgeons experience in diagnosis accuracy in the early stage of BAT.

387.2 Methods

387.2.1 Patients

Patients receiving surgical intervention for blunt abdominal trauma in China–Japan Union Hospital between March 2010 and March 2013 were retrospectively reviewed. Computer tomography was underdone in all the patients and final diagnosis was confirmed according to intra-operative exploration and post-operative pathological examination. Patients suspected blunt abdominal trauma without surgical intervention were excluded in this study.

387.2.2 Computer Tomography Examination

Light speed 64 slice spiral CT used in this study was made in USA (GE company). Patients received CT examination on the basis of stable life signs, and liquid transfusion and life sign monitoring were supplied during the examination.

387.2.3 Surgeons' Classification

Three senior surgeons who have more than 10 years experiences in reviewing CT and three junior surgeons who have less than 3 years work were asked to review the CT films independently with double blind method. The accuracy of diagnosis was got by the three surgeons' average value, and compared between senior and junior groups.

387.2.4 Injury Judgment and Classification

The viscera injury indications from abdomen CT include liquid collection, abnormal gas in the abdominal cavity (Fig. 387.1a), and morphology change of viscera [1–3]. Diagnosis was evaluated in three levels: (1) Viscera trauma exist or not; (2) Solid organ or hollow organs; (3) Accuracy in different solid organs.

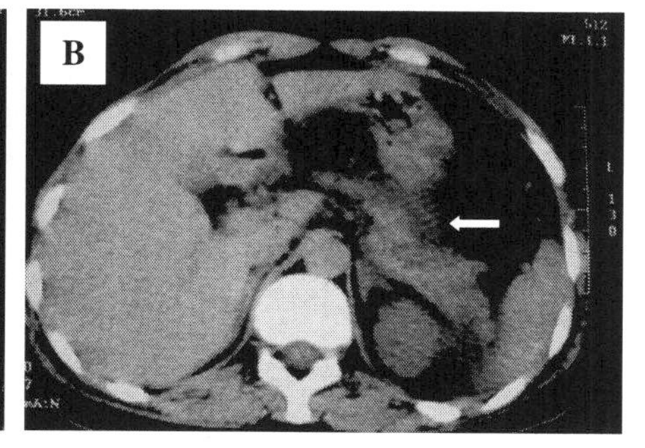

Fig. 387.1 Abnormal gas collection in the abdominal cavity for intestine perforation due to blunt abdominal trauma (**a**), The blurred margin of pancreas observed for pancreas injury (**b**)

387.2.5 Statistical Analysis

The data of patient's age, body index were presented as $\chi \pm$ s. Chi square test was used to compare the differences in accuracy. All statistical analyses were performed with SPSS software, version 11.0 (SPSS Inc, Chicago, United States).

387.3 Results

387.3.1 Patients' Characteristics

Altogether 82 patients were included in this study, the general data of patients' gender, age and injury site were listed in Table 387.1. Spleen was the most common injury site which occupied 41 % in the total injuries Incidence of pancreas injury was the most lower (Fig. 2), which was only 6.8 %. Six patients suffered from combined injuries of solid and hollow organs, so injury site was counted as 88.

387.3.2 General Accuracy of Injury Judgement in Senior and Junior Groups

Totally the accuracy of viscera injury judgement in the senior group was significantly higher than that in the junior group. The data were listed in the Table 387.2.

Table 387.1 Patients' general characteristics and injury site

Mean age (years, Mean ± SD	40.3 ± 12.5	
Male/Female	69:13	
Body mass index(kg/m^2, Mean ± SD)	35.6 ± 5.2	
Injury site		
Liver	17	19.3
Spleen	36	41
Pancreas	6	6.8
Intestine	23	26.1
Combined injury	6	6.8
Total number of injury site	88#	100

Six patients suffered from combined injury of both solid and hollow organs

Table 387.2 Comparison of viscera injury judgement from CT between the two groups

	Senior group	Junior group
Correct	65	30
Mistake	23	58
Total	88	88
Accuracy	73.9 %	34.1 %

Kappa analysis: K = 0.085, $P < 0.05$

387.3.3 Accuracy Comparison in Different Organs Between Senior and Junior Groups

The Senior group showed significant higher injury judgement accuracy in both solid and hollow organs. The accuracy of injury judgement of solid organ was higher than that of hollow organs in both Senior and Junior groups, but no significant difference was found (Table 387.3). Both groups showed lower accuracy in the judgement of pancreas injury, but no difference was found due to the fewer cases of pancreas injury.

Table 387. 3 Accuracy comparison in injuries of solid and hollow organs between senior and junior groups

	Senior group		Junior group	
	Solid organ	Hollow organ	Solid organ	Hollow organ
Correct	64	20	56	14
Mistake	7	4	15	10
Total	71	24	71	24
Accuracy	90.1 %#	88.4 %#	78.9 %	58.3 %

$P < 0.05$,difference comes from comparison in solid and hollow organs respectively between the senior and junior groups

387.4 Discussion

Abdominal trauma is increasing in clinic following the quick industry development especially traffic tools. The morbidity, mortality, and economic costs resulting from BAT are particularly substantial [2]. Besides clinical findings, diagnostic peritoneal lavage, Ultrasound examinations, and CT play important roles in the diagnosis and therapeutic strategy decision [3–5]. With the help of electric network, doctors in clinic can get the CT image in the early stage after examination. Therefore, the experiences and ability of doctors in reviewing CT image might influence the early diagnosis of BAT. In this study, senior surgeons showed more than two times accuracy in the diagnosis of BAT, suggesting that experienced surgeons are helpful in the early diagnosis, which may further influence the treatment.

Compared with solid organs, the early diagnosis of hollow organ injury is more difficult in BAT [6]. Some patients with hollow organ injuries showed only abdominal discomfort, and no acute peritonitis can be found in the early stage. However, in the early stage of BAT, abnormal gas collection, other than liquid collection in the abdominal cavity from CT scan, may be the only information, of which it is difficult for the junior surgeons to find. Though repeated CT and 64 slice CT could help to reduce the miss findings of CT [7, 8], the best way to increase the diagnosis accuracy of BAT is to combine CT and clinical findings [9, 10], because some injuries may not show any abnormal indications in the early stage. In this study both the senior and junior groups showed a lower accuracy in the diagnosis of hollow organ injury compared with solid organ injury. In our opinion, besides the experience factor, less signs in CT film in the early stage of hollow organ injury may be the factor of lower accuracy in the two groups.

Though difference could be found between the two groups in the judgement of solid organ injury from CT scan, both the senior and junior groups showed a relatively higher accuracy. This may be due to the liquid collection was common because of hemorrhage, and could be found easily by experienced surgeons. Liver and spleen injuries occupied more than 50 % of the BAT in this study. In BAT, the shape change of solid organ and relatively large amount of hemorrhage present clear information of injury from CT for clinicians [11–14]. The judgement of injury grade is the key point to choose treatment strategy [15–17], and in clinic the specialists in the injury site could present better evaluation than general emergency physicians [18], so the attendance of senior surgeon in abdominal surgery seems very necessary. The incidence of pancreas injury is very rare, but it is the most difficult organ to judge injury from CT scan [19, 20]. The reason may be due to pancreas' small size, special position, and stable hemodynamic after injury. In our experience, repeated CT combined with clinical and laboratory findings may increase the diagnosis accuracy of pancreas injury.

In conclusion, surgeon‘s experience in the reviewing of CT scan significantly influence the accuracy of viscera injury in BAT. Senior surgeon‘s attendance can help the diagnosis of viscera injury in the early stage of BAT.

References

1. Raza M, Abbas Y, Devi V, et al (2013). Non operative management of abdominal trauma–a 10 years review. World J Emerg Surg 8:14 [Epub ahead of print]
2. Soto JA, Anderson SW (2012) Multidetector CT of blunt abdominal trauma. Radiol 265:678–93
3. Holmes JF, McGahan JP, Wisner DH (2012). Rate of intra-abdominal injury after a normal abdominal computed tomographic scan in adults with blunt trauma. Am J Emerg Med 30:574–579
4. Wang YC, Hsieh CH, Fu CY et al (2012) Hollow organ perforation in blunt abdominal trauma: the role of diagnostic peritoneal lavage. Am J Emerg Med 30:570–573
5. Mihalik JE, Smith RS, Toevs CC et al (2012) The use of contrast-enhanced ultrasound for the evaluation of solid abdominal organ injury in patients with blunt abdominal trauma. J Trauma Acute Care Surg 73:1100–1105
6. Chichom Mefire A, Weledji PE, Verla VS, et al (2013) Diagnostic and therapeutic challenges of isolated small bowel perforations after blunt abdominal injury in low income settings: analysis of twenty three new cases Injury. 2 pii: S0020–1383 (13):00116–2 [Epub ahead of print]
7. Walker ML, Akpele I, Spence SD et al (2012) The role of repeat computed tomography scan in the evaluation of blunt bowel injury. Am Surg 78:979–985
8. Petrosoniak A, Engels PT, Hamilton P et al (2013) Detection of significant bowel and mesenteric injuries in blunt abdominal trauma with 64-slice computed tomography. J Trauma Acute Care Surg 74:1081–1086
9. Joseph DK, Kunac A, Kinler RL et al (2013) Diagnosing blunt hollow viscus injury: is computed tomography the answer? Am J Surg 205:414–418
10. Bhagvan S, Turai M, Holden A et al (2013) Predicting hollow viscus injury in blunt abdominal trauma with computed tomography. World J Surg 37:123–126
11. Uzkeser M, Sahin H, Ozogul B et al (2013) Defining the percentage of intra-abdominal hemorrhage in abdominal computerized tomography using stereology in patients with blunt liver injury and determining its relationship with outcomes. J Trauma Acute Care Surg 74:224–229
12. Jin W, Deng L, Lv H, Zhang Q et al (2013) Mechanisms of blunt liver trauma patterns: An analysis of 53 cases. Exp Ther Med 5:395–398
13. Boscak A, Shanmuganathan K (2012). Splenic trauma: what is new?. Radiol Clin North Am 50:105–122
14. Boscak AR, Shanmuganathan K, Mirvis SE, et al (2013) Optimizing Trauma Multidetector CT Protocol for Blunt Splenic Injury: Need for Arterial and Portal Venous Phase Scans. Radiol 28 [Epub ahead of print]
15. Radhiana H, Azian AA, Razali MR et al (2010) Computed tomography (CT) in blunt liver injury: a pictorial essay. Med J Malaysia 65:319–325
16. Huang YC, Wu SC, Fu CY, Chen YF et al (2012) Tomographic findings are not always predictive of failed nonoperative management in blunt hepatic injury. Am J Surg 203:448–453
17. Hassan R, Abd Aziz A, Md Ralib AR et al (2011) Computed tomography of blunt spleen injury: a pictorial review. Malays J Med Sci 18:60–67
18. Sokolove PE, Kuppermann N, Vance CW et al (2013) Variation in specialists reported hospitalization practices of children sustaining blunt abdominal trauma. West J Emerg Med F 14:37–46
19. Lee PH, Lee SK, Kim GU et al (2012) Outcomes of hemodynamically stable patients with pancreatic injury after blunt abdominal trauma. Pancreatol 12:487–492
20. Cigdem MK, Senturk S, Onen A et al (2011) Nonoperative management of pancreatic injuries in pediatric patients. Surg Today 41:655–659

Chapter 388
Analysis of Face Recognition Methods in Linear Subspace

Hongmei Li, Dongming Zhou and Rencan Nie

Abstract How to extract discriminant features from face images is a key problem to face recognition. Many methods have been proposed, and among these methods linear subspace analysis method has been given more and more attention owing to its good properties, since principal component analysis (PCA) was applied successfully. In this paper, all the linear subspace methods which have been successfully applied to face recognition and some good summaries will be given.

Keywords Face recognition · Linear subspace analysis · PCA

388.1 Introduction

In recent years, with the rapid development of computer science, in-depth study on the face recognition can greatly promote the development of the discipline [1]. Because of face recognition have direct, friendly and convenient features. It is applied to national security, military security, and many other fields.

In the face recognition field, the raw input image data, often have very high dimensionality comparing with the sample features [2]. It is very difficult to analyze the sample features of such data. Dimensionality reduction for input data provides a favorable way to analyze the sample features [3]. Feature extraction is a dimensionality reduction method [4]. Linear subspace analysis is a popular linear feature extraction method in the face recognition field.

Linear subspace analysis method includes PCA, LDA, ICA and NMF. PCA was first applied to recognize faces, which drastically reduces the dimensionality of the original space, and face identification are then carried out in the reduced space.

H. Li · D. Zhou (✉) · R. Nie
Information College, Yunnan University, Kunming, China
e-mail: zhoudm@ynu.edu.cn

S. Li et al. (eds.), *Frontier and Future Development of Information Technology in Medicine and Education*, Lecture Notes in Electrical Engineering 269,
DOI: 10.1007/978-94-007-7618-0_388,

However, it cannot guarantee the same classification rate when changing viewpoints. LDA was used to enhance the separation between different classes [5]. As PCA and LDA consider the second order statistics only but lack information on higher order statistics. ICA was used to accounts higher order statistics. When the input data is non-negative, NMF is an effective method in reducing the dimensionality of data and preserving the non-negative nature of data.

388.2 Linear Subspace Analysis

388.2.1 Analysis on Principal Component

The main idea of the PCA is to find the vectors which best account for the distribution of face images within the entire image space. Each vector is a linear combination of the original face images.

To obtain the eigenfaces for a training set, it is crucial to first determine the mean vector, deviation-from-mean vectors and the covariance matrix for the particular training set. Let the training set of face images be $\{X_1, X_2, \ldots, X_N\}$, the mean vector of the set is defined by $\bar{X} = \sum_{i=1}^{N} X_i$. The set of deviation-from-mean vectors are simply defined as: $\psi_i = X_i - \bar{X}$.

To obtain the eigenfaces description of the training set, we seeks a set of vectors, which significantly describes the variations of the data [6]. Mathematically, the principal components of the training set are the eigenvectors of the covariance matrix of the training set. The covariance matrix is given by:

$$S_t = \frac{1}{N}(X - \bar{X})(X - \bar{X})^T = \frac{1}{N}\sum_{i=1}^{n} \psi_i \psi_i^T \tag{388.1}$$

It is from the matrix that we are interested in finding the set of orthogonal vectors w_i and scalars λ_i that satisfy the relations:

$$S_t w_i = \lambda_i w_i \; i = 1, 2, \ldots, m \tag{388.2}$$

388.2.2 Analysis on Linear Discriminant

LDA optimizes the low dimensional representation of objects with focus on the most discriminant feature extraction. It's tries to "shape" the scatter in order to make it more reliable for classification [7].

Let the between-class scatter matrix be defined as:

$$S_b = \sum_{i=1}^{c} \frac{N_i}{N} (\mu_i - \mu)(\mu_i - \mu)^T \tag{388.3}$$

And the within-class scatter matrix be defined as:

$$S_w = \frac{1}{N} \sum_{i=1}^{c} \sum_{j=1}^{N_i} \left(x_i^j - \mu_i\right)\left(x_i^j - \mu_i\right)^T \tag{388.4}$$

If S_w is non-singular, the optimal projection $J_F(w)$ is chosen as the matrix with orthonormal columns which maximizes the ratio of the determinant of the S_b of the projected samples to the determinant of the S_w of the projected samples. They are simply defined as:

$$J_F(W) = \arg\max_w \frac{|W^T S_b W|}{|W^T S_w W|} = [w_1, w_2, \ldots, w_m] \tag{388.5}$$

where w_i is the set of generalized eigenvectors of S_b and S_w corresponding to the m largest generalized eigenvalues λ_i, they are simply defined as:

$$\mathrm{S_b} w_\mathrm{i} = \lambda_i S_w w_\mathrm{i} \; i = 1, 2, \ldots m \tag{388.6}$$

388.2.3 Analysis on PCA and LDA (Fisherfaces)

In order to make the S_w is non-singular. It has been proposed an alternative to the criterion in (388.5). It's achieved by using PCA to reduce the dimension of the feature space to $N-c$, and then applying the LDA to reduce the dimension to $c-1$. $\hat{W}$ is given by:

$$\hat{W} = W_{PCA} W_{LDA} \tag{388.7}$$

$$W_{PCA} = \arg\max_W \left|W^T S_t W\right| \tag{388.8}$$

$$W_{LDA} = \arg\max_W \frac{\left|W^T W_{PCA}^T S_b W_{PCA} W\right|}{\left|W^T W_{PCA}^T S_w W_{PCA} W\right|} \tag{388.9}$$

388.2.4 Analysis on Independent Component

ICA searches for a linear transformation to express a set of random variables as linear combinations of statistically independent source variables [8].

Let X representing an image, and the covariance matrix of X is defined as:

$$C = E\{[X - E(X)][X - E(X)]^T\} \tag{388.10}$$

ICA factorizes the C into the form: $C = A\Delta A^T$, where Δ is diagonal real positive and A transforms X into S, $X = AS$, and the new data S are independent.

Three operations: whitening, rotation and normalization used to derive the ICA transformation A. First, the whitening can be defined as:

$$X = \phi\Lambda^{1/2}U \tag{388.11}$$

The ϕ and Λ are derived by solving the following eigenvalue equation:

$$C = \phi\Lambda\phi^T \tag{388.12}$$

Second, the rotation operations, minimizing the mutual information approximated using higher order cumulants. Finally, the normalization derives unique independent components in terms of orientation, unit norm, and order of projections.

388.2.5 Analysis on Non-Negative Matrix Factorization

NMF is a matrix analytical method and described as: Given a non-negative $V(m \times n)$, find non-negative matrix factor $W(m \times r)$ and matrix factor $H(r \times n)$, so that

$V \approx WH$, where r is a smaller number than m and n.

The solution of NMF is equivalent to the following objective function:

$$\underset{W,H}{Min}\, D(V\|WH) = \sum\left(V_{ij}\log\frac{V_{ij}}{(WH)_{ij}} - V_{ij} + (WH)ij\right) \tag{388.13}$$

And the updating equation can be defined as follows:

$$W_{ia} \leftarrow W_{ia}\sum_{\mu}\frac{V_{i\mu}}{(WH)_{i\mu}}H_{a\mu} \quad W_{ia} \leftarrow \frac{W_{ia}}{\sum_j W_{ja}} \quad H_{a\mu} \leftarrow H_{a\mu}\sum_i W_{ia}\frac{V_{i\mu}}{(WH)_{i\mu}} \tag{388.14}$$

388.3 Experimental Results and Analysis

The experimental data, consisting of 40 distinct persons with ten images per person, comes from the ORL database. The images are taken at different time instances, with varying facial expressions and facial details.

- The number of training samples N1 and test samples N2 per person effects on recognition rate

In the experiments, we calls for from one to nine images per person sequentially chosen for *N*1, and the remaining 10-*N*1 as *N*2, the recognition rate as shown in Fig. 388.1; and calls for from one to nine images per person sequentially chosen for *N*1, 10 images per person as *N*2, the recognition rate as shown in Fig. 388.2.

Figure 388.1 not only describes the different number of training samples and test samples influence on recognition rate, also proves that the linear subspace method is availability and superiority used for face recognition. This shows when *N*1 gets bigger, the face recognition rate increases. If possible, training samples were obtained as much as possible, the recognition rate can be improved greatly.

Figure 388.2 describes the recognition rate under the same number of test samples, and the different number of training samples. This figure shows when *N*1 gets bigger, the face recognition rate increases. That is because the test samples contains all information of the training samples, and can be widely covered different posture, facial expression changes, so the recognition rate is higher, the recognition time and the complexity of the calculation is not increased.

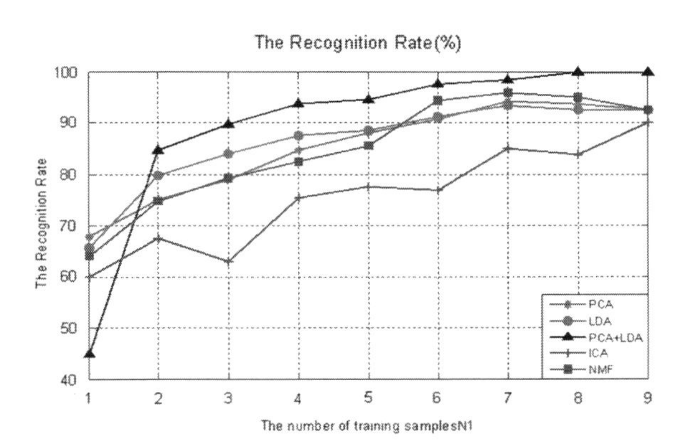

Fig. 388.1 Recognition rates (different number of N1 per person)

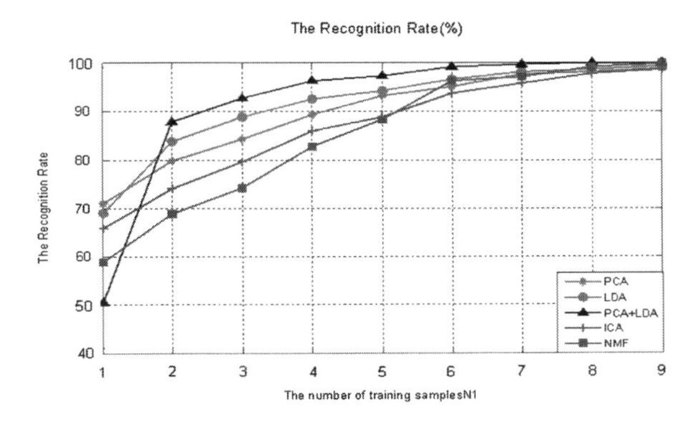

Fig. 388.2 Recognition rates (same number of N2 per person)

Fig. 388.3 The different size of data sets of recognition rates (%)

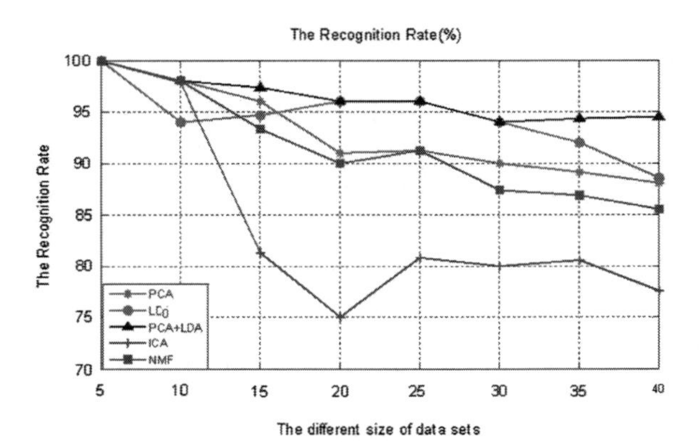

- The different size of data sets effects on recognition rate

The size of the training and test samples has a certain influence on the recognition rate. Figure 388.3 describes this influence. We select the first five images per person as the training samples, and the remaining five images as the test samples.

Figure 388.3 describes the effect of different training and test sample size on recognition rate. It shows that the recognition rate decreases with increasing the number of individuals, the training and test of only 40 people set the recognition rate is decreased. Therefore, for the reliability of face recognition of large scale and important must consider the recognition results and the number of samples.

388.4 Conclusions

For face recognition, the key problem is to extract discriminant features from face images. The subspace analysis has become one of the main methods of face recognition owing to its good properties. But because face recognition is an interdisciplinary challenge, so the current face recognition methods are mainly suitable for a particular environment, limit the number of application classes. Diversity of lighting conditions, facial expressions and facial details, will affect the recognition results, there are many places needs improvement.

Acknowledgments This work is supported by the National Natural Science Foundation of China (61065008), Natural Science Foundation of Yunnan Province (No.2012FD003).

References

1. Chen Y, Zheng W-S (2013) Discriminant subspace learning constrained by localli statistical uncorrelation for face recognition. Neural Netw 42:28–43
2. Shekar BH (2011) Face recognition using kernel entropy component analysis. Neurocomputing 74(6):1053–1057
3. Huang W, Yin H (2012) On nonlinear dimensionality reduction for face recognition. Image Vis Comput 30(4–5):355–366
4. Wang S-J, Zhou C-G (2011) Face recognition using second-order discriminant tensor subspace analysis. Neurocomputing 74(12–13):2142–2156
5. Kautkar SN, Atkinson GA, Smith ML (2012) Face recognition in 2D and 2.5D using ridgelets and photometric stereo. Pattern Recognit 45(9):3317–3327
6. Luh G-C, Lin C-Y (2011) PCA based immune networks for human face recognition. Appl Soft Comput 11(2):1743–1752
7. Shu X, Gao Y (2012) Efficient linear discriminant analysis with locality preserving for face recognition. Pattern Recognit 45(5):1892–1898
8. Deng W, Liu Y (2012) The small size problem of ICA: a comparative study and analysis. Pattern Recognit 45(12):4438–4450

Chapter 389
Energy Dispersive X-Ray Spectroscopy of HMG-CoA Synthetase During Essential Oil Biosynthesis Pathway in *Citrus grandis*

She-Jian Liang, Ping Zheng, Han Gao and Ke-Ke Li

Abstract Essential oil as one kind of terpenoid plays an important role in disease resistance and plant protection. In recent years, it becomes one of research hotspots in the field of plant secondary metabolism, but its synthetic site has been debated. Electron microscopic cytochemistry of 3-hydroxy-3-methylglutaryl coenzyme A (HMG-CoA synthetase) was introduced in biosynthesis pathway of essential oils in *Citrus grandis*. Using energy dispersive X-ray spectroscopy (EDS), the qualitative and quantitative analysis approved that the cytochemistry position of HMG-CoA synthesize is more accurate and reliable.

Keywords *Citrus grandis* · Essential oil · EDS · HMG-CoA synthetase · Terpenoid

389.1 Introduction

Terpenoid is made up of isoprenoid as the basic structural unit to build a class of compounds. Its biosynthesis is also known as isoprenoid biosynthetic pathway including two possible routes: the mevalonate (MVA) pathway in the cytosol and the methylerythritol phosphate (MEP) pathway in plastids. In recent years, a large number of molecular cloning researches mainly focus on the path of the biosynthesis of terpenoids. These two ways though exists in different locations in the plant cells, but the space is not absolutely independent, in which there are a small number of metabolites can interchange on plasmid membrane [1]. A small amount of products can enter the plasmids from MVA pathway in the cytoplasm, forming part of monoterpene and diterpene [2]. Monoterpene, sesquiterpene and diterpene

S.-J. Liang (✉) · P. Zheng · H. Gao · K.-K. Li
Center for Medicinal Plant Research, South China Agricultural University, Guangzhou 510642, China
e-mail: liangshejian@scau.edu.cn

S. Li et al. (eds.), *Frontier and Future Development of Information Technology in Medicine and Education*, Lecture Notes in Electrical Engineering 269,
DOI: 10.1007/978-94-007-7618-0_389,

are the main components of essential oils, including monoterpene as strong aroma and bioactive substances, sesquiterpene as volatile substances, and diterpene as important pharmacological active substances [3]. Essential oils of *Citrus* can be used as antibacterial, antitumor and medicinal materials [4, 5].

The synthesis and secretion pathways of essential oil in *Citrus* plant were studied by electron microscopy. Bosabalidis and Tsekos [6] pointed out that the essential oil was produced by plasmid, transferred by plasmid membrane to the surrounding of endoplasmic reticulum, later endoplasmic reticulum vesicles fused with the plasma membrane, releasing oil into the oil cavity. However, cytoplasm was partly involved in the synthesis process [7]. Terpenoid turned to be eosinophilic osmium drops in the cell fixed by osmium tetroxide. Usually according to the distribution of eosinophilic osmium drops the sites of terpenoids were determined [8]. For the combination of osmium tetroxide and terpenoid was not a specificity reaction, the sensitivity was not high. In addition, the distribution of osmium drops did not accurately show the changes of terpenoid transfer among organelles. In the process of sample preparation, terpenoid would be extracted from dehydration and fix. Therefore, it was necessary using enzyme cytochemistry method to study the synthetic process of terpenoid substances and secretory pathway. Energy dispersive X-ray spectroscopy (EDS) would examine which sediment was exact [9].

389.2 Materials and Methods

Fruits of *Citrus grandis* were collected from cultivated trees in campus of South China Agricultural University. The materials were cut into 0.5 × 0.5 × 1 mm blocks and fixed in 4 % formaldehyde and 1 % glutaraldehyde (0.05 mol/L sodium dimethyl arsenic acid buffer, pH 7.0), then washed in three changes of the same buffer, and incubated in 3.0×10^{-3} mol/L potassium ferricyanide (0.05 mol/L sodium dimethyl arsenic acid buffer, pH 7.0) at room temperature for 20 min. After

Table 1 composition of various incubation fluids

	Acetyl CoA sodium salt (0.8 mg/ml)	Acetyl-acetyl CoA sodium salt (1.6 mg/ml)	Potassium ferricyanide (2.0 mg/ml)	Uranium acetate (1.0 mg/ml)
Sample	+	+	+	+
Control 1	–	+	+	+
Control 2	+	–	+	+
Control 3	–	–	+	+
Control 4	+	+	+	+
Heating control	+	+	+	+

* + reagent adding; – no reagent adding; *Control 4* without post-fixed. *Heating control* tissue blocks were first disposed in 90 °C dimethyl sodium arsenate buffer for 20 min

the same buffer washing, the tissue blocks were incubated in different incubation fluids for 45 min at room temperature (Table 389.1).

After incubation, tissue blocks were post-fixed (except Control 4) in 2 % osmic acid (0.05 mol/L sodium dimethyl arsenic acid buffer, pH 7.0) for 1 h at room temperature. All above samples were washed with distilled water and dehydrated through a graded ethanol series (30, 50, 70, 50, 95, and 100 %), then infiltrated and embedded in Epon 812 (SPI Supplies Division of Structure Probe Inc., West Chester, USA). Ultra-thin sections were cut with a diamond knife on a Leica (Wetzlar, Germany) UCT ultramicrotome (slice thickness 90 nm), and then stained with uranyl acetate and lead citrate. The sections were examined and under Philip FEI-TECHNAI 12 transmission electron microscope (TEM) and INCA—Analyzer X-ray energy spectrum test (working conditions: 20 kV acceleration voltage, 1×10^{-10}A electron beam).

389.3 Results and Discussion

Synthetic precursor of terpenoid is isopentenyl diphosphate (IPP) producing by acetyl CoA through mevalonate (MVA) pathway [10–12]. In the process of generation of IPP, there are at least three steps producing coenzyme A: (1) acetyl CoA under the catalysis of acetyl CoA acetyl transferase generats acetyl-acetyl CoA; (2) acetyl CoA and acetyl-acetyl CoA under the catalysis of HMG-CoA synthetase generate HMG-CoA; (3) HMG-CoA under the catalysis of HMG-CoA reductase generates mevalonic acid. Coenzyme A can reduce potassium ferricyanide to potassium ferrocyanide. The reaction of potassium ferrocyanide and uranium acetate generates ferrocyanide uranium sediment which can be observed under transmission electron microscope. According to this principle, we added exogenous acetyl CoA and acetyl-acetyl CoA in incubation fluids. Under the catalysis of HMG-CoA synthetase, it produces HMG-CoA and release CoA. Adding potassium ferricyanide and uranium acetate, the ferrocyanide uranium sediment can generate which is on behalf of the locations of HMG-CoA synthetase [13]. Under the electron microscope, the sediment appeared like a black granule with relatively uniform shape. These sediments distributed in the cytoplasm, plastid, mitochondria and endoplasmic reticulum and other organelles (Fig. 389.1a). The same result described by Liang and Wu [9]. In order to verify the ferrocyanide uranium sediment, energy dispersive X-ray spectroscopy (EDS) was examined in a dense micro area (Fig. 389.1a, black circle). From the diagram of EDS (Fig. 389.2a), four main characteristic peaks of metal elements can be detected, respectively Cu ($K_\alpha = 8.04$ keV), Fe ($K_\alpha = 6.40$ keV), Pb ($L_\alpha = 10.55$ keV) and U ($L_\alpha = 13.61$ keV). By spectrum peak area calculating, the percentage weight of Cu, Pb, U and Fe are 88.6, 8.4, 1.7 and 1.3 % respectively (Fig. 389.3a). In Control 1 (Fig. 389.1b), black grains was not found in cells. EDS was examined randomly from a micro area (Fig. 389.1b, black circle). Only two peaks appeared in the spectral graph (Fig. 389.2b): the main characteristics of the metal elements

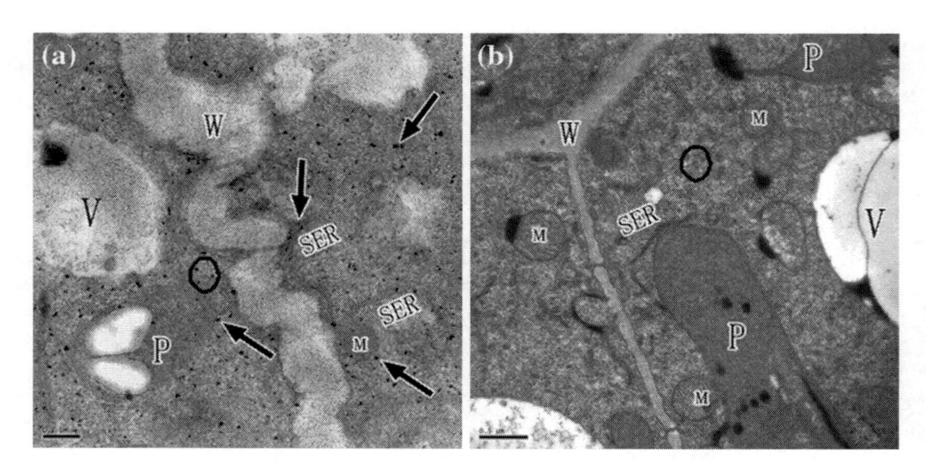

Fig. 1 Photos of enzyme cytochemistry in *Citrus grandis.* **a** *Black grains* appear in cytoplasm, plastids, mitochondria and ER. **b** No *black grains* appear in cytoplasm, plastids, mitochondria and ER. *M* mitochondria, *P* plastids, *V* vacuole, *W* cell wall, *SER* smooth endoplasmic reticulum, Bars = 0.5 μm

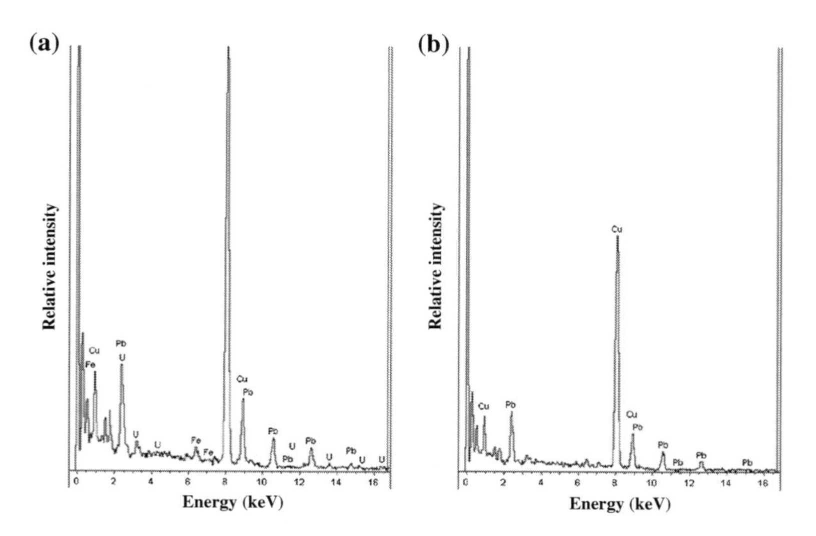

Fig. 2 Energy dispersive X-ray spectra acquired from different areas. **a** Area of *black circle* in Fig. 389.1a. **b** Area of *black circle* in Fig. 389.1b

were Cu ($K_{\alpha} = 8.04$ keV) and Pb ($L_{\alpha} = 10.55$ keV) whose percentage weights were 90.4 and 9.6 % respectively (Fig. 389.3b). Other controls were the same as the control 1 (Not shown). In the process of cytochemistry experiment, ultrathin slices are collected on copper grids and dyed by citrate. Therefore, two metal elements copper and lead both can be detected by EDS in Fig. 389.2a and b. From

(a)
100
80
60
40
20
0
Fe Cu Pb U

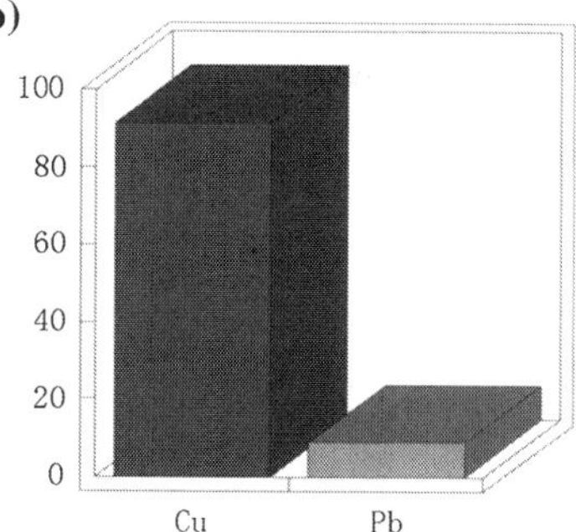

Fig. 3 Results of quantitative analysis acquired from different areas. **a** Area of *black circle* in Fig. 389.1a. **b** Area of *black circle* in Fig. 389.1b

quantitative analysis, the percentage weight of the copper (Cu) occupied absolute proportion (>88 %), and lead (Pb) was only about 8 %. The peak of Cu peak was very high. In addition, iron (Fe) and uranium (U) only appeared in Fig. 389.2a. It meant that these sediments were undoubtedly ferrocyanide uranium.

389.4 Conclusions

The qualitative and quantitative analysis of EDS accurately detects the reaction products of HMG-CoA synthetase. These sediments were mainly located in cytoplasm, plastids, mitochondria and endoplasmic reticulum. Plastids should be the main synthesis part of essential oils. These results could provide cytology evidences for molecule regulation in terpenoid biosynthesis.

References

1. Kasahara H, Hanada A, Kuzuyama T et al (2002) Contribution of the Mevalonate and Methylerythritol Phosphate Pathways to the Biosynthesis of Gibberellins in *Arabidopsis*. J Biol Chem 77:45188–45194
2. Arigoni D, Sagner S, Latzel C et al (1997) Terpenoid biosynthesis from 1-deoxy-D-xylulose in higher plants by intramolecular skeletal rearrangement. Proc Natl Acad Sci USA 94:10600–10605
3. [3] Ma L, Ding P, Yang GX et al (2006) Advances on the plant terpenoid isoprenoid biosynthetic pathway and its key enzymes, Biotech Bull (S):22-30
4. Suffredini IB, Paciencia MLB, Varella AD et al (2006) In vitro prostate cancer cell growth inhibition by Brazilian plant extracts. Pharmazie 61(8):722–724
5. Viljoen AM, Moolla A, van Vuuren SF et al (2006) The biological activity and essential oil composition of 17 Agathosma (Rutaceae) species. J Essent Oil Res 18:2–16

6. Bosabalidis Tsekos (1982) Ultrastructural studies on the secretory cavities of *Citrus deliciosa* Ten.I. Early stages of the gland cells differentiation. Protoplasma 112:55–62
7. Heinrich G, Schultze W (1985) Composition and site of biosynthesis of the essential oil in fruits of *Phellodendron amurense* Rupr. (Rutaceae). Israel J Bot 34:205–217
8. Fahn A, Benayoun J (1976) Ultrastructure of resin ducts in *Pinus halepensis* development, possible sites of resin synthesis, and mode of its elimination from the protoplast. Ann Bot 40:857–863
9. [9] Liang SJ, Wu H (2010) Energy Dispersive X-ray Spectroscopy in Cytochemistry of Key Enzyme during Terpenoid Biosynthesis Pathway. EMBB 18-21
10. Chappell J (1995) Biochemistry and molecular biology of the isoprenoid biosynthetic pathway in plants. Annu Rev Plant Physiol Plant Mol Biol 46:521–547
11. McGarvey DJ, Croteau R (1995) Terpenoid metabolism. Plant Cell 7:1015–1026
12. Chen DH, Ye HC, Li GF et al (2000) Advances in molecular biology of plant isoprenoid metabolic pathway. Acta Bot Sinica 42:551–558
13. Curry KJ (1987) Initiation of terpenoid synthesis in osmophorres of *Sanopea anfracta* (Orchidaceae): a cytochemical study. Am J Bot 74(9):1332–1338

Chapter 390
The Method Research on *Tuber* spp. DNA in Soil

Yong-jun Fan, Fa-Hu Li, Yan-Lin Zhao and Wei Yan

Abstract Truffles are ascomata of ectomycorrhizal hypogeous fungi associated with endemic *Pinus tabuliformis* in Mount Helan National Nature Reserve in Inner Mongolia, China, was investigated f in soil cubes taken from pure *P. tabuliformis* stands. The objectives of this study were (i) to develop a molecular method to detect mycelia of *Tuber* spp. in soil and (ii) to test for mycelial distribution around two truffle-bearing *P. tabuliformis* trees in a truffle orchard. Isolation of total DNA from soil was performed, followed by PCR amplification with *Tuber* spp.-specific primers and restriction analysis. To address the detection sensitivity level, soil samples were inoculated with known amounts of gleba of *Tuber* spp. Mycelium was detected primarily within the area defined by the truffle burn and within the top 35 cm of the soil in all directions from the trees.

Keywords *Tuber* spp · Soil mycelium · PCR–RFLP · Truffle orchard · ITS

390.1 Introduction

Tuber spp. hyphae are not visible to the naked eye, but its DNA can be selectively amplified by PCR from total soil DNA extracts using specific primers. Several authors have designed *Tuber*spp.-specific primers [1–4], but these primers were not adequate for our purposes because of weak or nonspecific amplifications. The objectives of this study were (i) to establish an accurate DNA isolation protocol applicable to soil samples (ii) to develop a PCR primer pair specific for *Tuber*spp.,

Y. Fan (✉) · F.-H. Li · Y.-L. Zhao · W. Yan
The Biology Science and Technology Department of Baotou Teacher's College,
Baotou, China
e-mail: fanyj1975@163.com

S. Li et al. (eds.), *Frontier and Future Development of Information Technology in Medicine and Education*, Lecture Notes in Electrical Engineering 269,
DOI: 10.1007/978-94-007-7618-0_390, © Springer Science+Business Media Dordrecht 2014

and (iii) to test the ability of these primers to detect the presence and distribu-tion of *Tuber*spp. Mycelium in soil surrounding two *Pinus tabuliformis* trees in a commercial truffle orchard.

390.2 Materials and Methods

390.2.1 Source of Fungal Material

Fruit bodies from 1 *Tuber* species and from 1 subspecies belonging to same genera were collected from under the *Pinus tabuliformis* in Mount Helan National Nature Reserve in Inner Mongolia, China. Fresh fruit bodies were freeze-dried and stored at −20 °C before use.

390.2.2 Soil Samples

Four soils were used to test the extraction procedure: (1) from nursery pots of truffle-inoculated *Pinus tabuliformis*; (2) from a wild truffle bed; (3) from a productive truffle orchard; and (4) from a cereal field adjacent to the truffle orchard. All samples were stored at −20 °C until use. Roots from nursery seedlings were examined under a light micro-scope to confirm the presence of *Tuber* Spp. ectomy-corrhizae, which were characterized by spinulae surface of the mantle and sheath ornamentations (Rauscher et al. [5]). Soil samples from the wild truffle bed and the truffle orchard were collected close to the base of truffle bearing trees.

390.2.3 DNA Isolation and PCR Amplification

DNA from 2 fruit bodies was isolated using Biospin Fungus Genomic DNA Extraction Kit. As Fungal DNA miniprep kit following the manufacturer's instructions. The soil DNA isolation protocol was based on a described hexade-cyltri–methylammonium bromide (CTAB) extraction method Karen et al. [6].

DNA extracted from fruit bodies and soils were amplified [7] with primers ITS1F/ITS4 [8, 9] to estimate the extraction efficiency and to confirm the presence of fungal DNA and the lack of Taq polymerase inhibitors.

390.2.4 Restriction Fragment Length Polymorphism

Five microlitres of the amplification products obtained with ITS1TM/ITS2TM were analyzed by RFLPs generated by *AluI, EcoRI, HinfI, MseI* (Invitrogen, Paisley, Scotland), and TaqI (Amersham). The fragments were resolved on 2 % agarose gels. Fragments smaller than 100 bp were not recorded.

390.3 Results

390.3.1 DNA Isolation and PCR Amplification

DNA extracts from soils gave $OD_{260/280}$ nm ratios between 1.0 and 1.5 and $OD_{260/230}$ nm ratios between 0.4 and 1.0. DNA extractions from fruit bodies were successfully ampli-fied with the fungal-specific primers ITS1F/ITS4, giving the expected ITS-size amplicons. Extractions from soils gave different bands after amplification with this primer pair, indicating the presence of multiple fungi (Fig. 390.1).

390.3.2 RFLP and Sequencing

The RFLP patterns from ascomata and soil mycelia were identical: *AluI*(<100, 120, 250 bp), *EcoRI* (double band around 230 bp), *HinfI* (219, 228 bp), *MseI* (370 bp) and *TaqI* (170, 185 bp). Since amplicons had the same digestion patterns, only one from soil mycelium and one from an ascoma were sequenced. Both of these sequences were identical and also to those of 100 other *Tuber* Spp. sequences in GenBank database.

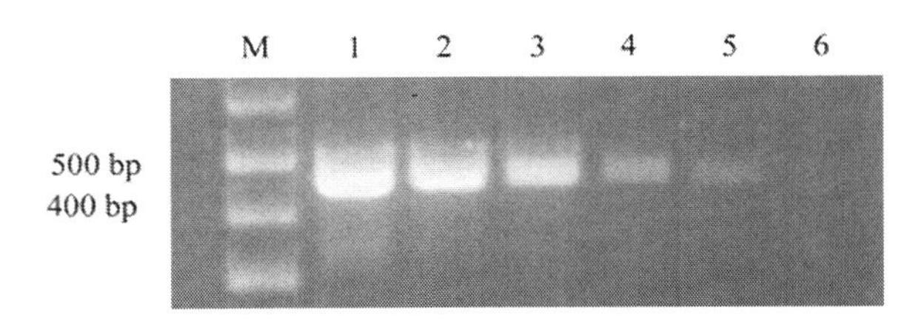

Fig. 390.1 Patterns of band-intensities of *Tuber* Spp. in soil extractions after amplification with ITS1F/ITS4. Lane M, 1 kb Plus Ladder marker. Lane1, DNA from a *Tuber* Spp. Ascoma (known standard), level [+++]; lanes 2–6, DNA from soil samples: lane 2, 70.92 % = [+++]; lane 3, 41.44 % = [++]; lane 4, 10.71 % = [+]; lane 5, 6.96 % = [(+)]; lane 6, undetectable = [−]. Intensity gradings corre-spond to percentages comparable with band intensity from the known standard. [+++] = 70–100 %; [++] = 40–70 %; [+] = 10–40 %; [(+)] o 10 %; [−] = undetectable

390.3.3 Detection Limit of Designed Protocol

DNA extractions from the noninoculated cereal field soil gave amounts of DNA of c.16 ugg^{-1} of soil with $OD_{260/280}$ nm of 1.2 and $OD_{260/230}$ nm near 0.7. Amplification with ITS1F/ITS4 yielded several bands, but no *Tuber* Spp. DNA was detected in the ITS1TM/ITS2TM amplifications. DNA extracted from inoculated soils could be amplified with ITS1F/ITS4 and ITS1TM/ITS2TM. DNA from samples with dilutions down to and including 8×10^{-2} mg of gleba had the expected 465 pb band. DNA extracted from gleba ground alone in buffer solution had the expected band in samples down to and including 8 mg of gleba. The amount of *Tuber* Spp. DNA inoculated into the soil, inferred from the amount of DNA obtained from the extraction of freeze-dried dilutions, suggests ~310 mg of DNA g^{-1} of gleba. PCR results from the extractions corre-sponding to the small volumes of supernatants showed that the expected band could be detected in dilutions containing down to and including 8×10^{-2} mg of gleba. Extractions performed with the remaining large volume of supernatant after first centrifugation, gave amplification with the specific.

390.3.4 Field-Testing of the Detection Techniques

Optical density $OD_{260/230}$ nm ratios ranged between 1.0 and 1.3 and OD260/280 nm between 0.4 and 1.0. The average amount of DNA recovered in crude preparations were of 24.68 ± 6.83, 17.57 ± 4.82 and 6.32 ± 1.23ug $g^{-1}$of soil in 5–10, 30–35 and 55–60 cm of depth soil cores respectively. The final DNA extracts were suitable for PCR and no additional purification was required. PCR reactions with primers ITS1F/ITS4 detected the expected band.

390.4 Discussion

The first objective, to develop a molecular tool to detect *Tuber* spp. mycelium in soil, was achieved, pro-viding a technique applicable for monitoring the presence of this fungus in truffle orchards even prior to truffle produc-tion. In our field testing, we did not obtain very pure DNA extracts, but the noninhibition of Taq polymerase indicated that our resultant DNA extractions were sufficiently pure for amplification without need for further purification, which is time-consuming and reduces the DNA yield (Kuske et al. 1998). In addition, extracts with the lowest ratios of $OD_{260/280}$ and $OD_{260/230}$ nm did not correspond to the lowest *Tuber* spp. detection levels after PCR reactions.

When using the *Tuber*-specific primers de-signed by other authors [1, 2]; Gande-boeuf et al. [3], we encountered problems of weak or nonspecific amplifications. The low level of genetic varia-bility found in *Tuber* spp. (Henrion et al. 1994; Gandeboeuf et al. 1997b; Bertault et al. 2001; [10]) and the high number of available sequences in GenBank, allowed us to design a specific primer pair for this fungus (ITS1TM/ITS2TM) and to test it with a relatively low number of *Tuber* spp. ascomata. The use of RFLP comparisons of the ITS region permits the confirmation of species-level identification (Henrion et al. 1994; Amicucci et al. 1996; Karen et al. 1997; [11]). We obtained amplifications with enough DNA for RFLP or sequencing analyses. The similar RFLP patterns from the soil mycelia and the ascomata amplicons allowed the identification of those from soil mycelium as *Tuber* spp. Sequences obtained confirmed the RFLP identi-fication.

It was not possible to utilize hyphal mycelia because of growth difficulties in pure culture (Fasolo-Bonfante and Fontana 1973), or hyphae from germinating spores because of the symbiotic nature of this fungus, which cannot grow well in the absence of a host. The minimum quantity of *Tuber* spp. DNA that we could detect from inoculated soil samples with our technique was 3.6 ngg^{-1} of soil corresponding to 11.4 mg of *Tuber* spp. hyphae g^{-1} soil. As only 1 ml of the 50 ml of the soil DNA extracts was used for PCR amplification, this value indicates that our PCR protocol has the potential to detect as little as 7.5 pg of *Tuber* spp. DNA. We observed a positive soil effect in DNA extraction procedures but a negative effect in PCR-amplifications. The positive effect of soil in extractions could be explained by additional abrasion of the soil particles increasing the lysis efficiency and subsequent DNA yield. The negative effect of soil in amplifications is probably because of the presence of Taq polymerase inhibitors. Differences in the minimum detectable DNA between samples from gleba without soil (ground in a standard mortar and pestle), and gleba ground in a 1.5 ml tube, also may be due to the effectiveness of cell disruption, which is greater with a pellet pestle in a 1.5 ml tube.

Acknowledgments This work was supported in part by the DMAH-GENCAT, by scholarship 2002FI-00711 to L.M. Suz from the DURSI-GENCAT, and by the research project FMI-REN2002-04068-CO2-01. We are indebted to M. Donate for the open access to his truffle orchard. The authors thank C.R. Fischer for helpful suggestions and English support.

References

1. Paolocci F, Rubini A, Granetti B et al (1997) Typing *Tuber melanosporum* and Chinese black truffle species by molecular markers. FEMS Microbiol Lett 153:255–260
2. Paolocci F, Rubini A, Riccioni C et al (2000) Cloning and characterization of two repeated sequences in the symbiotic fungus *Tuber melanosporum* Vitt. FEMS Microbiol Ecol 34:139–146
3. Gandeboeuf D, Dupr′e C, Roeckel-Devret P et al (1997a) Typing *Tuber* ectomycorrhizae by polymerase chain amplification of the internal transcribed spacer of rDNA and the sequence characterized amplified region markers. Can J Microbiol 43:723–728

4. Paolocci F, Rubini A, Riccioni C et al (2000) Cloning and characterization of two repeated sequences in the symbiotic fungus *Tuber melanosporum* vitt. FEMS Microbiol Ecol 34:139–146
5. Riousset LG, Chevalier G, Bardet MC (2001) Truffes d'Europe et de Chine (Institut National de la Recherche Agronomique Eds). Centre Technique Interprofessionnel des Fruits et L′egumes, Paris
6. Karen O, Jonsson L, Jonsson M et al (1999) Cook-book for DNA extraction, restriction analysis (RFLP), agarose gel electrophoresis, PCR and sequencing. Preconference workshop, Uppsala June 29–July 4 1998. DNA based methods for identification of ectomycorrhiza. http://www-mykopat.slu.se/Thesis/ola/protocol/pcrguide. html DNA% 20 extraction
7. Martın MP, Winka K (2000) Alternative methods of extracting and amplifying DNA from lichens. Lichenologist 32:189–196
8. White TJ, Bruns T, Lee S et al (1990) Amplification and direct sequencing of fungal ribosomal RNA genes for phylogenetics. In: Innis MA, Gelfand DH, Sninsky JJ, White TJ (eds) PCR protocols, a guide to methods and applications, pp 315–322
9. Gardes M, Bruns TD (1993) ITS primers with enhanced specificity for basidiomycetes—application to the identification of mycorrhizae and rusts. Mol Ecol 2:113–118
10. Mello A, Cantisani A, Vizzini A et al (2002) Genetic variability of *Tuber uncinatum* and its relatedness to other black truffles. Environ Microbiol 4:584–594
11. Grebenc T, Piltaver A, Kraigher H (2000) Establishment of a PCR-RFLP library for basidiomycetes, ascomycetes and their ectomycorrhizae on *Picea abies* (L.) Karst. Phyton (Austria) 40:79–82
12. Pacioni G, Comandini O (1999) *Tuber*. Ectomycorrhizal fungi key genera in profile. In: Cairney WG, Chambers SM (eds). Springer Verlag, Berlin

Chapter 391
The Impact of Modern Information Technology on Medical Education

Zifen Guo, Yong Feng and Honglin Huang

Abstract With the rapid development and deep penetration of multimedia and internet technology, some tremendous and profound changes have happened in educational content, teaching methods, teaching philosophy and mode, which make it easy for people to access to the knowledge and information of the higher medical education. The perfect combination of multimedia and network technology not only provides a convenient flexible learning space and time for students, but also enables them to master the forefront of medicine and broaden their professional knowledge. The information technology has promoted the modernization process of higher medical education reform and development, so that it will have extremely profound impact on high-quality medical personnel training in China.

Keywords Information technology · Medical education · Education reform

391.1 Introduction

Modern information technology based on computer technology includes digital information acquisition, processing, handling, storage, transmission and interaction dynamic technology [1]. And the modern educational technology naturally has become the hot issue on the contemporary education whose core is information technology. Compared to the other disciplines education, the traditional inculcation of the theoretical knowledge is not the only requirement, and more practice teaching to culture independent operation ability is also necessary. Furthermore,

Z. Guo (✉) · H. Huang
Department of Pharmacy, University of South China, Hengyang 421001, China
e-mail: guozifen@aliyun.com

Y. Feng
The Student Affairs Department, University of South China, Hengyang 421001, China

S. Li et al. (eds.), *Frontier and Future Development of Information Technology in Medicine and Education*, Lecture Notes in Electrical Engineering 269,
DOI: 10.1007/978-94-007-7618-0_391,

the student should understand the latest development of modern medicine. The emergence of the computer and the internet produce the possibility to improve medical education contents and enrich teaching methods, and the information technology will play an increasingly important role in modern medical education.

391.2 The Application of Modern Information Technology in Higher Medical Education

To comprehensively improve the quality of medical education for achieving high-quality medical personnel training objectives, the medical colleges seize the opportunity to deepen the educational reform and development and accelerate the application of modern information technology in medical education. The digital information technology revolution runs through the whole process of higher medical education not only from the medical multimedia course software development to the computer-aided teaching, but also from teaching database construction to the medical network resources sharing and from the local teaching network construction to medical education development remotization.

391.2.1 Application of the Multimedia Technology [2, 3]

For a medical student, the vivid graphic materials are more attractive than boring textbook knowledge. The important traditional teaching always uses flip charts or overhead projectors to display chart information, which requires teachers to take some time to replace the flip chart in class and then the students, attention are easy to disperse. Computer multimedia technology can integrate images, sounds and texts, and so it possesses unparalleled advantages on the vividness of lectures, stimulating study interest of students. Now the computer multimedia technology plays an increasingly prominent role in teaching. Medical colleges all have greater investment in computer hardware facilities to further develop medical multimedia curriculum software suitable for medical education teaching characteristics. Through teachers explaining with large-screen projection display system, the students repeatedly receive visual and auditory stimulus and their understanding and memory could be deepened to make the knowledge systematize.

391.2.2 Application of the Network Teaching Platform [3]

Owing to the uneven learning basis and different ability among students, it is difficult to teach students. The establishment of teaching network environment in higher medical colleges may promote the realization of network sharing the multimedia teaching courseware which can provide a convenient flexible learning space for students instead of particular teaching time and the existing teaching place. The network teaching platform shortens the temporal and spatial distance for education and is suitable for various professional students with uneven learning basis and different ability levels to increase achievement. The popularization and application of the network technology will provide them favorable support for the medical colleges to carry out remote medical education, consultation and services. Both the teachers can answer the off-site students' questions and the doctors can provide remote medical consultation and services for off-site patients by the network.

391.2.3 Application of the Virtual Reality Technology [4, 5]

Compared with other disciplines education, medical students need not only the traditional theoretical knowledge but also more practical teaching to enhance their independent operation ability. Due to the limitations of laboratory instruments, places and other reasons, the virtual reality technology came into being. By means of multimedia, simulation and virtual reality technology, the virtual simulation experiment creates experimental operation environment on the computer to replace or partially replace traditional experimental operation environment for medical experiment and clinical teaching demonstration. The results obtained from the virtual simulation experiment are equivalent or even better than from the real medical experiment, thus the virtual simulation experiment breaks a new way to reproduce a specific realistic medical environment in medical education, research and clinical treatment.

391.3 The Influence of Modern Information Technology on the Development of Higher Medical Education

With the rapid development and deep penetration of modern information technology, some tremendous and profound changes have happened in educational content, teaching methods, teaching philosophy and mode. The perfect combination of multimedia and network technology not only meets the requires of particular teaching time and existing teaching place, but also enables students to master the forefront of medicine and broaden their professional knowledge. The information technology has promoted the modernization process of higher medical education reform and development, and so it will have extremely profound impact on high-quality medical personnel training in China.

391.3.1 Change the Teaching Philosophy and Mode [6]

Since it emphasizes the teachers' cramming education and students' passive full record, the traditional medical teaching mode is conducive neither to play the subjective initiative of teachers, nor to mobilize the enthusiasm of students or to develop the thinking skills of students. The modern information technology improves medical education contents and enriches teaching methods, and forms a new teaching mode emphasizing on the subjectivity of student and the dominant of teachers in class.

391.3.2 Update the Content of Medical Education [7]

Differing from other disciplines, the medical education should closely follow the international preface and merge the latest medical advances into class. The well-planned teaching content always has more impact on learner satisfaction than the teaching means, and the internet has gradually grown as a resource for disseminating medical education curricula. With the appearance of the internet, networks provide convenient conditions to solve the problem how to grasp the objective and progress of related disciplines for teachers. The network is an important tool for teachers and students to conduct medical research and exchange information, and is also a significant way for teachers to comprehensively understand medical latest advances which could broaden their horizons and enrich the teaching content.

391.3.3 Share the Networked Educational Resources [8]

The modern medical education network is encouraged by the development of information technology. With the network growing, the educational resource of medical colleges is becoming increasingly influential, especially the well-known colleges and universities. As a consequence of the network disregarding the constraints resulted from temporal and spatial, all the students can enjoy the influential educational resource wealth. Educational courses and resources are shared by internet, which offers the students an accessible way to learn more medical education curriculum and master more advanced medical techniques and research means. Furthermore, they search and read literatures to understand the international dynamics and development of related disciplines. The popularization and application of information technology in medical education accelerate medical education to meet the international standards, and the international medical education development is the inevitable trend of modern information technology.

391.4 Summary

Networks gradually integrate into people's lives accompany with the advent of internet. The education informatization is a trend of the times, and the modern information technology based on computer technology is the major driving force for technological innovation in medical education. Correct understanding about the role of modern information technology in medical education and appropriate concern about the tremendous influence of modern information technology on future medical education must be owned. We should fully utilize the informationalized educational resources to promote the modernization process of higher medical education reform and development. The application of modern information technology not only accelerates the reform pace of medical education content and teaching method, but also strengthens teachers' practical teaching ability and enhances the quality of talent cultivation.

Acknowledgments The study is partially supported by the National Natural Science Foundation of China (Grant No. 81102516) and the construct program of the key discipline in Hunan province.

References

1. Uddin MJ, Hasan MN (2012) Use of information technology in library service: a study on some selected libraries in northern part of Bangladesh. Int J Libr Inf Sci 4(3):34–44
2. Luo J, Boland R, Chan CH (2013) How to use technology in educational innovation. The academic medicine handbook. Springer, New York, 117–123
3. Ruiz JG, Mintzer MJ, Leipzig RM (2006) The impact of e-learning in medical education. Acad Med 81(3):207–212
4. Kilmon CA, Brown L, Ghosh S et al (2010) Immersive virtual reality simulations in nursing education. Nurs Educ Perspect 31(5):314–317
5. Duncan I, Miller A, Jiang S (2012) A taxonomy of virtual worlds usage in education. British J Educ Technol 43(6):949–964
6. Yue HP, Liu G, Liu JP (2012) Discussion on mode of medical information education in the information times. China Sci Technol Inf 3:90
7. Sisson SD, Hill-Briggs F, Levine D (2010) How to improve medical education website design. BMC Med Educ 10(1):30
8. McGee JB, Kanter SL (2011) How we develop and sustain innovation in medical education technology: keys to success. Med Teach 33(4):279–285

Chapter 392
In the Platform of the Practice Teaching Link, Study on Environmental Elite Education

Yu Caihong, Huang Ying, Xu Dongyao, He Xuwen, Wang Jianbing and Yu Yan

Abstract In recent years, the environmental engineering of China university of mining and technology (Beijing) specialty carried out a series of reforms, aimed to improve the students' practical experience of innovative ability. This paper explores the practice teaching system of environmental engineering by combining with that practical experience. It is on the basis of the spirit that "Constructing energy industry elite education teaching system actively and explore diversified personnel training mode", which was put forward by our school. In addition, this paper also introduces the measures to integrate the advantage of research with the discipline's in environmental engineering, to highlight energy professional advantages of our school, to build practice teaching link in the field of coal disposal and to cultivate environmental professional elite talent.

Keywords Environmental engineering · Practice teaching · Elite education · Innovation capability

392.1 Introduction

Recent years, just that people pay increasing attention to harmonious development of environment protection and economy circumstance, the requirement of intellectual majoring in environmental engineering is growing.

The enrollment scale of environmental engineering in college is expanding. Facing to the situation of popularized higher education, the students majoring in environmental engineering are feeling much big pressure. The force of employment leads to utilitarian study and make a challenge to the traditional development

Y. Caihong (✉) · H. Ying · X. Dongyao · H. Xuwen · W. Jianbing · Y. Yan
College of Chemistry and Environment Engineering, China University of Mining and Technology (Beijing), 100083 Beijing, China
e-mail: caihongy@yahoo.com.cn

S. Li et al. (eds.), *Frontier and Future Development of Information Technology in Medicine and Education*, Lecture Notes in Electrical Engineering 269,
DOI: 10.1007/978-94-007-7618-0_392,

of perception and ability. Elite education emphasizes the intelligence and the base of educator, but, the ratio of those people who can accept elite education is very low in contemporary. Elite education aims at improving students comprehensive quality rather than raising the examination specialist. Practice teaching is a vital part in the whole environmental engineering teaching process, it can enhance students' comprehensive quality, analysis ability and problem solving ability [1]. Our school is attaching importance to practice teaching. It attempts to structure the practice teaching link in the field of coal disposal and has already made a great effect in personnel training. These years, the students of environmental engineering in our school have made some marvelous achievement in this field.

392.2 Setting of the Practice Teaching Link in Environmental Engineering

Practice teaching must start with a comprehensive application of knowledge for the purpose, and must aim at cultivating the innovative ability. A great practice teaching part can not only enhance the practice ability, but also improve students' ability of solving practical problems and innovation ability [2]. In the cultivation project of China University of Mining and Technology (Beijing), version 2012, the practice teaching link divides into traditional practice teaching link and innovation teaching link. The traditional one contains the following:

1. classroom experiment, which include validation experiment, comprehensive experiment and innovation experiment;
2. design, which include course design, comprehensive design, graduation design;
3. practice, which include acquaintance practice, productive practice and graduate practice;
4. thesis, which include design, experiment and paper;
5. social practice, which include vocation practice, public benefit activity, corporation activity, and so on. There are 42 credits in total.

Innovation practice teaching link contains undergraduate innovation experiment project, undergraduate course and technology competition, patents obtaining, experiments electing, creative design in environmental engineering, project research in environmental engineering, Chemistry innovation experiment design and so on. Students can get 3 credits through electing courses according to their own condition. The students in our school have been cultivated their skills by practice teaching link in recent years, which include experimental skills, operation ability, process design ability, engineering design, scientific research ability and innovation ability.

392.2.1 Attaching Importance to the Basic Operation Skills of Classroom Experiments

We made an overall plan to these normal practice parts. On one hand, we need assure students' basic experimental skills, on the other hand, we emphasize the cultivation of self-test experiment ability. Proving experiment is mainly about to develop practice skills, operate standard and the ability to analyze and solve problems. Basic chemical experiment and instrumental analysis experiment help students to grasp the chemical operating skills, the compound analysis method, and to be familiar with the principle and function of important instruments. Comprehensive experiment is mainly about to teach students how to prove relative theory and solve the actual problems by the knowledge they learn. Specialized experiments mainly include *Water pollution control engineering*, *air pollution control engineering*, *Mine solid waste treatment and disposal engineering*, and *Environmental Edaphology*. These experiments deeply discuss the environment problems, especially the control technology and principles of pollutants, by which students can learn specialty knowledge, and grasp the basic skills.

392.2.2 Emphasize the Cultivation of Project Design Ability in Internship and Practical Training

Design teaching links in our school environmental engineering include course design, integrated design and graduation design et al. The curriculum design link was arranged in some courses such as *Water pollution control engineering*, *Air pollution control engineering* to strengthen the students' ability for engineering and equipment design. In design teaching links, curriculum design pays attention to technological design and is guided by teacher. Integrated design is guided by professors who have much design experience, and requires to achieve degree of feasibility study report. Graduation design must to achieve preliminary design level, it is guided by hired experienced engineers who work on design institute.

Environmental engineering professional practice includes acquaintance practice, productive practice and graduate practice. Acquaintance practice is carried by combining with course teaching and course design. Students need to visit actual projects, to learn dispose methods of water pollution, air pollution and solid waste in production. By doing so, they can combine practice with theories. Trough productive practice, students could learn each productive part in an environmental enterprise, such as the management system, productive technology, operative procedure, costing benefit, pollution producing and prevention. Graduate practice is a comprehensive practice teaching before graduation. Our College actively conducts cooperation between higher vocational colleges and setup long-term, flexible, stable practice bases. It is ensured the internship effects by establishing stable cooperation relations with sewage treatment plant, companies in the field of energy and all kinds of environmental protection company.

392.2.3 Developing Innovation Ability in Innovation Link

As an environmental engineering and technical personnel training base, it is necessary to be adapt to the need of national development and to cultivate environment engineering professionals which one had innovative ability. Innovation ability is generally development, sublimation and integrated embodiment of manipulative ability. The students' ability of active initiative investigation is an important part of students' innovative ability. And the nature of academic is exploring innovation. Therefore, the academic training is the most important way to cultivate undergraduates' innovative qualities. Our innovative practice teaching links are arranged as following courses for students to choose from, such as *The college students innovation experiment program*, *The college students science and technology competition*, *The published academic papers and patents as it is approved*, *Scientific research project training*, *Chosen for experiment*, *Chemistry innovation experiment design*, *Environmental engineering innovative design* and *Environmental engineering research project* et al. It provides more academic opportunities for environmental engineering undergraduates to understand the academic frontier dynamic as early as possible, to inspire the academic interest and innovation potential. At the same time, students are encouraged to take part in all kinds of practice activities outside the curriculum and professional activities so that they can found problems, learn to observe and analysis and form their own understanding through extensive in-depth contact with a lot of different things. In this paper, the author has been introduced the teaching arrangement and concept of innovation practice teaching link in environmental engineering in China University of Mining and Technology (Beijing) [3, 4]. It will not repeat here.

392.2.4 Attaching Great Importance to Various Practices

Social practice is one part of the professional training program in Environmental Engineering. The students in our school are encouraged to participate in a variety of extracurricular activities besides courses and professional activities, so that they can learn to observe and analyze, and form their own original ideas in the process of extensive and in-depth exposure to different things.

Some of the teachers in our college guide students' social practice by combining professional courses with experience in the field of scientific research. In undergraduate summer social practice, the students could choose their theme freely and they are encouraged to combine into a team. The students concentrate the superior forces to research on energy environmental governance and social hot issues and other related topics, make classroom knowledge applied to social practice, especially make the theoretical system applied into practice. In their spare time. The undergraduates whose major is environmental engineering in our school had been took part in the summer social practice activities during the past three years. They were awarded a prize of 50 items, include all kinds of team awards and advanced individual awards.

These social practice activities achieved good effect. Some practice teams and practice units also reached to build and form a mechanism, came up with ideas and methods for the local energy and environmental governance problems, had been well received by a lot of practice units. It has also greatly improved students' interest in learning professional courses, consolidated the teaching achievement, and made the level of practice teaching up to a new level.

392.3 Prospect

The higher education in China has obtained the rapid development in recent years. But at the same time, there are also many difficulties and problems. Such as how to turn scale expansion to improve the quality of higher education.

China University of Mining and Technology (Beijing) adheres to high standards and high starting point, focuses on building an elite teaching system of Chinese energy industry, and explores diversified talent cultivation model. Environmental engineering in our school also closely around its teaching theory. It highlights the characteristics of mine environmental protection in the practice teaching and pays attention to the development of students' innovative ability and study ability by integrating with scientific research advantage. We also know that the connotation construction of education cannot be realized in short time. We need to start from each teaching link, each course and each course, to changing teaching idea, then make great efforts to reform and explore curriculum system, teaching contents and teaching methods. Finally push forward personnel training work of our environmental engineering undergraduate.

References

1. Jia M, Qian R, Xu Y et al (2010) Study on the practice teaching in research-based teaching. Research and exploration in laboratory
2. Chang W, Xing P, Zhao Z (2004) China higher education
3. Yu C, Wang R, Xu D et al (2012) In the platform of Innovation experiment plan, to explore environmental innovative talent cultivation. Meitan higher education
4. Yu C, Wang J, Yu Y et al (2012) Exploration of innovative courses system construction in mining characteristics of environmental specialty. Environmental science and management

Chapter 393
The Application of a Highly Available and Scalable Operational Architecture in Course Selection System

Yanxia Li, Zhang Yu, Peng Yu, Chun Yu and Zhenglong Shao

Abstract To improve service quality and reduce costs, we design and practice a highly available and scalable operational architecture of Web applications. This architecture provides a stable and scalable operational environment for information systems. Its application in the course selection system at Tsinghua University greatly improves the overall performance of the system by adopting flexible deployment of applications and dynamic allocation of operational resources.

Keywords Operational architecture · High availability · High scalability · High load · Course selection system

393.1 Introduction

With regard to the operational environment of information systems, in the past people pay more attention to the construction of infrastructural facilities like servers, databases, networks and laboratories. However, with the maturing of information systems, it is increasingly recognized that the performance and effectiveness of information systems do not rely solely on the capabilities of infrastructural facilities, but on the full use of operational resources, the well-designed operational architecture, and the stable, efficient and secure operational environment.

The course selection system, a major application in Tsinghua digital campus, is characterized by high load and periodicity. During a course selection session, once a system failure happens, students will not be able to register their courses online, and the entire educational administration system will malfunction. When dealing

Y. Li (✉) · Z. Yu · P. Yu · C. Yu · Z. Shao
Information Technology Center, Tsinghua University, Room 220, Central Building, Beijing 100084, China
e-mail: liyx@cic.tsinghua.edu.cn

S. Li et al. (eds.), *Frontier and Future Development of Information Technology in Medicine and Education*, Lecture Notes in Electrical Engineering 269,
DOI: 10.1007/978-94-007-7618-0_393,

with high concurrency, people take common approaches such as introducing high-performance servers and databases, adopting high-efficiency programming languages as well as using high-performance Web containers. However, these approaches are not sufficient to settle the issues of high load and high concurrency. The design and implementation of operational architectures also plays a very important role [1, 2].

393.2 Common Operational Architecture of a Web Application

The most commonly adopted operational architecture of Web applications is a three-tier architecture consisting of a Web server, an application server, and a database server. The Web server receives and processes HTTP requests, and returns views to the user. The application server handles business logic. The database server stores and manages application data [3, 4].

Figure 393.1 depicts the architecture.

This architecture meets common operational needs of a Web application. But it is highly susceptible to single point failures. Server failure at any tier will lead to breakdown of the whole application. This architecture is not well scalable. When the server at a certain tier is overloaded, it is infeasible to add additional resources to that tier. Under high application load, any one of the three tiers is likely to become a bottleneck, so as to form a domino effect, bringing down the entire operational environment and leading to an application breakdown.

393.3 A Highly Available and Scalable Operational Architecture

The design goal of the new architecture is to make full use of existing resources, and to realize predictable, stable, and dynamically scheduled operation of Web applications. The architecture must first ensure the high availability of the

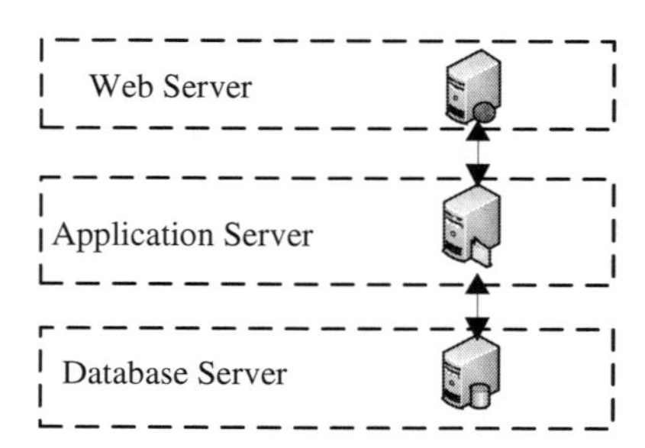

Fig. 393.1 Common operational architecture of a web application

operational environment, i.e., to ensure that failure at a certain tier does not affect the normal operation of the entire environment. And it should also provide sufficient flexibility and scalability, i.e., when operational resources at a certain tier are running out, similar resources can be quickly added, so as to ensure the normal operation of the Web application.

The architecture we design is shown in Fig. 393.2. Techniques adopted include clustering, load balancing, dynamic server clusters, and shared storage. Under this architecture we achieve the high availability and high scalability of Web servers, application servers, database servers and other infrastructural facilities.

We introduce a load balancing tier on top of the Web server tier. The load balancer dispatches HTTP requests to the web servers according to their availability and real-time load, avoiding single point failure at the Web server tier, as well as balancing their load pressure. The Web server tier is altered to ensure load balancing in the application server tier, avoiding single point failure at that tier. On each application server may deploy one or more Web application instances. Shared storage technology ensures program and data sharing among application servers. And mirroring enables program and data synchronization. To reduce the load of database servers, cache is used at the application server tier. Caches are synchronized among application servers through multicast or by introducing dedicated cache servers. At the database server tier, clustering is used to ensure reliability and stability [4].

Under this architecture, single point failures do not affect the normal operation of the Web application. When operational resources at a certain tier are running out, similar resources can be quickly added. For example, when the web server tier is overloaded and cannot be further optimized by adjusting runtime parameters, a new web server can be added by simply making a duplication of the software configurations and registering the new server at the load balancing tier. Likewise, when the application server tier is running short of resources and cannot be optimized by adjusting parameters or by adding application instances, a new

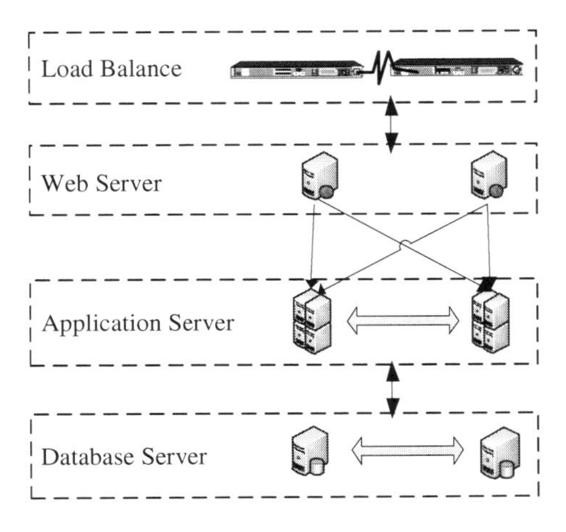

Fig. 393.2 A highly available and scalable operational architecture

application server can be added by making a duplication of the software configurations, deploying an application instance of the same version, and registering the new server at the Web server tier. The dynamic allocation of database resources is made available by clustering technology.

393.4 Application and Results

The course selection system at Tsinghua University has a huge number of concurrent accesses, especially at the time the course selection switch is turned on, when students compete for the few popular courses, and during the complementing and withdrawing phase of course selection, when students stay up online and constantly search for available courses that other students withdraw. However, this happens only three or four times in a year and each time it takes only a few days. It is uneconomical to have a long-term possession of large operational resources just to cope with high concurrency in a short period. In fact, the funding of the construction and operation of information systems at the university is relatively scarce, and operational resources run short now and then. It is discovered that peak periods of information systems do not overlap but take place in a serial manner. Therefore, to make full use of existing resources, we adopt the highly available and scalable operational architecture mentioned above. Just before the peak period, we allocate additional resources to the course selection system to cope with high load and high concurrency. When the peak passes, resources are freed immediately for use in other systems.

The course selection Web application at Tsinghua University runs under Apache, Resin, and Oracle. It operates in two different environment: one during the course selection period and the other during normal times. The former focuses on dealing with high load and high concurrency; while the latter emphasizes

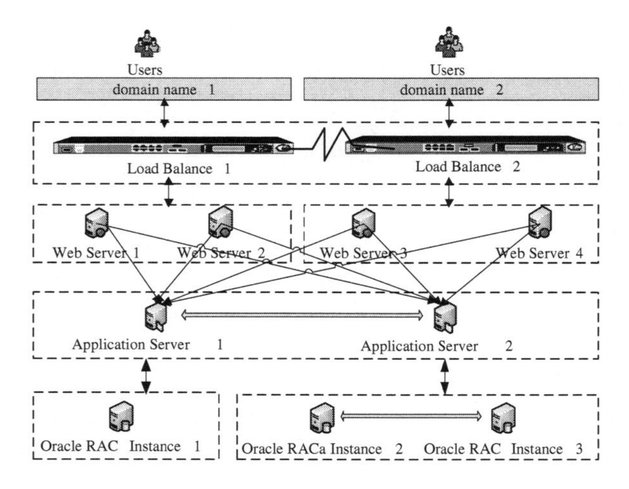

Fig. 393.3 The operational environment during the course selection period

security, stability, and availability of the application. The architecture of the former environment is shown in Fig. 393.3.

The environment is established and configured based on our assessment of history statistics and performance evaluation of the running program. During the course selection period, the operational environment uses an independent domain name, a separate Web server group, and a separate database instance. The application server group used is shared with other web applications. Two independent application instances are deployed in the group. Caches are synchronized by multicasting between the instances. Cashes are refreshed by scheduled tasks, user operations, or administrator operations. F5 is used at the load balancing tier. Apache runs on the Web servers and is configured to enable load balancing of the Resin instances at the application server tier. Oracle RAC ensures high availability and load balancing at the database server tier. Furthermore, operational status of each tier is monitored on a central platform, which will send out alarm by e-mail or SMS as soon as any potential problem is discovered [4].

Server configurations are listed in Table 393.1.

The number of users allowed into the system per unit time is strictly controlled. When the load at a certain tier is about to reach its maximum, the operational parameters will be adjusted and the number of concurrent users will be restricted, so that operations of the already entered users can be safeguarded. If the maximum of concurrent users is reached, new arrivals will be given a friendly reminder at the entrance of the system. After corresponding resources are added to the environment, new users will be again allowed into the system.

The entire process of course selection is closely monitored, including login, course search, course registration and other phases. Abnormal operations and malicious behaviours are strictly prohibited and effectively prevented. Captcha is used in the login process to counter login automators. After login, excessively frequent operations will be considered malicious and the user will be forced to logout.

The current version of the course selection system at Tsinghua University has been operating online since April 2009. It has gone through many rounds of pre-selection, regular selection, and complementing and withdrawing selection. During each round, an average of 32,000 students access the system and successfully register their courses. The peak period during the complementing and withdrawing

Table 393.1 Server configurations of the operational environment during the course selection period

Server	Configurations	Remarks
Web server	HP Blade system,Intel Xeon E5110 CPU ×1,4 GB Memory	Two independent servers during peak periods
Application server	Sun X4450 Intel Xeon E7320 CPU ×4,64 GB Memory	Two servers shared with other applications during peak periods
Database server	SunV490 SPARC IV + CPU ×4,32 GB Memory	Two independent servers during peak periods

selection lasts no more than 20 min. The load pressure closely relates to user behaviours, therefore we make estimations in advance and prepare contingency plans and make operational resources ready for use.

In autumn 2010, during the complementing and withdrawing phase of course selection, the Web server tier became overloaded immediately after the course selection switch was turned on. According to the pre-arranged contingency plan, we timely adjusted the number of concurrent users allowed into the system, added backup servers to the Web server tier and ensured stable and efficient operation of the system. Under previous architectures, such operations would require a shutdown of the system to reallocate operational resources. Users would not be able to access the system during the operation. Under the highly available and scalable operational architecture, adding servers to the environment took only a few minutes. It was done by adjusting configurations of the load balancing tier and user operations were not affected.

During normal times, the system load is relatively low. After each round of course selection, resources are freed for use in other systems and the standalone environment is switched off and merged with the educational administration system. Portal users can roam into the system in a single-sign-on fashion. During course selection period, the only entrance into the course selection system is at the portal system. This makes the entrance easier to find. What's more, the number of concurrent users could be monitored and controlled more effectively.

393.5 Summary

To improve service quality and reduce costs, we design and practice a highly available and scalable operational architecture of Web applications. This architecture is designed to serve the full life-cycle of projects and is overall planning-oriented. It realizes predictable, stable, and dynamically scheduled operation of Web applications. Under this architecture, the course selection system at Tsinghua University has been operating stably and efficiently since its launching in April 2009. System load is closely monitored and operational resources are dynamically allocated. The course selection and other significant activities at the University are well supported.

References

1. Liu N, Yu P, Wang X, Fu X (2011) Research and implementation performance optimization of elective course system at Tsinghua University. Exp Technol Manag 28(5)
2. http://hi.baidu.com/918165239/item/9bebf42e84b06e59c28d5945
3. Wang X, Li Y, Liu N, Yu C (2012) Research and application of operation strategy optimization based on web application. Exp Technol Manag 29(12)
4. Liu N, Wu H, Cheng Z (2008) Research and practice on high available architecture for web application in colleges and universities. Exp Technol Manag 25(8)

Chapter 394
Network Assisted Teaching Model on Animal Histology and Embryology

Xin Ma, Yunjiao Zhao, Limin Wang, Aidong Qian and Winmin Luan

Abstract As an effective type of educational resources, network-assisted teaching has become effective approaches to boost the creativity of education and to enhance the self-learning abilities of students. Taking the network-assisted teaching mode targeting for Veterinary Medicine depending on the campus network, the paper is aiming at evaluating the teaching effectiveness through comparative analysis of test results and questionnaire on this teaching mode. It is shown that the network-assisted teaching mode is superior to the single traditional classroom teaching mode and can improve the teaching effect significantly. Therefore, it is important to break through the limitations of traditional classroom teaching and contribute to the independent learning for students in terms of network-assisted teaching mode.

Keywords Network assisted teaching · Animal histology · Embryology

394.1 Introduction

Animal histology and embryology, is an important morphology in Veterinary Medicine of agricultural schools. However, there were various problems to be solved in this subject, such as large capacity, tedious and abstract content, a wide range of knowledge, tight teaching hours and so on. On the other hand, it is more difficult to teach and to learn for the teachers and students respectively. Therefore, it is necessary to come up with a new teaching method as a useful complement to traditional teaching mode. As a result, network-assisted teaching has become an unalterable trend and main direction in the background of teaching reform. Given to

X. Ma · Y. Zhao · L. Wang · A. Qian · W. Luan (✉)
College of Animal Science and Technology, Jilin Agricultural University, Changchun, Jilin, China
e-mail: maxin3202@aliyun.com

S. Li et al. (eds.), *Frontier and Future Development of Information Technology in Medicine and Education*, Lecture Notes in Electrical Engineering 269,
DOI: 10.1007/978-94-007-7618-0_394, © Springer Science+Business Media Dordrecht 2014

its fully use of network and teacher resources, network-assisted teaching could provide an open, interactive, shared learning environment for students, which realizes the student-centered teaching and brings off the modern teaching methods and means. Furthermore, network-assisted teaching will be conducive to the reform of teaching content and teaching methods, there is bound to be positive impact on the transformation of teaching concepts, improving the quality of teaching and promoting quality education in all ways (1). This paper is going to explore out a new teaching model of network teaching as complementary of classroom teaching through establish the histology and embryology website based on the campus network. The new teaching model, network-assisted teaching used in animal histology and embryology will improve the quality of teaching in colleges and universities by promoting the integration between the network technology and curriculum.

394.2 Research Object and Methods

394.2.1 Research Object

The control group: 120 students in 2010 Veterinary Medicine. The experimental group: 120 students in 2011 Veterinary Medicine. The two groups of students have no significant difference in admission results, basic knowledge, ages, gender, etc. Both of the two groups enrolled in the Animal Histology and Embryology course in the first semester. Choosing the Animal Histology and Embryology as the textbook, published by China Agriculture Press, under the general editorship of Shen Xiafen.

394.2.2 Teaching Methods

The control groups were accordance with the teaching plan strictly: there are 60 total hours including 40 h of theory classes and 20 h of experimental courses in traditional classroom teaching manner. The same teaching plan applied in the experimental group, but the content of teaching would be cut and compressed: 20 % of the hours (12 h) for network teaching, including 10 h of theory classes, carrying out the network independent study under the instructor of teacher in the interactive lab; the other 2 h were arranged in the experimental class, for watching the video that was related to the experiments on Animal histology and embryology.

It is essential to establish a network teaching platform that was involved in the pictures, animation and excellent course video on this course, making the platform to be an interactive platform with 9 plates: syllabus, courseware, excellent courses, experimental courses, practice tests, tutoring, answering questions, relevant literature and open forum.

394.2.3 Evaluation Method

394.2.3.1 Test Results

Students were forced to take an exam after ending the course. Carrying out the experiment skills assessment by site operation, recording the assessment results in the light of 4 grades: fail, pass, good, excellent. Carrying out the comprehensive test by selecting the sample of the item bank in the computer, recording the exam results according to 4 grades: fail, pass, good, excellent. With the efforts of all the teachers and experts, both the comprehensive exam papers in grade 2010 and grade 2011 have the same degree of difficulty. Moreover, the number of questions and the type of questions are exactly the same. SPSS13.0 statistical software were used in the analysis of skill results and theory results that were making by the two groups of students.

394.2.3.2 Questionnaire

The anonymous questionnaire survey was performed targeting for grade 2011 after the course ending. The questionnaire was designed according to the teaching characteristics of our school and the course itself. There were 10 questions altogether including the attitude towards the network-assisted teaching mode, learning content of network courses, improvement of the ability of independent learning, efficiency of positive learning and so on. The main purpose is to provide a practical basis to reform the traditional teaching mode through investigating the teaching situation and existing problems of animal histology and embryology teaching during the network-assisted teaching in a questionnaire manner.

394.3 Results and Discussion

As for the students of grade 2011, the testing scores rates of fail, pass, good, excellent were 1.67 % (2/120), 25 % (30/120), 40.83 % (49/120), 32.5 % (39/120) respectively in the comprehensive results, compared with 2010, the difference of fail rate (1.61/10.1 %) and excellent rate (32.5/8.3 %) was statistically significant (Fig. 394.1). ($P < 0.01$).

120 questionnaires were distributed to the students of Veterinary Medicine 2011, and got 113 replies, 108 questionnaires were available, the response rate was 90 %. Network-assisted teaching mode and traditional classroom teaching mode were compared by students in this questionnaire investigation, the results showed that 88.5 % students thought good of the network assisted teaching mode, students' reaction was overwhelmingly favourable. So it's necessary to induce network-assisted teaching mode in animal histology and embryology.

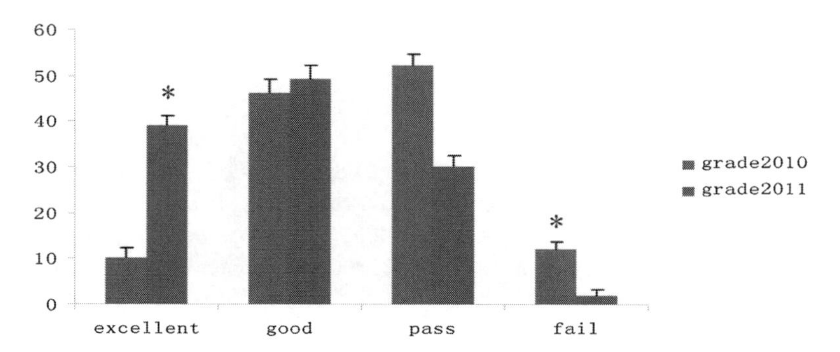

Fig. 394.1 The results of comprehensive assessment in different grades

394.4 Discussion

Currently, Animal histology and embryology teaching mainly include two parts, basic theoretical teaching using multimedia courseware, and experimental class using optical microscope to observe histological slice. In the process of the basic theoretical teaching, a large number of pictures, images, flash and model which are two-dimensional were used, but the real histological structure is three-dimensional, so the students need to be cultivated the ability of thinking in images step by step. However, for the basic theoretical class is very large, good teaching results will not be achieved in the basic theoretical courses of university. The blackboard, wall charts, models, and multimedia courseware were generally used in traditional teaching methods, which is boredom, rather dismaying, especially for the complex, fine, abstract contents can not be displayed visually, the students often had difficulties in understanding. Multimedia courseware can provide a lot of clarity, high resolution pictures and flash, enriched the teaching content, but also raised some problems: such as fast teaching pace, fail to keep up with the idea of teachers and easy to produce visual fatigue. This is dangerous, as it can foster negativity and adversely effect on learning efficacy and quality. With the development of teaching reform in our college, the latest research results and scientific research dynamic have been paid more and more attention in classroom teaching, but the teaching hours were further compressed, so students need to learn more in classroom teaching than before. It is difficult to understand and master the knowledge deeply only in classroom teaching, computer assistant instruction must be induced (2). Network-assisted teaching mode is a new educational philosophy with the main body of the students studying which is lying on student-oriented, it will be help to stimulate students' interest in learning and to develop students' awareness of innovation and practice, and also it can well solve the problems, such as too much lecture, little practice, too much content and fewer classroom hours. Network-assisted teaching based on the campus network, is truly achieved the traditional teaching and online teaching complementing each other with advantages (3).

We constructed the teaching mode which made the lecture-based classroom primary and the network classroom supplementary. In this mode, about 80 % of the lessons were for the traditional teaching in the classroom, and 20 % of the lessons were for the network classroom teaching in digital interactive laboratory. The teaching mode was practiced by students of animal medical 2011, the results showed that the scores both in skills test and theory test was significantly improved than the control group, students of animal medical 2010. In the network-assisted teaching mode, experimental abilities and theoretical knowledge can be enhanced significantly. The majority of students tended to have a more favourable attitude towards the network-assisted teaching mode of animal histology and embryology using questionnaire survey in students of animal medical 2011. And it was generally believed that the net-based assisted teaching mode improved their interest in major study and practiced their confidence. Meanwhile this net-based assisted teaching mode does cultivate the student's thinking power and capacity to solve problems.

Network-assisted teaching model combines the advantages of traditional teaching mode and network teaching mode, showed an immense superiority in modern teaching, and improved the quality and efficiency of teaching. The preliminary practice also shows that this teaching model is valid in China's current full-time college which is in the traditional classroom based education system.

However, the innovation of teaching model has its diversity and complexity, network-assisted teaching mode need to be further researched and practiced to make it more systematic and standardized.

Acknowledgments This work was supported by Veterinary Medicine "Eleven Five-Year" Featured Specialty Foundation (20070502) and Science Technology Foundation of Jilin Province Education Department (Jilin Province Education Department Contract 2012 No. 56) in China.

References

1. Xia Y (2008) Network model with the traditional classroom model of complementarity in mathematics teaching, Ph.D. Central China Normal University
2. Hu Q, Ma J, Yuan Z et al (2010) Research and realization of multifunctional, active network teaching platform of medical genetics. Sci Technol Inf Comput Netw 16:637
3. Lim CP (2001) The dialogic dimensions of using a hypermedia learning package. Comput Educ 36(2):133–150

Chapter 395
Research on Application of Artificial Immune System in 3G Mobile Network Security

Dongming Zhao

Abstract Currently, 3G communication technology develops very rapidly. Ensuring the security of 3G communication, monitoring network attack and avoiding risk become a hotspot concerned by the academic circle. This paper puts forward an intrusion detection algorithm based on artificial immunity, which is an important development direction of the improvement of security and reliability of 3G mobile network and detects network attack and real-time risk of mobile communication network with a good monitoring effect and high accuracy. Compared to RBF method, it has more accurate risk prediction of communication network and such characteristics as distributivity, diversity, auto-answer, self-maintenance, high accuracy and short time.

Keywords Artificial immunity · 3G · Network security

395.1 Introduction

With the extensive use of mobile communication technology in the daily life and constant expansion of its related network, how to ensure the information security of wireless network effectively while improving communication quality and providing diversified and personalized services and various wireless data services has become a key problem restricting the development of mobile communication technology [1].

Compared to the first and second generations of mobile communication network, 3G mobile communication has made great progress in security [2]. However, due to 1P structural feature of its own network, various security

D. Zhao (✉)
Langfang Teachers College, Langfang, 065000 Hebei, China
e-mail: dzhaoongming2013@yeah.net

S. Li et al. (eds.), *Frontier and Future Development of Information Technology in Medicine and Education*, Lecture Notes in Electrical Engineering 269,
DOI: 10.1007/978-94-007-7618-0_395,

problems based on IP network will pose a threat to 3G network to different extents [3]. Security risk caused by network openness, if not avoided effectively, will impose a great impact on the normal operation of 3G network based on IP network.

There is a great similarity between biology immune system and computer security system [4]. The former protects organism from being damaged by pathogenic organism, while the latter protects the computer system from hostile attack by hacker [5]. This paper puts forward a real-time monitoring algorithm with the method of artificial immunity based on immunology principle of organism, which can monitor network attack and communication risk in 3G mobile communication network in real time and ensure the security of communication system.

395.2 Artificial Immune Technology

Artificial immune system (AIS) is an umbrella name of various intelligent systems developed by researching, imitating and using the principle and mechanism of biology immune system. Intrusion detection and proactive protection based on immunology are research hotspot in the security field such as computer, communication and data processing, as well as an important development direction of the improvement of security and reliability of 3G mobile network [6].

Biology immune system (BIS) is a distributed adaptive complex system with self-organization and dynamic balance ability. For invading antigens, different kinds of lymphocyte distributed in the whole body can produce corresponding antibodies. It aims at ensuring that basic physiological functions of the whole biological system can maintain normal operation.

AIS is an umbrella name of various intelligent systems such as various information and computer technologies developed by researching, imitating and using the principle and mechanism of biology immune system. Immune algorithm has a good system responsiveness and independency and a strong ability of maintaining self-balance of system for interference.

395.3 Application of Artificial Immune System in Security Maintenance of 3G Mobile Network

According to theories mentioned above, this paper puts forward a real-time risk monitoring algorithm of 3G network based on immunology, which imitates the immune system of human body. Table 395.1 shows the mapping relation between the immune system of human body and this algorithm.

In the process of immunological surveillance, when the host is not attacked, the number of antibodies on the host keeps relatively invariant; when the host is

Table 395.1 Mapping relation between immune system of human body and risk monitoring algorithm based on immunology

Immune system of human body	Risk monitoring algorithm based on immunology
Antigen	Binary string after feature extraction of IP package
T cell, B-cell	Antibody expressed by binary string
Binding	R-bit consecutive bit matching algorithm
Auto-tolerance	Negative selection algorithm
The number of antigens of B cell conjugation exceeds affinity threshold	Matching exceeding activation threshold
Cell clone	Antibody copying
Human body	3G mobile network
Lymph gland	Mobile terminal in 3G mobile network

attacked, the number of antibodies on the host will increase sharply due to clone of memory antibody and activated mature antibody. When the attack disappears, the number of antibodies on the host will decrease and tend to be stable due to the life cycle of mature antibodies. Table 395.2 shows the main parameters in this algorithm.

This algorithm is imitated in MATLAB software. First, make the type of network attack synflood type and danger of attack 0.8. Table 395.3 shows the actual synflood attack power suffered by a terminal (A, importance of terminal 0.6) in 3G mobile network terminal. The attack power is expressed by hundred-mark system.

Make the type of network attack land type and danger of attack 0.6. Table 395.4 shows the actual land attack power suffered by a terminal

Table 395.2 Main parameters of detection algorithm based on immunology

Parameters	Significance	Size or composition
Antigen	Binary string obtained after feature extraction of IP package	Source/destination address, port, protocol type, TCP/UDP/ ICMP domain
Activation threshold of mature antibodies	The accumulated affinity of mature antibodies reaches this value and they are activated as memory antibodies.	10
Life cycle	Existence time of mature antibodies	100
Antibody appreciation	Number of new added antibodies in every generation	5
Number of terminals	Number of terminals in 3G network	20
Importance of terminal	Degree of importance of this terminal	0.5–0.8
Type of attack	Type of network attack	Synflood, land, teardrop etc.
Danger of attack	Danger level of network attack	0.5–0.8

Table 395.3 Actual synflood attack power suffered by mobile terminal A

Time (s)											
	0	10	20	30	40	50	60	70	80	90	100
Attack power	25	30	40	45	75	80	70	70	65	50	30

(A, importance of terminal 0.6) in 3G mobile network terminal. The attack power is expressed by hundred-mark system.

Make the type of network attack teardrop type and danger of attack 0.5. Table 395.5 shows the actual teardrop attack power suffered by a terminal (A, importance of terminal 0.6) in 3G mobile network terminal. The attack power is expressed by hundred-mark system.

Tables 395.6, 395.7 and 395.8 are risk changing curves of risk monitoring algorithm based on immunology under three different network attacks. Risk value 0 indicates "as safe as a house" and risk value 1 indicates "very unsafe". The higher the risk value, the higher the risk suffered by 3G mobile network.

Table 395.9 shows the overall security risk faced by 3G mobile communication network.

Table 395.4 Actual land attack power suffered by mobile terminal A

Time (s)											
	0	10	20	30	40	50	60	70	80	90	100
Attack power	22	36	41	35	28	42	51	22	18	30	32

Table 395.5 Actual teardrop attack power suffered by mobile terminal A

Time (s)											
	[illegible]	10	20	30	40	50	60	70	80	90	100
Attack power	11	24	32	20	37	48	67	40	59	46	29

Table 395.6 Changing curve of 3G network security under synflood attack

Time (s)											
	0	10	20	30	40	50	60	70	80	90	100
Risk	0.23	0.31	0.40	0.47	0.81	0.84	0.72	0.73	0.61	0.48	0.33

Table 395.7 Changing curve of 3G network security under land attack

Time (s)											
	0	10	20	30	40	50	60	70	80	90	100
Attack power	0.20	0.35	0.40	0.36	0.30	0.43	0.50	0.20	0.20	0.32	0.30

Table 395.8 Changing curve of 3G network security under teardrop attack

Time (s)	0	10	20	30	40	50	60	70	80	90	100
Attack power	0.10	0.25	0.30	0.22	0.35	0.45	0.65	0.41	0.60	0.45	0.30

Table 395.9 Overall security risk faced by 3G mobile communication network

Time (s)	0	10	20	30	40	50	60	70	80	90	100
Attack power	0.42	0.45	0.52	0.55	0.77	0.82	0.63	0.51	0.65	0.52	0.50

395.4 Discussion

(1) The algorithm based on immunology has monitored the influence of three network attacks on 3G network security risk. Its relative size is basically consistent with the actual network attack power. This indicates that the real-time risk monitoring algorithm of network providing immunology can effectively monitor communication risk and ensure communication security.

(2) Its corresponding risk increases rapidly with the increase of attack power. When the attack power decreases, its corresponding risk reduces. However, its descending slope is lower than that of attack power. The descending slope is determined by the life cycle of mature antibodies. This has important meanings under real mobile communication environment. When an attack recurs in a short time, network can still maintain a high alert.

To conclusion, this paper puts forward a real-time risk monitoring method of network in 3G mobile communication network with organic combination of 3G network, intrusion detection system and artificial immune model. It has a good monitoring effect and high accuracy for common network attacks (such as synflood, land and teardrop). Compared to RBF method, the monitoring method based on immunology has a more accurate risk prediction of communication network, greatly improved design of network model and training speed, short time consumed and realistic feasibility.

References

1. Wang F, Liu Z, Li J (2003) A computer security system model imitating biological immunity. Mini Micro Comput Syst 4:698–701
2. Tang J (2004) An architectural design of intrusion detection system based on computer immunology. Comput Knowl Technol 11:70–72
3. Xiao R, Wang L (2002) Artificial immune system: principle, model, analysis and prospect. Chinese J Comput 12:1281–1291

4. Li B (2007) Computer network security strategies based on artificial immune system. Appl Technol 8:94–95
5. Fu H, Yuan X (2008) Artificial immune model based on bilayer defense architecture. Comput Eng 1:178–180
6. Run Q, Jiang Y, Wu J (2005) Antibody forming and detection component of network intrusion detection system based on immune mechanism. Chinese J Comput 10:1601–1606

Chapter 396
Neuromorphology: A Case Study Based on Data Mining and Statistical Techniques in an Educational Setting

F. Maiorana

Abstract The importance of neuromorphology cannot be underestimated since knowledge of the brain supports interesting and disparate applications ranging from obtaining an insight into mental diseases to try a comprehension of the human cognitive processes while performing complex tasks. Indeed, it is widely recognized that the knowledge of the morphological structure of the neurons is a fundamental step towards studying neurons and understanding their functions and interactions. This paper presents a case study of an engineering course provided with a data mining module whose final projects were dedicated to manage computational tools for neuron morphology. The results suggest how such tools may be reused in neuroscience and bioengineering courses as a basis for the important and difficult task of neuron modeling and understanding.

Keywords Neuromorhpology · Data mining · Medical education · Matlab

396.1 Introduction

The importance of neuroscience has been growing in recent years. Applications in this field range from electrophysiological and functional recordings such as EEG and fMRI to neuronal morphology. This kind of study must be well represented in medical education and in bioinformatics courses. Training in this field is complex and requires teaching and presenting materials ranging over different domains: first the medical knowledge of the domain in question which could span from anatomy to genes and to pathways regulating the biological process. On top of this

F. Maiorana (✉)
Department of Electrical, Electronic and Informatics Engineering, University of Catania, Viale A. Doria, 6 95125 Catania, Italy
e-mail: francesco.maiorana@dieei.unict.it

S. Li et al. (eds.), *Frontier and Future Development of Information Technology in Medicine and Education*, Lecture Notes in Electrical Engineering 269,
DOI: 10.1007/978-94-007-7618-0_396,

knowledge it is required to have a deep understanding and knowledge of computational methods, statistical techniques, data mining algorithms and so on.

In the medical domain the importance of neuron morphology in understanding brain function has been widely recognized. The morphological characteristics of the neuron have an influence on its function. It is widely reported in literature that the nervous system's organization and behavior depend critically on size, position, and shape of the neuron [1].

The focus of this work will be on the presentation of a case study on neuromorphology that, by making use of data mining and statistical techniques as well as neuron anatomy, provides the ground to practically apply knowledge on different fields into a project fostering the possibility of a deeper understanding by engaging students in practical activities.

The work presents the educational setting of the experience by giving the course context and its content in Sects. 396.2 and 396.3 briefly presents the neuromorphology field; Sect. 396.4 describes the educational experience and finally Sect. 396.5 draws conclusions and proposes further work.

396.1.1 Educational Context and Course Content

The educational experience was performed within a master course in Information Systems. Half of this 60 h course was centered on data mining and its application in different domains with a particular emphasis on the medical domain. The data mining applications in the medical domain ranged from document classification and association discovery as proposed in [2–4], macro array data analysis [5], brain computer interfaces, protein structure and so on.

The course was held for 6 years and its content varied over the years. All the students in the same semester had to attend a mandatory course on statistics. For a description of the course, with its particular emphasis on the data mining module, its main teaching objective and its content design the reader can refer to [6].

In the last part of the course, after the main topics were presented, discussed and practically applied, the students had to complete a project. The project was concerned with practical data mining and statistical analysis. Also, the project was considered as a capstone to the module. The driving factor of the project was to give to the students the possibility to practically apply all the knowledge learned in the course and in parallel courses, such as the statistics course, and to analyze a dataset and to solve a non-trivial problem. The project could be undertaken by a single student or by a group of students.

This work describes a medical data mining application in the emerging domain of digital reconstruction of neuron morphology. The aim of the work is to present a practical case study to be managed, as a proof of concept, by statistical and data mining process, in order to foster other applications in the same domain, but with different techniques or neuronal cell datasets. The experience can be applied to students on other courses such as bioinformatics or other medical domains.

The experience allowed non-medical students to be exposed to a medical domain problem, grasp the main features essential to its understanding, and apply the knowledge learned in the course to the medical domain under study.

The students had the possibility to explore a pool of final projects performed by previous students and organized as a shared memory of projects [7, 8]. By looking at this set of projects the students had the opportunity to improve their knowledge, to obtain inspiration, and in many cases to start from one project thus increasing and improving the overall quality of the elaboration.

396.1.2 Neuromorphology and Computational Models

According to [9] "the importance of neuronal morphology in brain function has been recognized for over a century". In this field morphological "digital reconstructions" of neurons has gained a paramount importance and has inspired many research works in literature bringing about the development of different tools for "data acquisition, anatomical analysis, three-dimensional rendering, electrophysiological simulation, growth models, and data sharing" [9].

The research works have been collected on the portal [10, 11]. NeuroMorpho.org, a "centrally curated inventory of digitally reconstructed neurons associated with peer-reviewed publications".

For a recent review on morphological metrics used in analysis and development of computational models the reader can refer to [12], where the authors point out the importance of understanding the pattern of neuron growth since it provides an insight into their function.

The computational model of the neuron morphology as proposed by Donohue et al. [13, 14] tries to simulate the morphological structure of the neurons as a tree where each branch has a bifurcation probability that depends on the diameter of the branch and on the length of the segment. The model is based on a set of parameters such as:

- the diameter ratio, defined as the ratio between two diameters such as:
- the parent daughter ratio, defined as the ratio between the diameter of the parent and the diameter of the larger daughter;
- the daughter ratio, defined as the ratio between the larger daughter diameter and the smaller daughter diameter
- the probability of bifurcation
- the branch path length, defined as the length between two consecutive bifurcations
- the tape rate defined as the ratio between the start diameter and the end diameter of a segment between two bifurcations

A possible algorithm proposed by Ascoli and colleagues to compute a model of a neuron is reported in Fig. 396.1.

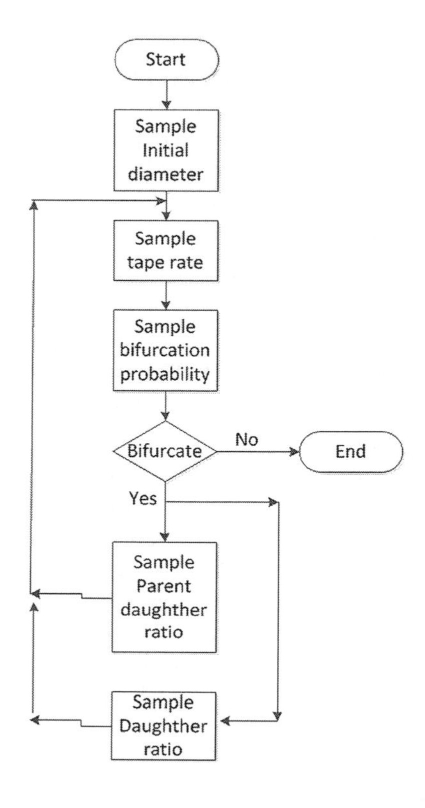

Fig. 396.1 Flowchart of the algorithm to compute the neuron model

The ramifications of the neuronal cell model will start from the first branch and will follow a series of bifurcations on the basis of the above rules.

396.1.3 The Educational Experience

The education experience was, with regard to a data mining project presented by the student, on a morphological reconstruction of a pyramid cell CA3B of the Hippocampus of a rat. The dataset was available on the Neuromorpho.org portal and was provided by Ascoli. The didactic experience aimed at obtaining a good understanding of the problem at hand and could be an object of further study, e.g., in a master thesis.

The dataset is composed of 4,287 rows describing the segments or cylinders of the cell. Each row is composed of 7 fields, namely:

- An identifier of the cylinder
- The type of the cylinder
- x, y and z coordinates of the end extremity of the cylinder
- the radius of the cylinder section
- the identifier of the parent, if it exists.

The study performed by the students comprised the following steps:

- General statistical analysis of the data distribution
- Computation and analysis of statistical indicators
- Univariate analysis
- Bivariate analysis
- Model construction and simulation in order to obtain a synthetic model of the neuronal cell.

The project was developed with the Matlab software suite. The students after loading the dataset on the Matlab environment started with a statistical analysis of the bifurcation by computing basic indices such as number and overall rate of bifurcation. The analysis was repeated for the length of each segment with statistical analyses such as average, total, minimum and maximum length. The analysis proceeded performing the computation of statistical indices for each type of segment: soma, axon, apical and basal dendrite. For the analysis of the radius length the radius values were clustered in 4 classes and the probability of a segment having a radius in each class is computed.

The univariate analysis was performed in order to study the symmetry of each attribute, by computing indexes such as kurtosis, asymmetry and other moments as well as descriptive data indicators such as minimum, maximum, mean, standard deviation and so on.

One of the goals of the bivariate analysis was to find correlations between different variables such as between the type of segment and the radius.

The model construction part is the most interesting experience towards the construction of a cell model on the basis of the available data.

One approach followed by the students was to use a negative exponential model to approximate the probability of bifurcation on the basis of the analysis of the distribution of the aleatory variable representing the number of bifurcations. This represents a first trial approximation but can be used as starting point for further analyses. Starting from the model of the probability of bifurcation the student constructed the model of the other parameters such as taper rate, branch path length, diameter ratio in order to produce a simulation of the branching path of the neuronal cell.

Finally the produced model was compared with the original model using many aggregate measures such as number of bifurcations, length of the structures, diameter, section, area and volume. This has been done by comparing aggregate measures such as total, minimum, maximum, average, standard deviation and so on. The 3D representation of the model and of the original dataset were also visually compared.

Other machine learning techniques such as neural networks could be used in order to practically apply the concepts developed in the course and to construct a model of the main parameters describing the neuron as presented above.

Overall, although students do not possess medical expertise, they obtained a good level of performance in relation to the described didactic theme. In particular we tested that all the students gained a satisfactory understanding of the basic concepts of the neuromorphology and an excellent ability in managing the computational tools needed for morphological reconstruction. In particular the 3D model of the neuron was comparable, taking into account the didactic nature of the experience compared with a relevant research project, with the one available in the portal neuromorpho.org. Similar results were obtained for overall summative indices such as number of bifurcations, percentage of bifurcated segments, total length of the structure, mean, minimum and maximum length of the segments, mean, minimum and maximum diameter, mean, minimum and maximum section, mean, medium and maximum area, mean, minimum and maximum volume, parent daughter ratio, and so on.

The results obtained can be used as a starting point for further improvements of the didactic experience and for better measurement of the gained skills.

396.1.4 Concluding Remarks and Further Work

In this work we have presented a case study of an educational data mining project in the neuron morphology analysis domain and in the development of its computational model.

Although the case study reports a didactic experience to train students without prior medical or bioinformatics knowledge in an interesting and important medical domain, it can be used in other contexts to train students with a medical or a non-medical background.

This study represents an initial step in the complex and variegated domain of neuromorphology. The portal neuromorpho.org offers a rich set of data that can be used in further didactical projects to obtain an insight into the described problems and to deepen understanding of how data mining and statistical knowledge may be applied to real medical cases.

In the future we plan to interlink the student projects in the neuromorphology domain in order to generate an organizational memory of student projects in such a way that the students can easily find the mining results of other students on the same dataset allowing them to reuse the computational experience and to take advantage of the textual and graphical annotations inserted by the previous learners [15–17]. It can be useful an eye tracker study to obtain an objective indication of the difficulty of a morphological analysis performed by an expert using monitors with different sizes as in [18, 19].

References

1. Kaiser M, Hilgetag CC, van Ooyen A (2009) A simple rule for axon outgrowth and synaptic competition generates realistic connection lengths and filling fractions. Cereb Cortex 19(12):3001–3010
2. Faro A, Giordano D, Maiorana F, Spampinato C (2009) Discovering genes-diseases associations from specialized literature using the grid. IEEE Trans Inf Technol Biomed 13(4):554–560
3. Faro A, Giordano D, Maiorana F (2011) Mining massive datasets by an unsupervised parallel clustering on a GRID: novel algorithms and case study. Future Gener Comput Syst 27(6):711–724
4. Giordano D, Faro A, Maiorana F, Pino C, Spampinato C (2009) Feeding back learning resources repurposing patterns into the "information loop": opportunities and challenges. In: 9th International conference on information technology and applications in biomedicine ITAB 2009, pp 1–6. IEEE
5. Faro A, Giordano D, Spampinato C (2012) Combining literature text mining with microarray data: advances for system biology modeling. Briefings Bioinform 13(1):61–82
6. Maiorana F (2012) A teaching experience on a data mining module. In: 2012 Federated conference on computer science and information systems (FedCSIS), pp 871–874. IEEE
7. Faro A, Giordano D (1998) Concept formation from design cases: why reusing experience and why not. Knowl Based Syst J 11(7):437–448
8. Faro A, Giordano D (2003) Design memories as evolutionary systems: socio-technical architecture and genetics. In: IEEE Proceedings international conference on systems, man and cybernetics, vol 5. Washington, D.C. USA, pp 4288–4293, IEEE
9. Parekh R, Ascoli GA (2013) Neuronal morphology goes digital: a research hub for cellular and system neuroscience. Neuron 77(6):1017–1038
10. http://neuromorpho.org/neuroMorpho/index.jsp
11. Ascoli GA, Donohue DE, Halavi M (2007) Neuromorpho.Org: a central resource for neuronal morphologies. J Neurosci 27(35):9247–9251
12. Gillette TA, Ascoli GA (2012) Measuring and modeling morphology: how dendrites take shape. In: Computational systems neurobiology. Springer,Dordrecht, pp 387–427
14. Donohue DE, Ascoli GA (2005) Local diameter fully constrains dendritic size in basal but not apical trees of CA1 pyramidal neurons. J Comput Neurosci 19(2):223–238
13. Donohue DE, Ascoli GA (2008) A comparative computer simulation of dendritic morphology. PLoS Comput Biol 4(6):e1000089
15. Giordano D (2002) Evolution of interactive graphical representations into a design language: a distributed cognition account. Int J Human Comput Stud 57(4):317–345
16. Ahmed S (2005) Encouraging reuse of design knowledge: a method to index knowledge. Des Stud 26(6):565–592
17. Faro A, Giordano D (1998) Story net : an evolving network of cases to learn information systems design. IEEE Proc Softw 145(4):119–127
18. Giordano D, Maiorana F, Leonardi R (2012) Effects of monitor size on accuracy and time needed to detect cephalometric radiographs landmarks. Displays 33(4–5):206–213
19. Maiorana F, Leonardi R, Giordano D (2012) Eye-tracker data analysis in cephalometric land marking. In: 2012 International conference on computer and information science (ICCIS), vol 2, pp 1025–1029

Chapter 397
Construction and Practice of P.E. Network Course Based on Module Theory in University

Xin-Ping Zhang and Dong-Hai Wu

Abstract Network course provides a new form in developing new teaching resources and extending classroom teaching, offers a positive and practical significance in optimizing the quality of teaching and transmitting education information. The modular design of Physical Education (P.E.) network course constitutes an integrated teaching system, which includes an overall plan on teaching system, special module development, and systematic integration of teaching topics, teaching system evaluation and testing. It will fully integrate the content of different areas of expertise to improve the scientificity, relevance and effectiveness of teaching. The P.E. program which was developed based on the internet framework software platform has the functions of course management, curriculum development and course research. Through one semester teaching experiment, the results of final exam and fitness tests indicated that the network course assisting P.E. teaching got better performance than traditional teaching.

Keywords P.E. course · Network course · Modularity · Teaching platform

397.1 Introduction

The latest advances in technology are inevitably making their way into schools and gymnasiums across the country [1]. Current multimedia and network technology as the core of modern educational technology boom is the rapid rise and violently hitting schools of various subjects, especially in colleges and universities. P.E. course is a compulsory course for all the college and university students in China. Since the computer was introduced into classroom to assisting classroom teaching, many P.E. teachers and researchers trying to use it to help students to grasp motor

X.-P. Zhang (✉) · D.-H. Wu
School of Education, Sun Yat-sen University, Guangzhou 510275 Guangdong, China

S. Li et al. (eds.), *Frontier and Future Development of Information Technology in Medicine and Education*, Lecture Notes in Electrical Engineering 269,
DOI: 10.1007/978-94-007-7618-0_397,

skills, sports drills and to better understand the knowledge of sports. With the internet explored on the campus rapidly, many courses have introduced a network course to build a new one teaching mode. This study discoursed features of P.E. network course, implemented network teaching of P.E. course,it pointed that the network course assisted teaching can improve the education effect by optimizing the teaching content.

At present, the development of modern educational technology in teaching time and space to break the boundaries, changing the teaching environment and teaching methods, teaching contents, teaching methods and the quality of teaching had a positive impact [2]. It promotes the integration and optimization curriculum resources, curriculum resources, the presentation had a fundamental impact: (1) hypertext technology breaks through the traditional teaching of the subject content of the logical structure, convenient for students to self-search, retrieval, analysis, composition and exploration, to knowledge acquisition and preservation of providing a great convenience; (2) network technology has greatly enriched the scientific information resources to a more open curriculum resources, and practical issues and the development of modern science and technology more closely linked; (3) multimedia technology to optimize the presentation of scientific knowledge way to meet the visual learners, auditory and other sensory needs of students can be mobilized to maximize non-intelligence factors and perception activities; (4) information technology has the highly interactive nature of which was more convenient for students in independent study, communication, can fit Student personality development, the formation of a democratic and harmonious relationship between teachers and students. Thus, modern educational technology to conduct our own inquiry learning based teaching mode, students explore the ability of independent study learning activities provides a convenient and powerful information and technology platform. For the modern education technology environment for students to study independently explore the ability of research and practical exploration of teaching has a positive and practical significance and potential value.

Technological advancements have challenged educational institutions to expand upon traditional teaching methods in order to attract, engage crud retain students. One strategy to meet this shift from educator-directed teaching to student-centered learning is greater computer utilization as an integral aspect of the learning environment [3]. The purpose of the present study was to introduce the construction of P.E. network course and to assess the effectiveness of utilizing the network course into swimming class.

397.2 Research Methodologies

In this paper, we mainly study on the effectiveness of applying network course in swimming class. The methodologies of literature, experimental studies and logical analysis are applied.

397.2.1 Literature Data

To meet the needs of the study, a lot of literature about computer, technology and internet and the P.E. teaching were collected and reviewed carefully. Through carefully reading the results of previous studies we got the basic understanding of relevant background knowledge and formatted a theoretical foundation.

397.2.2 Experimental Study

To compare the effectiveness of traditional teaching and the network course assisted teaching, 6 classes (175 students) enrolled in swimming course were randomly assigned to the control ($n = 90$) and or experimental ($n = 85$). Each participant completed a pre-test (knowledge and skills of swimming) and computer literacy. Students then attended the course in the designated medium and took a post-test at the end of the semester.

397.2.3 Logical Analysis

The researchers followed the logical rule to analyze the information from the literature and the results of experiment, and use inductive and deductive method to draw the conclusions of this study.

397.3 Construction of P.E. Network Course

397.3.1 The Features of P.E. Network Course

For introduction P.E. network course, we focus on the user-friendly designing. The practicality was highlighted during interface design, course content system design and learning activities and evaluation feedback link. Based on a modular rules, network course achieved functional integration of systems integration. The teaching module integration process is actually functional integration process of the content of the course, consisted of the number of both independent and interrelated thematic teaching module. This system is not simple accumulation of teaching topic, but need to integrated each teaching module in a unified operating platform, on which the teaching topic information can be shared and integrated, various teaching thematic modules can run coordinately, thus, to the function of system can be played overall. Knowledge integration also can be achieved in the process of integration based on the design rules. Through formal or informal relations, individuals and organizations promote knowledge sharing and communication, and integrate individual knowledge into organizational knowledge. Knowledge integration process is dispersed in the minds of classroom teachers, professional knowledge and explicit knowledge dispersed in the inter-organizational integration, sharing, through the connection of knowledge to achieve the integration of the "Course" system function. Knowledge integration process of knowledge transfer, the process of production, can effectively break through the limitations of the different teachers' professional background to improve the speed and efficiency of organizational learning.

397.3.2 The Contents of P.E. Network Course

Combining with the characteristics of physical education, the constituted elements of the static system in the physical education course resources includes several aspects [4]; the organization of physical education curriculum content includes: arrange the elements of physical education content at different segment and grade through a certain way, form the elements of physical education content to a scientific and complete knowledge system, thus contribute to promote the effective accumulation and continuity of the physical education [5]. In the curriculum interface design, following the principles of concise and practical, the network of the swimming course is divided into three parts: network assisting study, teaching resources, module management and class management. Network assisting study divided into 3 parts: individual study, teacher introduced study and group discussion. Variety teaching resources are supplied to students in second module, which includes teaching plan, courseware, video of swimming course, and the link of swimming website. The module management and classroom management teachers and curriculum assist student to use teaching resources effectively [6]. The information of class and teacher, and the notification of class, and selection of course integrated into this management system (Fig. 397.1).

397.3.3 The Module Design of P.E. Course

Figure 397.2 illustrated the procedure of P.E. network course design, at eh beginning of the course, we should set up the goal, and then analyze students and study environment, design the interface and navigation, introduction of course, organize contents of course, and finally implement and manage course. Every step can be modified through feedback from both teachers and students.

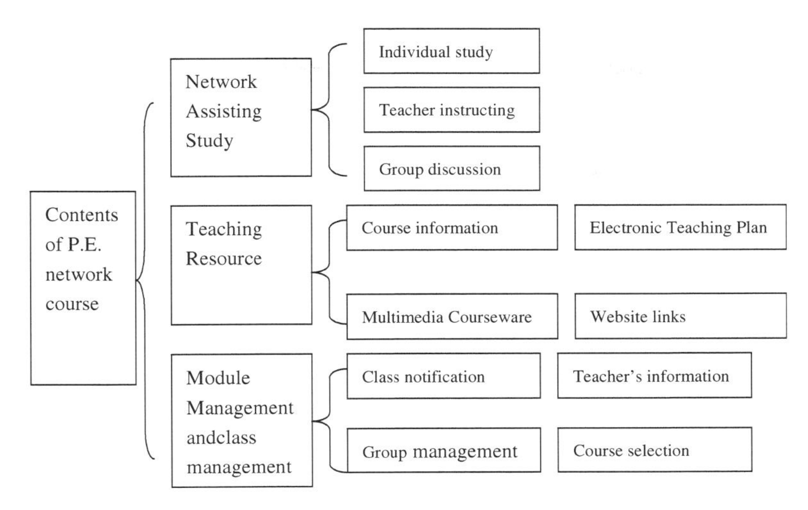

Fig. 397.1 The contents of P.E. network course

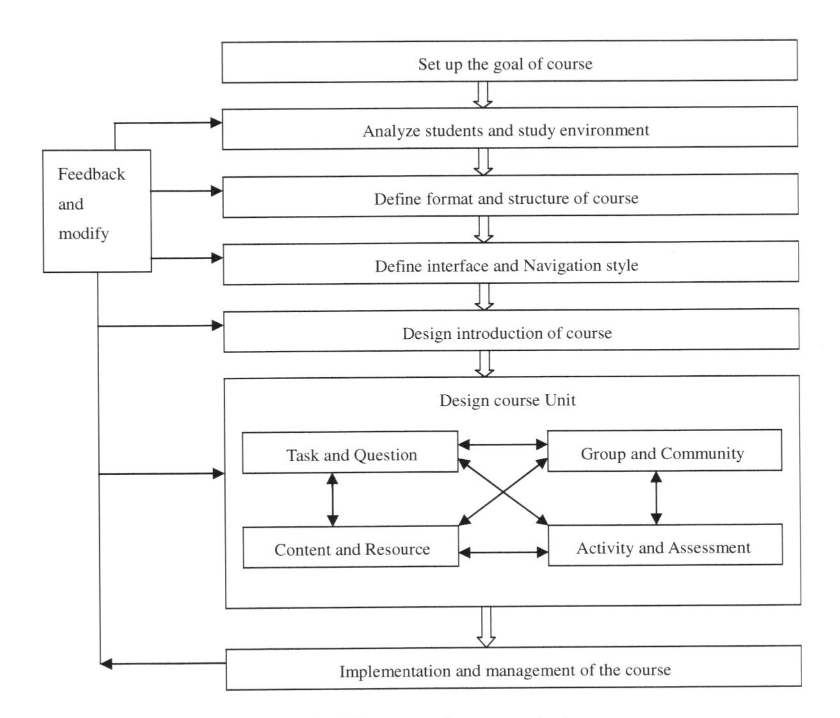

Fig. 397.2 The procedure of Module P.E. network course design

397.4 The Implementation and Effectiveness the of P.E. Network Course

397.4.1 The Implementation of P.E. Network Course

As Module Learning Management System using widely at home, the teacher will face the problem how to design and implement the network course based on Module in teaching. The thesis summarizes the designing modes of the network course and three kinds of typical informatization teaching modes, in order to provide the majority of teachers with use and reference. First one is the auxiliary teaching style teaching mode, which gives full play to the advantages of traditional classroom teaching, but makes up for the defects of the traditional classroom teaching resources, promoted asynchronous communication, multi-channel interaction, and student subjectivity play party; second one is the network independent study course teaching mode. In module learning environment, with the help of others, students in consultation with others, conversation, exchange, access to knowledge through the initiative of the construction of meaning, and teachers' role is only for the help and guidance. The third one is Group network courses collaborative teaching mode, in this mode teaching contents is well-designed for each task, students learn in the form of a group or team, each play a role together to accomplish a task or solve a problem.

397.4.2 The Effectiveness of Introducing Network Course into P.E. Teaching

As can be seen through the results of experimental data (Tables 397.1, 397.2 and 397.3), compared experimental group with control group, pre-test results of the basic knowledge of swimming, swimming skill and fitness showed no significant difference both groups. But the test scores of post-test shows significant difference. Comparing the results of experimental classes and control classes in the mastery of basic knowledge of swimming, swimming skill test and fitness test, there are significant differences in performance of the experimental group, which indicated

Table 397.1 Fundamental knowledge of swimming test results

	n	x	s	t	p
Experimental group pre-test	90	56.23	6.87		
Control group pre-test	85	57.02	8.41	1.56	0.21
Experimental group post-test	90	70.27	6.02		
Control group post-test	85	75.23	8.48	3.43	0.00

Table 397.2 Swimming skill test results

	n	x	s	t	p
Experimental group pre-test	90	56.72	3.65		
Control group pre-test	85	58.63	4.87	0.55	0.59
Experimental group post-test	90	87.67	5.81		
Control group post-test	85	82.89	4.53	3.25	0.00

Table 397.3 Fitness test results of experimental group and control group

	n	x	S	t	p
Experimental group pre-test	65	72.57	7.43		
Control group pre-test	66	75.88	8.51	1.87	0.42
Experimental group post-test	65	85.23	7.02		
Control group post-test	66	78.25	10.48	3.54	0.00

that through introducing network teaching mode, progress amplitude of experimental students was significantly higher than that of the control group ($p < .01$).

As it mentioned earlier, network course provides a new idea and form in developing new teaching resources, extending classroom teaching, offers a positive and practical significance in optimizing the quality of teaching, and spreading education information. It provides a good platform to student sharing the experience and promoting interactivity with teachers. The PE network course allow students to provide updates on their progress to other students in the group, provide a platform for coordinating group activities, create platforms for the building and sharing of ideas, and post drafts of projects and reports for others in the group to see. If the instructor or students is absent or the instruction is not finished, students can get instruction online. So the students in experimental group are able to get more study material and more instruction than those studying at the control group. And the students in experimental group gathered in several group, and the member of group practice more after class. All the advantages of applying network course contribute to the better performance of the experimental group.

397.5 Conclusions

While there are many good reasons to use technologies to facilitate P.E. teaching, it is important to recognize that these are merely aiding measures. There may be group assignments and collaborative learning assignments for which face-to-face interaction is a necessary and valued component of the education process. The discussion about internet-learning technologies should focus on the attributes of the tools that can help students and teachers to facilitate the process and product of group work, and not about whether one set of tools is fundamentally better than the other. That said, as teachers contemplate the potential value of network course, as well as their drawbacks for both students and faculty, they should consider how they might better use the tools that are at their disposal to manage the process more effectively.

References

1. Oleg S (2012) A using the iPad in a sport education season journal of physical education, recreation and dance. Pro Quest Res L 83(1):39
2. Wu PI (2006) The expansion of instrumental rationality in China's education system and reflections. Xuzhou Inst Technol 21(2):72–75
3. Hyland, MR, Genevieve P-Z, Valerie O, Lichtman SW (2010) A comparative analysis of computer-assisted instruction and management topics in physical therapy education. J College Teach Learn June 2010:1–13
4. Zhi Z, Nan Z (2011) Research on the construction of the physical education course resources system theory IT in medicine and education (ITME). Int Symp Volume 1:151–155
5. Nan Z, Zhi Z (2011) Research on the organization of the contents for physical education based on computer IT in medicine and education (ITME). Int Symp Volume 1:61–65
6. Liu GN, Liu RG, Liu XQ (2008) Design and implementation of the network course based on moodle are explored. Modern Educ Technol 18(6):66–69

Chapter 398
Application and Practice of LAMS-Based Intercultural Communication Teaching

Bin Long and Jinxi Li

Abstract Optimization Theory, proposed by Бабанский, emphasizes that ideal teaching and learning outcomes depend on how to bring the best performance out of current condition. On the one hand, this theory requires the concordance f teaching objectives, teaching contents, teaching approach and teaching form; on the other hand Бабанский puts emphasis on learner's activities and their interactions with teachers. As far as what Optimization Theory is concerned, LAMS, featuring learners' activities arrangement, just satisfies the need of the Optimization Theory. The author believes that combination of LAMS and Optimization Theory is bound to promote current teaching outcomes. Therefore, this paper intends to take intercultural communication course for example to further explain the application of LAMS under the guidance of Optimization Theory.

Keywords Optimization theory · LAMS · Intercultural communication course

398.1 Introduction

The most important and brilliant innovation of e-learning no doubt lies in the development of learning design software, among which Learning Activities Management System (LAMS) might be most successful in terms of application and feedback. Learning design software has evolved from Course Management

This paper is sponsored by the Project of Research on the Cultivation of Chinese College Students' Intercultural Communication Competence

B. Long (✉) · J. Li
Tianmu College, Zhejiang A & F University, Hangzhou, Zhejiang, China
e-mail: pennylonda@hotmail.com

S. Li et al. (eds.), *Frontier and Future Development of Information Technology in Medicine and Education*, Lecture Notes in Electrical Engineering 269,
DOI: 10.1007/978-94-007-7618-0_398,

System (featuring websites-presented form of teaching content), Leaning Management System (highlighting online management of teaching content as well as learners) to Learning Activities Management System (emphasizing online management of learning process). The transformation from pure learning content management to learning process management makes LAMS gain universal compliments among teachers and students.

LAMS is developed by a team led by James Dalziel, a professor at Macquarie University. It is taken as a revolutionary tool for designing, managing and delivering online collaborative learning activities. It provides teachers with a highly intuitive visual authoring environment for creating sequences of learning activities. To put it in detail, as a learning activities management tool, teachers could monitor learners' learning process as well as control teaching contents by designating and arranging activities sequences, like Forum, Notice board, Multiple Choice etc. One of the most typical advantages brought by LAMS is learners are not limited to time and space. Besides, with teachers' macro-guidance, learners could gain more freedom in the course of learning. To be exact, there are no exact learning contents designated by teachers. In other words, while approaching the same topic, learners gain more freedom for options.

398.2 Rationale

Optimization Theory is proposed by Бабанский who takes teaching as a complicated system with all kinds of elements actively and interactively involved. Ac-cording to him all elements relevant to teaching and learning are connected to a certain degree and their joint functions result in teaching outcome. Therefore, to bring the best out of each element in teaching as well as in learning is critical to teaching outcome. In other words, given both teachers' and learners' condition in time, Optimization Theory highlights how teachers and learners could make the best use of their time and efforts to achieve optimal teaching and learning outcomes. According to Бабанский, Optimization Theory is not a teaching approach, rather it is a wise teaching decision based on a good understanding of teaching principles and a good knowledge of learners' learning level. In addition, Optimization Theory can not always remain the same, as it changes with concrete teaching conditions. That's why teaching condition is put on the priority all the time. Therefore the ap-plication of Optimization theory depends on concrete teaching condition. In real cases, to create an ideal teaching outcome, concordance of teaching objectives, teaching contents, teaching approach as well as teaching form should be taken into consideration. On the other hand, students' activities should also be emphasized. According to Бабанский, without teaching interactions between teachers and students, an ideal teaching outcome cannot be achieved. Concerning learners' activities, LAMS is no doubt a good choice in helping teachers' organizing activities. With careful activities arrangement, teachers could repeatedly refine and perfect their teaching objectives, teaching contents, teaching approach as well as teaching form. In the following part, the author is going to present an intercultural communication class with the application of LAMS to achieve optimal teaching and learning outcomes.

398.3 An Example of Intercultural Communication Class Based on LAMS

The following intercultural communication course design will be revolved around the topic "cultural values and Hofsted's four value dimensions". Subjects are 30 non-English major students of advanced level in their second year study. And characteristics of non-English major students just decide this intercultural communication course cannot be too theory-focused and stressful. The teaching objective covers four levels: (a) knowledge level: to understand cultural values and Hofsted' four value dimensions; (b) skill level: to be able to exemplify cultural values and the four value dimensions;(c) emotional level: to show empathy to different cultures and to be more understandable and tolerable to other cultures; e) cultural level: to understand and appreciate American cultural values. Teaching contents are intended to cover topic approach, theory discussion and exemplification, from theory to practice. Teaching form involves group discussion, individual work with online presentation.

In the first period, the teacher is going to lead students into the learning environment by giving the activities of "voting", "chat and forum" and "share resource". Studens are required to vote on "what is cultural value?" and the following options are provided: (a) It is kind of enduring belief; (b) It can be translated into actions; (c) It is broad-based consensus; (d) It is norms of a culture. e) others. In addition to casting a vote, students are also required to share and exchange their opinions in forum. The aim of doing this is to provoke students' interests, widen their thinking on this topic. After discussions in forum, the teacher may give academic explanation for cultural values by sharing the following website: http://en.wikipedia.org/wiki/Value_(personal_and_cultural). Of course, in the whole LAMS-based English class, access to internet is provided all the time to students. That is to say, if they have any trouble in discussing and debating online, they can refer to online dictionary for help. Besides they can discuss their language problems online with teachers and their classmates as well.

The second period is intended to explore the theory, and activities of "group", "submit files", "notice board" and "notebook" will be adopted. With the activity of "group", the teacher can divide the class into 7 groups in the principle of better ones working with the poors according to their autonomous learning abilities. Teacher could post the following requirements on "notice board": (a) Read Hofsted's value dimensions in your textbooks. While reading, please make some notes; (b) Work in groups to find out examples to illustrate each value dimension; (c) Submit results of group discussion. Exploring theory involves both individual efforts as well as group work. What's more important is teacher's involvement in group discussion to clear learners' puzzles about the theory.

When operating the third and the fourth period in real classes, the two periods have to go together, as these two periods aim to combine theory with practice and it indeed takes longer time. The activities of "notice board", "chat and forum", "share resource" and "submit files" will be adopted. To begin with, teacher could publish the following tasks on "notice board"—watch the video and explore Chinese and American cultural values based on the video. Then the following wetsites will be shared with students: (a) http://www.iqiyi.com/zongyi/20120921/d65954328a8fbc3b.html, (b) http://v.youku.com/v_show/id_XNTUxMzk2NTg4.html. These two video clips are The Voice of China and The Voice of America. The Voice is a hot TV show, enjoying great popularity among college students. Their familiarity and preference of this program will easily emerge themselves in doing this comparatively serious task. Further more, with regard to the content of this program, both versions highlight talent shows among average people, whose behaviors on stage are typically representative of their culture behind. Students are required to watch these two versions of programs and voice their opinions about cultural values in forum at the same time. Of course, the teacher is supposed to take part in their discussions in forum and voice his or her opinions when clarification and explanations are needed. In the end, students are required to write a composition on their understanding about one of the four value dimensions quoting examples from The Voice.

The fifth period featuring "exhibit" is to adopt the activities of "Q&A" and "submit files". Questions in this part will be closely linked to the understanding of the theory and Chinese and American cultural values based on the TV program.

The sixth period is for reflections. To help students look back on what they have learned. The activities of "multiple choices" and "Q&A" will be employed to help reflections. By checking students' compositions and students' answers in "Q&A" and their results in "multiple choices" plus the whole process of monitoring their involvement in discussing, chatting and debating, teachers will easily assess students' learning performance and make relatively fair judgement on evaluation.

Taking into account Optimization Theory and typical features of LAMS, this learning design is bound to best bring out advantages of the theory as well as the software. Therefore there is no doubt that the optimal learning outcomes would turn out when this learning design is put into practice properly.

398.4 Conclusion

This paper takes Optimization Theory as theoretical framework proposing a practical intercultural communication course design with using LAMS. LAMS with its unique feature of learning-process-orientation well perform and realize what Optimization Theory is calling for. However, no learning design is perfect and so are theory and software. While arousing learners' interest in learning, the problem of easily directing learners' attention to irrelevant information is unavoidable. Except that, there are flaws on theories too, so constant perfection for learning design and content upgrade for learning management software are called for all the time. There is one principle for improvement: Creating designs for experiences that are motivating, enjoyable and productive for students and teachers alike. Teaching serves learning and design is always learning-oriented.

References

1. Boud D, ProsserM (2001) Key principles for high quality student learning in Higher Education—from a learning perspective. Paper presented at a workshop held on April 27, 2001 for the AUTC funded project: information and communication technologies and their role in flexible learning. Sydney, Australia
2. Dalziel J (2003) Implementing a learning design: the learning activity management systems (LAMS). In: Crisp G, Thiele D, Scholten I, Barkerand S Baron J (Eds) Interact, Integrate, impact: proceedings of the 20th annual conference of the australasian society for Computers in learning in tertiary education. Adelaide, 7–10
3. George W, Gagnon Jr Michelle CG Constructivist Learning Design
4. Gibbs D, Philip R (2005) Really Changing Teaching and Learning. Prof Educr 4(4):
5. Harper B Oliver R (2002) Reusable learning designs: information and communication technologies and their role in flexible learning. Presentation for the "AUTC Reusable Learning" designs: opportunities and challenges" conference, UTS, Sydney
6. Koper R, Tatersall C (2005) Learning design: a handbook on modeling and delivering networked education and training, Springer. Retrieved from http://books.google.co.uk/books?id=MNQxDKbTpisC&dq=what+is+learning+design&pg=PP1&ots=dlP0osJPNg&sig=6cfACk_AC4JXh9HSrDvIBck81Rg&prev=http://www.google.co.uk/search%3Fhl%3Dzh-CN%26q%3Dwhat%2Bis%2Blearning%2Bdesign&sa=X&oi=print&ct=result&cd=1#PPP1,M1
7. Manon M, Bulk D (n.d.) Phoebe: a pedagogical planner tool. Tall University of Oxford, http://wiki.cetis.ac.uk/uploads/8/84/PheobeCetisLiverpool.ppt#256,1,Phoebe a pedagogical planner tool, 29 May 2007
8. What Is Lams? http://www.lamsfoundation.org/

Chapter 399
A Study on Using Authentic Video in Listening Course

Yan Dou

Abstract This paper reports a case study investigating and comparing the usage of authentic video in public English teaching and English major teaching. The study has been undergone in both classroom conditions and autonomous learning. By observing the participants, including teachers and students, findings suggest that teachers hold a systematic cognition which shapes their practice.

Keywords Authentic video · Handling materials · Teachers' cognition

399.1 Introduction

Language teaching in the twenty-first century is characterized by frequent changes, innovation, competing language teaching ideologies and by the development of technology. The method concept in teaching—based on the theories of language teaching—is quests for better methods of many teachers in this century. In listening course, the traditional method of playing cassette tapes and video cassette has been taken place of by multimedia, among which, authentic video has been gaining more attention from teachers and researchers.

This paper is sponsored by Project of Study on English Teaching Modals for Experimental Class in Independent College, Zhejiang A&F University

---

Y. Dou (✉)
Tianmu College, ZheJiang A&F University, Lin'an 311300 Zhejiang, China
e-mail: Douyan_2006@126.com

S. Li et al. (eds.), *Frontier and Future Development of Information Technology in Medicine and Education*, Lecture Notes in Electrical Engineering 269,
DOI: 10.1007/978-94-007-7618-0_399,

399.2 Studies on Using Authentic Video

Some studies have been conducted to investigate the use of authentic video in second language teaching. We have been particularly influenced by Sherman [5], Flowerdew and Miller [2], Helgesen and Brown (2007) and some Chinese scholars. We have also benefited from our own teaching experience and studies. Various studies on using video were carried out by adopting different perspectives.

399.2.1 The Motivation of Using Authentic Video

Sherman [5], Flowerdew and Miller [2], Helgesen and Brown (2007) concluded that the compelling power of video in the classroom is an inducement—there is a special thrill in being able to understand and enjoy the real thing. Videos often promote the motivation to listen and provide a rich context for authenticity of language use. Moreover, the paralinguistic features of spoken text become available to the learners and it aids learners' understanding of the cultural contexts in which the language is used.

399.2.2 The Ways of Using Authentic Video

Sherman's [5] research contains a systematic account of using specific kinds of video materials (e.g. feature films, soaps, documentaries, the news, etc.). Flowerdew and Miller's [2] study focuses on active viewing done as part of private study time and provides some issues for teachers to follow up to exploit the material. While, Helgesen and Brown (2007) described some detailed steps that supplemented Sherman's suggestions.

399.2.3 The General Guidelines for Video Activities

As Sherman [5] noted, "the supply is enormous and the materials are…cheap and constantly renewed. Audio-visual input is now as accessible as print. It's a resource we can't ignore, and our students certainly won't." On the one hand, we found it appealing and promising. On the other hand, we realized that we should have 'teacher cognition' on using authentic video. These experts provide some precautions and suggestions on proper video watching so that this language learning method in and out of classroom cannot be overused and misused.

In the past decade, researchers in China have also investigated the use of authentic video in the Chinese students' listening. For example, Zhou and Yang

(2004) explored "the effects of visual aid on EFL listening comprehension". Their statistical results revealed that "The students listening comprehension is positively related to the use of visual aid. Specifically, students of a lower proficiency benefit more from it." The results also suggest "that the use of visual aid has no significant effect on the comprehension of difficult words and the information to which the visual images bear no relation".

On the basis of multimodalities, Zhang [6] explored the selection of modalities in EFL. As a part of multimodalities, video is discussed briefly. He pointed out that the teaching conception, teaching design and teaching practice should serve to teaching aim and teaching content.

The above review surveys the researches related to use of authentic video in EFL in these 10 years. Generally, these studies shed light on the key aspects of application and some activities in English teaching. As to the selection of materials in different stages, out-class study and advanced-level study in listening course are still to be further investigated.

399.3 Research Design

399.3.1 Research Purpose and Research Questions

This research is intended to investigate the use of authentic video in action both in classroom conditions and automatic learning. Two research questions are to be addressed in this study:

- What are the types of video actually used in listening? Specifically, what materials are selected by teachers, what principles do they follow? And do they overuse or underuse some types in a certain period?
- What approaches are "proper" ones to build up a repertoire of activities in different sessions of class time, different stages of a term and different levels of school years? In sum, when employing authentic video in listening courses, what and how do those teachers do and what "should" be kept up and improved in the future work?

399.3.2 Participants

It is well-known that the listening ability changes with age and language proficiency. Therefore, this study investigated students in different ages and proficiencies and teachers who teach in different school years.

5 teachers and 50 students were chosen as participants in the investigation. As for the students, each 10 of them were chosen from these five teaching classes respectively and randomly. All of the teachers are going in for English listening teaching. The first participant was a young female teacher who taught freshmen

College English. The second male teacher taught the sophomore College English. Other three teachers were English major teachers from first to third year, of which the second one is male and the other two are female. For the sake of following description, the five teachers were named T_1 to T_5. One reason for choosing them was that they differed from each other in teaching experiences and teaching objectives. Another reason was that they were under pressure of nationwide English Tests.

This involved selection would provide a basis for comparison in terms of variables within and across the two divisions and the 3 years.

399.3.3 Methods

399.3.3.1 Data Collection

In order to gain a full picture, class observation, interview, questionnaire and teaching journal were used as study methods. These five teachers' classes were observed, from which some reports were made thereby. The teachers were interviewed individually and asked to explain their teaching practice and views on using video. Then, the students were interviewed in groups, meanwhile, the questionnaire were distributed to them to fill out. The researchers, as both observers and participants, wrote some teaching journals and observation notes for the reflective purpose. All of the related questions were as mentioned in 3.1.

399.3.3.2 Data Analysis

Teacher Cognition

All of the teachers' aim was to attempt to get students to develop their intensive and extensive listening skills by way of authentic video programs and they believed that viewing videos were beneficial in helping learners develop their listening skills. Another belief they held was that it was a window into culture, it was a nice change of regular listening exercises and it added a good variety to the structured teaching format. They said in short, students wanted it and it consequently brought about a good classroom atmosphere and active learning.

Handling Materials

According to the data, among the large amount of video resources, the rank of selected frequency was as following: daily news, sitcoms, popular films, music video, documentaries, interviews and cartoons, etc. As regards the time of playing video in class, these teachers had some common preferences. For example, they often put latest news at the beginning of class, arranged music video, sitcoms and popular films during the breaks or at the end of second section, while, they usually scheduled the documentaries and interviews to be interwoven with the related topic of lessons. In addition, we found many differences in their teaching.

(i) Different Attitudes to Video Importance

As is well-known, teacher beliefs about language teaching proved to be the critical factor influencing their decisions. These decisions were clearly consistent with individual teaching practices. That was evident in how these teachers chose and organized the video materials. The two College English teachers, in a way, regarded the use of authentic video to be an optional task. They viewed audio for improving listening ability as central in listening course, while, video was dispensable and supplementary. But the English major teachers held different views. They also admitted that listening by ears was the essential and indispensible activity. Meanwhile, they didn't think that video was only a spice to the routine or a way to enliven the class. They realized that viewing authentic videos—news, films, ads and talk show, etc.—was one of the students' major goals in learning English and in all fairness. So, in classroom, those English major teachers provided a lot of up-to-date materials, but the College English teachers didn't do like that.

(ii) Different Preferences to Types of Materials

These 5 teachers who came from different grades were well aware of their teaching objectives. Therefore, they selected different types of materials in hierarchy: elementary, lower-intermediate, intermediate, lower-advanced. For instance, T_1 and T_3 selected short news from BBC or Special VOA for elementary classes. They adapted the news for the exercises of spot-dictation and short questions. Contrastively, T_3 spent longer time on more types of video than T_1 did in class. This case was the same as T_2 and T_4 in the corresponding grades at lower-intermediate level. T_5 was very different from the other four colleagues in using videos. She chose relatively difficult materials for her course "Advanced Listening and Speaking". The materials, including news, films, sitcoms, interviews, were a set of variations, which were an advance both in length and depth.

It could be seen that English major teachers adopted more types of materials and paid greater attention to the contents, which was a reflection of their belief and attitude to the use of video.

(iii) Different Procedures of Using Videos

Another important aspect of organization within a method is what we will refer to procedure. It encompasses the actual techniques, practices and behaviors that operate in language teaching. According to Richards and Rodgers (2001), a common procedure might consist of:

- resources in terms of time, space and equipment used by the teacher
- interactional patterns observed in lessons
- tactics and strategies used by teachers and learners when the method is being used.

Here is a description of typical procedural aspects observed in the participants' classes:

- Lead-in: vocabulary
  The teacher presented words or proper names on PPT. These words were chosen from the video materials. Firstly, the teacher explained some key words. Then, the students read the words aloud, sometimes in chorus, sometimes individually, and sometimes in silence.
- Lead-in: background knowledge
  The teacher moved PPT to next page. This page included some background information. The teacher would raise some related questions, asked the students to answer orally, and give some brief comments.
- Viewing
  The teacher played the video once. Next, he (she) showed the prepared exercises to the students and let them try to complete the tasks. Then, the teacher replayed the video to ensure the students to find the answer.
- Tasks
  The teachers arranged a wide range of exercises, such as questions, blank-fillings, note-taking, discussion, comments, story-retelling, even role-play.
  We found that not all the teachers followed above procedures. Of course, viewing was the only compulsory one. Comparatively, T_3, T_4 and T_5 did it "more earnestly", but in their classes, the observing teachers felt the tough questions and the tense atmosphere as well. There was another thing that could be considered as the procedural factor. The evidence showed that male teachers were better at operating computers than female ones. They were more skillful in controlling the video facilities and making the programs colorful. We had the experience of watching those female teachers try to solve technical problems.

(iv) Different Procedures of Using Videos

Another issue to be considered relates to the students' independent study. Field [1] noted, in a whole-class situation, it is the teacher who determines which parts of a recording to focus on. So it is with video uses. At times, the teacher dwelt overlong on sections that the individual learner had been able to match and interpret accurately; at other times, the teacher took for granted areas that the learner found problematic. There are some limits to how much can be achieved through whole-class listening practice. Teachers therefore need to supplement class work by seeking ways of promoting independent learning. Nowadays, our language labs enable teachers to spare a short period of time to the students and encourage them to carry out the tasks in class by themselves, but no one did in this way. Nor did they give much attention to the after-class assignment in forms of video.

It is possible today to give students some listening homework to finish after class. In our university, most students have their own computers and get easy access to internet. It thus becomes a practical and useful proposition to provide materials with some tasks for independent listening. In addition, teachers had better give some instructions on listening strategies and help students find some resources on websites for independent viewing outside classroom.

Students' Responses

Students reported in the questionnaire that their exposure to a series of authentic videos granted them to see language-in-use and allowed them to look at situations far beyond their classrooms. This was especially useful to sense the cultural differences. Video was a necessary component in a long lesson sequence. But they also complained that the lesson format used by teachers in using video was a relatively rigid one and sometimes the impact of videos on their listening skills were not so much as expected.

399.4 Discussion

We've taken brief account of using authentic video in listening course. The changes have been extensive, but it can be argued that we still need more extensive changes. For example, the current approach—Comprehension Approach- did not serve teaching purpose adequately, or we can say it restricted the listeners' role to perform. We should rethink the teaching approaches. We can find some of its weakness:

- More practice than better listening
- Showing understanding by answering questions
- More comprehension than communication.

Generally, viewing video became a question-based format of listening tasks. In fact, teachers may combine comprehension tasks with integrative tasks and communicative tasks.

We've also found some problems with using video in teaching listening. It comes to dealing with the reform of teaching approaches. Field [1] proposed that CA be treated not as the centerpiece in listening practice but as the means of an end. We should bear in mind that the gist of listening is "teaching not testing". We shouldn't lie so much in the approach to obtaining information as in the use we make of the answers.

399.5 Conclusion

In this study, we have described various aspects of using authentic videos in listening course. We have also identified several factors that play an important role in teaching with video. However, some relevant information need to be illustrated and discussed fully and systematically. We will turn to those special kinds of information in the forthcoming study.

References

1. Field J (2003) Listening in the language classroom. Cambridge University Press, Cambridge
2. Flowerdew J, Miller L (2005) Second language listening. Cambridge University Press, Cambridge
3. Harmer J (2001) The practice of english language teaching. Pearson Education Limited
4. Lei H, Yang S (2004) The effects of visual aid on EFL listening comprehension. J PLA Univ Foreign Lang
5. Sherman J (2003) Using authentic video in the language classroom. Cambridge University Press, Cambridge
6. Zhang D (2010) Preliminary investigation into the concept of design and the selection of modalities in multimodal foreign language teaching, Foreign Languages in China

Chapter 400
Comparison of Two Radio Systems for Health Remote Monitoring Systems in Rural Areas

Manuel García Sánchez, Rubén Nocelo López and José Antonio Gay-Fernández

Abstract Real time health remote monitoring systems require the use of radio networks to transmit data from patients to a health center where that data are analyzed. However, the required radio networks may not have a good coverage (or even not exist) in rural areas, where often an important number of elderly people with chronic diseases live. The performance of two remote monitoring systems based on two different radio networks (digital cellular network for mobile phones (GSM/UMTS) and Digital Mobile Radio (DMR)) to provide remote monitoring services in rural areas are compared and results and conclusions of the comparison are presented in this paper.

Keywords Aging · Patient monitoring · Home monitoring · Rural/frontier counties · Remote monitoring · Radio coverage

400.1 Introduction

During the last years there has been a growing interest on the development of health remote monitoring systems for patients with chronic diseases [1–6]. These systems would present several advantages for the patients that could be under real time continuous survey while remaining at their homes, but also for the Health

---

M. G. Sánchez · R. N. López (✉) · J. A. Gay-Fernández
VigoDepartamento de Teoría de la Señal y Comunicaciones, Universidad de, 36210 Vigo, Spain
e-mail: rubennocelo@uvigo.es

M. G. Sánchez
e-mail: manuel.garciasanchez@uvigo.es

J. A. Gay-Fernández
e-mail: jagfernandez@uvigo.es

S. Li et al. (eds.), *Frontier and Future Development of Information Technology in Medicine and Education*, Lecture Notes in Electrical Engineering 269,
DOI: 10.1007/978-94-007-7618-0_400,

Authorities, that could optimize the health resources. Elderly people, with increasing chronic medical conditions, are often the candidates for the use of these systems.

Thanks to the radio communication networks the information regarding patients health parameters can be transmitted continuously in real time to a remote center for analysis. With radio networks this can be done even while the patient develops daily life moving at home or around home.

However, radio coverage may not be adequate or even may not exist in rural areas. This would be a problem particularly if an important percentage of population in rural areas is aging population living alone and requires the use of these systems.

Two health remote monitoring systems are compared in this paper. The first one is based on digital cellular networks for mobile phones: second (GSM) and third generation (UMTS) systems, but it is GSM the network that should exhibit better coverage, mainly due to the lower operating frequency.

The second is based on Digital Mobile Radio (DMR) an open digital radio standard for professional mobile radio (PMR). Two frequency bands were considered for this DMR network, Very High Frequency (VHF) and Ultra High Frequency (UHF). Theoretically the lower frequency network (VHF) should provide better coverage.

Several remote monitoring systems were built to test and compare the radio networks, but the sensors used to gather information were the same: a wearable hearth rate meter, a portable blood pressure meter, and a Global Positioning System (GPS) receiver. In this way the difference between the systems is the radio technology used, but not the type or amount of information.

400.2 System Description

400.2.1 Digital Cellular Network for Mobile Phone

The system to test the coverage was built around a 3G mobile phone, a Samsung Galaxy S-II, with integrated GPS and Bluetooth. Heart rate meter was a wearable Zephyr model HxM BT connected to the mobile phone through the wireless Bluetooth link. The portable blood pressure sensor was an Omron model 708-BT, also connected to the mobile through the Bluetooth link.

An Android application was developed to gather the information from the sensors and the GPS and transmit the information through the GSM/UMTS network to a remote server where the information is stored.

400.2.2 Digital Mobile Radio

Digital radio terminals MOTOTRBO from Motorola with Bluetooth and GPS were used to build this system (see Fig. 400.1). The same sensors for hearth rate and

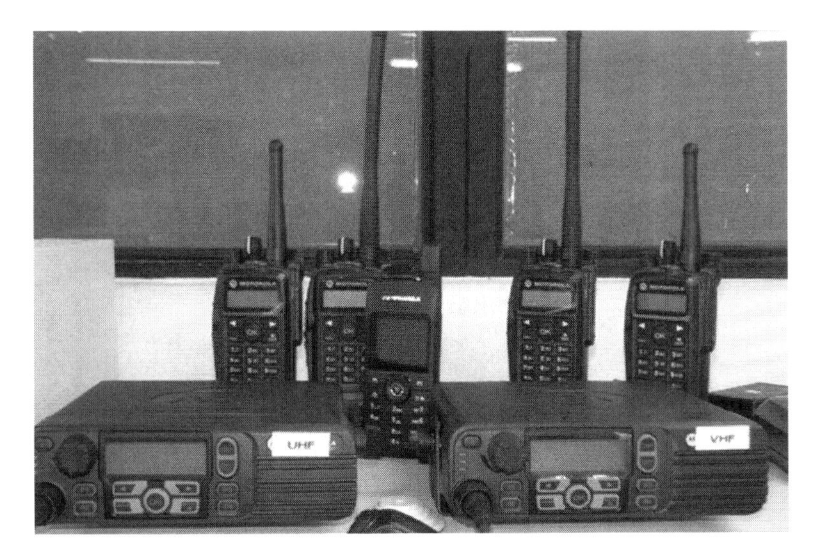

Fig. 400.1 DMR terminals

blood pressure were connected to the DMR terminals through the Bluetooth wireless link. The information from the sensors and the terminal was transmitted to the remote database through the DMR network.

As DMR is a Private Mobile Radio system, and there are not commercial public networks available, a DMR base station was built both for VHF and for UHF. The corresponding radio licenses to get the privative use of the portion of the radio spectrum needed for the experiment were obtained from the Spanish Radio Spectrum Management Authority. The base station, which is shown in Fig. 400.2a, b, was installed at University of Vigo.

Finally the system was completed with another application to consult the data base from mobile phone, and to receive alarms in case the monitored patient leaves

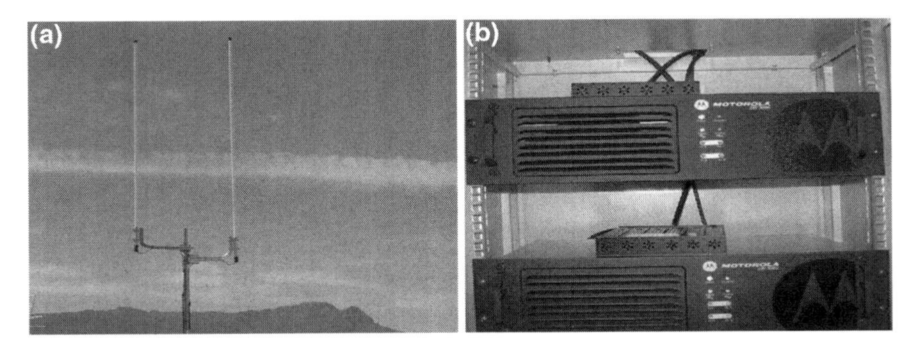

Fig. 400.2 **a** DMR base station antennas. **b** DMR base station

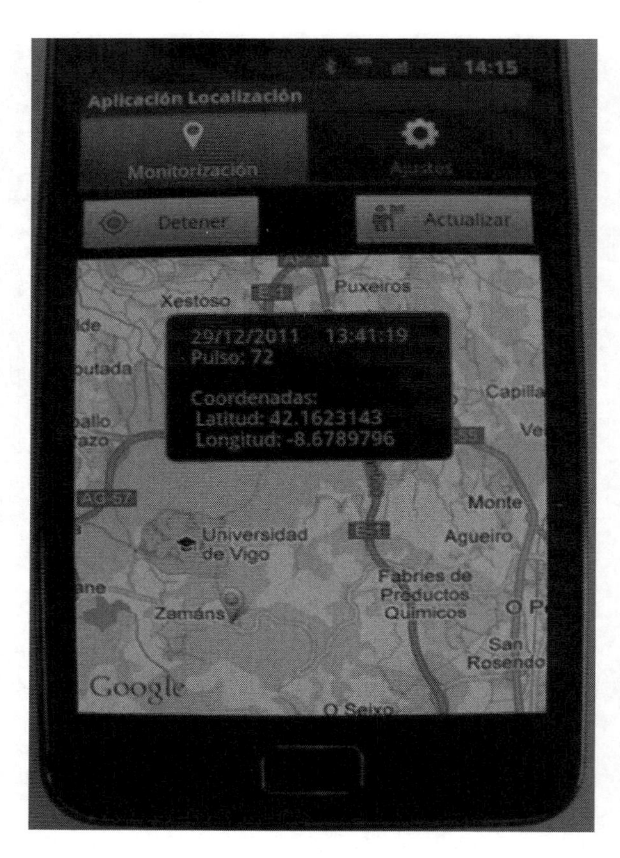

Fig. 400.3 Application to access the database

a predetermined area, or in case a health parameter falls out of predetermined limits. Figure 400.3 shows the mobile phone application with the location of the patient and the heart rate information.

A complete diagram of the whole system is shown in Fig. 400.4.

400.3 Measurement Setup and Results

To compare the coverage area of the systems under study, the system terminals were carried in a car that was driven around the DMR base station at University of Vigo. The surroundings of the campus correspond to a mountainous rural area.

For this experiment, together with the sensors and GPS information, also the Receive Signal Strength Indication (RSSI) at the terminal was measured and transmitted to the database. Figure 400.5 shows an example of the path followed by the car with the received power in the DMR-VHF terminal. Received power by the GSM, DMR-VHF and DMR-UHF terminals are compared in Fig. 400.6.

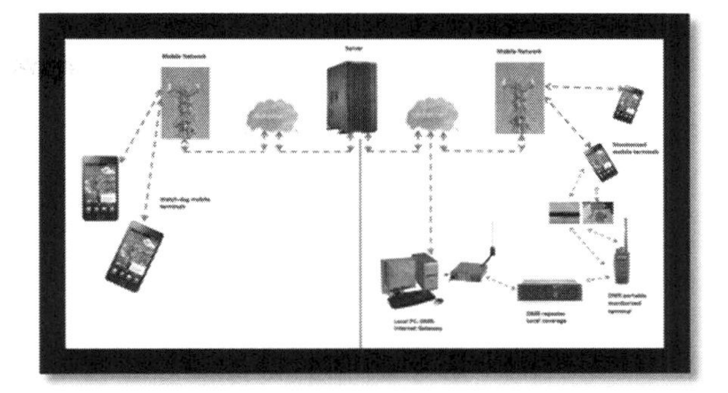

Fig. 400.4 Diagram of the health remote monitoring system

With this information an analysis was carried to calculate the corresponding Bit Error Rate (BER) of the radio link and the probability of receiving a wrong packet of information. It should be noted that, despite the signal levels are similar, GSM requires more signal level than DMR to achieve the same BER. This is mainly due to the different modulation schemes of both systems. While GSM uses a modulation known as Gaussian Minimum Shift Keying (GMSK) and a bit rate of 271 Kbps DMR uses 4-FSK (4 level Frequency Shift Keying) and a bit rate of 9.6 Kbps.

Results of this analysis are plotted in Fig. 400.7, where the probability of having a BER below certain value is given for the GSM, DMR-UHF y DRM-VHF systems.

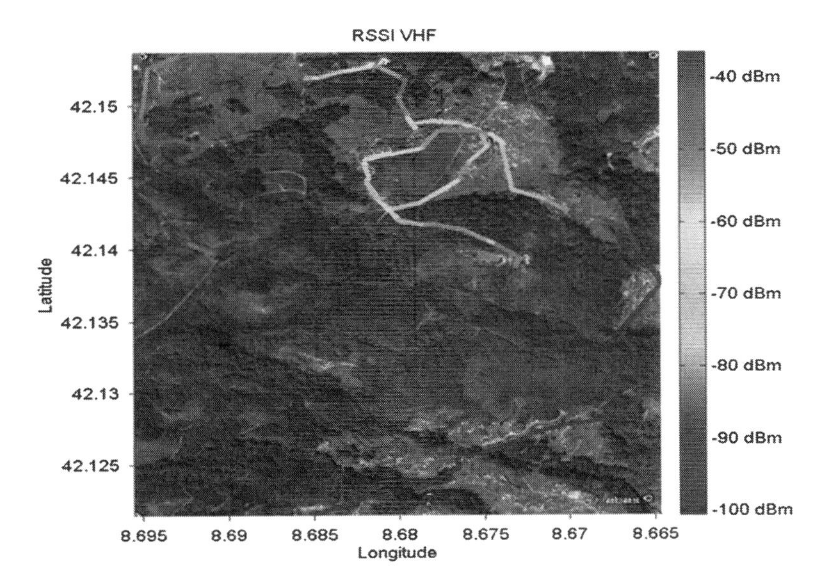

Fig. 400.5 An example of coverage measurement

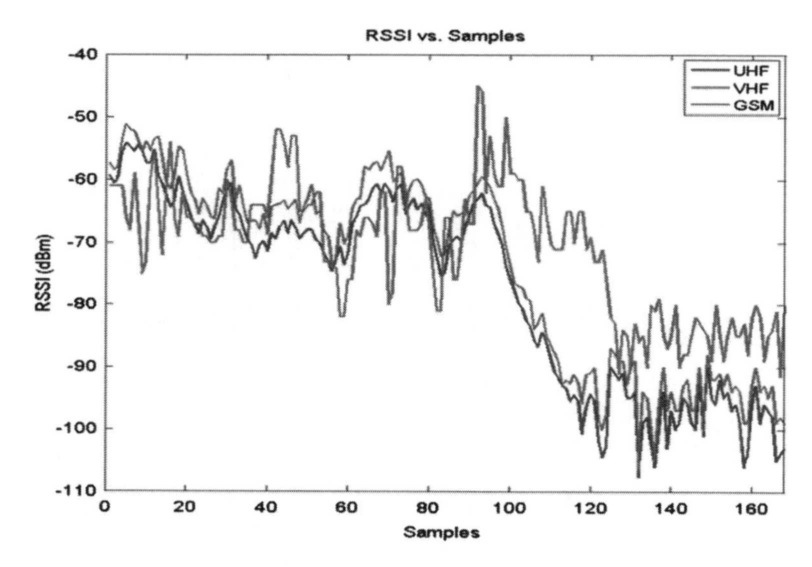

Fig. 400.6 An example of coverage measurement

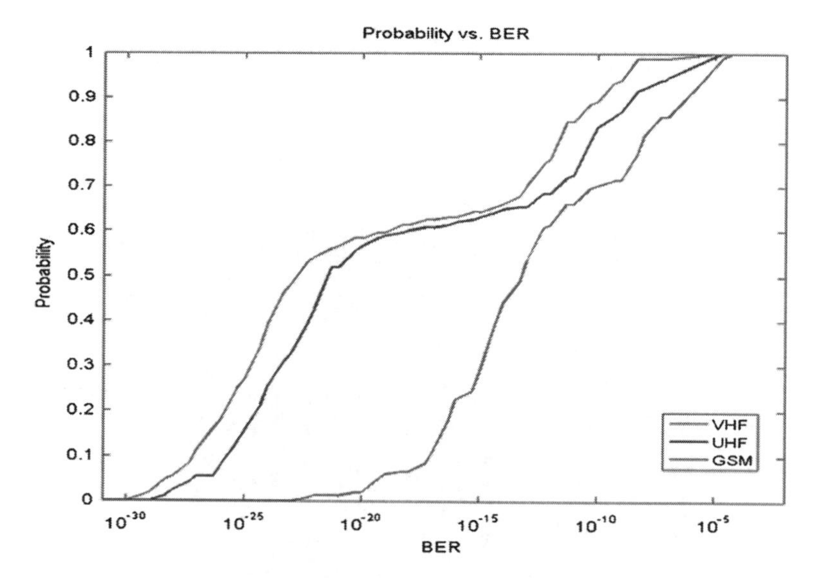

Fig. 400.7 Comparison of the BER probability

As can be seen the three systems have a high probability of having a low BER below 10^{-5}, so all three will be adequate for health remote monitoring. However, the DRM-VHF shows the better performance. As the information packet from the heart rate sensor is made of 480 bit and is transmitted at a rate of 1 packet/s, this means that we could have an erroneous packet every 30 s for GSM, every 102 s for DMR-UHF and every 266 s for DMR-VHF.

400.4 Conclusions

For health remote monitoring in rural areas where no commercial mobile phone networks are available Digital Mobile Radio may be an alternative radio network that would guarantee at least as good performance as mobile phone networks.

A DMR network, however, would require the deployment of a specific base station but this may be compensated by the large DMR base station coverage areas. Depending on the base station power and the environment, the DMR coverage area could be extended tens of kilometers away from the base station.

Acknowledgments Research supported by the European Regional Development Fund (ERDF) and the Galician Regional Government under project CN 2012/260 "Consolidation of Research Units: AtlantTIC" and project 10SEC322021PR.

References

1. Weeg S (2004) Home health and home monitoring in rural and frontier counties: human factors in implementation. In: engineering in medicine and biology society. IEMBS '04. 26th annual international conference of the IEEE, vol. 2, pp. 3264–3265, 1–5 Sept 2004 Doi: 10.1109/IEMBS.2004.1403918
2. Mitra M, Mitra S, Bera JN, Gupta R, Chaudhuri BB (2007) Preliminary level cardiac abnormality detection using wireless telecardiology system. In: Digital society. ICDS '07. First international conference on the vol, pp. 14, 2–6 Jan 2007, doi: 10.1109/ICDS.2007.34
3. Fong B, Pecht MG (2010) Prognostics in wireless telecare networks: a perspective on serving the rural Chinese population. In: Prognostics and health management conference. PHM '10, pp 1–6, 12–14 Jan 2010 doi: 10.1109/PHM.2010.5413506
4. Kappiarukudil KJ, Ramesh MV (2010) Real-time monitoring and detection of "Heart Attack" using wireless sensor networks. In: Sensor technologies and applications (SENSORCOMM), 2010 fourth international conference on, pp 632–636, 18–25 July 2010, doi: 10.1109/SENSORCOMM.2010.99
5. Ramesh MV, Anand S, Rekha P (2012) Mobile software platform for rural health enhancement. In: Proceedings of the 2012 international conference on advances in mobile network, communication and its applications (MNCAPPS), pp 131–134, 1–2 Aug 2012, doi: 10.1109/MNCApps.2012.34
6. Rajasekaran MP, Radhakrishnan S, Subbaraj P (2009) Elderly patient monitoring system using a wireless sensor network. In: Telemed JE Health 15(1):73–79, doi: 10.1089/tmj.2008.0056

Chapter 401
3D Ear Shape Feature Optimal Matching Using Bipartite Graph

Xiaopeng Sun, Wang Xingyue, Guan Wang, Feng Han and Lu Wang

Abstract In this paper, we present an optimized matching algorithm based on bipartite graph for 3D ear shape key points. Comparing with the graph matching algorithm of key points, our algorithm avoid the 2D Delaunay triangulation on 3D key points, then has less accuracy error; and our complexity is lower because our matching algorithm is basing on the bipartite graph. And then we optimal the bipartite graph matching work by weighting the edge between the key points. Experiments show that, our optimal matching on bipartite graph of ear key points can get a higher matching accuracy and a better matching efficiency.

Keywords Ear matching · Keypoints · Shape feature · Bipartite optimal matching

401.1 Introduction

The research on the automatic recognition using human ear shape is an emerging hot topic in the field of biologic characteristic identification. With the mature of 3D laser scanning technology, it has become possible to obtain the 3D point cloud data of ear real-time and the analysis and identification of the ear point cloud shape features has become the latest issue. There are several bottlenecks in 3D ear recognition: the convenience and stability of data acquisition devices, the robustness and the accuracy of 3D feature extraction algorithm, the complexity of shape feature matching algorithm and the accuracy of matching [1, 2].

The problem of Graph Matching is to find the correspondence between the given vertex or edge, and compare the similarities, its fundamental purpose is to determine the maximum or optimal corresponding relationship between the two

---

X. Sun (✉) · W. Xingyue · G. Wang · F. Han · L. Wang
Liaoning Normal University, No.850 Huanghe Road, Dalian, China
e-mail: cadcg2008@gmail.com

S. Li et al. (eds.), *Frontier and Future Development of Information Technology in Medicine and Education*, Lecture Notes in Electrical Engineering 269,
DOI: 10.1007/978-94-007-7618-0_401,

graphs' vertices [3, 4]. Isomorphism is the most stringent graph matching problem, i.e., if there was a one-to-one mapping between two vertices of tow graphs, the necessary and sufficient conditions of two vertices connected in one graph is that, their mapping vertex is connected in another graph. The subgraph isomorphism requires the vertices of the two graphs exists a single-shot relationship only, but it is still an NP-complete problem [5, 6]. The approximation algorithms, such as propagation algorithm, spectral algorithm and optimization algorithm, allow edges missing, so they match graphs with the lowest constraint strength, and look for the max-common subgraph based on edges approximately, rather than the public-induced subgraph basing nodes. The common algorithms of bipartite graph matching include multiple matching, maximum matching (the Hungarian algorithm of BFS and DFS, Hopcroft-Karp algorithm, and Ford-Fulkerson network flowing algorithm), and the Kuhn-Munkras optimal matching algorithm [7, 8].

In this paper, we propose a novel feature weighted optimization bipartite matching for the key points of 3D ear: First, we improved the work in [9], our algorithm match the key points by bipartite graph, that avoiding the projecting 3D key points into 2D, meshing the 3D dataset into a graph by the Delaunay triangulation, and reverse projecting the 2D graph back into 3D, thereby avoiding the extra accuracy error. Second, comparing with the graph-based feature matching, the complexity of our algorithm is lower because it is basing on the bipartite graph match. Third, our algorithm did an optimal matching by weighting the edge of the bipartite.

401.2 Local Shape Feature of Ear

We set an arbitrary 3D ear model as $V = \{v_i | v_i = (x_i, y_i, z_i), i = 1, 2, \ldots, n\}$, and select a point $v_i = (x_i, y_i, z_i)$ randomly, make a sphere centered on v_i with a radius of R, then we note R_i as the set of all the points in the sphere, and note the mean and covariance matrix of R_i as m and C respectively [9]. We apply *PCA* to C and get the eigenvector matrices L and eigenvalue matrix D, and note Lx and Ly as the eigenvectors corresponding the bigger two eigenvalues, then we project all points in R_i onto Lx and Ly. We note the difference between the maximum and the minimum of projection values in Lx direction as dx and denote the difference between the maximum and the minimum of projection values in Ly direction as dy. Then let $d = |dx\text{-}dy|$, if d is bigger than a given threshold a, then we accept v_i, and note it as a key point kv_i. We repeating this process till get enough number of key points. Our experiments show that the number of 200 can get a good result. Finally we note the key points set of the ear as $KV = \{kv_i | kv_i = (kx_i, ky_i, kz_i), i = 1, 2, \ldots, 200\}$.

For a key point kv_i in set KV, let $N(kv_i, 2\sigma)$ be its neighborhood with a radius of 2σ, and it is a set of all those points with a distance to kv_i less than 2σ. Basing on the work in [10], we give a single value surface fitting on all the points within the neighborhood $N(kv_i, 2\sigma)$. The fitting patch on the product parameter domain uv is single-valued projection in a rectangular area. Firstly, we make uniform nu and nv sampling along the u and v parameter plane respectively, to obtain a uniform $nu \times nv$ parameter distributing sampling points. Calculate the depth coordinate value Zuv of the $nu \times nv$ sampling point, then we note the set $\{Z_{uv}\}$ consisting of $nu \times nv$ sampling depth as partial shape feature on kv_i, and denot it by $LSF_i = \{Z_{uv}, u = 1, 2,\ldots, nu, v = 1, 2,\ldots, nv\}$, so we can get the local shape feature set $\{LSF_i, i = 1, 2,\ldots, 200\}$ on the key points set KV.

401.3 Bipartite Optimal Matching of Global Feature

Let the local shape feature vector of two ear V_1 and V_2 as $LSF_1 = \{LSF_{1i}, i = 1, 2, \ldots, 200\}$ and $LSF_2 = \{LSF_{2j}, j = 1, 2, \ldots, 200\}$, where LSF_{1i} and LSF_{2j} are the 5-dimension feature vectors of the i-th and j-th key points of the ear V_1 and V_2 respectively, which denoted as $kv_{1i} = (kx_{1i}, ky_{1i}, kz_{1i}), kv_{2j} = (kx_{2i}, ky_{2i}, kz_{2i})$. The similarity metric between $kv_{1i}$and kv_{2j} is defined as $d_{ij} = w_{Pos} \times S_{Pos} + w_{LSF} \times S_{LSF}$, where w_{Pos} and w_{LSF} are the weight coefficient of location and local shape features, $S_{Pos} = \left|\left|kv_{1i} - kv_{2j}\right|\right|^2$ is the space distance difference between key points $kv_{1i}$and key points kv_{2j}, and $S_{LSF} = \arccos\left(LSF_{1i}(LSF_{2j})^T\right)$ indicates the local shape feature vector difference between kv_{1i} and kv_{2j}.

Let $M \subseteq E$, then we call M is a bipartite match of G, and for each edge e_{ij}, its two endpoints V_i^p and V_j^g are matched by M. Obviously, a bipartite match of G is composed of a subset of E. Denote $|M|$ as the size of M, that is the number of edge in M. Construct a new edge between the key points V_i^p and V_j^g, and make sure V_i^p and V_j^g have not been used by other matching edges before, iterate this procedure till unable to construct a new edge. Each edge e_{ij} in M is given a non-negative weights $w(e_{ij})$ and the match corresponding to the maximum of total weight value is known as the Optimal Matching. The ear key point matching problem is to seek the Optimal Matching between $V_i^p$and V_j^g.

For a weighted graph $G = \{V^p \cup V^g, E\}$, denote the weight of edge $e_{ij} = \left(V_i^p, V_j^g\right)$ as $w(e_{ij})$. We define a real function $L(V_i^p)$ and $L\left(V_j^g\right)$ on each vertex in V^p and V^g respectively. Then $L(V_i^p)$ is initialized as the maximum weight of all vertex V_i^p associated side, and $L\left(V_j^g\right)$ is initialized as zero. If for any $V_i^p \in V, V_j^g \in V^g$ in G, the non-equality of $L(V_i^p) + L\left(V_j^g\right) \geq w(e_{ij})$ always is right, we call the real function $L(V)$ is Feasible Vertex Labeling of G. Let $M = \{e_{ij} | e_{ij} \in E(G), L(V_i^p) + L\left(V_j^g\right) = w(e_{ij})\}$, a G's spanning subgraph, which M is its edge set, we called it equality subgraph, note as *GM*, and then, a perfect match of *GM* is an optimal matching of *G*. Here we describe our bipartite optimal matching algorithm as follows:

Step 1 Initialize the value of Feasible Vertex Labeling

Step 2 Search the perfect match in the subgraph using Hungary algorithm

Step 3 If don't find the perfect match, then update the Feasible Vertex Labeling as follows: $L(V_i^p) = L(V_i^p) - \Delta L$, $L\left(V_j^g\right) = L\left(V_j^g\right) + \Delta L$, where $\Delta L = \min\left\{L(V_i^p) + L\left(V_j^g\right) - w\left(e_{ij}\right)\right\}$

Step 4 Repeat step 2 and step 3 till we find a perfect match of the equality subgraph. Then we can get an optimal matching.

Assuming the node number of *G* is *n*, and its edge number is *m*, then the complexity of searching the augmenting-path from each vertex is $O(m)$. We can find an augmenting path within *n* times, and need to find up to *n* augmenting path, so the complexity of modifying Feasible Vertex Labeling is $O(n^2)$, and the overall complexity can be $O(n^3)$ by adding the slack variable.

401.4 Experimental Results and Analysis

The similarity metric between kv_{1i} and kv_{2j} has been defined as d_{ij} in [0, 1], the larger the d_{ij} is, the similar the key points kv_{1i} and kv_{2j}. When $d_{ij} = 1$, the two local shape on kv_{1i} and kv_{2j} are exactly same. When d_{ij} is less than a specified threshold δ, kv_{1i} and kv_{2j} fail to match, and there is no edge between kv_{1i} and kv_{2j} in the bipartite graph. In this paper $\delta = 0.8$. We compare our algorithm with other matching algorithms, such as Hungarian with BFS (H-BFS), Hungarian with DFS (H-DFS), Hopcroft-Karp (HK), and the graph matching (GM) algorithm in [9].

Figure 401.1 gives the matching results of two different ears, and the same ear with different scanning angles, with algorithms H-DFS, H-BFS, HK and our algorithm. Because of the high of random with the 3D scanning data, the key points of the different ears cannot achieve perfect matching, even the different scanning data of the same ear. The less the green lines, the greater the difference between the local shape features on two ears' key points there are, and the less successful the matching is. The more declining the green lines, the worse the matching is and the lower similarity.

In Fig. 401.2, 001, 002 and 003 are the 3D point cloud data that taken from different angles of the same ear. Same is 010, 1567 and 1563, but from another ear. We match them with H-BFS, H-DFS, HK, GM and our optimal matching algorithm. And the numbers on the bar are the correct match. We can see that, the correct matching number get by our algorithm is higher than anyone of other four matching algorithms. Figure 401.3 shows the running time comparison of the H-DFS, H-BFS, HK, GM and our optimal matching algorithm; we can see that the

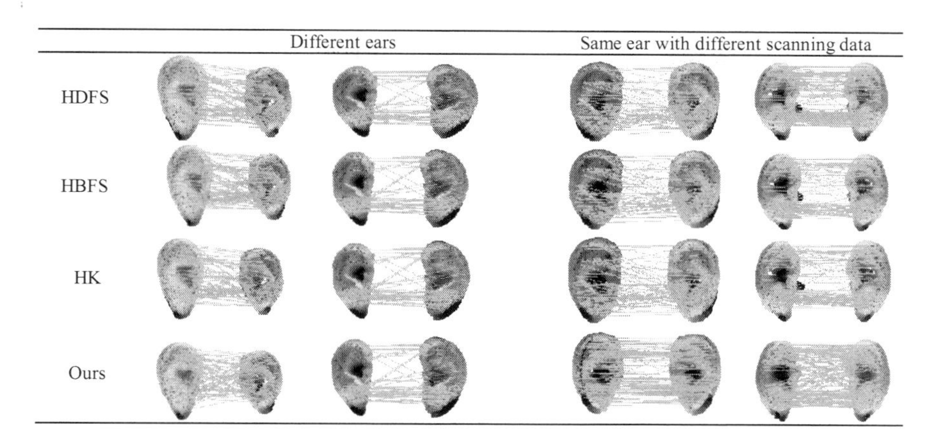

Fig. 401.1 Some of match results with four algorithms

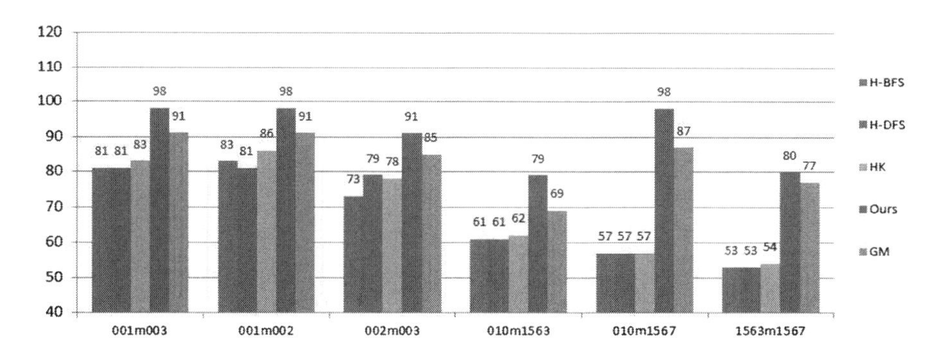

Fig. 401.2 Comparison of match accuracy

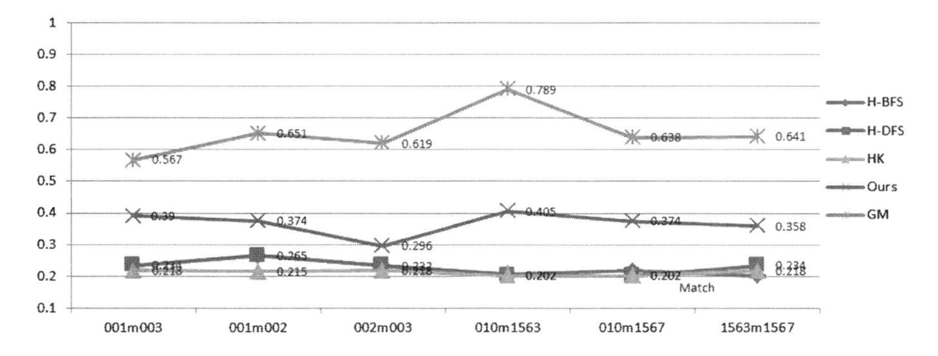

Fig. 401.3 Comparison of match time

time complexity of our algorithm is not the biggest while its accuracy is the highest, so our optimal matching algorithm is superior to other matching algorithm.

401.5 Conclusion and Future Works

We present a novel optimal matching method for local shape features on random selected key from 3D ear scanning point cloud. Experiments show that our algorithm is faster and has a higher accuracy.

In the future, we intend to explore some novel algorithm on real-time and highly efficient dynamic matching to further improve the 3D ear shape matching.

Acknowledgments This work is supported in part by National Natural Science Foundation of China with projects No. 61170143 and No. 60873110.

References

1. Burge M., Burger W (2000) Ear biometrics in computer vision. In: Proceedings 15th international conference on pattern recognition, vol 2, pp 822–826. doi: 10.1109/ICPR.2000.906202
2. Torresani L, Kolmogorov V, Rother C (2008) Feature correspondence via graph matching: models and global optimization. In Proceedings 10th European conference computer vision, pp 596–609. doi: 10.1007/978-3-540-88688-4_44
3. Bhowmick P, Pradhan R, Bhattacharya B (2009) Approximate matching of digital point sets using a novel angular tree. IEEE Trans Pattern Anal Mach Intell 31(5):769–782. doi: 10.1109/TPAMI.2007. 70812
4. Leordeanu M, Hebert M (2009) Unsupervised learning for graph matching. In: IEEE conference on computer vision and pattern recognition, pp 864–871. doi: 10.1109/CVPRW.2009.5206533
5. Caetano T, Caelli T, Schuurmans D, Barone D (2006) Graphical models and point pattern matching. IEEE Trans Pattern Anal Mach Intell 28(10):1646–1663. doi: 10.1109/TPAMI.2006.207
6. Mcauley J, Caetano T, Barbosa M (2008) Graph rigidity, cyclic belief propagation and point pattern matching. IEEE Trans Pattern Anal Mach Intell 30(11):2047–2054. doi: 10.1109/TPAMI.2008.124
7. Mikolajczyk K, Schmid C (2004) Scale and affine invariant interest point detectors. J Int J Comput Vis 60, 1:63–86. doi: 10.1023/B:VISI.0000027790.02288.f2
8. Weiss Y, Freeman W (2001) On the optimality of solutions of the max-product belief-propagation algorithm in arbitrary graphs. IEEE Trans Inf Theory 47(2):736–744. doi: 10.1109/18.910585
9. Mian AS, Bennamoun M, Owens R (2008) Keypoint detection and local feature matching for textured 3D face recognition. Int J Comput Vis 79(1):1–12. doi: 10.1007/s11263-007-0085-5
10. SasiKanth (2010) Bi-dimensional empirical mode decomposition. MATLAB central file exchange select

Chapter 402
Research on Anti-Metastasis Effect of Emodin on Pancreatic Cancer

Haishuai Yu

Abstract To investigate the anti-metastasis effect of emodin on the pancreatic cancer in vitro and in vivo. Human pancreatic cancer cell line SW1980 was treated with different concentrations of emodin (10, 30, 40 μmol·L^{-1}) for 2 h, the effects of emodin on migration and invasion of SW1980 cells were examined by using wound assay. Western blot was used to detect the protein expression of NF-κ and MMP-9 in SW1980 cells after various concentrations of emodin (10, 30, 40 μmol.L^{-1}) treatment for 48 h. Eight weeks after implantation, the presences of metastasis were evaluated respectively after the mice were sacrificed. Immuno-histochemistry was used to detect the positive expression of CD41, NF$_{-\kappa}$B and MMP-9 in the tumors. Emodin suppressed the migration and invasion of SW1980 cells in a dose-dependent manner. Western bolt assay indicated that emodin downregulated the expression of NF-κ and MMP-9 proteins. The incidences of metastasis were de-creased significantly in L-EMO group and H-EMO group as compared with that in control group. The percentage of CD41, NF$_{_\kappa}$and MMP-9-positive cells in the tumors were significantly reduced by the administration of emodin.

Keywords Pancreatic tumors · Emodin · Transfer

402.1 Introduction

Emodin as a method of psychological intervention clinical application in various fields will help ease the patient tense psychological pressure, lower blood pressure. Studies have shown that emodin on patients rebuild the emotional activities,

---

H. Yu (✉)
Jilin Vocational College of Industry and Technology, Jilin 132013, China
e-mail: yuhaishuai@126.com

S. Li et al. (eds.), *Frontier and Future Development of Information Technology in Medicine and Education*, Lecture Notes in Electrical Engineering 269,
DOI: 10.1007/978-94-007-7618-0_402,

motivate thinking, increased interest in the surrounding, to motivate behaviours, improve retreat tend to have a positive effect. Especially in the field of cancer treatment, because cancer patient anxiety, depressive disorder incidence of up to 48 %, 45 %. Cancer is a treatment and recovery a long illness, it will make the patient is subjected to the pain of the different stages of treatment and quality of life have also been varying degrees of impact. In recent years, the quality of life of cancer patients there is a growing trend, on this basis; we explore the application of emodin on the quality of life of cancer patients.

402.2 Materials and Methods

Clinical data 2004 January 2007-April sick patients, diagnosed with cancer, and more than a primary school education, no previous history of mental illness and disturbance of consciousness, Karnofsky Functioning Scale (Karnof-sky performance status, KPS) score\ 60. Into the group of patients with a total of 38 cases, of which 15 cases of nasopharyngeal carcinoma, lung cancer in 11 cases, six cases of breast cancer after six cases of liver cancer; youngest 19 years old, maximum 76 years, an average of 45.56 years.

402.2.1 Rating Scale

Cancer patients quality of life scale (Quality of Life Questionnaire-Core 30 QLQ-C30), a total of 30 projects, functional subscale physical functioning (PF), role function (RF), cognitive function (CF), emotional function (EF), social function (SF), 3 symptom subscales (fatigue, pain, nausea, vomiting), an overall health subscale (GH) and a single measurement projects (difficulty breathing constitute, insomnia, lack of appetite, constipation, diarrheal, financial difficulties). The Functioning Scale the PF, RF and GH higher the score, the better quality of life; CF, EF, SF and symptom scale and individual measurements project the higher the score, the worse the quality of life. The questionnaire was comparable with that in different countries and regions, its reliability and validity and sensitivity has been validated in a number of countries, successfully used in the clinical studies of cancer patients. Questionnaire by the researchers under the unified guidance language.

402.2.2 Cartesian Functioning Scale

KPS into 10 grades, according to the assessment of the functional status of patients given the range of 0 to 100 points, the higher the score, the better physical function. Up to 100 points, followed by 90 points, 80 points, 70 points, which means that researchers different assessment of the patient's physical condition from high to low. 100 indicating normal, with 10 indicating critically ill dying, with 0 representing death. Space environment to a certain extent affect the patient's therapeutic effect, and should therefore be avoided noisy interference environment. We choose a single area of 26 m^2, and from the wards, offices at some distance from a dedicated treatment room; built-in with living flowers and murals with health education, information, and as warm as possible, so that the patient is relaxed, natural and comfortable environment .

402.2.3 Music Selection

The principles of the "symptomatic soundtrack", based on the patient's level of cultural enrichment, music appreciation and hobby selections. Nervousness, irritability patients election relaxation, quiet music, such as the "Palace Moon" "cold duck swimming" "mysterious circle"; dizziness, weakness, fatigue, physical decline the patients selected cheerful kind of music, such as" Clouds Chasing the Moon "Red Beans Love" "Minuet"; upset, palpitations, chest tightness patients choose the soft, beautiful, lyrical music, such as "Spring Song" "Gorillas in the Mist"; the depression patients election cheerful kind of music, such as "step by step" "radiant," "Swan Lake Waltz". Based on content classification in compiling the music CD, each music CD playback time of 30 min.

402.2.4 Interfere with the Preparation and Methods

Before the intervention, the patient emptying urine, lying in bed, eyes closed, in a natural state of relaxation. Music player, stereo space surround playback, and in order to avoid the interference of others, each time only one person, per day, each time 30 min, 5 times a week for 4 weeks for an intervention treatment. All patients studied before and after the intervention test of the quality of life; 1st measurement time after the patient is admitted to the acoustic space around the player, in order

Table 402.1 The intervention QLQ-C30 in function subscale scores

Time	Number of cases	Physical function	Role and function	Cognitive function	Emotional function	Social function
Before intervention	38	7.84 ± 1.44	3.65 ± 0.73	3.52 ± 1.63	7.76 ± 2.47	5.24 ± 2.15
After intervention	38	7.77 ± 1.45	3.64 ± 0.62	3.54 ± 1.29	7.80 ± 2.22	5.25 ± 1.86
t		0.175	0.465	−0.865	−1.499	−0.634
p		0.862	0.645	0.394	0.144	0.531

Table 402.2 QLQ-C30 score of six individual measurement items

Time	Number of cases	Difficulty breathing	Insomnia	Lack of appetite	Constipation	Diarrhea	Economic difficuities
Before intervention	38	1.65 ± 0.86	2.11 ± 0.98	1.67 ± 1.02	1.87 ± 1.03	1.11 ± 0.30	3.02 ± 1.15
After intervention	38	1.63 ± 0.79	1.51 ± 0.62	1.70 ± 1.06	2.21 ± 0.76	1.21 ± 0.42	3.05 ± 1.12
t		1.099	2.516	−0.229	−1.871	−1.68	−1.648
p		0.28	0.017	0.82	0.071	0.103	0.11

Table 402.3 QLQ-C30 symptom subscale and overall health subscale score

Time	Cases	Fatigue	Pain	Nausea and Vomiting	Overall health
Before intervention	38	5.05 ± 2.69	3.25 ± 1.93	2.89 ± 1.305	9.21 ± 2.21
After intervention	38	5.06 ± 2.59	3.13 ± 1.86	2.88 ± 0.987	9.23 ± 1.95
t		−0.205	1.928	1.222	−0.316
p		0.839	0.190	0.231	0.754

to avoid the interference of others, each time only one person, once a day, each time for 30 min per week 5 for 4 weeks for an intervention treatment. All the patients studied in the test of the quality of life before and after the intervention; first measurement time of patients admitted to hospital after receiving radiation therapy and chemotherapy before intervention. Second measurement time second after the end of the intervention applied again QLQ-C30 quality of life assessment situation.

402.3 Statistical Results

SPSS 10.0 statistical package for statistical analysis using the t test was used to compare the before and after intervention quality of life (Tables 402.1, 402.2 and 402.3).

Shown in the table, after the intervention the insomnia score is lower than before the intervention ($P < 0.05$), other quality of life and overall health evaluation before the intervention were not statistically significant ($P > 0.05$).

402.4 Conclusion

According to foreign Derogates (1983) reported that 47 % of cancer patients have significant psychological stress response or psychological disorders. As Hang said, fear of cancer is global, because cancer means extreme suffering and death. Due to the incidence of cancer usually does not cause people's attention, so many patients are diagnosed in the late often accompanied by other symptoms, such as pain, insomnia, indigestion, and most patients; and the long duration of treatment, the patient need to face treatment the emergence of side effects, such as chemotherapy, nausea, vomiting, constipation, fatigue, mouth ulcers, these factors could materially and adversely affect the patient's overall quality of life. This study is based cancer patients psychological and disease characteristics, the implementation of the principle of mainly symptomatic soundtrack. When people get sick, the rhythm of the body is in an abnormal state, choose the appropriate music, harmony through music audio, allows the body to a variety of vibration frequency coordination of activities, to the benefit of the patient back to health. The results of this study show that emodin has a good effect to improve the quality of sleep in patients with cancer, statistically significant ($P < 0.05$) before and after the intervention. Due to the application of nature music easily beat the promotion of sound waves of sleep, the sleep center of the brain gradually relaxed, and goes to sleep. Johnson and abroad personalized music for insomnia in elderly women (age > 70 years) is similar to the findings, both of which can improve the patient's quality of sleep. On the positive side, the music as a wonderful sound waves, the role of the human brain, people feel the life force from the natural world, in order to stimulate the love of life; the other hand, it can enrich people's imagination, people with good ideas and vision for the future. For cancer patients, to arouse their courageous battle with cancer, recognizing the value of self-existence, face reality, cherish every second of life, actively cooperate with treatment, improve treatment compliance, you can improve the patient's quality of life.

References

1. Min L, Xu H, Xia Y (1999) Cancer patients with anxiety and depression survey. Chin Ment Health J 13(3):187
2. Zhang H, Chen R (2000) Fang tumor, nursing. Tianjin Science and Technology Press, Tianjin, p 261
3. Wang J, Cuijun N, Chen Z et al (2000) Cancer patients quality of life and related factors. Chin J Clin Psychol 8(1):23–26
4. Huang Y, Wang K (2004) Ovarian cancer quality of life survey and analysis. J Nurs 19(10):938
5. Olschewski M, Schulgen G, Schumacher M et al (1994) Quality of life assessment in clinical cancer research. Br J Cancer 70(1):1–5
6. Hang X, Butow PN, Mciscr B et al (1999) Attitudes and information needs of Chinese migrant cancer patients and their relatives. Aust NZ J Med 29:207–213

Chapter 403
Research on Chronic Alcoholic Patients with Nerve Electrophysiology

He Wei

Abstract The clinical characteristics of the study in patients with chronic alcoholism, peripheral neuropathy and nerve electrophysiological testing analysis. The method detected 80 cases of patients with chronic alcoholism median nerve, nerve, perennial motor nerve conduction velocity (MCV) and F-wave, tibiae nerve, median nerve, ulnas nerve sensory nerve conduction velocity (SCV) and F-wave and 78 cases of healthy people without drinking hobby as control. 80 patients with chronic alcoholism MCV decreased abnormal rate of 65.6 %, SCV decline, abnormal rate of 81.8 %. Significant difference compared with the control group ($P < 0.01$), the SCV involvement more MCV. Detection of neurons physiological abnormalities is earlier than clinical symptoms. The electrical nerve is detecting early diagnosis of chronic alcoholism and guide treatment.

Keywords Chronic alcoholism · Electrophysiology · Peripheral neuropathy

403.1 Introduction

As people socialize frequently and social pressures increase, the population of alcohol dependence has continued to increase. The incidence of chronic alcoholism is gradually increasing trend. Chronic alcoholism insidious on set manifestation. Involving the central and peripheral nervous system, the highest incidence of peripheral neuropathy, and more for the initial performance. Nerve electrophysiological testing can accurately reflect the early lesions of peripheral nerves, and provide a basis for the timely diagnosis and treatment. August 2001–June

H. Wei (✉)
Affiliated Hospital, Beihua University, Jilin 132013, China
e-mail: hewei@126.com

S. Li et al. (eds.), *Frontier and Future Development of Information Technology in Medicine and Education*, Lecture Notes in Electrical Engineering 269,
DOI: 10.1007/978-94-007-7618-0_403,

2005, 80 cases of patients with chronic alcoholism, the clinical features of peripheral neuropathy and nerve electrophysiological testing analysis. The results reported below.

403.2 Materials and Methods

Mental disease classification schemes and diagnostic criteria based on the Chinese Medical Association Psychiatric Association developed in 1995 to confirm the diagnosis of chronic alcoholism 80 patients were set in the observation group. 78 males, two females, age 32–65 years, mean 46.5 years. History of drinking 5–35 years, an average of 20 years, each meal daily drinking, drinking in high spirits. The amount of daily drink liquor (200–800) ml, average daily drinking is about as 250 ml, more than a brief history of alcoholics. Clinical manifestations of upper limb parentheses 46 cases, 58 cases of lower limb parentheses, numbness, lower limbs step on the cotton-like feeling, shoes do not know who, vibratory sensation subsided. 12 cases of muscle weakness and diminished tendon reflexes, muscle atrophy eight cases. Sleep disorders, near thing memory loss, and decreased attention in 30 cases. Limb tremor in 36 cases. Ataxia in three cases. Admission delirium or drowsiness consciousness disorder patients. Jaundice in 12 cases. The chest of spider veins and facial telangiectasia 16 cases. Control group, 78 cases no drinking hobby healthy persons, 75 cases were male and three females, aged 29–64 years, mean 40.6 years, no nervous system diseases and signs.

403.2.1 Rating Scale

Cancer patients quality of life scale (Quality of Life Questionnaire-Core 30 QLQ-C30), a total of 30 projects, functional subscale physical functioning (PF), role function (RF), cognitive function (CF), emotional function (EF), social function (SF), three symptom subscales (fatigue, pain, nausea, vomiting), an overall health subscale (GH) and a single measurement projects (difficulty breathing constitute, insomnia, lack of appetite, constipation, diarrheal, financial difficulties). The functioning scale the PF, RF and GH higher the score, the better quality of life; CF, EF, SF and symptom scale and individual measurements project the higher the score, the worse the quality of life. The questionnaire was comparable with that in different countries and regions, its reliability and validity and sensitivity has been validated in a number of countries, successfully used in the clinical studies of cancer patients. Questionnaire by the researchers under the unified guidance language(Fig. 403.1).

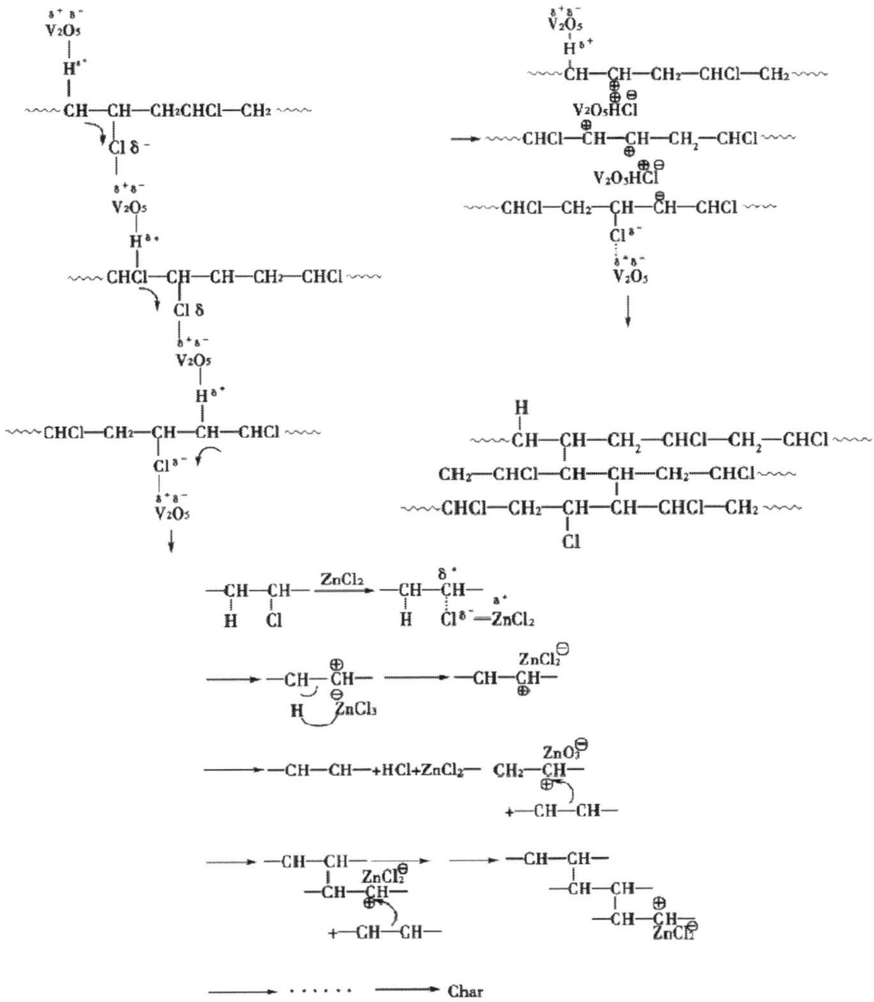

Fig. 403.1 Wine suppression mechanism model

403.2.2 Cartesian Functioning Scale

KPS into 10 grades, according to the assessment of the functional status of patients given the range of 0–100 points, the higher the score, the better physical function. Up to 100 points, followed by 90 points, 80 points, 70 points, which means that researchers different assessment of the patient's physical condition from high to low. 100 indicating normal, with 10 indicating critically ill dying, with 0 representing death. Space environment to a certain extent affect the patient's therapeutic

Table 403.1 observation group and control group MCV, SCV determination ($x \pm s$) (m/s)

		MCV			SCV		
Groups	Cases	Median nerve	Ulner nerve	Peroneal nerve	Tibial nerve	Median nerve	Ulnar nerve
Observation group	80	43.69 ± 6.68	46.36 ± 5.64	38.65 ± 6.82	34.56 ± 6.72	42.56 ± 7.82	38.55 ± 8.92
Control group	78	58.89 ± 6.10	56.62 ± 4.69	53.35 ± 5.98	46.56 ± 5.68	72.56 ± 6.58	56.52 ± 7.63
T		14.92	12.42	14.39	12.11	26.06	13.59
P		<0.01	<0.01	<0.01	<0.01	<0.01	<0.01

Table 403.2 case group compared with the control group F wave (x ± s) in m/s

Seized nerve	Observation items	Observation group	Observation group	*T*	*P*
Observation items	F Wave Velocity (m/s)	62.21 ± 3.25	64.65 ± 3.01	17.99	<0.001
Median nerve	F Wave Velocity (m/s)	53.28 ± 2.98	56.06 ± 2.9	18.26	<0.001
Tibial nerve	F Wave latency (ms)	25.78 ± 1.16	23.62 ± 1.80	79.07	<0.001
Wave velocity	F Wave latency (ms)	40.88 ± 1.24	38.86 ± 1.98	50.65	<0.001

effect, and should therefore be avoided noisy interference environment. We choose a single area of 26 m^2, and from the wards, offices at some distance from a dedicated treatment room; built-in with living flowers and murals with health education, information, and as warm as possible, so that the patient is relaxed, natural and comfortable environment.

403.3 Statistical Results

SPSS 10.0 statistical package for statistical analysis using the t test was used to compare the before and after intervention quality of life (Tables 403.1, 403.2).

403.4 Conclusion

According to foreign Derogates (1983) reported that 47 % of cancer patients have significant psychological stress response or psychological disorders. As Hang said, fear of cancer is global, because cancer means extreme suffering and death. Due to the incidence of cancer usually does not cause people's attention, so many patients are diagnosed in the late often accompanied by other symptoms, such as pain, insomnia, indigestion, and most patients; and the long duration of treatment, the patient need to face treatment the emergence of side effects, such as chemotherapy, nausea, vomiting, constipation, fatigue, mouth ulcers, these factors could materially and adversely affect the patient's overall quality of life. This study is based cancer patients psychological and disease characteristics, the implementation of the principle of mainly symptomatic soundtrack. When people get sick, the rhythm of the body is in an abnormal state, choose the appropriate music, harmony through music audio, allows the body to a variety of vibration frequency coordination of activities, to the benefit of the patient back to health. The results of this study show that music therapy has a good effect to improve the quality of sleep in patients with cancer, statistically significant ($P < 0.05$) before and after the intervention. Due to the application of nature music easily beat the promotion of sound waves of sleep, the sleep center of the brain gradually relaxed, and goes to sleep. Johnson and abroad personalized music for insomnia in elderly women (age >70 years) is similar to the findings, both of which can improve the patient's quality of sleep. On the positive side, the music as a wonderful sound waves, the role of the human brain, people feel the life force from the natural world, in order to stimulate the love of life; the other hand, it can enrich people's imagination, people with good ideas and vision for the future. For cancer patients, to arouse their courageous battle with cancer, recognizing the value of self-existence, face reality, cherish every second of life, actively cooperate with treatment, improve treatment compliance, you can improve the patient's quality of life.

References

1. Lu M, Xu H, Xia Y (1993) Cancer patients with anxiety and depression survey. Chin Ment Health J 13(3):187
2. Zhang H, Chen R, Fang T (2000) Nursing. Tianjin Science and Technology Press, Tianjin, p 261
3. Wang J, Nan C, Chen Z et al (2008) Cancer patients quality of life and related factors. Chin J Clin Psychol 8(1):23–26
4. Huang Yao ball (2004) Wang Kai ovarian cancer quality of life survey and analysis. J Nurs 19(10):938
5. Olschewski M, Schulgen G, Schumacher M et al (1994) Quality of life assessment in clinical cancer research. Br J Cancer 70(1):1–5

Chapter 404
Genetic Dissection of *Pax6* Through GeneNetwork

Hong Lu and Lu Lu

Abstract To introduce a new method about analysis of gene expression, upstream or downstream gene regulation, genetic regulatory network from the Analysis Tools of GeneNetwork (http://www.genenetwork.org). To better illustrate this approach, *Pax6* were selected as an example. The analysis of *Pax6* includes the revealing variation in expression of *Pax6*, expression quantitative trait locus (eQTL) mapping for *Pax6*, screening and positioning upstream gene of *Pax6* and finally constructing genetic regulatory network of *Pax6*. Such dissection of *Pax6* provides new direction and clues for further in-depth study of *Pax6* function.

Keywords Genenetwork · Genetic regulatory network · *Pax6*

404.1 Introduction

The scope and depth of medical research progress rapidly with the growth of computer science and Internet. Although traditional experimental methods still play an important role, with the help of medical informatics, Internet resources and some special animal models, the development of some entirely new fields and research methods of medical science and biology emerged and matured gradually. The purpose of this paper is to introduce a research method about analysis of gene expression, genetic regulatory network, filtering pathogenic related genes by means of gene expression data and expression quantitative trait locus (eQTL) analysis [1–3] from GeneNetwork (http://www.genenetwork.org). To better

H. Lu (✉)
Nantong University, 20 Xisi Road, Nantong, Jiangsu 226001, China
e-mail: adanlu2000@yahoo.com.cn

L. Lu
Jiangsu Key Laboratory of Neuroregeneration, Nantong University, Nantong 226001, China

S. Li et al. (eds.), *Frontier and Future Development of Information Technology in Medicine and Education*, Lecture Notes in Electrical Engineering 269,
DOI: 10.1007/978-94-007-7618-0_404,

illustrate the advantages of this approach and make it easier to understand and operate, the analysis of gene *Pax6* should be an example.

Pax6 has a wide range of expression during the development of vertebrates and invertebrates and has important regulatory roles during embryonic development [4]. *Pax6* mutations have been associated with a wider spectrum of eye and brain defects including Peter's anomaly, corectopia with nystagmus, macular, foveal hypoplasia, anophthalmia, absence or hypoplasia of the anterior commissure, absence of the pineal gland, auditory processing defects and anosmia [5]. Analysis of *Pax6* differentially expression in different organs, looking for the genes which expression and function closely related with *Pax6*, and further establish the gene regulatory networks of *Pax6* can help to understand the exact role and regulatory pathway of pax6 in development and disease.

404.2 Methods and Results

404.2.1 Enter Pax6 into GeneNetwork

GeneNetwork is public web service and open source project for systems genetics with 10 active mirror and production sites. Its service is used to study genetic causes that influence gene expression and that control phenotypes and disease susceptibility. GeneNetwork combines 30 years of open data generated by hundreds of scientists with sequence data (SNPs and indels) and massive transcriptome data sets (array and RNA-seq). This paper used the source and analysis tools of GeneNetwork to get the gene expression information of *Pax6* in BXD recombinant inbred (BXD RI) mice [6, 7]. And then a series of analyzes including eQTL analysis were carried out to dissect systematic the vinculum of *Pax6* with other genes and build the genetic regulatory network.

After open the website of GeneNetwork, Set up the pull-down menu fields of Find Records: Choose Species = Mouse, Group = BXD, Type = Eye mRNA, Database = Eye M430v2 (Sep08) RMA. Enter the search term "*Pax6*" and click on the "Search" button. A Search Results window will open with a list of five probe sets, one of which, probe set 1452526_a_at (located on Chr 2 @ 105.531755 Mb, exons 5, 6, 7, and 8) was selected because of the comprehensive consideration of the location of probe set, the level of expression and the maximum locus had significant linkage scores (LRS). Click the blue text of the 1452526_a_at to generate a new window called the Trait Data and Analysis Form. The top of this window shows basic information of *Pax6* and the probe set 1452526_a_at; the middle position offers Analysis Tools; and the lower part provides a set of editable boxes that contain the gene expression averages.

404.2.2 Variation in Expression of Pax6

After open the Trait Data and Analysis Form mentioned previously, select the "Basic Statistics" button; choose Includ = BXD only. The data of variation in expression of *Pax6* and its bar graph display by the corresponding button. For the probe set 1452526_a_at, the expression level in eye varied across 68 BXD RI strains, their parental strains (C57BL/6 J and DBA/2 J), and F1 individuals (B6D2F1 and D2B6F1). Figure 404.1 showed the expression variation of 1452526_a_at across the BXD RI strains. The average expression level of 1452526_a_at in the BXD strains is 11.245, with range from a low of 10.312 in BXD29 to a high of11.802 in BXD24; the expression level in C57BL/6 J is 11.303 while in DBA/2 J is 11.143.

404.2.3 Expression QTL (eQTL) mapping for Pax6

In the Trait Data and Analysis Form, select the "Mapping Tools" button; and then select the "Interval" button; choose Chromosome = All, Mapping Scale = Megabase, Permutations = 2000; click the blue "Compute" button. This will initiate the analysis and display the whole-genome interval map for *Pax6*. The mapping was carried out by marker regression and interval mapping to define the chromosome regions associated with expression difference at a genome-wide significance level of 0.01. The probe set 1452526_a_at showed that the locus had significant linkage scores (LRS) of 15.800 ($p < 0.01$). The QTL interval for 1452526_a_at is located on chromosome 19, at 20 $\sim$ 30 Mb (Fig. 404.2). This QTL was mapped in another chromosome of the transcript (*Pax6*, located on chromosome 2). In general, this type

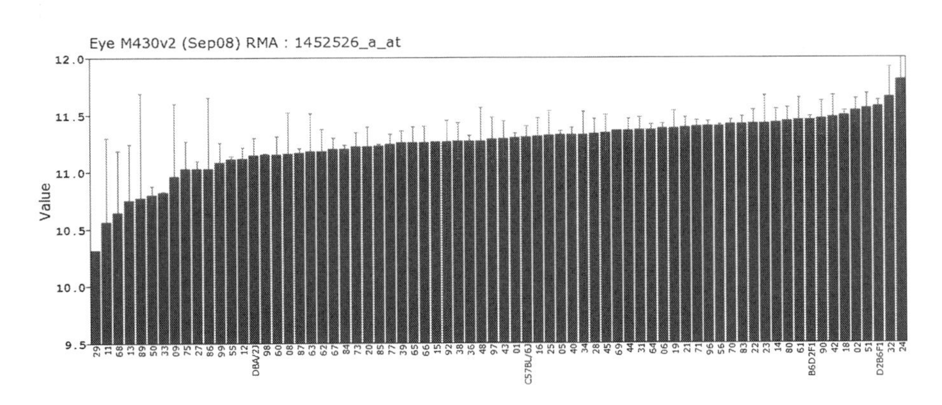

Fig. 404.1 The variation in expression level of the probe set 1452526_a_at of *Pax6* across 68 BXD RI strains and their parental strains. Value denotes normalized relative expression level. The x-axis indicates strain names or numbers, while the y-axis indicates expression on a log2 scale. Bars are standard errors of the mean

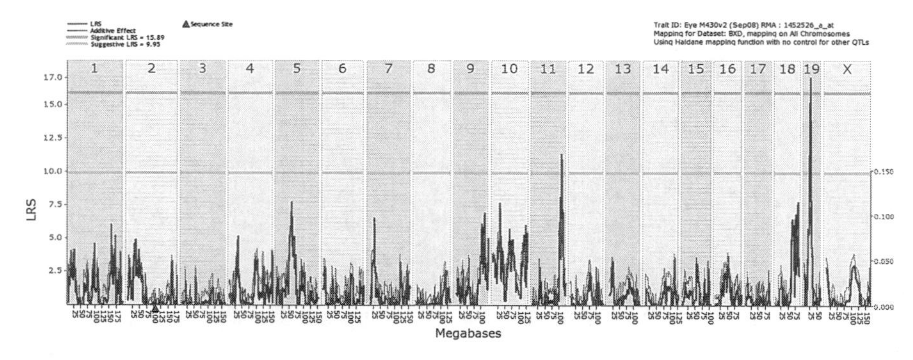

Fig. 404.2 Graphics of LRS scores for *Pax6* expression QTL in eye for BXD mice. The solid blue line indicates LRS scores across the genome. A positive additive coefficient (*green line*) indicates that DBA/2 J alleles increase trait values, whereas a negative additive coefficient (*red line*) indicates that C57BL/6 J alleles increase trait values. Horizontal lines mark the transcript-specific significance thresholds for significant (*red*) and suggestive (*grey*) based on results of 1,000 permutations of the original trait data. The y-axis denotes the level of linkage and the x-axis denotes genetic markers along the different chromosomes (autosomes 1–19 and X)

of QTL in expression genetics is defined as a trans-acting QTL. And then click on the chromosome numbers (Chr 19) along at the top of the plot to zoom in the single chromosome.

404.2.4 Upstream Gene of Pax6

The significant eQTL of *Pax6* locates at 23.5 Mb to 24.5 Mb of chromosome 19 (Fig. 404.3). A total 20 transcripts were located in this region. Among them, five genes whose mean expression level was more than 7 were cis-action with significant eQTL, high SNP counts. Only the gene phosphatidylinositol-4-phosphate 5-kinase, type 1 alpha (*Pip5k1a*) which is cis-action with LRS of 27.345 had significant correlation to *Pax6* (p = 1.676E − 09). Thus *Pip5k1a* was identified as a candidate upstream gene of *Pax6*.

404.2.5 Genetic Regulatory Network of Pax6

Still in the Trait Data and Analysis Form, select the "Calculate Correlations" button; and then select the "Sample r" button; choose Database = Eye M430v2 (Sep08) RMA, Reture = top 100, Samples = BXD Only; click the blue "Compute" button. A Correlation Table is constructed listing the top 100 correlates associated with the *Pax6* expression variation in the eye. Click on the top 30 of the correlates. After the probe sets are chosen, select the 'Add to Collection' function.

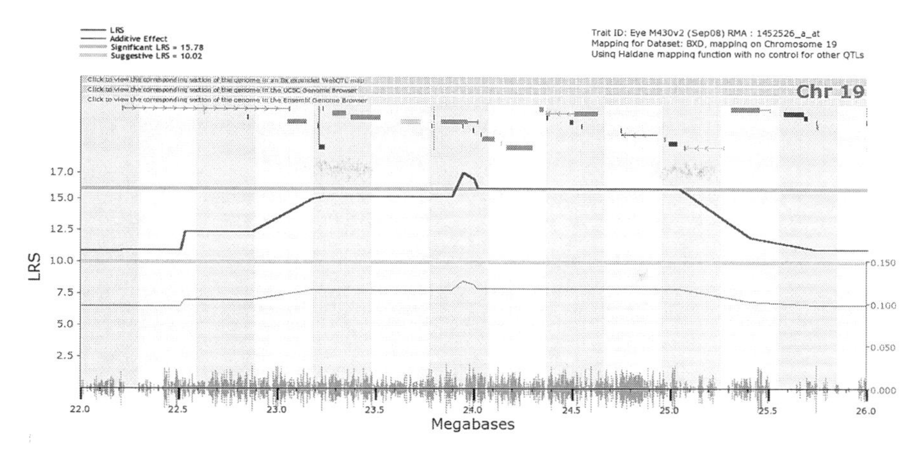

Fig. 404.3 The significant eQTL region of *Pax6* at 22 Mb to 26 M of chromosome 19. The solid blue line indicates LRS across the genome. Horizontal lines mark the transcript-specific significance thresholds for significant (red, $p \leq 0.05$) and suggestive (grey, $p \leq 0.63$) based on results of 1,000 permutations of the original trait data. The y-axis denotes the level of linkage and the x-axis denotes genetic markers. Yellow histogram: frequency of peak LRS (bootstrap analysis). Orange seismograph marks indicate SNP density

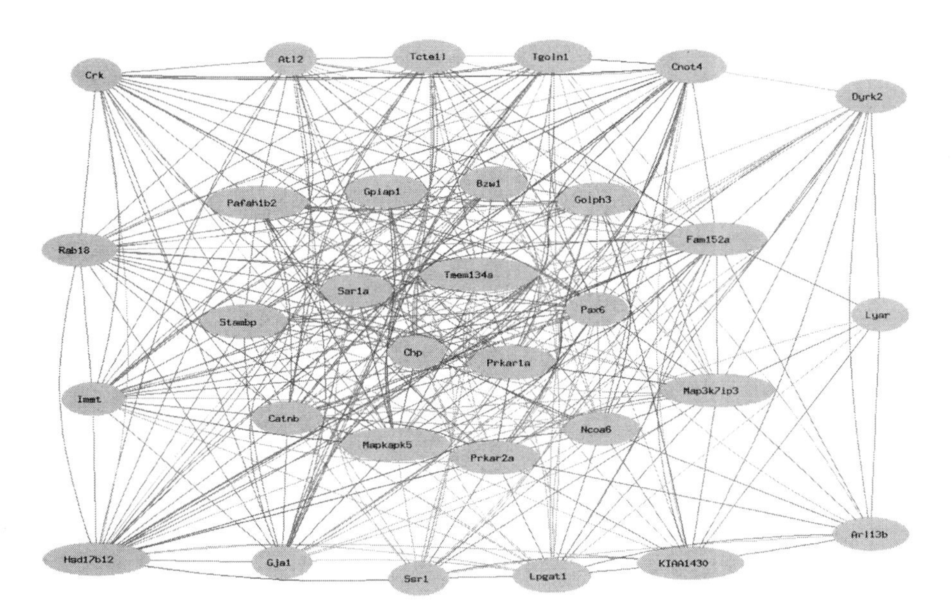

Fig. 404.4 Genetic regulatory network of *Pax6* using Pearson Correlation for the BXD RI mouse eye. The top 30 genes showed Pearson correlation coefficients greater than 0.6 (*red* and *orange lines*) or less than −0.6 (*blue* or *green lines*). Genes (*blue box*) are connected to their most likely regulator by edges. *Pax6* Located in the central of the network

At the BXD Trait Collection page, select *Pax6* and all the top 30 genes and select the "Network Graph" function. The network is drawn using certain default parameters that can easily be changed.

The 30 genes in the network are co-regulated with *Pax6* gene expression in eyes of BXD RI mice (Fig. 404.4). The correlation analysis revealed the mean genetic correlation between the 30 genes with *Pax6* is 0.720; the mean literature correlation is 0.271; the mean tissue correlation is 0.151.The mean expression level is 10.282. All these genes in the network are closely related with *Pax6*. These genes provide the new direction and clues for further in-depth study of *Pax6* function.

404.3 Conclusion

The gene analysis and dissection by means of the Analysis Tools of GeneNetwork providing new opportunities for the investigation of the biological mechanisms of selected genes such as *Pax6*. Certainly, it is essential to verify the interaction between *Pax6* and other genes in the pathway through experiments. We conclude that all these analysis may be a powerful tool for future identifications of candidate genes and for the pathway analysis for some disease.

References

1. Jansen RC, Nap JP (2001) Genetical genomics: the added value from segregation. Trends Genet 17:388–391
2. Chesler EJ, Lu L, Shou S et al (2005) Complex trait analysis of gene expression uncovers polygenic and pleiotropic networks that modulate nervous system function. Nat Genet 37:233–242
3. Schadt EE, Monks SA, Drake TA et al (2003) Genetics of gene expression surveyed in maize, mouse and man. Nature 422:297–302
4. Simpson TI, Price DJ (2002) *Pax6*; a pleiotropic player in development. BioEssays 24:1041–1051
5. Hever AM, Williamson KA, van Heyningen V (2006) Developmental malformations of the eye: the role of PAX6, SOX2 and OTX2. Clin Genet 69:459–470
6. Peirce JL, Lu L, Gu J et al (2004) A new set of BXD recombinant inbred lines from advanced intercross populations in mice. BMC Genet 5:7
7. Williams RW, Gu J, Qi S et al (2001) The genetic structure of recombinant inbred mice: high-resolution consensus maps for complex trait analysis. Genome Biol 2:RESEARCH0046

Chapter 405
Impact of Scan Duration on PET/CT Maximum Standardized Uptake Value Measurement

Qiuping Fan, Minggang Su and Luyi Zhou

Abstract Although readily available and convenient to use on PET/CT, SUV measurements are influenced by biologic and technologic factors like injected activity and scan duration. The aim of this study was to investigate the effect of varying scan duration on SUV using standard clinical activities of ^{18}F-FDG. Patient PET/CT images were acquired in list-mode for 6 min in forty ^{18}F-FDG oncology patients with known tumor. For each patient, data were sorted into 10 images of different durations (from 10 s to 6 min). SUVmax were measured for the lesions in the images. Tumor SUVmax were statistically analyzed taking the low-noise 6 min SUVmax as standard. For each of the nine scan duration from 10 s to 5 min, the normalized SUVmax were 1.080 ± 0.1611, 1.041 ± 0.1043, 1.005 ± 0.0732, 1.004 ± 0.0696, 1.005 ± 0.0456, 0.995 ± 0.0452, 0.996 ± 0.0299, 1.001 ± 0.0233, and 1.0002 ± 0.0144, respectively. One-sample *t* test revealed that the SUVmax biases for scan durations greater than 40 s were not statistically significant. It was concluded that scan duration as short as 40 s could be applied without compromising the quality of SUVmax measure.

Keywords PET/CT · Standardized uptake value · Maximum standardized uptake value · Quantification · Scan duration

405.1 Introduction

^{18}F-FDG PET/CT imaging of tumor cell glycolysis has emerged as the most accurate tool for diagnosing, staging, restaging, and treatment monitoring of many malignancies. To quantify radiotracer accumulation, standardized uptake value

Q. Fan · M. Su · L. Zhou (✉)
Department of Nuclear Medicine, West China Hospital,
Sichuan University, Chengdu, Sichuang 610041, China
e-mail: zhouluyi@scu.edu.cn

S. Li et al. (eds.), *Frontier and Future Development of Information Technology in Medicine and Education*, Lecture Notes in Electrical Engineering 269,
DOI: 10.1007/978-94-007-7618-0_405,

(SUV) analysis [1] of ^{18}F-FDG PET images is increasingly applied as a practical and effective method to characterize lesions and monitor response to therapy. Although readily available and convenient to use on commercial PET/CT, SUV measurements can be influenced by a variety of biologic and technologic factors [2], including injected activity and scan duration. Shorter scan durations can not only improve the patient throughput, which is critical for high capacity departments where 30–40 scans are performed daily on a single scanner, but also reduce the risk of motion artefacts, patient discomfort, complications from potential sedation and cost of ^{18}F-FDG supply. The purpose of this study was to investigate the effect of varying scan duration on SUV measurements using standard clinical activities of ^{18}F-FDG, to find out whether further shortening of scan duration could be applied without compromising the quality of SUV measurement.

405.2 Materials and Methods

405.2.1 Data Acquisition and Image Reconstruction

A Gemini GXL PET/CT system (Philips Healthcare) was used to acquire image data for 40 patients with known malignancies in the chest. Patients were prepared according to a standard oncology protocol, and data were acquired approximately 1 h after administration of 295 MBq-445 MBq of ^{18}F-FDG. Image data were acquired in list mode over the tumor site using a single PET bed position for 6 min. CT data were acquired over the same scan range using 16-slice multichannel CT, with 120 kVp voltage and 100 mA current. The 6 min list mode data were sorted to form multiple images of ten different durations (10, 20, 40 s, and 1, 1.5, 2, 3, 4, 5, 6 min). All images are reconstructed routinely using the line-of-response (LOR) based row-action maximum-likelihood algorithm (LOR-RAMLA) [3].

405.2.2 SUV Measurement

Maximum standardized uptake value (SUVmax) [4] were measured for the target lesion in the images of different scan durations.

The basic formula to calculate the SUV is as following:

$$SUV(g/mL) = activity\ concentration\ in\ the\ tumor\ (Bq/mL) \times body\ weight(g)/injected\ activity\ (Bq) \tag{405.1}$$

To measure SUVmax, a large, spherical region of interest (ROI) was defined so as to encapsulate the entire tumor, and used the maximum pixel within the ROI as the “activity concentration in tissue”.

405.2.3 Data Analysis

To account for variations in the absolute magnitude of the tumor SUVmax between the different patients, the SUVmax determined from the low-noise 6 min data were used to normalize each of the corresponding SUVmax from the shorter-scan-duration images. One-sample t test was done against the value of 1 using the normalized SUVmax data from all patients at each scan duration at 95 % confidence level, with SPSS for windows 11.0 (SPSS inc.).

405.3 Results

The normalized SUVmax was demonstrated in Fig. 405.1.

The normalized SUVmax, as well as the corresponding t and P value of the one-sample t-test were presented in Table 405.1.

As the figure and table revealed, there were obvious biases (8.0–4.1 %) for SUVmax of 10 and 20 s scan durations. However, the biases for SUVmax of scan duration greater than 40 s were less than 0.5 %, and one-sample t-test revealed that those biases were not statistically significant.

405.4 Discussion

SUVmax is the most widely used method of analyzing tumors in quantitative ^{18}F-FDG oncology studies [5]. Because SUVmax is derived from the maximum pixel within the ROI, as mentioned above, concern regarding its vulnerability to image noise remains [6]. Image noise can be reduced by improving the total counts with the modification of two parameters: the injected activity or the scan duration.

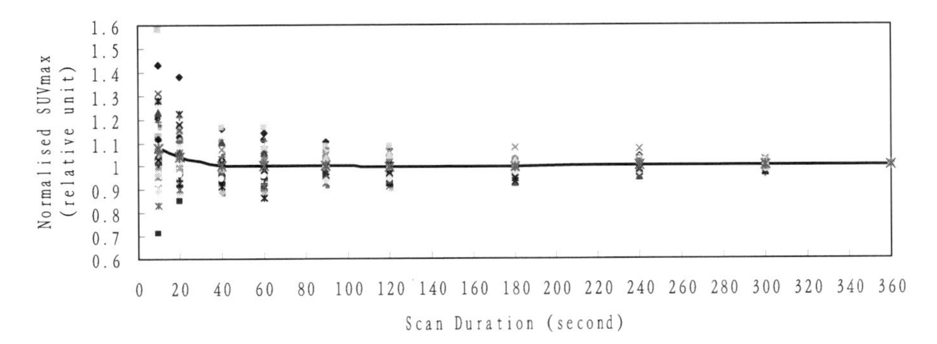

Fig. 405.1 Effect of varying scan duration on tumor SUVmax. Each colored data series represents normalized SUVmax for particular patient. Solid line is the average for all patients

Table 405.1 The normalized SUVmaxs, with t and P value of the one-sample t-test

Scan duration	10 s	20 s	40 s	1 min	1.5 min	2 min	3 min	4 min	5 min
SUVmax (mean ± SD) [1]	1.080 ± 0.1611	1.041 ± 0.1043	1.005 ± 0.0732	1.004 ± 0.0696	1.005 ± 0.0456	0.995 ± 0.0452	0.996 ± 0.0299	1.001 ± 0.0233	1.0002 ± 0.0144
T	3.159	2.483	0.436	0.333	0.703	−0.736	−0.779	0.271	0.1
P value (two tailed)	0.003	0.017	0.665	0.741	0.486	0.466	0.441	0.788	0.921

[1] Normalize to the 6-min SUVmax

Several guidelines have been published [7–9], recommending the ^{18}F-FDG activities to be administered in adults and children to ensure good quality images, but optimal scan duration per bed position is still not well established. Furthermore, it has been found that above a certain level, an increased injected activity does not necessarily improve the image quality [10–12], so scan duration becomes an very important parameter to study in order to attain good image quality, as well as good SUV measurement. Reports have been published to study the image quality in term of image quality scale, lesion detection rate and SUV, in patient[13, 14] or phantom[15] under various conditions such as scan duration and the results for SUVmax measurement are by no means concordant. In real patient images, Lodge et al. [14] reported that relative to the low-noise 15-min images, SUVmax had significant positive biases of 30, 18, 12, and 4 % for the 1, 2, 3, and 4-min images respectively, but a non- significant bias of 5 % for the 5-min images, for patients with malignancies in the chest or abdomen. Also in real patient images, Goethals et al. [13] reported that for 0.5, 1, 2, 3, 5, 7 and 10-min PET images of patients with head and neck cancer, SUVmax was not significantly different between images with various scan duration and the reference, except for the 0.5-min PET image. The present study augments the study of Goethals et al. with the finding that the biases for SUVmax of scan duration greater than 40 s were less than 0.5 %, and those biases were not statistically significant, in real images of patients with chest cancer. It is generally agreed that quantitative measurement of tracer uptake in a tumor is influenced by a number of factors and SUV values obtained under different conditions must not be compared directly. However, our results showed that, in chest tumors, using the same scanner and under identical scanning and image reconstruction conditions, shorter scan duration as 40 s could be applied without compromising the quality of SUV measurement. Shorter scan duration can not only improve the patient throughput, but also reduce the risk of motion artefacts, patient discomfort, complications from potential sedation and cost of ^{18}F-FDG supply. Further more, the finding that SUVmax does not change with the scan duration longer than 40 s imply that ^{18}F-FDG uptake in chest tumors can be semi-quantitatively compared independent of scan duration. This could enhance the confidence of tumor treatment response monitoring, because the change in SUVmax values on sequential PET/CT scans is frequently used as a parameter of tumor treatment response.

References

1. Thie JA (2004) Understanding the standardized uptake value, its methods, and implications for usage. J Nucl Med 45(9):1431–1434
2. Adams MC, Turkington TG, Wilson JM et al (2010) A systematic review of the factors affecting accuracy of SUV measurements. Am J Roentgenol 195(2):310–320
3. Hu Z, Wang W, Gualtieri EE, et al (2007) An LOR-based systematic and fully-3D PET image reconstruction using a blob-basis function. In: IEEE nuclear science symposium conference record, 2007 (NSS'07), vol 6. pp. 4415–4418)

4. Borst GR, Belderbos JSA, Boellaard R et al (2005) Standardised FDG uptake: a prognostic factor for inoperable non-small cell lung cancer. Eur J Cancer 41:1533–1541
5. Wahl RL, Jacene H, Kasamon Y, et al (2009) From RECIST to PERCIST: evolving considerations for PET response criteria in solid tumors. J Nucl Med 50(suppl):122S–150SS
6. Soret M, Bacharach SL, Buvat I (2007) Partial-volume effect in PET tumor imaging. J Nucl Med 48(6):932–945
7. Delbeke D, Coleman RE, Guiberteau MJ et al (2006) Procedure guideline for tumor imaging with 18F-FDG PET/CT 1.0. J Nucl Med 47(5):885–895
8. Barrington SF, Begent J, Lynch T et al (2008) Guidelines for the use of PET–CT in children. Nucl Med Commun 29(5):418–424
9. Boellaard R, O'Doherty M, Weber W et al (2010) FDG PET and PET/CT: EANM procedure guidelines for tumour PET imaging: version 1.0. Eur J Nucl Med Mol Imaging 37(1):181–200
10. Tatsumi M, Clark P, Nakamoto Y et al (2003) Impact of body habitus on quantitative and qualitative image quality in wholebody FDG-PET. Eur J Nucl Med Mol Imaging 30(1):40–45
11. Halpern B, Dahlbom M, Quon A et al (2004) Impact of patient weight and emission scan duration on PET/CT image quality and lesion detectability. J Nucl Med 45(5):797–801
12. Watson C, Casey M, Bendriem B et al (2005) Optimizing injected dose in clinical PET by accurately modeling the counting-rate response functions specific to individual patient scans. J Nucl Med 46(11):1825–1834
13. Goethals I, D'Asseler Y, Dobbeleir A et al (2010) The effect of acquisition time on visual and semi-quantitative analysis of F-18 FDG-PET studies in patients with head and neck cancer. Nucl Med Commun 31(3):227–231
14. Lodge MA, Chaudhry MA, Wahl RL (2012) Noise considerations for PET quantification using maximum and peak standardized uptake value. J Nucl Med 53(7):1041–1047
15. Brambilla M, Matheoud R, Secco C et al (2007) Impact of target-to-background ratio, target size, emission scan duration, and activity on physical figures of merit for a 3D LSO-based whole body PET/CT scanner. Med Phys 34(10):3854–3865

Chapter 406
16-Slice Spiral Computer Tomography and Digital Radiography: Diagnosis of Ankle and Foot Fractures

Hanqing Zhang, Liangzhou Xu, Peng Wang, Huang Bo, Jian Liu, Xiaojun Dong, Nianzu Ye, Wang Fei and Peng Gu

Abstract Acute ankle and foot fracture is one of the most common injuries seen in trauma departments. It is not easy to diagnose subtle occult fracture or fracture displacement using Digital Radiography (DR) because of the complex anatomical structure of the ankle and foot, and overlapping structure of DR. Computed Tomography (CT) technologies provides 3-dimensional (3D) visualization of the anatomical structure and eliminates overlapping structures, makes it easier for diagnosis purposes. Seventy-three ankle and foot injuries patients were examined using both DR and CT. The results showed that the diagnosis of fracture using DR was 68.5 % and 100 % using CT. The study showed that CT has better diagnosis rate than DR ($P < 0.01$). The 3D reconstruction of the CT images provides a better tool showing the position and type of fracture lines and free sheet position clearly for diagnosis purposes. Therefore 16-slice spiral CT has a clear advantage over DR in the diagnosis, especially on the subtle occult fracture and fracture displacement, treatment and evaluation purposes in clinical intervention.

Keywords 16-slice spiral CT · Digital radiography · Ankle and foot fractures · Diagnosis

H. Zhang · X. Dong
Department of Orthopaedics, Wuhan Hospital of Traditional Chinese Medicine, Wuhan 430014, China

L. Xu (✉) · P. Wang · H. Bo · J. Liu
Department of Radiology, Wuhan Hospital of Traditional Chinese Medicine, Wuhan 430014, China
e-mail: 215850880@qq.com

N. Ye
Department of Radiology, 2nd hospital of Wuhan, Wuhan 430010, China

W. Fei · P. Gu
Class of Seven-Year Orthopaedics Program of Hubei University of Chinese Medicine, Wuhan 430060, China

S. Li et al. (eds.), *Frontier and Future Development of Information Technology in Medicine and Education*, Lecture Notes in Electrical Engineering 269,
DOI: 10.1007/978-94-007-7618-0_406,

406.1 Introduction

The acute ankle and foot fracture is one of the most common injuries seen in trauma departments. X-ray or Digital Radiography (DR) is a common routine examination in the diagnosis and treatment of fracture. Due to the complex bone anatomical structure and overlapping structure of the X-ray film, it is difficult to diagnose the fractures in the ankle and foot injuries resulting in increasing oversight and wrong diagnosis. With the advent of isotropic 16-slice spiral CT, which provided improved image quality and 3D reconstruction of the volume scan, it effectively compensates the overlapping structure issue of DR images and the non-distinct crack fracture showing in a two-dimensional (2D) image. Thus greatly improve the diagnosis, the treatment and prognosis evaluation of ankle and foot fracture in the clinical setting.

406.2 Material and Method

406.2.1 Material

Between January 2011 and December 2012, there were 325 out-patients with pain and swelling of ankle and foot caused by falls and traffic accident injuries were accepted for examination and treatment. 73 patients (50 males, 23 female), mean age 43.6 yeas (15–80 years old) who took the DR examination also agreed to taking the 16-slice spiral CT scan. This study compares DR images with the reconstruction of the 3D CT scan.

406.2.2 Method

The following DR images were acquired using the Toshiba DR, on the ankle joint: antero-posterior, lateral and oblique views; on the foot: antero-posterior and oblique views; and on the calcaneal: lateral and axial views. 16-sliced spiral CT (Toshiba Aquillion 16) was performed with the following variables: pitch: 0.938, 120 kV, 50 mAs, scanning with 0.5 mm reconstruction. The data was transferred to the Vitrea workstation for post-processing and reconstruction, using multiple planar reconstruction (MRP), 3D volume rendering (VR) features, to generate the 2D images and 3D model.

A senior radiologist and a doctor of Orthopedics Department compared with plain X-ray and CT image, and observed fracture line, bone fragments position, joint alignment and surrounding soft tissue injury, through the CT 3D image,so as to further clarify the diagnosis.

406.2.3 Statistical Analysis

All the data were analyzed with the SPSS 18.0 software (X^2 test or Chi square test), result was considered to be significant difference while P value <0.05

406.3 Results

The results showed that the diagnosis of fracture was concordant between DR and CT in 50 patients (68.5 %). 15 cases of the fracture were deemed suspicious,and 8 cases were missed on the 2D DR whereas all of the fractures were detected by 3D CT. The accuracy rate of CT was 100 %, and was significantly higher than that of DR. Comparing of two methods, the difference was statistically significant ($X^2 = 27.301$, P value < 0.01) (see Table 406.1).

In this group of 73 cases, 3D CT showed that there were medial malleolar fracture in 15 cases, lateral malleolar fractures in 13 cases, double ankle fracture in 6 cases, three ankle fractures in 4 cases; 12 cases of calcaneal fractures, Calcaneus comminuted fractures of the lateral malleolus fracture in 2 cases, comminuted calcaneal with avulsion of talus rim in 1 case, calcaneal fracture of anterior lateral margin combined with the base of the 34 metatarsal bone fracture in 1 case, 3 cases of calcaneal protrusion avulsion, 2 cases of calcaneal protrusion with lateral malleolar fractures, 4 cases of talar fracture of talus, 1 case of trailing edge avulsion of talar; 3 cases of navicular bone fracture; first cuneiform bone fracture in 1 case; 1 cases of fracture of cuboid, 2-4 metatarsal bones, third cuneiform with hip fracture in 1 case, multiple fractures including the first metatarsal metatarsal, first, 2-4, 3 cuneiform, navicular bone, cuboid in 1 case. 3D CT shows the anatomy of the ankle and foot, fracture line position, fracture type, displacement and fracture involved articular surface allowing for clinical diagnosis and treatment.

406.4 Discussion

The ankle joint is the body's largest flexion weight-bearing joints, composed of the lower end of tibial and fibula and talus; foot includes calcaneus, talus,navicular bone, cuneiform, phalanx, metatarsal,and so on [1]. In the joint of all body, foot

Table 406.1 Comparison of 16-slice spiral CT and DR in diagnosing ankle and foot fractures

	Definite	Suspicious	Missed	Total	Accuracy (%)
DR	50	15	8	73	68.49
16-slice spiral CT	73	0	0	73	100[a]

[a] Compare with DR,P < 0.01

and ankle fractures are very common; the complex anatomical structure and bone composition resulted in the complexity and diversity of the fracture types. The conventional 2D DR is a simple and convenient routine examination method, but the DR image cannot display the fractures clearly due to the overlapping structure. Additional views of the fractures were taken to compensate for the overlapping structure of DR images. The patients sometimes need to be position specially for the different views, for example navicular is taken the internal oblique, calcaneal taking lateral, axial. However these views only provide preliminary diagnosis for the occult fractures. It is still very challenging to diagnose most of the occult fractures without obvious fracture displacement, resulting in increasing oversight and wrong diagnosis.

CT and high-resolution Magnetic Resonance Imaging (MRI) overcomes the shortcoming of the DR diagnosis of this kind of fracture [3, 4]. MRI is the best modality for diagnosis of occult fracture, is considered as the gold standard [5]. But the examination time is very long, costly, and it is difficult to manage with the emergency patients. On the other hand, high resolution MSCT is more feasible and practical. The postprocessing such as multiplanar reconstruction (MPR), shaded surface display (SSD) and volume rendering (VR) provides the clinicians with an intuitive overall, comprehensive observation of the fracture and dislocation of the ankle from the 3D model [2, 6]. CT scanning with thinner slice parameter increase the density and the spatial resolution of the image, improving the visualization to show the subtle fractures, more conducive to the complex fracture and anatomical structure display [7]. 3D reconstruction eliminates the overlapping structure issue allows the visualization of the occult fracture, especially the complex fracture and anatomical structure. It also helps to determine the location of the fracture, the type

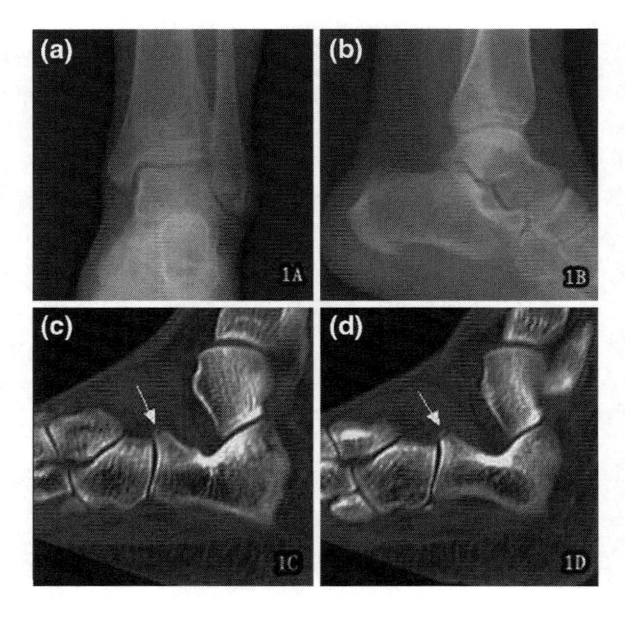

Fig. 406.1 A 26-year-old female with pain caused by an acute left ankle sprain after 5 h (**a**, **b**); R showed no fracture (**c**, **d**); CT showed fracture of anterior superior process of calcaneus (*white arrow*)

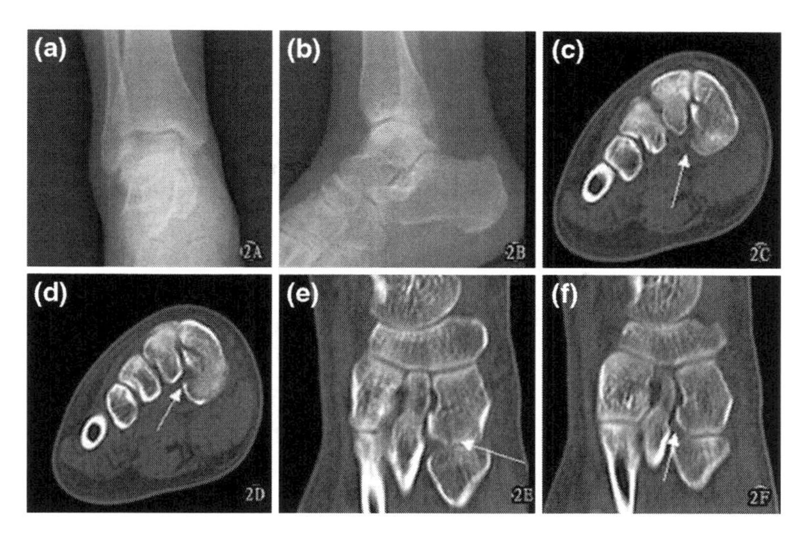

Fig. 406.2 A 44-year-old female with pain caused by an acute right ankle sprain (**a**, **b**) DR showed no fracture (**c–f**); CT showed fracture of first cuneiform bone (*white arrow*)

and extent of the fracture, and the anatomical relationship with the surrounding tiusse, the size and quantity of the fracture, the distribution of the fracture, the shift direction and extent of the fracture; the length and direction of the fracture line. Therefore provide the clinicians with the tool for more accurate diagnosis to increase the diagnosis rate and prevent oversight and wrong diagnosis (see Figs. 406.1 and 406.2).

In summary, although DR is the conventional means of ankle trauma examination, it is very difficult to diagnose ankle and foot injuries, especially occult fracture or fracture displacement, because of the ankle's complex anatomical structure, and the overlapping structure of DR imaging. On the other hand, the postprocessing and reconstruction of CT provides the clinicians with a better visualization tool for more accurate diagnosis of the fracture. It makes it easier for diagnosis, especially in occult fracture or subtle fracture displacement, treatment planning and evaluation purposes. Therefore 16-slice spiral CT has a clear advantage over 2D DR in the diagnosis of subtle ankle and foot fracture, treatment and evaluation purposes in the clinical setting.

References

1. Bo S, Ying D (2011) Descriptive anatomy [M]. Beijing. People's Medical Publishing House, Chinese, pp 56–58
2. Choplin RH, Buckwalter KA, Rydberg J et al (2004) CT with 3D rendering of the tendons of the foot and ankle: technique, normal anatomy, and disease [J]. Radiographics 24(2): 343–356

3. Frahm R, Wimmer B, Bonnaire F (1991) Computed tomography of the superior and inferior ankle joint [J]. Radiologe 31(12):609–615
4. Haapamaki VV, Kiuru MJ, Koskinen SK (2004) Ankle and foot injuries: analysis of MDCT findings [J]. AJR Am J Roentgenol 183(3):615–622
5. Kiuru MJ, Pihlajamaki HK, Hietanen HJ et al (2002) MR imaging, bone scintigraphy, and radiography in bone stress injuries of the pelvis and the lower extremity [J]. Acta Radiol 43(2):207–212
6. Magid D, Michelson JD, Ney DR et al (1990) Adult ankle fractures: comparison of plain films and interactive two- and three-dimensional CT scans [J]. AJR Am J Roentgenol 154(5):1017–1023
7. Shi L, Tian J, Wang P et al (2003) Evaluation of multi-slice spiral CT in diagnosing trauma of bones and joints: a comparison between different reconstructions [J]. J Clin Radiol 22:772–774

Chapter 407
Structural SIMilarity and Spatial Frequency Motivated Atlas Database Reduction for Multi-atlas Segmentation

Yaqian Zhao and Aimin Hao

Abstract Multi-atlas segmentation has been proved to be an effective approach in biomedical images segmentation. In this approach, all atlases in atlas database participate in segmentation process. This results in the fact that the computational cost and the redundancy bias will increase correspondingly with the size of atlas database. To decrease the computational cost, many researches proposed atlas selection which selects limited atlases to register with the query image. This strategy effectively reduces the number of atlases in registration, but is ineffective in reducing redundancy bias. To address this problem, we propose a novel strategy that improving segmentation quality through analyse of atlas database. Our contributions are summarized as follow: (1) define optimal minimum reduced atlas database (MinRAD); (2) give an algorithm of constructing optimal MinRAD based structure similarity and spatial frequency; and (3) demonstrate validity of our strategy by experimental results.

Keywords Multi-atlas segmentation · Atlas database reduction · Structural SIMilarity (SSIM) · Spatial Frequency (SF)

407.1 Introduction

Atlas-based segmentation is a common and powerful approach in brain MR image segmentation [1]. Its main advantage is that labels are transferred as well as the segmentation. In this method, the atlas image is registered to the query image,

Y. Zhao (✉) · A. Hao
State Key Laboratory of Virtual Reality Technology and Systems,
Beihang University, Beijing, China
e-mail: ms.zhaoyq@gmail.com

A. Hao
e-mail: ham.vrlab@gmail.com

S. Li et al. (eds.), *Frontier and Future Development of Information Technology in Medicine and Education*, Lecture Notes in Electrical Engineering 269,
DOI: 10.1007/978-94-007-7618-0_407,

yielding a transformation which allows the atlas segmentation to be transformed and treated as a segmentation result. To obtain more high accuracy, recent approaches use multi-atlas, instead of a single atlas. In Heckemann et al. [2], have demonstrated that segmentation accuracy can be improved as more atlases are combined. However, when the atlas database is too large multi-atlas segmentation has its own limits. Firstly, the computational cost of segmentation increases linearly with the number of atlases. Secondly, segmentation precision maybe decreases due to the redundancies in atlas database.

To decrease the computational cost, a number of recent studies have proposed atlases selection methods aimed at selecting the atlases most similar to the query image [3–6]. These proposed methods effectively reduce the number of atlases in registration, but ignore the redundancy bias. To address this problem, we propose a novel strategy to simultaneously reduce the size of atlas database and the redundancy bias, named atlas database reduction. In the next section, we define the optimal Minimum Reduced Atlas Database, and give an algorithm of structural similarity and spatial frequency motivated reduction. Experimental results in Sect. 407.3 show the redundancy bias can decrease the our strategy produced a more.

407.2 Optimal Reduced Atlas Database

Redundancy bias results from the strong correlations among atlases. For instance, if an atlas is duplicated multiple times in the atlas database, segmentation result will bias towards the repeated atlases for its weight value increase several-fold. This maybe produces bad result. To reduce the redundancy bias, we propose an atlas database reduction method motivated by Structural SIMilarity (SSIM) and Spatial Frequency (SF).

407.2.1 Definition of Optimal MinRAD

Definition 1 For a given threshold θ and correlation function *CF*, a subset *R* of atlas database *D* is defined RAD, if it satisfies the following condition:

$\forall\ atlas_i \in R$, there is at least a $atlas_j \in D$, and $CF(atlas_i, atlas_j) \geq \theta$.

Definition 2 For a given threshold θ, a similarity measure function *CF* and an optimal function *OF*, a subset *R* of atlas database *D* is defined optimal MinRAD about *OF*, if it satisfies the following conditions:

(1) $\forall\ atlas_i \in D$, there has only one $atlas_j \in R$, and $CF(atlas_i, atlas_j) \geq \theta$

(2) $\forall\ atlas_i \in D$, if $CF(atlas_i, atlas_j) \geq \theta$, and $atlas_j \in R$, then $OF(atlas_j) \geq OF(atlas_i)$

For easy to compare the performance among different MinRADs derived from the same database, we define two evaluation indices: size of MinRAD and ratio of segmentation accuracy based MinRAD to that based the whole atlas database [7].

$$N = |RAD| \tag{407.1}$$

$$RA = accuracy_R / accuracy_D \tag{407.2}$$

where |·| represents pixel counts. For two MinRADs about the database D, R_1 and R_2, if RA_{R_1} is larger than RA_{R_2}, R_1 is superior to R_2, if RA_{R_1} is equal to RA_{R_2} and N_{R_1} is larger than N_{R_2}, R_1 is inferior to R_2.

407.2.2 Construction of Optimal MinRAD

In this paper, we suppose the strong correlation between atlases mainly results from their structure similarity. Therefore, we select SSIM as correlation function [8, 9]. Since the atlases in reduced database should contain more spatial features, SF is considered as the optimal function [10]. The algorithm of constructing SSIM and SF based MinRAD is described as follows.

Algorithm of constructing the optimal MinRAD about SSIM-SF:

Step 1 Initialize the optimal MinRAD R as null

Step 2 Calculate the structure similarity between $atlas_i$ and $atlas_j$, denote $SSIM(atlas_i, atlas_j)$, $i \neq j$

Step 3 Put these atlases satisfied $SM(atlas_i, atlas_j) \geq \theta$ into the same Group k, $k = 1,2,\ldots,K$

Step 4 *if length* (Group k) = 1 Directly put the atlas in Group k into MinRAD*else*Calculate the Spatial Frequency of each atlas in Group $k$$SF(atlas_m)$, $atlas_m \in$Group k;Select the atlas with highest value of SF to MinRAD

Step 5 Repeat *Step* 4 until all Groups are carried out, the final result of R is the desiring reduced database.

From the above description of algorithm, it is obvious that the optimal MinRAD is independent with the query image. Therefore, database reduction can be carried out in pre-processing.

407.3 Experimental Results and Analysis

In this section, we demonstrate existence of redundancy bias and the validity of our technique in reduction the size of database and redundancy bias by experimental results.

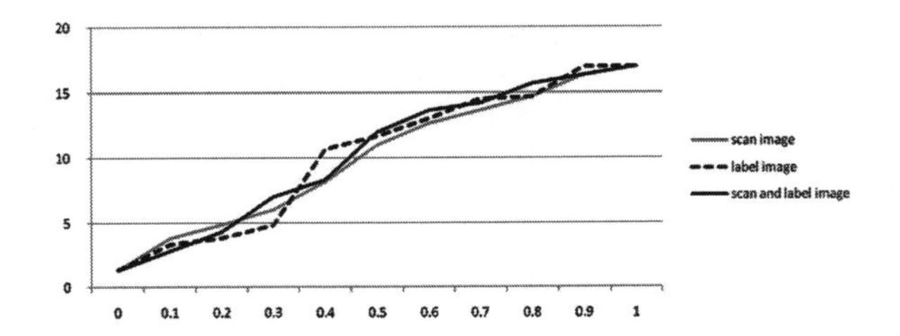

Fig. 407.1 Comparison of size of optimal MinRAD between different SSIM withθ

Since an atlas is a couple of scan image and label image, we use three kinds of SSIM: SSIM of scan image, SSIM of label image, and SSIM of scan and label image. We carry out the same multi-atlas segmentation method on brain database and its three optimal MinRADs. To compare atlas database reduction method with similarity based atlas selection method, we also compute the accuracy ratio of atlas selection and all atlases using the same registration and label fusion method. All 18 brain images are obtained from IBSR database. In our work, the cross validation leave-one-out approach was employed. The results in Figs. 407.1 and 407.2 are the average value of ten examinational results.

From the comparison results in Figs. 407.1, 407.2, 407.3, we can draw the following conclusions:

(1) There exits redundancy bias produced by the correlations between atlases.
(2) Optimal MinRAD can effectively reduce the size of database and the redundancy bias.
(3) With the increasing of threshold, the size of MinRAD surely increases, but accuracy ratio not always increases, such as results appeared in Fig. 407.2b. This demonstrates the fact that strong correlation between atlases can result in segmentation errors.
(4) Optimal MinRAD based SSIM of scan and label image produced a better result.
(5) When number of atlases ranges from 7 to 11, atlas selection method is inferior to atlas reduction because of the effect of correlations among atlases.

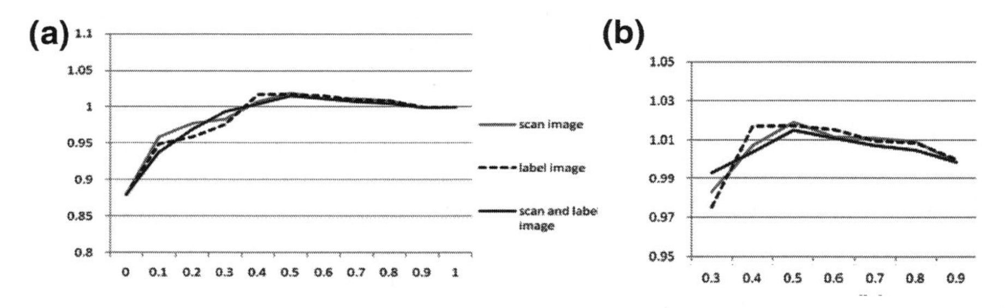

Fig. 407.2 Comparison of accuracy ratio of optimal MinRAD between different SSIM with θ **b** is the part of **a** with θ range from 0.4 to 0.9

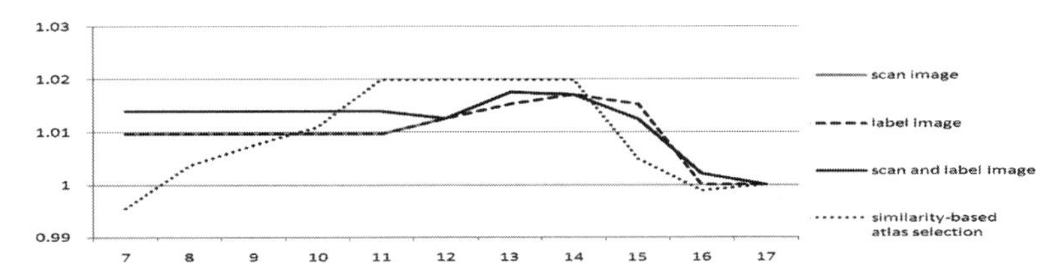

Fig. 407.3 Comparison of accuracy ratio between atlas database reduction and similarity based atlas selection with number of atlases range from 7 to 17

(6) Highest value of *SF* does not mean highest value of similarity, so these atlases most similar to query image may be abandoned in reduction process. This leads to the fact that atlas selection method gets more accurate result when number of atlases ranges from 11 to 14, as shown in Fig. 407.3.

407.4 Conclusions

In this paper, we proposed the SSIM and SF motivated atlas database reduction method, which is a novel strategy of reducing the computational cost and the redundancy bias. Comparing with these recent atlas selection methods, atlas database reduction has three advantages: (1) simultaneously reduce the size of atlas database and the redundancy bias; (2) can be carried out in pre-processing; (3) can combine with atlas selection to further decrease the computational cost when atlas database is extremely large. In future work, we will try to find more suitable construction of optimal MinRAD methods.

References

1. Cuadra MB, Pollo C, Bardera A, Cuisenaire O, Thiran JP (2003) Atlas-based segmentation of pathological brain MR images. ICIP 573–576:2003
2. Heckemann RA, Hajnal JV, Aljabar P, Rueckert D, Hammers A (2006) Auto-matic anatomical brain MRI segmentation combining label propagation and decision fusion. Neuroimage 33(1):115–126
3. Aljabar P, Heckemann RA, Hammers A, Hajnal JV, Rueckert D (2009) Multi-atlas based segmentation of brain images: atlas selection and its effect on accuracy. Neuroimage 46(3):726–738
4. Lötjönen JM, Wolz R, Koikkalainen JR, Thurfjell L, Waldemar G, Soininen H, Rueckert D (2010) Fast and robust multi-atlas segmentation of brain magnetic resonance images. Neuroimage 49(3):2352–2365
5. Akinyemi A, Plakas C, Piper J, Roberts C, Poole I (2012) Optimal atlas selection using image similarities in a trained regression model to predict performance. In: Biomedical Imaging (ISBI), 2012 9th IEEE International Symposium on IEEE, pp 1264–1267

6. Tong T, Wolz R, Coupé P, Hajnal JV, Rueckert D (2013) Segmentation of MR images via discriminative dictionary learning and sparse coding: application to hippocampus labeling. Neuroimage 76(1):11–23
7. Dice L (1945) Measures of the amount of ecologic association between species. Ecology 26:297–302
8. Wang Z, Bovik AC, Sheikh HR, Simoncelli EP (2004) Image quality assessment: from error visibility to structural similarity. IEEE Trans Image Process 13(4):600–612
9. Łoza A, Mihaylova L, Bull D, Canagarajah N (2009) Structural similarity-based object tracking in multimodality surveillance videos. Mach Vis Appl 20(2):71–83
10. Eskicioglu AM, Fisher PS (1995) Image quality measures and their performance. IEEE Trans Commun 143(12):2959–2965

Chapter 408
Some Reflections on Undergraduate Computer Graphics Teaching

Shanshan Gao and Caiming Zhang

Abstract This paper analyzes the discipline status of computer graphics and some problems in the teaching and the effect of scientific research in the course teaching and the teacher itself. In order to solve these problems, some teaching suggestions are given. Especially a new systematic and overall case-centered teaching mode is proposed, and the promoting use of various competitions for students is analyzed. Proven by practice, the efficiency and quality of teaching can be improved.

Keywords Computer Graphics · Scientific Research · Case teaching · Teaching mode · Competitions for college students

408.1 Introduction

Computer graphics(CG) is a discipline using computers to research the representation, generation, disposition and display of graphics, and is one of the branches that are most active and widely used in the current computer science [1]. This course is one of the important courses of computer and related professions, and is the foundation course of digital media technology, computer-aided design, scientific computing visualization, 3D animation technology, etc. This course aims to enable students to master the basic knowledge, principles and methods of generation and dispose technology of CG, cultivate students' ability of development of software related to graphics [2].

At present, almost all colleges and universities have set up the CG course and some related courses for the computer or digital media specialty. However, there are still many unresolved issues in the CG teaching. First of all, this course has a

S. Gao (✉) · C. Zhang
School of Computer Science and Technology,
Shandong University of Finance and Economics, Jinan 250014, China
e-mail: gsszxy@yahoo.com.cn

S. Li et al. (eds.), *Frontier and Future Development of Information Technology in Medicine and Education*, Lecture Notes in Electrical Engineering 269,
DOI: 10.1007/978-94-007-7618-0_408,

characteristic of strong theoretical and practical, the contents are abstract and the algorithms are elusive. Secondly, as to the teachers and students, some of the teachers themselves have a little understanding about the course. So the students have to accept knowledge negatively without understanding the learn purpose. Therefore, it would be difficult to absorb knowledge, not to mention to use the knowledge. The course characteristic is fixed, and the students are passive recipients, so the key to solve the teaching problems is the teacher.

Therefore, this paper analyzes the disciplinary status of CG and the problems in teaching. In view of these problems above, we propose some corresponding recommendations based on the role of scientific research and a variety of competitions played on the course, as well as the application of the holistic case-centered teaching mode in the teaching of the course.

408.2 Understanding of CG Course

We will introduce CG and analyze the problems in the current teaching firstly.

408.2.1 The Knowledge Points of CG

At present, according to the international customary, all fields of vision design and production using computer are generally known as CG technology. The concept of CG is still expanding, and has been formed a considerable economic industry. Beginning with Ivan Sutherland's sketchpad program in 1962, the needs of industries have promoted the development of CG technology, which is also a strong support for these industries, especially in the digital media industry which develops rapidly, CG has brought considerable economic benefits. For example, in the film and television animation industry, all kinds of cartoon characters, impressive stunts we see in the film all rely on CG technology.

The contents of CG are very extensive, however, at the stage of undergraduate, it is more important to explain how to use computer to generate pleasing real graphics and achieve the perfect combination of technology and art. Simply speaking, realistic 3D graphics rendering can be divided into two stages, one is geometry processing including coordinate transformation, clipping, illumination calculation, and the other one is rasterization processing, including scan conversion, visible surfaces determination, texture mapping and so on. According to its process, realistic 3D graphics rendering also can be summarized as follows: (1) Graphical representation, or modeling. (2) Graphics calculation and processing using computer, including geometric transformation, clipping, projector, visible surfaces determination, and illumination calculation, etc. (3) Display of graphics.

408.2.2 Reasons for Existing Problems in the CG Teaching Process

The problems in the CG teaching and learning are due to the characteristic of the course itself as well as the limitations of the teaching process.

(1) The course is comprehensive, its content and applications are very broad. (2) The course is rich in content and algorithms, and is highly theoretical. (3) The course is a comprehensive curriculum which is both theoretical and practical. However, most of the current experimental courses still only focus on the confirmatory test. (4) At present, the teaching method of the course makes it difficult to understand the knowledge. In many universities, the teaching modes and methods are as same as that of other courses, which does not reflect the special characteristics of the CG. As to case teaching method widely concerned at present, it only presents the implementation result of each algorithm to students.

408.3 Suggestions

408.3.1 Importance of Scientific Research

As mentioned above, the development of CG would thank to its applications. For example, the classic forms of surface in the course such as Bezier, Coons, NURBS and so on, are proposed by some well-known masters like Bezier to solve surface modeling problems encountered in the producing and designing process. The entire creative industries related to digital media originated from CG, and benefit from the achievements in scientific research of higher colleges. Courses of such colleges generally emphasize on CG theory, the principle of algorithm operations, as well as man–machine interface and its applications, the most representative one of which is the College of Number Crunching of University of Utah. In the field of CG and digital media, almost every influential figure has a specific contact with this famous college in some way, for instance, the founders of some industrial giants like Adobe, Netscape, E&S, SGI, etc., all come from this college. Obviously, new achievements and technologies brought by these industrial giants and their teams have become the important content of CG and its related courses, enriching the teaching content and keeping the frontier position of the teaching content.

Therefore, achievements in scientific research on the one hand can promote the development of related industries in the CG field, while on the other hand can bring the course with fresh teaching content and cutting-edge technology. Hence, scientific research is very important for a CG teacher. Enhancing teachers' abilities of scientific research will allow both themselves and the students to get a better understanding of this subject. Secondly, scientific research can keep the frontier position of the teaching content, and encourage students to innovate.

408.3.2 Case-Based Teaching Model

It is concrete and vivid to explain the content of the course with cases, and helpful for students to understand and master basic theories. Case-based teaching has been widely used in the teaching of various courses because of its obvious advantages, including CG.But in terms of the application instances in many colleges, designs of the case are limited to the integration of independent experiments, that is, simply put a large number of sub-projects of the rendering algorithms of graphic elements under a procedural framework, which are still independent in actual [2–4], or concentrate on the visualization of algorithms implementing process [5]. Unfortunately, these methods, to some extent, alleviate the difficulties of understanding the CG course and its abstract algorithms, but for the students still do not know what role it plays, and it is still difficult to stimulate students' interest and scientific exploration passion of initiative thinking and solving problems.

We design dancing robots on the stage as the graphic scene, associating the key steps and knowledge points, which the 3D CG display involved, to the generation process of the case scene(see Fig. 408.1). This case scene enables students to completely understand of the entire knowledge structure, master and use the knowledge of the course, and we form a new teaching model which is systemic and holistic case-centered in the teaching process.

(1) At first, build a model of the robot. We simulate robot's head and body with simple sphere and cube. These basic geometries are easy to model, for example a cuboid is easily modeling by its eight vertices and their connection relationship.
(2) The contour of the robot, such as arm, the contour of the stage, can be drew by some classic algorithms, and each robot surface can be filled or changed by a variety of polygon filling algorithms. Then students can understand the ideas of the classical algorithms commonly used in graphics, such as DDA, Bresenham straight line/arc algorithm, all kinds of polygon fill algorithms, etc.

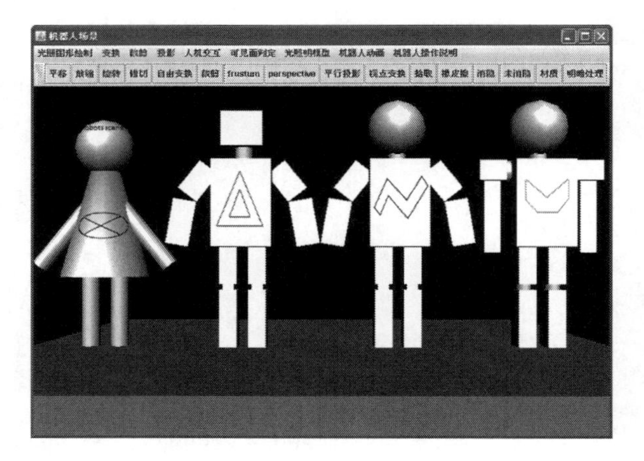

Fig. 408.1 Robots scene

(3) In order to obtain different observations, we transform the framing and observing method of the object. This process will put the classical algorithms like cutting, projection, and visual surface determine into use, and allow students understand the entire transforming process from a three-dimensional object space coordinate system to the two-dimensional window pixel coordinate system.
(4) Use illumination model to add the illumination on the robot to form the realistic graphics. This process can help students understand local illumination model.
(5) Transformation can complete a series of actions which make the robot become more vivid, you can change robot so that it can complete a series of actions.

408.3.3 The Application of Knowledge

As mentioned above, just because they do not know where the knowledge can be used, students are out of touch with practice, and gradually lost interest in the course. In addition to case-based teaching, various competitions for students [6] are a good way to make up for this deficiency, such as virtual reality software development, software design contest, game design contest and so on. In 2007, "Quality Project File" of the Ministry of Education has fully affirmed the importance of competitions in the respect of promoting education quality and cultivating innovative talents, and clearly put forwards that contests should be added into the content of practice teaching and talent training model reform.

In the teaching practice, on the one hand, based on the integration of classroom teaching knowledge and the comprehensive application, we should use various competitions as media to guide students to find problems, solve problems, and practice what they have learned through the completion of competitions. This will help to stimulate students' interest and potential, consolidate the knowledge learned, enhance students' initiative of learning and researching, and cultivate the students' team cooperation consciousness and innovation capability. On the other hand, we should also make the competition become a useful supplement of the daily teaching. Put some knowledge related to the contest into teaching plan, and combine the course and practical application to achieve a goal that contest would promote the teaching content, and teaching reform would support the contest.

408.4 Summary

According to the characteristics of CG course, and the existing difficulties encountered in the process of teaching and learning, this paper proposes some teaching suggestions. The importance of scientific research for the course and the teacher is analyzed, a cases-centered teaching model is proposed which can help the students intuitively understand the knowledge point and the role it played in the practical application. So that it is easy for students to get a complete understanding of the entire knowledge structure and digest the knowledge, and obtain the experience of project management and teamwork. The teaching practice has proved that this new teaching model significantly improved the efficiency and quality of teaching.

Acknowledgments This project is supported by Shandong provincial higher education teaching reform project "Construction of quality early warning system of personnel training in Colleges and Universities" and "Study on the mode of cultivating creative talents centered on digital media platform system "and Shandong finance and economics university teaching and research project"research and practice of the training model of innovative talents platform based on technology competitions".

References

1. Jiaguang Sun (2004) Computer Graphics. Tsinghua University press, Beijing
2. Wang Q (2010) The use of case teaching in computer graphics. J Shanxi Coal-Min Adm Coll:3
3. Zhang S, Li H (2008) Systematic case teaching in Computer Graphics, Career Horizon p 12
4. Wang G, Guo C, Lu D (2012) Case design for computer graphics case teaching, education teaching forum p 16
5. Luo S (2011) Research and implementation of visualization teaching for computer graphics algorithm. J Guangdong Polytech Norm Univ:1
6. Jin R,Wan Z,Liu Y-P (2011) Promoting Reform of the Course "Basic Digital Media Technology"through contests and case studies. J Zhejiang Wanli Univ:3

Chapter 409
The Application of the Morris Water Maze System to the Effect of Ginsenoside Re on the Learning and Memory Disorders and Alzheimer's Disease

Tie Hong, Shunan Liu, Liangjiao Di, Ning Zhang and Xiangfeng Wang

Abstract Aim The aim of this study was to evaluate the effect of Ginsenoside Re on the learning and memory disorders and Alzheimer's disease (AD) by using the Morris Water Maze (MWM) system. Method: Scopolamine was used to induce learning and memory disorders, AD was induced by the D-galactose and chronic aluminum toxicities. The MWM was performed to measure the escape latency, the times to cross the platform and the ratio of the platform quadrant's path length to the total path length. Result: The results showed that the escape latency was prolonged, the ratio of the platform quadrant's path length to the total path length and the times to cross the platform were decreased in the model group as compared with the control group. However, the administration of Ginsenoside Re reversed the prolongation of the escape latency, the decrease of the ratio of the platform quadrant's path length to the total path length and of the times to cross the platform in the scopolamine-treated mouse, while the high-dose administration of Ginsenoside Re reversed those indicators in the D-galactose and chronic aluminum toxicities-treated mouse. Conclusion: It suggested that Ginsenoside Re had a strong effect on the learning and memory disorders and on AD. The application of MWM system provided a reliable method of studying the cognitive function. The data collected by the tracking software was more accurate and convincible than the manual record, which proved that the computerization of MWM could improve the efficiency of MWM and evaluate the mouse's learning and memory ability more comprehensively and objectively.

Keywords The Morris water maze · Computerization · Tracking software · Learning and memory disorders · Alzheimer's disease

T. Hong (✉) · S. Liu · L. Di · N. Zhang
Department of Pharmacology, School of Pharmacy, Jilin University, Changchun, China
e-mail: hongtie@jlu.edu.cn

X. Wang
The Second Hospital, Jilin University, Changchun, China

S. Li et al. (eds.), *Frontier and Future Development of Information Technology in Medicine and Education*, Lecture Notes in Electrical Engineering 269,
DOI: 10.1007/978-94-007-7618-0_409,

409.1 Introduction

The MWM test was used as a primary method of behavioral observation which was designed by a British psychologist Richard GM Morris on early 1980s. Nowadays, the MWM was often used as a general assay for cognitive function [1], such as various disturbances of the nervous system, aging, neurodegenerative disease, or for evaluating the effect of novel therapeutic drugs on some kinds of cognitive disorders. The task had also inspired computational neuroscientists and roboticists interested in navigation [2]. Many tracking software were developed based on the MWM and similarly composed of a computer tracking program and an image processing system, which could track and analyze the movement of the mouse. The movement was reflected mainly by three indicators: the escape latency, the ratio of the platform quadrant's path length to the total path length, and the times to cross the platform. Compared with the manual record, the most advantage of the computerization was that the path length in total or in each quadrant was measured. The computerization can also improve the efficiency and the degree of accuracy of the experiment.

Learning and memory disorders were the major manifestations of aging. AD was a chronic and progressive degenerative disease of nervous system. Because of the complex pathogenesis, AD was very difficult to cure clinically and the toxicity of the western medicine was more than the efficacy. Therefore, to explore a specific Chinese medicine was a valuable task.

In this study, the improvement effect of Ginsenoside Re which was an active component of Ginsenoside on the learning and memory disorders and on AD was investigated with the MWM system.

409.2 Materials and Methods

409.2.1 The Morris Water Maze Test

409.2.1.1 Apparatus

Morris water maze system consisted of a stainless-steel circular tank which was 100 cm in diameter and 38 cm in height, a platform, a camera which was placed above the center of the tank to capture images and connected to a computer, and the tracking software. The Morris water maze system was manufactured by Thai Union Technology Co., Ltd in Chengdu, Sichuan Province.

409.2.1.2 The Preparation of the Test

The Morris water maze test was performed in a circular tank filled with water at the temperature of 22 ± 1 °C. The water was colored opaque with titanium dioxide. The tank was placed in a quiet room with dimly light and ample surrounding visual cues, and was divided into four quadrants. The platform was fixed in the same position of the tank and submerged to 2 cm below the water surface.

Before the test, some parameters should be set in the tracking software. First, opened up a new project, meanwhile, the sample number and the maximum trial time are set. Additionally, loaded the tank calibration into the tracking software. Third, programmed the platform location to remain in the same position throughout all trials. To exclude the interference color which was as bright as the maker color painted onto the mouse's head, the recognizable level of the target should be regulated in the program. The instruction set was shown in Fig. 409.1.

409.2.1.3 Measurement of the Escape Latency

The place navigation test had been done 30 min after the administration during which the platform was placed in the same position and the references around the pool (cues outside the pool), including the experimenter's position was unchanged. In the place navigation test, the mouse was released into the water gently from every quadrant respectively, facing the sidewall of the tank. The time during which the platform was found by the mouse within 120 s was recorded as the escape latency. The average escape latency of the four quadrants was compared between the groups.

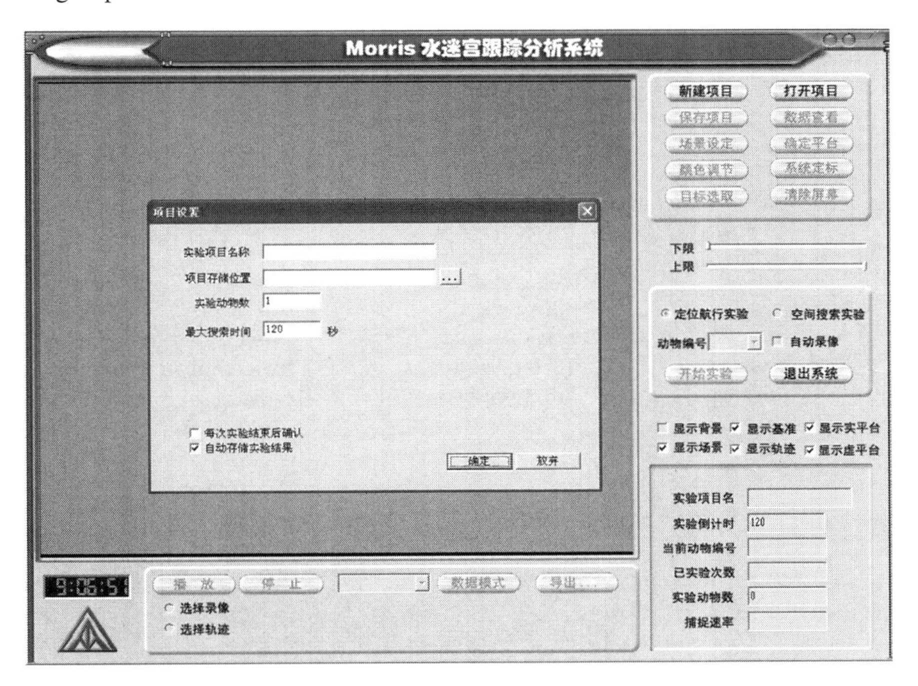

Fig. 409. 1 Open up a new project

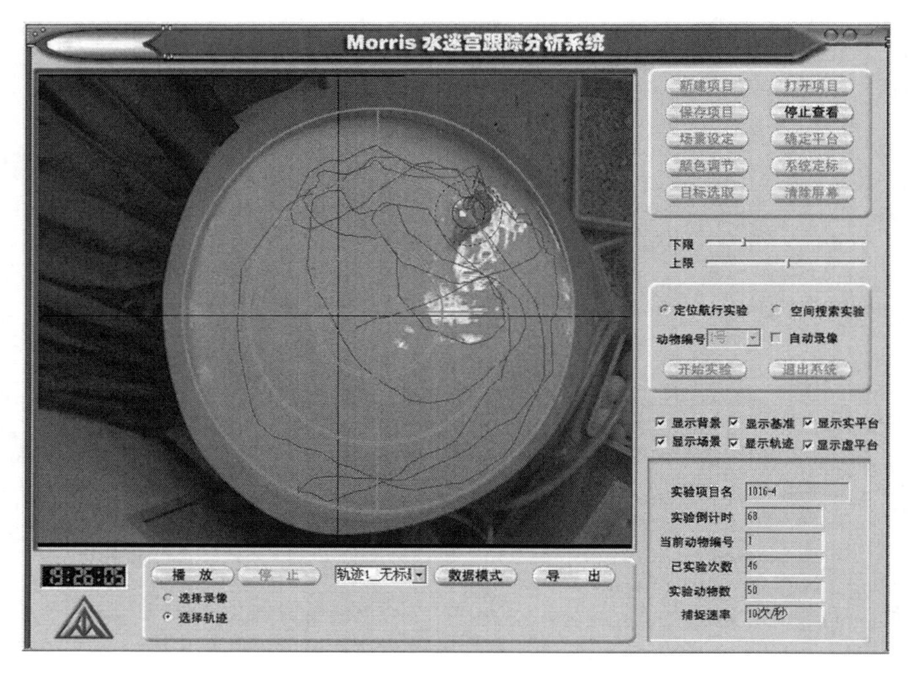

Fig. 409. 2 The place navigation test

There were two protocols in this software: the place navigation test and the spatial probe test. First, chose *the place navigation test* option. Second, ran the computer tracking program and the timer started as the experiment begin. When the mouse reached or touched the platform, the timer stopped automatically, the time was recorded by the computer as the escape latency. Before the test, a time cut-off was set as 120 s by the option of *the maximum trial time*. When the time reached 120 s, the computer tracking program stopped automatically, and the escape latency was recorded as 120 s. At this time, the mouse should be guided to the platform and stayed on it for at least 10 s, which allowed it to remember the position of the platform in relation to surrounding cues. The operation interface of the place navigation test was shown in Fig. 409.2.

409.2.1.4 Records of the Times to Cross the Platform

24 h after the last trial of the place navigation test, the spatial probe test was conducted. In the spatial probe test, the platform was removed, the mouse was arranged to search for it in 120 s. The times to cross the platform were recorded by the computer. The operation interface of the spatial probe test was shown in Fig. 409.3.

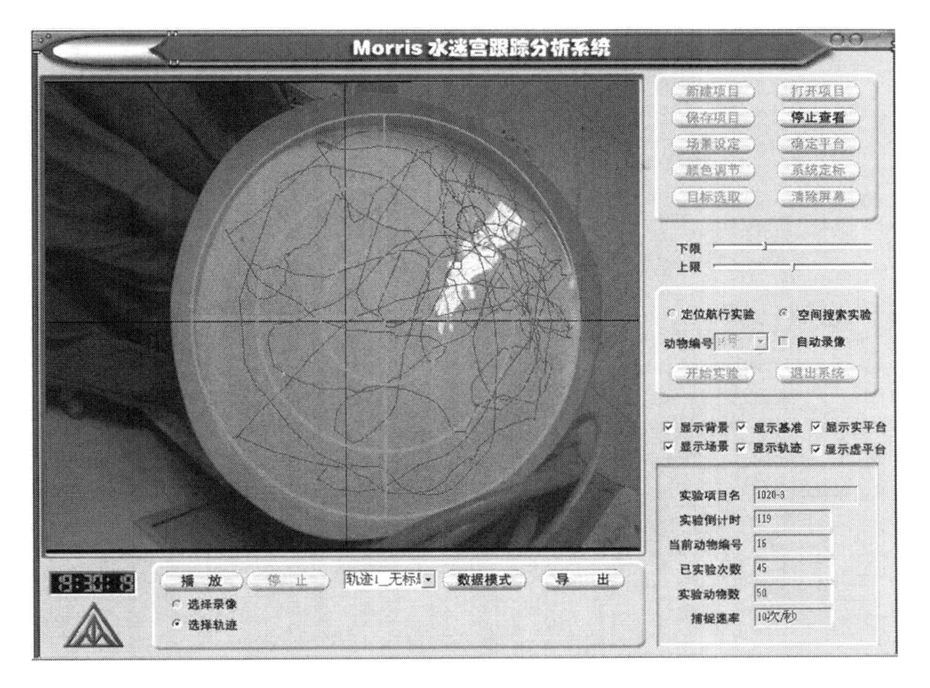

Fig. 409. 3 The spatial probe test

409.2.1.5 The Video of Typical Behavioral Traces

The total path length and platform quadrant's path length were measured. The platform was in the 2nd quadrant, thus the ratio of the 2nd quadrant's path length to the total was calculated. The video recording was optional in the program. The camera detected the trace of the mouse at a rate of 10 times per second automatically, the trace was painted on the screen with the background optional.

409.2.1.6 Derivation of the Data and Trace from the MWM Tracking Software

Choose *data checking* to enter the interface which displayed the trace of the test. Choose *data mode* to check the data.

The escape latency, the ratio of the 2nd quadrant's path length and the total path length, and the times to cross the platform were shown on the interface. The interface of checking the data was shown in Fig. 409.4.

409.2.2 *Animals*

Kunming mice, male, weight 18–22 g, attained by the Experimental Animal Center of Jilin University, the certificate number: 2003-0001.

409.2.3 *The Modeling and Experimental Procedures*

409.2.3.1 The Effect of Ginsenoside Re on Scopolamine-Induced Obtained Learning and Memory Disorder

The place navigation test was performed 30 min after the administration on the 5th day. In addition to the control group, other groups were intraperitoneally injected with scopolamine (2 mg·kg^{-1}) before the place navigation test. The time during which the platform was found by the mouse within 120 s was recorded as the escape latency. The spatial probe test was performed on the 6th day. The times to cross the platform in 120 s were recorded by the computer.

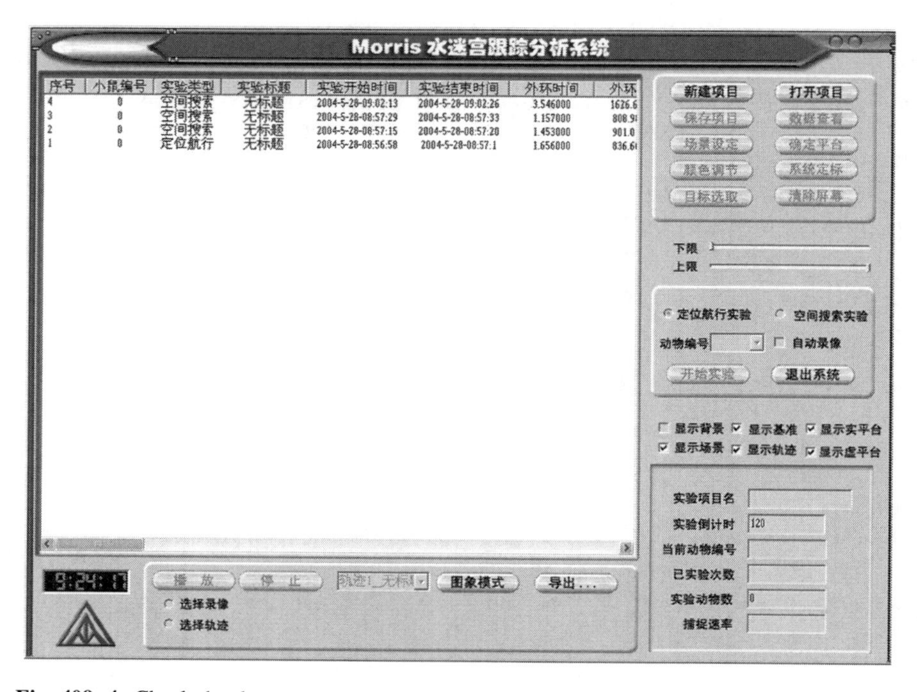

Fig. 409 .4 Check the data

409.2.3.2 The Effect of Ginsenoside Re on D-galactose and Chronic Aluminum Toxicities-Induced Alzheimer's Disease

In addition to the control group, other groups were orally administrated with the aluminum chloride 10 mg·kg^{-1} for consecutive 106 days, the control group was given the same amount of distilled water. From the 45th day, in addition to the control group, other groups received intraperitoneal injection with the D-galactose 120 mg·kg^{-1}·d^{-1}, the control group was injected with the same amount of saline.

The learning and memory ability of the mouse was investigated by the MWM test. The place navigation test has been done 30 min after the administration every other day, for 97 consecutive days. The time, during which the platform was found by the mouse within 120 s, was recorded as the escape latency. 24 h after the last trial of the place navigation test, the spatial probe test was conducted. The times to cross the platform in 120 s were recorded by the computer.

409.3 Results

409.3.1 The Effect of Ginsenoside Re on Scopolamine-Induced Obtained Learning and Memory Disorders

Compared with the model group, the escape latency of the low-dose, middle-dose and high-dose Ginsenoside Re group were significantly shortened on the 5th day ($P < 0.01$ or $P < 0.05$), the ratio of the 2nd quadrant's path length to the total path length on the 5th day of the high-dose, middle-dose and low-dose Ginsenoside Re group were significantly improved ($P < 0.01$ or $P < 0.05$), the times to cross the platform of those groups were significantly increased on the 6th day ($P < 0.05$), as shown in Table 409.1.

409.3.2 The Effect of Ginsenoside Re on D-galactose and Chronic Aluminum Toxicities-Induced Alzheimer's Disease

Compared with the model group, the escape latency of the high-dose Ginsenoside Re group was significantly shortened on the 5th day, the ratio of the 2nd quadrant's path length to the total path length on the 5th day of the high-dose Ginsenoside Re group was significantly improved and the times to cross the platform of the high-dose Ginsenoside Re group were significantly increased on the 6th day ($P < 0.01$ or $P < 0.05$), as shown in Table 409.2.

Table 409.1 The effect of Ginsenoside Re on scopolamine-induced obtained learning and memory disorders

Groups	The escape latency on the 5th day (s)	The times to cross the platform on the 6th day	The 2nd quadrant's path length/ the total path length on the 5th day (%)
The control group	15.36 ± 4.21**	3.7 ± 0.4**	60.85 ± 2.98**
The model group	91.86 ± 14.16	1.3 ± 0.4	27.56 ± 2.53
The Ginsenoside Re group (1 mg·kg^{-1})	51.99 ± 14.03*	2.8 ± 0.5*	40.38 ± 2.97*
The Ginsenoside Re group (2 mg·kg^{-1})	52.06 ± 13.04*	2.7 ± 0.5*	40.72 ± 2.63*
The Ginsenoside Re group (4 mg·kg^{-1})	40.00 ± 10.32**	2.7 ± 0.5*	46.08 ± 3.19**

Table 409.2 The effect of Ginsenoside Re on D-galactose and chronic aluminum toxicities-induced Alzheimer's disease

Groups	The escape latency on the 5th day (s)	The times to cross the platform on the 6th day	The 2nd quadrant's path length/ the total path length on the 5th day (%)
The control group	18.77 ± 14.12**	6.1 ± 3.0*	58.47 ± 2.66**
The model group	51.04 ± 33.07	3.1 ± 2.8	28.87 ± 2.16
The Ginsenoside Re group (1 mg·kg^{-1})	33.35 ± 40.58	4.2 ± 4.2	34.60 ± 2.12*
The Ginsenoside Re group (2 mg·kg-1)	33.12 ± 27.53	4.9 ± 3.2	35.84 ± 2.51
The Ginsenoside Re group (4 mg·kg-1)	24.19 ± 14.68*	5.9 ± 3.4*	39.05 ± 2.48**

409.4 Conclusions

In the past, the data of the MWM test were recorded by the experimenter; the process of the data collection was complex and time-wasting, while the results were liable to the experimenter's subjectivity. It only provided indicators in terms of time including the escape latency, the times to cross the platform, but the path length can not be measured.

The computerization of the MWM test promoted the data collection of MWM system, especially the measurement of the path length. The learning and memory abilities could be evaluated by comparing the ratio of the platform quadrant's path length to the total path length between the groups; the ratio was in direct proportion to the ability.

Statistics suggested that Ginsenoside Re has a strong effect on the learning and memory disorders and AD. In this study, the escape latency, the times to cross the platform and the ratio of the 2nd quadrant's path length to the total path length were measured. The result of the time was coherent with that of the path length, which indicated the path length evaluate the learning and memory abilities objectively.

In general, the computerization of the MWM test could provide more indicators than the manual work, comprehensively observe the process of the mouse's spatial cognition and memory, objectively evaluate the level of learning and memory ability, simplify the operation of MWM system and reduce the data error.

References

1. Brandeis R, Brandys Y, Yehuda S (1989) The use of the morris water maze in the study of memory and learning. Int J Neurosci 48(1–2):29–69
2. Krichmar JL, Seth AK, Nitz DA (2005) Spatial navigation and causal analysis in a brain-based device modellingcortical-hippocampal interactions. Neuroinformatics 5:197–222

Chapter 410
The Application of HYGEYA in Hospital's Antimicrobial Drugs Management

Xiangfeng Wang, Xiujuan Fu, Dasheng Zhu, Yadan Chen, Tie Hong, Shunan Liu, Liangjiao Di and Ning Zhang

Abstract *Purpose* We evaluate the impact of clinical drug analysis software (HYGEYA),which is embedded in the hospital information system (HIS) in the Second Hospital of Jilin University, in order to control overuse and abuse antimicrobials. *Method* HYGEYA is embedded in HIS with drugs basic information and set using rights limit in the HIS. The pharmacists could monitor the use of antimicrobial drugs in real time. *Result* The software which is embedded in HIS is able to control total antimicrobial use density, reduce medical treatment costs and the number of unnecessary antimicrobial prescriptions. *Conclusion* These results suggest that HYGEYA to control the use of antimicrobials is a feasible, cost-saving, suppressing the incidence of drug-resistant bacteria new modality that may help reduce the number of unnecessary antimicrobial prescriptions.

Keywords HIS · HYGEYA · Antimicrobial drugs

410.1 Introduction

Nowadays, the usage of antimicrobial drugs exits a lot of problems in many hospitals. Such as antibiotics use density (AUD) and daily drug number (DDDs) are too high, the clinical rational use ability is insufficient and increased drug-induced diseases. We know that antimicrobial drugs inappropriate use often leads to sudden outbreaks of resistant bacteria. The health administrative departments

X. Wang · X. Fu (✉) · D. Zhu · Y. Chen
The Second Hospital, Jilin University, Changchun, China
e-mail: fxj462003@163.com

T. Hong · S. Liu · L. Di · N. Zhang
School of Pharmacy, Jilin University, Changchun, China

S. Li et al. (eds.), *Frontier and Future Development of Information Technology in Medicine and Education*, Lecture Notes in Electrical Engineering 269,
DOI: 10.1007/978-94-007-7618-0_410,

have promulgated the policies and regulations which related clinical application of them in recent years.

The Second Hospital of Jilin University takes use of hospital information system (HIS) platform efficiently. The medication analysis software (HYGEYA) is embedded in it. Antimicrobial drugs management can be carried out by four aspects: ① antimicrobial drugs classification management ② hospital patients antimicrobial drug usage ③ outpatient antimicrobial drug usage ④ DDDs. We can implement dynamic monitoring for antimicrobial drug, and then effectively strengthen the management of hospital antimicrobial agents.

410.2 The Establishment of the Basic Information

410.2.1 The Maintenance of the Drug Dictionary

On the basis of HIS "drug dictionary", we added the pharmacological classification, dosage, defined daily dose (DDD) and antimicrobial drug classification and other fields. DDD value's maintenance is according to the World Health Organization (WHO) issued DDD value (2011 edition). The rest of the drug information is input, which in accordance with the "New Materia Medica" (version 17) or instruction book.

410.2.2 Make Evaluation Standard for the Rational Use of Drugs

With reference to "Clinical application of antimicrobial drugs guiding principles" [1], "The guide of perioperative preventive application of antimicrobial drugs", "On the notice on the management of clinical application of antimicrobial drugs" (for short "No. 38 document") and the guidelines and instructions of related disease treatment etc. We make evaluation standard for the rational use of drugs. Detailed information is shown in Table 410.1.

Table 410.1 The reasonable evaluation standard of antimicrobial drugs

Item	HYGEA prompt standard (green)	HYGEA warning levels (red)
Outpatient antibiotic drug usage	≤20 %	>20 %
Hospitalized patients antibiotic drug usage	≤60 %	>60 %
Antibiotics use density	≤40	>40
The percentage of drug cost accounts for the total cost	≤40 %	>40 %

410.2.3 On-line Monitoring of Antimicrobial Drugs Classification Management

Based on the antimicrobial drugs hierarchical management rulers established by the Hospital Pharmacy Administration Committee, we maintain drugs information of all the antimicrobial classification properties in the dictionary of the HIS [2]. According to the physicians title rank list provided by the medical department, we maintain the related physician authority information in the dictionary and connect the properties of antimicrobial drugs classification to title of doctor. We forbid primary title doctor opens "restrictions on the use of drugs", "special use of the drug" and ban intermediate title doctor opens "special use of the drug". Related information is shown in Fig. 410.1.

410.2.4 The Warning of Dynamic Monitoring for Antimicrobial Drug Use Index

The Second Hospital of Jilin University introduced the HYGEYA and embedded it into the HIS. Real-time monitor the indicators of antimicrobial drug use in the hospital, which include antimicrobial single variety sales amount, sales volume ranking, DDDs sort of antimicrobial drugs within the same variety, average using variety of antibiotics per inpatients, inpatients using antimicrobial percentage, the percentage of antimicrobial drug cost accounts for the total cost. According to the condition of department reach and out of the indicators, HYGEYA system will give red warning. And it will provide data support for the management of the hospital. Related information is shown in Fig. 410.2.

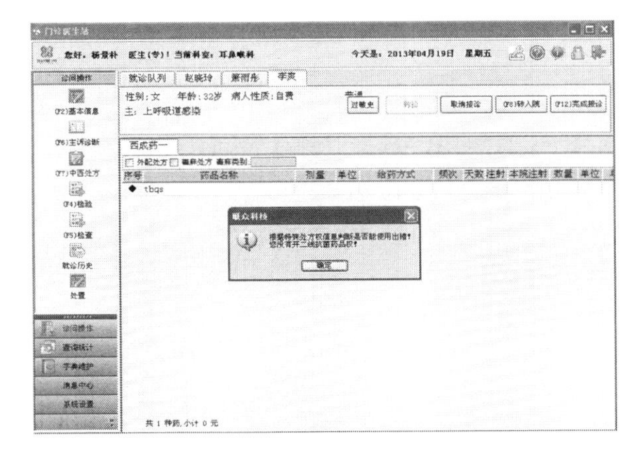

Fig. 410.1 The warning hints of primary physicians prescribe restrictions on the use of antimicrobial drugs

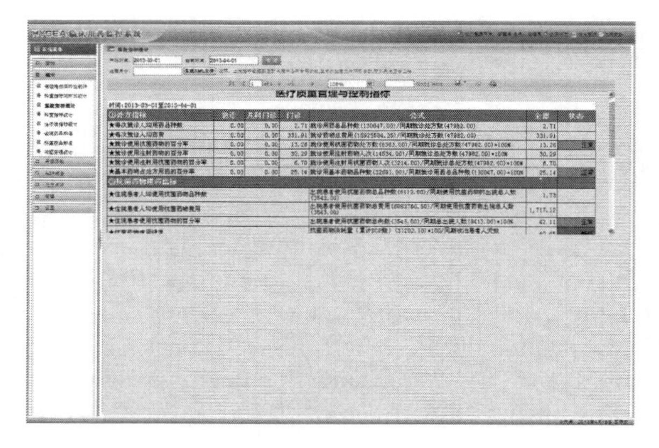

Fig. 410.2 The condition of department reach the indicators monitored by HYGEYA

410.3 The Query of Usage of Antimicrobial Drugs

410.3.1 The Query of Antimicrobial Drugs Index on Year-on-Year Basis

Statistics of outpatient pharmacy of antimicrobial drugs sales amount, DDDs, antimicrobial drug ratio in March. We found that sales amount of antimicrobial drugs decreased significantly in March 2013. Compared with 2012, we realize that antimicrobial drug ratio reduced from 9.60 to 6.42 % in 2013. And at the same time DDDs significantly reduced. Detailed information is shown in Fig. 410.3.

410.3.2 The Query of Usage of Antimicrobial Drugs in Chain Relative Ratio

Basing on the data of all kinds of antimicrobial drugs and DDDs were monitored by HYGEYA. Collate the results of DDDs are shown in Table 410.2.

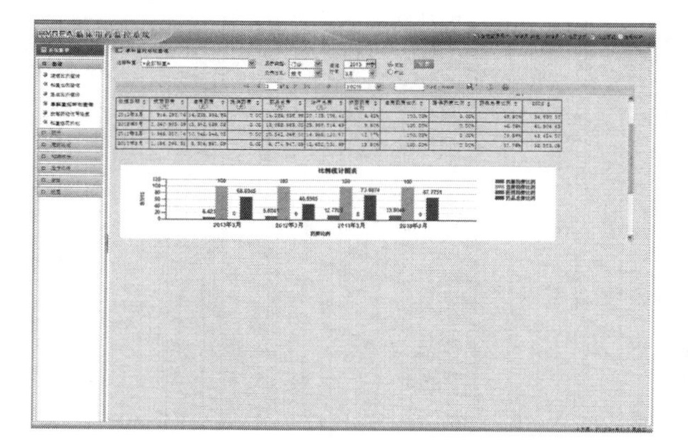

Fig. 410.3 The query results of sale amount and DDDs of outpatients' antimicrobial drugs on year-on-year basis in March 2013

Table 410.2 The order of the top ten antimicrobial drugs and amount sorted by DDDs in March 2013

Drug name	DDDs	Amount of order
Ceftezole Sodium for injection	3407.4	1
Moxifloxacin Hydrochloride tablets	2886.3	8
Erythromycin delayed-Release capsules	2878.2	15
Roxithromycin capsules	2782.7	26
Clarithromycin sustained release tablets l	2759.1	9
Terbinafine hydrochloride tablets	2710.8	2
Cefdinir capsules	2697.1	17
Itraconazole capsules	2134.9	7
Amoxicillin and clavulanate potassium tablets	1771.4	16
Cefuroxime axetil tablets	1442.6	25

410.4 The Effect and Experience of System Implementation Monitored by HYGEYA

The hospital early use of antimicrobial drugs application monitoring method was through regular sampling outpatient prescription and hospitalization records. Then we calculated various kinds of drugs use indicators and monitored the key part of the clinical departments. But the statistical process of this approach was trival, work efficiency was low, there was considerable error rate, and the results of the analysis were laggard.

When we introduce HYGEYA software embedded it on the basis of HIS and implement it. We find that it will accurate statistics and use indicators of antimicrobial drugs and then play an important role in application of antimicrobial drugs monitoring. In this way hospital administrators and medical workers can inquire antimicrobial drugs use indicators, comprehend dynamic application of various clinical departments and the whole hospital departments. Administrators targeted for the department which is out of indicators in application. They will take effective intervention to promote the rational use of antimicrobial drugs.

410.5 Conclusion

The application of this software has the important significance for standardizing prescription behavior, improving the quality of management and researching for the using of antibacterial and suppressing the incidence of drug-resistant bacteria and promoting the function of pharmacist. It could provide some practical experience for exploring the antimicrobial drug monitoring mode, establish the unified normal and practical standards, and realize the clinical monitoring of antibiotics with automation, information, and intelligence ways.

References

1. Xia G (2004) The guiding principles of clinical application of antimicrobial drugs. Chinese Medicine Press, Beijing, pp 12–159
2. Hong T, Fu X (2012) The application of information technology in the hospital pharmacy management based on HIS. ITME 604–607

Chapter 411
The Analysis of Wavelet De-Noising on ECG

Dongxin Lu, Qi Teng and Da Chen

Abstract The wavelet analysis is very popular in ECG de-noising as one of the most powerful tool to analysis or deal with different problems. This paper describes the generation and characteristics of ECG signals, and the origin of its three major noises. Estimating the original signals from the noise has always been an important part in the field of ECG signal processing. Some key methods of traditional de-noising based on Fourier transform and wavelet de-nosing are presented in this paper; the basic idea of the wavelet de-noising and wavelet de-noising method description show that the features and advantages of wavelet de-nosing are better than the traditional ways. Because of wavelet can simultaneously analyze signals in time-frequency, it can effectively distinguish the mutation and noise of useful signal so to realize de-noising of non-stationary signal and remain useful transient signal without loss, so we can find that wavelet de-noising not only reduces cost but also has better result than traditional methods.

Keywords ECG signals · Noise · Traditional de-nosing · Wavelet de-nosing

D. Lu (✉) · Q. Teng
Software College, Nanchang University, Nanchang 330000, China
e-mail: lu.dongxin@zte.com.cn

Q. Teng
e-mail: qianxuntq@163.com

D. Chen
International Education College, Jiangxi Normal University, Nanchang 330000, China
e-mail: 312035611@qq.com

S. Li et al. (eds.), *Frontier and Future Development of Information Technology in Medicine and Education*, Lecture Notes in Electrical Engineering 269,
DOI: 10.1007/978-94-007-7618-0_411,

411.1 The Characteristics of ECG Signals

ECG is a performance of the heart activities over the human body surface; it's a weak signal of MV-level with the changes of the state of human detection and time. ECG is a typical strong noise of non-stationary signals with obvious characteristics of non-stationary, micro energy and signal-to-noise is relatively small. Highly vulnerable to environmental impacts of ECG, it's often accompanied by noises in the course of acquisition, amplification, transmission. These noises mixed with ECG signals distort the ECG waveforms and make the waveforms are so blurred that directly affect the reliability of the ECG waveforms and diagnosis. Therefore, effective de-noising needs to be processed before the ECG automatic diagnosis. As shown in Fig. 411.1 is a typical ECG signals.

411.2 The Origin of ECG Noise

Due to the instrument, the human body and other aspects, the noises in ECG are divided into the following categories [1, 2]:

- Power line interference: Power line interference is interference caused by power system which constituted by the 50 HZ harmonics. In addition, the ambient electromagnetic interference is also an important factor. This interference may obscure the small twist in the ECG and affect the diagnosis of ECG. Figure 411.2 shows the ECG signals with power line interference.
- EMG interference: EMG (electromyography interference) is an interference caused by human activities muscle tension. The nervous, clod stimulus or certain diseases, etc. will also generate high-frequency EMG noise. Figure 411.3 shows the ECG signals with EMG interference.
- Baseline drift: baseline drift is caused by low-frequency interference like the movement of electrode or human breathing. This interference is lower than 1 HZ, is a periodic drift with human breathing. Figure 411.4 shows the ECG signals with baseline drift.

ECG is used to measure the rate and regularity of heartbeats, as well as the size and position of the chambers, the presence of any damage to the heart, and the effects of drugs or devices used to regulate the heart, such as a pacemaker. Most ECGs are performed for diagnostic or research purposes on human hearts, but may also be performed on animals, usually for diagnosis of heart abnormalities or research. However, these noises mixed with ECG distort the ECG waveforms, and generate errors on diagnosis. The ECG signal de-noising is very important and significative.

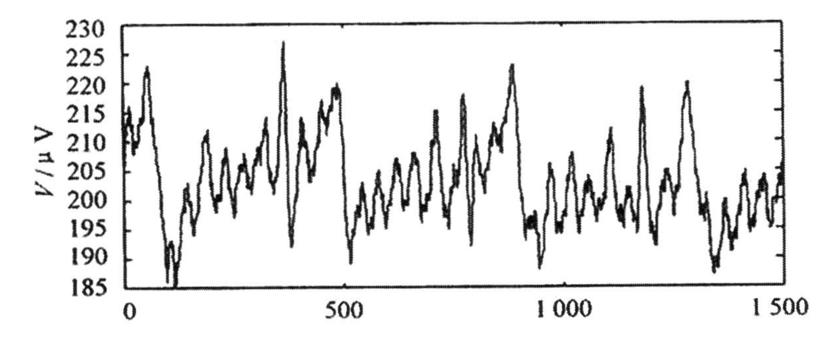

Fig. 411.1 ECG signals

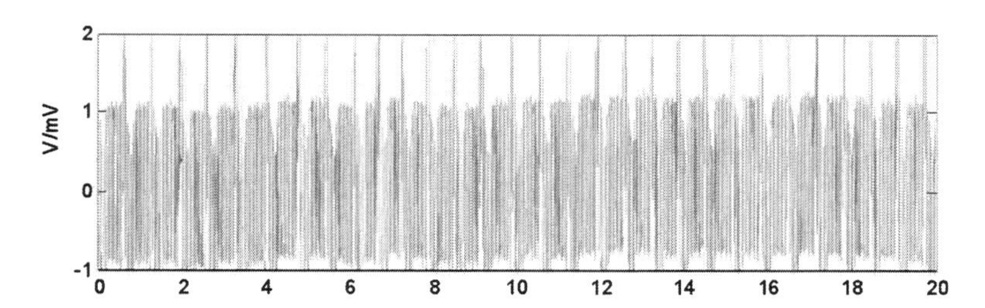

Fig. 411.2 The ECG signals with power line interference

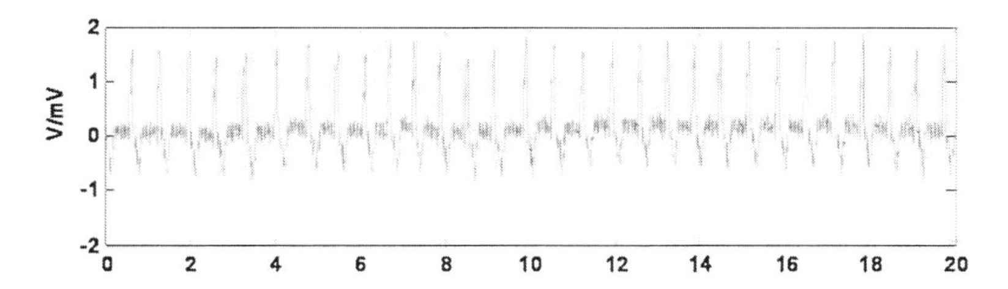

Fig. 411.3 The ECG signals with EMG interference

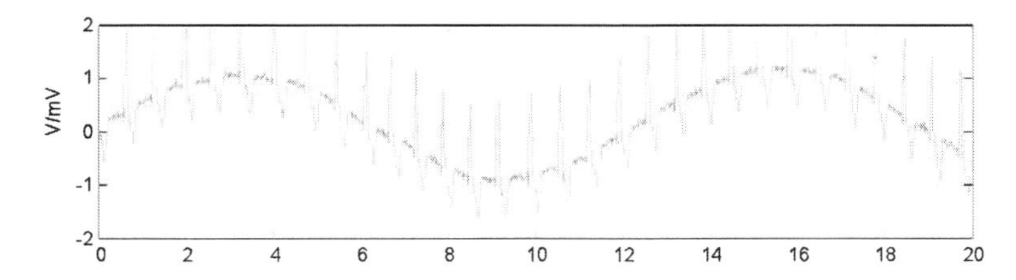

Fig. 411.4 The ECG signals with baseline drift

411.3 The Shortcomings of Traditional De-Noising

The traditional de-noising is mainly based on Fourier transform [1], distinguish different frequency spectrum signals and noises and then design of a digital filter to filter noises. According to the characteristics of time domain impulse response on the digital filters [3], the filters can be divided into infinite impulse response filter (IIR) and finite impulse response filter (FIR).

- Infinite impulse response (IIR) is a property of signal processing systems. IIR systems have an impulse response function that is non-zero over an infinite length of time. This filter has an exponential impulse response characterized by an RC time constant. Because the exponential function is asymptotic to a limit, and thus never settles at a fixed value, the response is considered infinite.
- Finite impulse response (FIR) filter is a filter whose impulse response is of finite duration. It has internal feedback and may continue to respond indefinitely. They can easily be designed to be linear phase by making the coefficient sequence symmetric; linear phase, or phase change proportional to frequency, corresponds to equal delay at all frequencies.

Since the Fourier analysis of the signals is in the frequency domain, it cannot give the changes of signals at a point in time, so each point mutation of the signals on the time axis will affect the entire domain, resulting in the ECG signals distortion, the judgment of certain diseases, and the cost is also high. It is not very satisfactory to filtering the ECG signals. Figure 411.5 shows the ECG signals after de-noising by traditional filtering.

411.4 Wavelet De-Noising

411.4.1 The Basic Ideas of Wavelet De-Noising

Wavelet de-noising is defined as follows: taking advantage of Multi-resolution time-frequency localization characteristics to disintegrate different frequency components of signals into different spatial scales. And further processing of corresponding scales of wavelet coefficients will be conducted [4]. The principle is to eliminate the wavelet coefficients caused by noise, reserve or even strengthen the wavelet coefficient caused by desired signals. Finally, the de-noised signals will be obtained after reconstruction of the treated wavelet coefficient, as shown in Fig. 411.6.

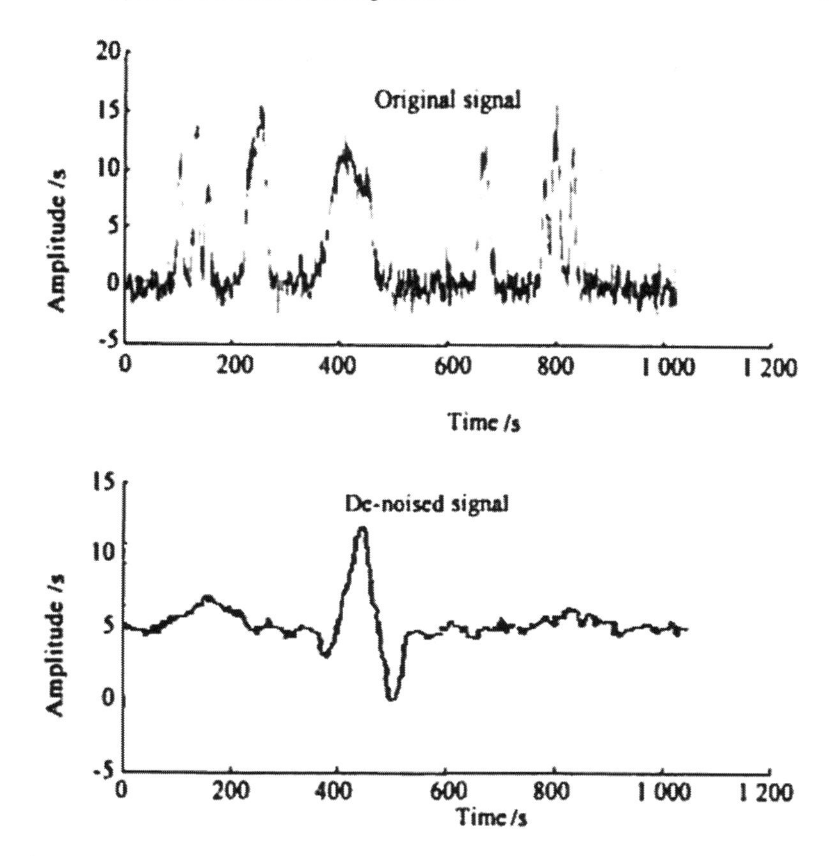

Fig. 411.5 The ECG signals after de-noising by tradition filtering

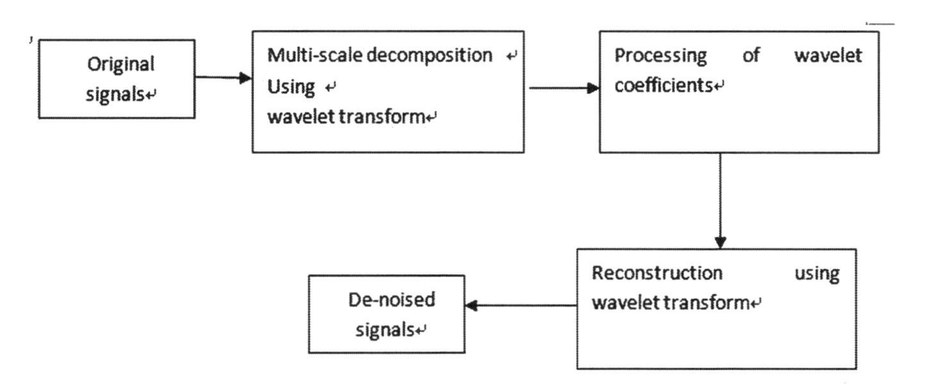

Fig. 411.6 Wavelet de-noising

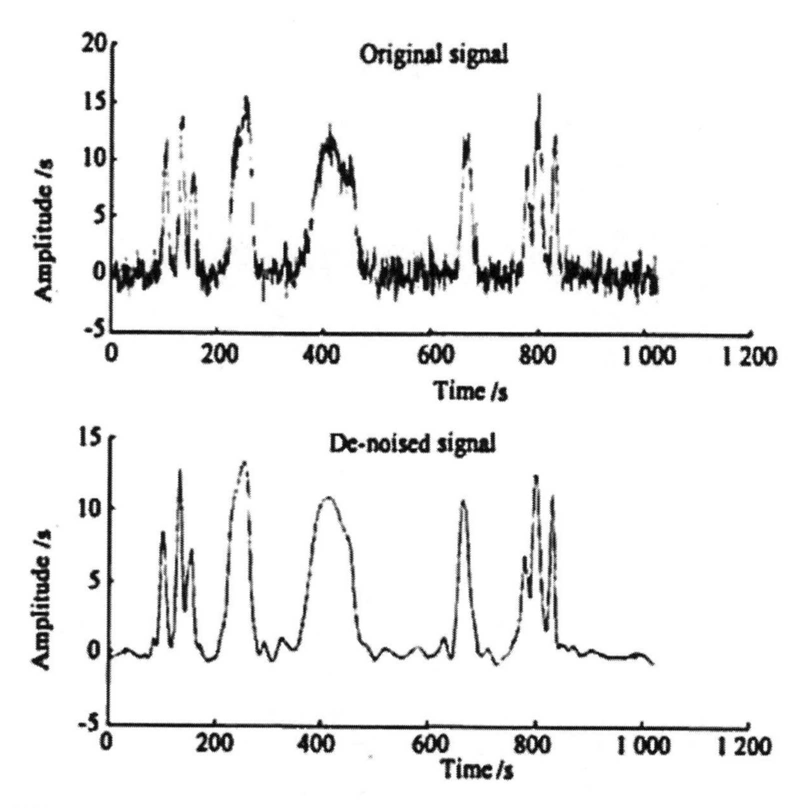

Fig. 411.7 The ECG signals after de-noising by wavelet de-noising

411.4.2 Methods of Wavelet De-Noising

Wavelet modulus maxima de-noising: it's a de-noising approach developed by the different propagation laws of the WT modulus extremum that signals and noises have on multitude scale spaces. Observe the laws of WT modulus maximum swinging on different scales, eliminate the amplitude points (corresponding noise extreme points) decreasing with higher scales, keep the amplitude points (corresponding extreme points of useful signal), then through replacement and projection method, reconstruct on kept wavelet modulus extremum, we can finally reach our goal of de-noising.

Related de-noising: transformed by wavelet, the wavelet modulus of signal has relatively strong relation, especially when it is around the margin of the signal, while the wavelet modulus of noise in the same case does not. In addition, the effect is more obvious on small scale than on big scale (Senhadji 1990; [5]).

Thresholding de-noising: Thresholding de-noising is setting modulus of lower absolute modulus zero but keeping or shrinking those modulus of higher absolute modulus so to get estimated wavelet modulus and then directly reconstructs signal in order to de-noise.

411.5 Summaries

Because wavelet can simultaneously analyze signals in time-frequency, it can effectively distinguish the mutation and noise of useful signal so to realize de-noising of non-stationary signal and remain useful transient signal without loss. As shown in Fig. 411.7, we can see the ECG signals after de-noising by wavelet de-noising can effectively discriminate signals form noise and achieves pretty good performance and we can know wavelet de-noising not only reduces cost but also has better result than traditional methods.

References

1. Singh BN, Tiwari AK (2006) Optimal selection of wavelet basis function applied to ECG signal denoising. Digital Signal Proces 16:275–287
2. Ercelebi E (2004) Electrocardiogram signal de-noising using lifting-based discrete wavelet transform. Comput Biol Med 34:479–493
3. Nazan PA (1997) Online digital filters for biological signals: some fast designs for a small computer. Med Biol Eng Comput 15:534–540
4. Mallat SA (1998) A wavelet tour of signal processing, California. doi: 10.1007/s001090000086
5. Mallat S. A (1989) A theory for multircslution signal decomposition: The wavelet represention. IEEE Trans PAMI 11:674–693

Chapter 412
Research of Education Training Model by Stages for College Students' Information Literacy

Jinyuan Zhou and Tianling Zhou

Abstract As the required knowledge and ability for humans, information literacy has gained more and more widespread attentions from the domain of international education. It's one of the important goals for personnel training of higher education to provide college students information literacy education. Efforts have been made to develop the students' information consciousness, information skills, information morality and to improve college students' ability of creative thinking and problem-solving skills. Based on the information literacy questionnaire for undergraduates from Jiangsu University and Yangzhou University, and the citation analysis of master thesis in Vehicle Engineering, Jiangsu University from 2010 to 2012, this research is aiming to put forward the new training model by stages for college students' information literacy, and to construct a complete training system which is adapted to the present domestic university development and the training focus of different stages.

Keywords Information literacy · Questionnaire survey · Citation analysis

412.1 Introduction

Information literacy is the required knowledge and ability during human's information activities in modern society, which is an important part of one's cultural cultivation. To develop good information literacy is the primary target of

J. Zhou (✉) · T. Zhou
Institute of Science and Technology Information of Jiangsu University, 301 Xuefu Road, Jiangsu 212013 Zhenjiang, China
e-mail: 1000007163@mail.ujs.edu.cn

T. Zhou
e-mail: zhoutianling923@126.com

S. Li et al. (eds.), *Frontier and Future Development of Information Technology in Medicine and Education*, Lecture Notes in Electrical Engineering 269,
DOI: 10.1007/978-94-007-7618-0_412,

information education and important part of cultivating innovative talents. The State Education Commission issued documents in 1984, "Literature Retrieval and Utilization" course is required to offer in colleges and universities with two purposes: to enhance students' information intelligence consciousness and to improve students' information retrieval skills [1]. During the next 20 years, the vast majority of colleges and universities setup the corresponding courses, to provide students training of information retrieval and utilization. However, the models and contents were different with each other, and the common consensus was not reached.

We are trying to make the combination of the existing research results with information literacy characteristics of college students in different grades by observing the situation of students' information literacy in different stages, based on the summarization of predecessors' information literacy training, to put forward the new training model by stages for college students' information literacy.

412.2 Objects and Methods

412.2.1 Survey on Information Literacy of Undergraduates

412.2.1.1 Survey Objectives

The survey is to acquaint the basic situation of the information literacy of undergraduate students at campus, to clarify the direction for university undergraduate information literacy training, also to provide basis for the establishment of college undergraduate information literacy training strategy [2].

412.2.1.2 Respondents

The respondents of this survey are full-time undergraduates from Jiangsu University and Yangzhou University. These two universities are in different types with distinguished characteristics. Jiangsu University is a polytechnic college, who is good at Vehicle Engineering, Mechanical Engineering, Material Science, etc., while Yangzhou University is a comprehensive university covering Humanities, Natural Science, Social Science, Technical Science, and so on.

412.2.1.3 Survey Methods

This survey used three methods including questionnaire survey, interview survey and literature survey to meet the requirements of the quantitative and qualitative research.

412.2.1.4 Status of the Questionnaire Survey

There were totally 1000 copies questionnaires provided, 500 copies for Jiangsu University and 500 for Yangzhou University, covering most undergraduate disciplines and specialties of these two universities. 637 questionnaires were returned, the recovery rate was 63.7 percentages.

412.2.2 Survey on Information Literacy of Postgraduates

412.2.2.1 Data Sources

In this article, 191 excellent master theses in Vehicle Engineering, Jiangsu University from 2010 to 2012 were retrieved via CNKI database and Wanfang database. Among them, 21 were from CNKI and 170 came from Wanfang, 167 articles remained by removing the duplicated. Finally, these 167 articles from Jiangsu University Vehicle Engineering were used for citation analysis in this article.

412.2.2.2 The Observation Indexes

Observed the quotation number, the literature types and proportion adopted in the dissertations, the number of literature types, the ability to use references and keywords standardization of 167 master theses from Vehicle Engineering, Jiangsu University.

412.3 Results and Analysis

412.3.1 Information Literacy of Undergraduates

412.3.1.1 Information Consciousness and Information Requirements

50.92 % of the fresh undergraduates in the respondents went to library more than 3 times a week, showing clear dependency on library, while only 6.78 % would never go library. 72 % undergraduates above first grade went to library 1–2 times each week in comparison, but none of them said has never been to the library. The results showed that the undergraduates above first grade had stronger desire for information than fresh undergraduates, on the other side indicated there is a lack of the current library information service system, which is not attractive enough for fresh undergraduates.

412.3.1.2 Information Query Behaviour and Information Skills

The paper library resources utilization was up to 92.49 % among the fresh undergraduates in the respondents, while 80.20 % undergraduates above first grade used e-journal database as their common resources. It showed that the library should continue to strengthen the construction of paper resources, and should also strengthen the propaganda service of resource on the other hand, to provide a powerful resource support for users' information literacy training [3].

412.3.1.3 Information Use Behaviour and Information Morality

Only 35.53 % of the fresh undergraduates in the respondents would always indicate the attribution when they referred to the contents of other's work, on the whole, the intellectual property right consciousness was not strong. On the other hand, there was a stronger intellectual property right consciousness during undergraduates above first grade, but the number was still only 65.24 %, which has become a hidden trouble of the protection for the library intellectual property.

412.3.1.4 Information Communication Behaviour

From the aspect of information communication, only 45.09 % undergraduates would use the method of group learning in the learning process. There were several factors that affect user group discussion from the results of the survey, 41.92 % of the fresh undergraduates thought the chief factors were no need to communicate and lack of communication skills and experience. So we need to start with training of communication skills to promote college students' group communication model, inspiring the users' information consciousness, increasing the users' information knowledge and improving the user's information ability, to constraint information ethical behaviour in group communication culture environment, which will benefit the improvement of information literacy fully.

412.3.2 Investigation of Postgraduate Information Literacy

412.3.2.1 Contrastive Analysis of Amount Quotation

Table 412.1 shows that the quotation number of students' references was keep in a stable state on the whole, however, Chinese literature utilization rate was about three times as much as the utilization rate of foreign literature during the three years from 2010 to 2012, which indicated that further improvement was needed for the foreign language level and ability of postgraduates in Vehicle Engineering. In addition, 2045 foreign references were all in English for the 167 master theses,

Table 412.1 Distribution table of the master thesis quotation amount in vehicle engineering from 2010 to 2012

Years	Article number	Total quotation	Chinese amount	Foreign amount	Percentage in Chinese (%)	Percentage in foreign (%)
2010	55	2883	2188	695	75.81	24.11
2011	56	2807	2099	708	74.78	25.22
2012	55	3003	2361	642	78.62	21.38
Total	167	8693	6648	2045		

none of them used second language besides English in the references, which reflected the reading range of foreign literature was narrow for postgraduates, and reading ability was poorer for other languages.

412.3.2.2 Analysis of all the Types of Literature Quotation

From Table 412.2, there was consistency in the types of literature referenced in the master theses of Vehicle Engineering 2010–2012 from the aspects of number and type; the postgraduates had preference for journals, monographs and dissertations when they wrote the master theses, which illustrated the postgraduates focused more on the frontier academic achievements in their research field. Furthermore, the newspaper and reports were at the last with 0.05 %, showing the ability was not strong for the postgraduates in literature retrieval and only limited to retrieve the literature easier to access, which the phenomenon was not conducive to the postgraduates to have a comprehensive understanding of the knowledge and scientific researches in their research field.

412.3.2.3 Number of the Adopted Literature Types

From Table 412.3, there was only 1 dissertation referenced all 7 types of literature in the 167 master theses in the research, and the number was 121 which referenced three to four types of literature, which accounted for 72.5 % in the researched samples. There are totally dozens of types of literature, which indicated the postgraduates were lack of the ability to collect knowledge and literature, only applied to certain kinds of literature one-sidedly and few students could make use of various literatures correctly for scientific research.

412.3.2.4 Ability to Use References and Keywords Standardization

There existed various types of format error in partial references of the dissertations, mainly for the following: duplicated and missing of serial number, missing of literature type and mark error, missing of published date and missing of author.

Table 412.2 Types of literature quotation distribution table of the master thesis in vehicle engineering from 2010 to 2012

Type Years	J	D	M	N	C	P	S	R	EB/ OL	Z	Total
2010	1562	508	625	2	56	14	65	12	18	11	2883
2011	1541	543	589	1	65	11	12	20	17	8	2807
2012	1633	651	564	1	84	6	33	11	18	2	3003
Total	4736	1702	1788	4	205	31	110	43	53	21	8693

Note *J* for Journal, *D* for Dissertation, *M* for Monograph, *N* for Newspaper, *C* for Collection/Conference Proceeding, *P* for Patent, *S* for Standardization, *R* for Report, *EB/OL* for Electronic Bulletin and Online, *Z* for Undefined

Table 412.3 Distribution table of the number of references types (The letter N in the table = 1, 2, 3, 4, 5, 6, 7)

References types(Type)	1	2	3	4	5	6	7
N of literature referenced in 2010	0	0	16	19	17	4	0
N of literature referenced in 2011	0	2	20	25	5	4	0
N of literature referenced in 2012	0	1	20	20	10	3	2
Total	0	3	56	65	32	11	1

Standardize the references format of dissertation is not only beneficial to come into the uniform format and neat appearance, and easy to retrieve and utilize the related literature for those who will use the dissertation, but also embodies the information literacy level the dissertation's author.

In the objectives researched in this article, parts of postgraduates did not understand the definition of key word, extracted from the passage and the topic optionally, which makes the key words extraction cannot accurately grasp the centrepiece of academic papers, which is also against the retrieval and utilization for others.

412.4 Discussions

412.4.1 Construction of College Students' Information Literacy Training System

According to the survey, the demands for information literacy were not totally the same between fresh undergraduates, undergraduates above first grade and postgraduates. So we advocate building the college students' information literacy training model by stages, to construct complete training system.

412.4.2 Key Points of Information Literacy Training in Every Stage

412.4.2.1 Key Points of Information Literacy Training by Stages for Fresh Undergraduates

The information consciousness of fresh university students is not strong, to educate them about "How to Make Use of Library in Colleges and Universities" is an effective way to rapidly improve the situation. The entrance education of the library should not only contain the readers' rules and regulations, services and the basic book classification and retrieval method, but also include the improvement of college students' information literacy, linkage of theory and practice and equal attention paid to knowledge and application.

412.4.2.2 Key Points of Information Literacy Training by Stages for Undergraduates Above First Grade

After a year's study of some common courses and basic courses, the fresh undergraduates almost adapt to campus study and life, and also have some foundational knowledge. This period is an initial stage for the students to construct their knowledge framework, so it's necessary to offer courses for science and technology literature retrieval based on the characteristics of different specialties, contents can include basic knowledge of the information retrieval, information retrieval system of commonly used Chinese-foreign language, the special literature and network information resource retrieval, etc. The students could use the knowledge of literature retrieval to access information, from which they can enhance their retrieval skills, and expand their professional knowledge.

412.4.2.3 Key Points of Information Literacy Training by Stages for Postgraduates

The postgraduates have the basic skills of information retrieval, with the gradual improvement of their cognitive level, it is particularly important for postgraduates to set up courses in utilization of literature at this time. In the meantime, teachers from each discipline must cooperate with the information literary education according to the characteristics of their own specialized courses, to arrange the necessary professional information ability trainings, mainly include the innovation of scientific research and information analysis, related information evaluation of scientific research, the main information resources at home and abroad, the applications of scientific research fund and related information retrieval, the forms of research result and preparation of public information, and so on. Need to give the students more questions and let themselves think to resolve. The students can do creative work by analyzing, utilizing, evaluating and organizing the specialized literature information they retrieved from different disciplines, to make the students not only consolidate the knowledge they learnt, but also carried on the creative practice [4].

References

1. Liu J, Ye Y, Xun S (2007) The development of university library service mode. Libr Inf Serv 51(12):66–69. [In Chinese]
2. Xin W (2007) Study on status quo and cultivation strategies of il with university students under net work environment (Master Thesis). Tongji University, Shanghai [in Chinese]
3. Yun L (2003) Research on user education of academic libraries under the network environment (master thesis). Sichuan University, Chengdu [In Chinese]
4. Zhou J (2009) An advanced tutorial of information literacy for postgraduates. Jiangsu University Press, Jiangsu [in Chinese]

Chapter 413
Effect of Bufei Granules on the Levels of Serum Inflammatory Markers in Rats with Chronic Obstructive Pulmonary Disease Stable Phase

Sijia Guo, Zengtao Sun, Enshun Liu, Jihong Feng, Wei Liu, Peng Guan and Jingshen Su

Abstract *Objective* To observe the effect of Bufei Granules on the levels of serum inflammatory markers in rats with chronic obstructive pulmonary disease (COPD) stable phase. *Methods* 60 health male Wistar rats were randomly divided into the control group (CG, n = 24) and the COPD stable phase model group (MG, n = 36). The rats in the CG breathed the fresh air for 30 days. However the rats in the MG were given by cigarette smoke 30 min daily for 30 days and we also instilled the lipopolysaccharide (LPS) into their airways on the 1st and the 14th day during the period. After that, we selected 12 rats from the two groups respectively to assess whether the COPD stable phase rat model was made successfully or not by observing the pathological slices of the lung tissue, and to detect the levels of serum interleukin-6 (IL-6), interleukin-8 (IL-8), tumor necrosis factor-α (TNF-α) and high-sensitivity C-reactive protein (hs-CRP) by the method of enzyme-linked immunosorbent assay (ELISA). Then the 24 rats remained in the MG were divided into the control treatment group (CTG) and the Bufei Granules intervention group (BGIG) randomly, 12 rats each group. Hereafter, the rats in the CG and the CTG were given by saline, and the rats in the BGIG were treated by Bufei Granules solution. Treatment lasted for 90 days. At last, we used ELISA to detect the levels of serum IL-6, IL-8, TNF-α and hs-CRP in the rats. Results: We could find the pathological features of chronic bronchitis and emphysema in pathological slices of the lung tissue in the MG, and the levels of IL-6, IL-8, TNF-α and hs-CRP in the MG were higher ($P < 0.05$) than those in the CG. After treatment, the serum levels of IL-8, TNF-α and hs-CRP lowered significantly ($P < 0.05$) in the BGIG. Conclusions: Bufei Granules might be an effective drug to mitigate the severity of inflammation in COPD stable phase.

S. Guo · Z. Sun (✉) · E. Liu · J. Feng · W. Liu · PengGuan · J. Su
The Second Affiliated Hospital of Tianjin University of Traditional Chinese Medicine, Tianjin 300150, China
e-mail: sunzengtao20042@sina.cn

S. Li et al. (eds.), *Frontier and Future Development of Information Technology in Medicine and Education*, Lecture Notes in Electrical Engineering 269,
DOI: 10.1007/978-94-007-7618-0_413,

Keywords Bufei granules · Chronic obstructive pulmonary disease · Stable phase · IL-6 · IL-8 · TNF-α · Hs-CRP

413.1 Introduction

Chronic obstructive pulmonary disease (COPD) is a preventable and treatable disease characterized by not fully reversible airflow limitation, it develops gradually and relates to inflammatory response induced by cigarette smoke and other harmful gases or particles in the lung [1]. In the process of COPD, there is micro-inflammatory state characterized by elevated inflammatory cytokines in the systemic circulation. Therefore, reducing the levels of serum inflammatory markers is beneficial to alleviate the micro-inflammation in treatment of COPD stable phase. In this study, we used Wistar rats as research subjects to make COPD stable phase model, so as to observe the effect of Bufei Granules on the levels of serum interleukin-6 (IL-6), interleukin-8 (IL-8), tumor necrosis factor-α (TNF-α) and high-sensitivity C-reactive protein (hs-CRP). It helped us explore and understand the treatment mechanism of Bufei Granules.

413.2 Materials and Methods

413.2.1 Experimental Materia

413.2.1.1 Experimental Animals

Sixty healthy and clean Wistar rats, male, weighing 180 $\pm$ 20 g, were purchased from Tianjin mountains and red Laboratory of Animal Science and Technology Co., Ltd [license number: SCXK (Tianjin) 2009-0001]. Rearing conditions: Clean-level, indoor temperature 18–22 °C, relative humidity 50–70 %, fixed illumination time, daytime lighting time: 8:00 am–8:00 pm, water and food ad libitum. All rats were acclimatized to new environment of laboratory for 1 week.

413.2.1.2 Treatment Drugs

Bufei Granules solution: Pharmaceutical Centre of the Second Affiliated Hospital of Tianjin University of Traditional Chinese Medicine provided the crude drug and made them into decoction (Bufei Granules, Production batch number: 200702003; composed by *Radix Codonopsis, Radix Rehmanniae Praeparata, Fructus Corni, Herba Ephedrae, and Pericarpium Citri Tangerinae,* etc.). We added 10,000 ml distilled water into 1,000 g crude drug, extracted twice for 1 h each time, filtered, and concentrated to 2,000 ml under the atmospheric pressure. At last, the concentration of crude drug of Bufei Granules solution was 0.50 g/ml, refrigerated in 4 °C.

413.2.1.3 Reagents

Lipopolysaccharide (LPS) was provided by SIGMA. IL-6, IL-8, TNF-α and hs-CRP enzyme-linked immunosorbent assay (ELISA) detection kits were provided by the eBioscience.

413.2.2 Experimental Methods

413.2.2.1 Animal Groups

Sixty health male Wistar rats were randomly divided into the control group (CG, n = 24) and the COPD stable phase model group (MG, n = 36). At the end of the modeling, we selected 12 rats from the two groups respectively to assess whether the COPD stable phase rat model was made successfully or not. Then the 24 rats remained in the MG were divided into the control treatment group (CTG) and the Bufei Granules intervention group (BGIG) randomly, 12 rats each group.

413.2.2.2 Method of Making Control and Disease Model

We used the method of cigarette smoke exposure combined with LPS airway instillation to make COPD stable phase model. The rats in the MG breathed cigarette smoke in toxin exposure glass box (30 × 40 × 50 cm), a cigarette for a rat, 10 rats once time, 30 min daily for 30 days. Meanwhile we instilled 200 μl LPS aqueous solution (1 mg/ml) into their airways in the case of ether inhalation anesthesia on the 1st and the 14th day during the period of making model. Then we bred them conventionally for 2 weeks in order to achieve the COPD stable phase. However, the rats in the CG breathed the fresh air for 30 days, and we instilled 200 μl saline into their airways alternatively.

413.2.2.3 Trial Treatment

After making model, the rats in the CG and CTG were given by saline orally, 1 ml/100 g, one time daily, and the rats in the BGIG were treated by Bufei Granules solution orally, 0.01 ml/(g . day), one time daily. The treatment lasted for 90 days.

413.2.2.4 Specimen Collection and Preparation

At the end of modeling, we selected 12 rats from the CG and MG respectively to collect the lung tissue and serum. Specific methods: With 3 % aqueous solution of sodium pentobarbital 80 mg/kg intraperitoneal anesthesia, we opened the chest to take the middle of the right lung tissue, placed them in 10 % neutral formalin to fix and make hematoxylin-eosin staining (HE staining) pathological slices. Then we opened the abdominal cavity and separated the abdominal aorta after alcohol disinfection, so as to exsanguinate 2 ml blood from abdominal aorta. After that, we centrifuged it under the condition of 4 °C for 10 min at 3,000 r/min to obtain the serum. After treatment, all 36 rats in the CG, CTG and BGIG were drawn to collect serum by the same method.

413.2.3 Outcome Measures

413.2.3.1 General States of Rats and Lung Tissue Biopsy

413.2.3.2 Detection of the Levels of Serum IL-6, IL-8, TNF-α and hs-CRP by the Method of enzyme-linked immunosorbent assay (ELISA)

413.2.4 Statistical Analysis

Quantitative data were summarized as mean ± standard deviation ($\bar{x} \pm s$). Paired *t* test was used for before and after treatment comparisons within the CG, CTG and BGIG, while independent samples *t* test was used between the CG and MG. We applied one-way ANOVA in comparing the data of three groups. Non-parametric test was used when data were not normally distributed. Statistical analysis was performed using SPSS 11.5 software and $P < 0.05$ was considered statistically significant.

413.3 Results

413.3.1 General States of Rats

Observing in the process of making model, the rats in the CG were well developed, lively, responsive, strong and stout. They had glossy leather and good appetite. The weight increased gradually. However, the rats in the MG coughed and wheezed. The intake of water and food reduced, so their weight decreased significantly.

Observing in the process of treatment, there was no significant change in the CG and CTG, while the rats in the BGIG improved significantly, such as increased activity and intake of water and food, relief of shortness of breath, etc.

413.3.2 Lung Histopathological Changes

We could find the pathological features of chronic bronchitis and emphysema in pathological slices of the lung tissue in the MG after making model.

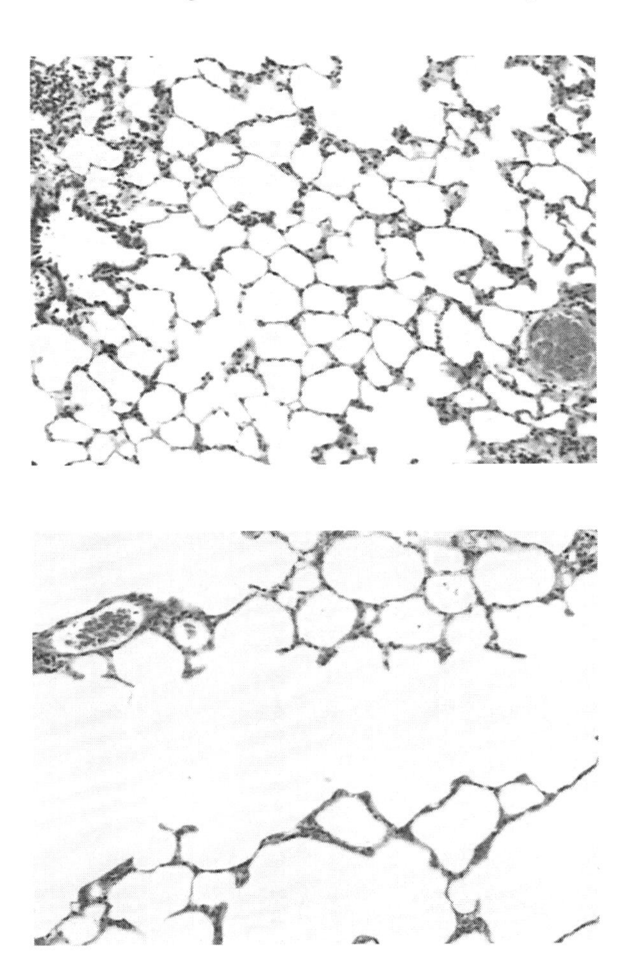

Table 413.1 Serum levels of inflammatory markers after modeling ($\bar{x} \pm s$, *Unit* ng/l)

Groups	hsCRP	IL-6	IL-8	TNF-α
Control group	724.82 ± 24.61	478.43 ± 92.37	315.56 ± 92.33	482.67 ± 67.99
Model group	1825.70 ± 101.77[a]	1321.87 ± 56.56[a]	1268.40 ± 82.60[a]	1423.13 ± 74.54[a]

[a] Compared with the control group, $P < 0.05$

413.3.3 Serum Levels of Inflammatory Markers After Making Model

After making model, the serum levels of IL-6, IL-8, TNF-α and hs-CRP of the rats in the MG increased significantly ($P < 0.05$) (Table 413.1).

413.3.4 Serum Levels of Inflammatory Markers Before and After Treatment

In comparison of between before and after treatment, the serum levels of IL-8, TNF-α and hs-CRP of the rats in the BGIG decreased significantly ($P < 0.05$), while there was no statistical difference ($P > 0.05$) in the serum level of IL-6 of the rats in the BGIG. Also, there was no statistical difference ($P > 0.05$) in the serum levels of IL-6, IL-8, TNF-α and hs-CRP of the rats in the CG and CTG (Table 413.2).

After treatment, there were significant differences ($P < 0.05$) in the serum levels of IL-8, TNF-α and hs-CRP between the rats in the CTG and BGIG, while we could not observe significant differences ($P > 0.05$) in the serum levels of IL-8, TNF-α and hs-CRP between the rats in the CG and BGIG. There was no statistical difference ($P > 0.05$) in the serum level of IL-6 between the rats in the CTG and BGIG, while there was significant differences ($P < 0.05$) in the serum level of IL-6 between the rats in the CG and BGIG.

413.4 Discussion

Chronic inflammatory response plays an important role in the pathogenesis of COPD, and widely involves the airway, the lung parenchyma, and pulmonary vascular. In our study, we found that Bufei Granules could lower the serum levels of IL-8, TNF-α and hs-CRP in rats with COPD stable phase significantly, while maintain the serum level of IL-6. TNF-α is a central and crucial factor in the process of inflammation, it can activate TNF-α receptor to promote the release of IL-6 and IL-8. IL-8 causes migration of inflammatory cells to the location of

Table 413.2 Serum levels of inflammatory markers before and after treatment, ($\bar{x}\pm s$, *Unit* ng/l)

Groups		IL-6	IL-8	TNF-α	hsCRP
Control	Before treatment	478.43 ± 92.37	315.56 ± 92.33	482.67 ± 67.99	724.82 ± 24.61
	After treatment	473.97 ± 24.76	320.36 ± 18.36	479.76 ± 26.85	732.42 ± 20.34
Control treatment	Before treatment	1321.87 ± 56.56	1268.40 ± 82.60	1423.13 ± 74.54	1825.70 ± 101.77
	After treatment	1334.58 ± 23.74	1206.22 ± 23.85	1463.29 ± 32.13	1831.85 ± 101.36
Bufei granule intervention	Before treatment	1321.87 ± 56.56	1268.40 ± 82.60	1423.13 ± 74.54	1825.70 ± 101.77
	After treatment	1252.87 ± 23.44	333.47 ± 13.23	475.99 ± 23.86	742.70 ± 23.23

inflammation especially in neutrophils, providing a binding capacity for neutrophils to the inflammatory spots, and also amplifies the effect of airway inflammation. IL-6 might enhance the pulmonary immune function and up-regulate the local immune response to reduce the inflammatory response. CRP is the most important acute phase response protein, so it is an ideal inflammatory marker to reflect the severity of inflammation response.

In traditional Chinese medicine (TCM), COPD is similar to the diseases named "lung-distention", "dyspnea syndrome", "phlegm retention" and "internal injury cough", etc. From the perspective of TCM theory, COPD mainly affects the lung in the early stage of pathophysiology, and with the progression of the disease, eventually leads to Ben deficiency Branch excess syndrome characterized by Yangqi deficiency of the lung, spleen and kidney, accompanied with retention of phlegm and blood stasis. The pathogenesis of COPD stable phase is more deficiency and less evil, so we use the treatment principle of strengthening Zhengqi primarily combined with dispelling blood stasis, resolving phlegm and relieving wheeze to treat it. Bufei granule is formulated based on the above treatment principle, thus it could enhance the immune function of the lung, improve the function of Zangfu, and alleviate the severity of inflammation.

Acknowledgments The research was supported by the International Cooperation Project of Science and Technology of National Ministry of Science and Technology (2011DFA32750).

Reference

1. Chinese Society of Respiratory Diseases, Chronic obstructive pulmonary disease study group (2007) Chronic obstructive pulmonary disease treatment guidelines (2007 Revision). J Intern Med 46(3):254–261

Chapter 414
Design of Remote Medical Monitoring System

Dongxin Lu and Yuanbo Qin

Abstract This paper first introduces the background and technologies of telemedicine briefly. Then it introduce the development and status of remote medical monitoring system and sums up their deficiencies. In response to these deficiencies, it introduces a remote medical monitoring system, which is consist of data collecting module, pre-processing module and monitoring module. By collecting and processing three physiological data–ECG, pulse and body temperature, they system can achieve the health care of the users. This paper focuses on the pre-processing module, an Android application, installed on your smart phone based on Android platform, which can realize real-time processing of data, display it to user and give a certain degree of warning.

Keywords KDD · AI · HIS · Medical industry · Information system

414.1 Telemedicine and Remote Medical System

Traditional remote medical monitoring system has equipment limitation, space limitation and time limitation. In other words, the patient can only be checked in a particular place in particular time. However, the survival time of most diseases ' onset' physiological data is usually very short, such as heart disease, epilepsy and so on. It takes a long time to guard patients in order to capture data.

However, the inadequacies of existing portable remote medical monitoring equipment has limit its development. 1. The cost is generally expensive. 2. The

D. Lu (✉) · Y. Qin
Software College, Nanchang University, Nanchang 330000, China
e-mail: lu.dongxin@zte.com.cn

Y. Qin
e-mail: qin.chamber@gmail.com

S. Li et al. (eds.), *Frontier and Future Development of Information Technology in Medicine and Education*, Lecture Notes in Electrical Engineering 269,
DOI: 10.1007/978-94-007-7618-0_414,

volume of equipment is quiet large and has so many sensors that it's not convenient for patients to carry. 3. The transmission of data still rely on human. Family members need to copy data to hospital using U disk manually. 4. Large number of redundant data and worthless data will waste our limited medical resource.

414.2 The Overall Design of Remote Medical Monitoring System

Take the remote medical monitoring as a starting point, the system consists of three modules, namely data collecting module, pre-processing module and monitoring module. The system architecture is shown in Fig. 414.1.

Data collecting module, also called the portable data collecting device, consists of signal collection module, Bluetooth module, control module and other modules.

Pre-processing module, also called the monitoring system consists of network module, data module, DB module, display module, alert module and so on.

Monitoring module, also called the monitoring platform consists of DB module, communicate module, diagnose module, expert system and other modules. The system architecture is shown in Fig. 414.2.

414.3 Data Collecting Module

The structure of data collecting module is shown in Fig. 414.3.

Data collecting module, which is the portable data collecting device, an wrist-mounted embedded device, allowing users to measuring the body's resting ECG, pulse and temperature, is responsible for collecting user's physiological information. After collected, data will be transmit to pre-processing module using Bluetooth at 2.4 GHz band.

Signal collect module is divided into two parts, one is the ECG signal acquisition circuit, pulse signal acquisition circuit and body temperature signal

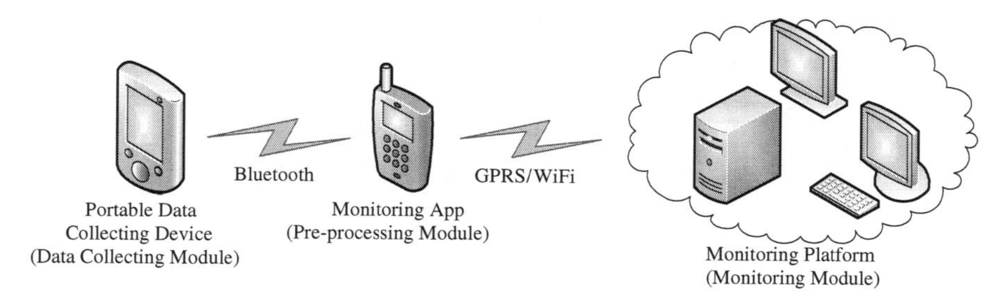

Fig. 414.1 The architecture of remote medical monitoring system

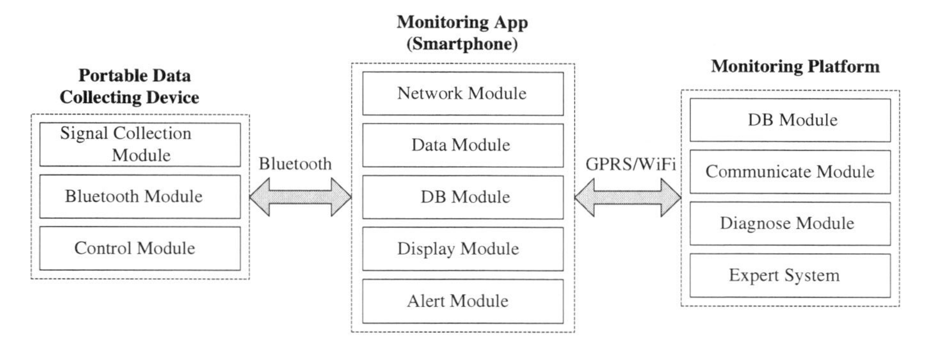

Fig. 414.2 The architecture of remote medical monitoring system

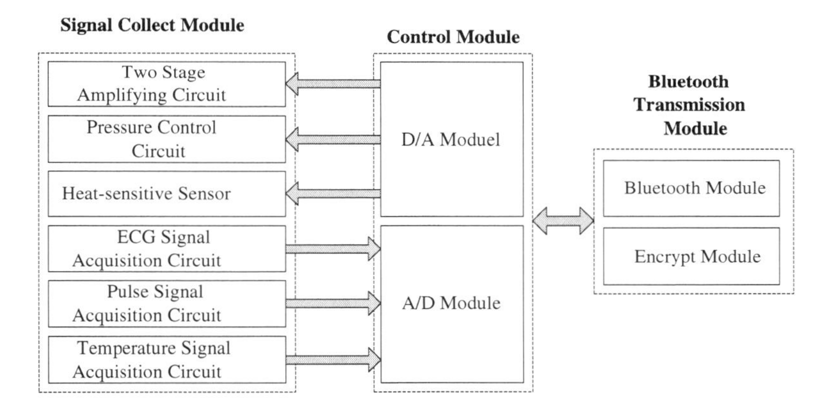

Fig. 414.3 The structure of data collecting module

acquisition circuit, the other part is the two stage amplifying circuit, pressure control circuit and heat-sensitive sensor. The former transmits data to the acquisition module, the later receives data from the control module.

Control module mainly has the A/D converter module and the D/A converter module, which is responsible for receiving and sending data and commands. It's also responsible for transmit the three physiological information.

Bluetooth transmission module mainly has Bluetooth module and encrypt module. The former transmit data to smart phone, while the later encrypts the data.

414.4 Pre-processing Module

Pre-precessing module, which is the monitoring application, installed on user's smart phone, can formate data, filter data, transmit data, store data, display user's body information, make preliminary diagnosis and work as sirens. The diagnosis

Fig. 414.4 The structure of pre-processing module

Network Module	GPRS Module
	WiFi Module
Data Module	Data Analysis
	Data Formation
	Smart Diagnose
Display Module	ECG Display
	Pulse Display
	Temperature Display
Alert Module	Message Module
	Mail Module
LDB Module	Query
	Save

result of ECG is displayed oscillometricly, while the diagnosis result of pulse and temperature is displayed in number. The monitoring application connects to Internet using GPRS/WiFi and then send filtered data to monitoring module in order to make further process. Take advantages of the portability and high performance of smart phone, the system will have a lower cost, high usability and scalability, it has positive effect for the popularization of the system.

The modules of the pre-processing module is shown in Fig. 414.4.

There are five main functional modules of the pre-processing module–network module, data module, display module, alert module and LDB module. Data module is the key one.

Data module is responsible for processing data after ECG, pulse and body temperature data are transmitted from data collecting module. First, the module will amplify signals and reduce the impact of noise information. Then, data will be formatted on the premise. It not only maintains the integrity of data, but also make it easier for user to handle. Then the three data will be analyzed according to its features.

414.5 Monitoring Module

Monitoring module, also called monitoring platform, consists of high performance servers and related equipment. The user group of this module is doctors and nursers. The platform receives pre-processed and filtered ECG, pulse and body temperature data from the pre-processing module and save it to electronic medical records.

For those data which is special and worth studying, the system will mark it, offer it to doctors and nurses and apply for diagnosis, consultation automatically using AI technology, expert system and DM in particular. For those data which is common and regular, the system will compress it and store it for future use. For patients with normal physiological data, the system will send an e-mail and a message to them and their families and notify them to go to hospital for further and a more comprehensive examination.

Monitoring module consists of DM module, communicate module, diagnose module, expert system and so on.

414.6 Conclusions

Bluetooth technology and its application is quiet mature today. Also, the appearance of various products related to ECG sensor, pulse sensor, body temperature sensor and related control circuit is a piece of good news. The difficulty lies in the low-cost integrated circuit design with high efficiency and low consumption. With the popularity of smart phone, the Android platform has become more sophisticated. The continuous development and improvement of the system design theory and the development of physiological data is progressive. Factors above is quiet supportive to the realization of remote medical monitoring system.

However, the study of KDD and agent of medical industry is far from mature. There are many difficulties for large and complex HIS to overcome, which is exactly the key point of future medical industry. It's expected that, in the next 5–15 years, the theory of computer science and technology related to medical industry will achieve a breakthrough. It will change our life greatly. We will live in a smarter life in the future.

References

1. Fayyad U, Piatetsky-Shapiro G, Smyth P (1996) From data mining to knowledge discovery in databases. Retrieved 2008-12-17
2. Cannataro M, Talia D (2003). The knowledge grid: an architecture for distributed knowledge discovery. Commun ACM 46 (1): 89–93. doi:10.1145/602421.602425. Retrieved 17 Oct 2011
3. Bouckaert RR, Frank E, Hall MA, Holmes G, Pfahringer B, Reutemann P, Witten IH (2010) WEKA experiences with a java open-source project. J Mach Learn Res 11: 2533–2541. The original title, practical machine learning, was changed [...] The term data mining was [added] primarily for marketing reasons
4. Data mining curriculum. ACM SIGKDD. 2006-04-30. Retrieved 2011-10-28
5. Clifton C (2010).Encyclopædia britannica: definition of data mining. Retrieved 2010-12-09
6. Witten IH, Frank E, Hall MA (2011). Data mining: practical machine learning tools and techniques (3rd edn). Elsevier, ISBN 978-0-12-374856-0
7. Kantardzic M (2003). Data mining: concepts, models, methods, and algorithms. Wiley. ISBN 0-471-22852-4. OCLC 50055336
8. Proceedings, International conferences on knowledge discovery and data mining. ACM, New York

Chapter 415
Development of University Information Service

Chun Yu, Fang Yuan and JunYang Feng

Abstract The current situation and existing problems in university informationisation was given briefly, with object of university information service development. It proposed the development content of both model design and technology realization of information service and practice the method of information service development. A system, which covers the core data resource of the university and providing one-stop comprehensive information service has been designed and realized. It provides comprehensive inquiry and statistical analysis service of all kinds of information for all the teachers, students and all levels of managerial staff, which serves talents training, the basic task of universities.

Keywords Information service · Data resource · Data management

415.1 Information Service System

Nowadays, universities pay special attention to the informationisation-supported education both at home and abroad. They start to develop the comprehensive information service which provides deep support to education processes. With the use of information technology and according to the integrated planning and design of data resource centre as well as the current situation of data resource

C. Yu (✉) · F. Yuan · J. Feng
Information Technology Center of Tsinghua University, Beijing, People's Republic of China
e-mail: yuchun@cic.tsinghua.edu.cn

F. Yuan
e-mail: yf@cic.tsinghua.edu.cn

J. Feng
e-mail: fjy@cic.tsinghua.edu.cn

S. Li et al. (eds.), *Frontier and Future Development of Information Technology in Medicine and Education*, Lecture Notes in Electrical Engineering 269,
DOI: 10.1007/978-94-007-7618-0_415,

development, abundant and accurate information resource service can be provided to teachers and students, including comprehensive inquiry and statistical analysis of all kinds of information. The development objectives of information service system are listed as follows.

First, to complete information service model: By analyzing the information service requirements of different users and in terms of teachers and students, complete information service model can be designed, upon which the comprehensive information service system can be established, covering the core data resources of the university and providing one-stop service can be established. The system is able to provide in-time decision-making support service to all levels of leaders, enabling in-time, complete and accurate information acquisition of users.

Second, to build a flexible and secure information service architecture: With the basis of data resource basic environment and comprehensive inquiry data model, with the help of integrated technology architecture design, the relevance of business and technology can be separated, providing flexible, customized, universal and effective data service to all kinds of users. Various presentation forms of result are allowed and strict visit permission control can be realized according to the role of user, providing secure data protection.

According to the integrated planning of data resource centre as well as the current situation of data resource development and with the use of information technology, integrated data resource basic environment, complete comprehensive inquiry service model as well as flexible and secure information service technology platform can be established.

415.2 Main Database Construction

The main database is an important component of data resource system and it provides unified shared basic data for all information systems. The main database is consisted of subject database and code database and it extracts and synchronizes data from corresponding information system. Meanwhile, the main database provides data inquiry and search service to other systems or users from the information service platform.

Comprehensive information service is designed according to integrated plan and organized according to subjects. It extract the main and core business data of the university and design the main database including business subject such as public code, teacher subject, student subject, enrolment, educational administration, personnel and etc. Data are then converted and standardized. The deployment and realization of the main database are completed via data share and exchange, which establishes the integrated data resource basic environment.

415.3 Technology Platform Construction

The information involved in comprehensive information system is massive and in various forms. Therefore, it is required yet very complicated to control the visit of information. Robust, effective and secure management mechanism is employed for comprehensive information service, which supports the permission management of multiple types of users and multiple levels of data, guarantees the legal use of data and prevents the illegal information acquisition and demolition.

Closed combination has been realized between comprehensive information service system and the Portal. The Portal is the integrated window for releasing information of the university and the information service system provides background preparation for information release. Comprehensive information service realizes the systematic integration of individual users, role permission and the Portal. According to the requirements of users, useful information can be extracted from the subject database and then released to the user terminal via the Portal as shown in Fig. 415.1.

As flexible and convenient release function is provided by the comprehensive information system, when basic data resource is ready in the main database, it can provide instant and efficient inquiry and statistic service, which meets the new requirements continuously proposed by users.

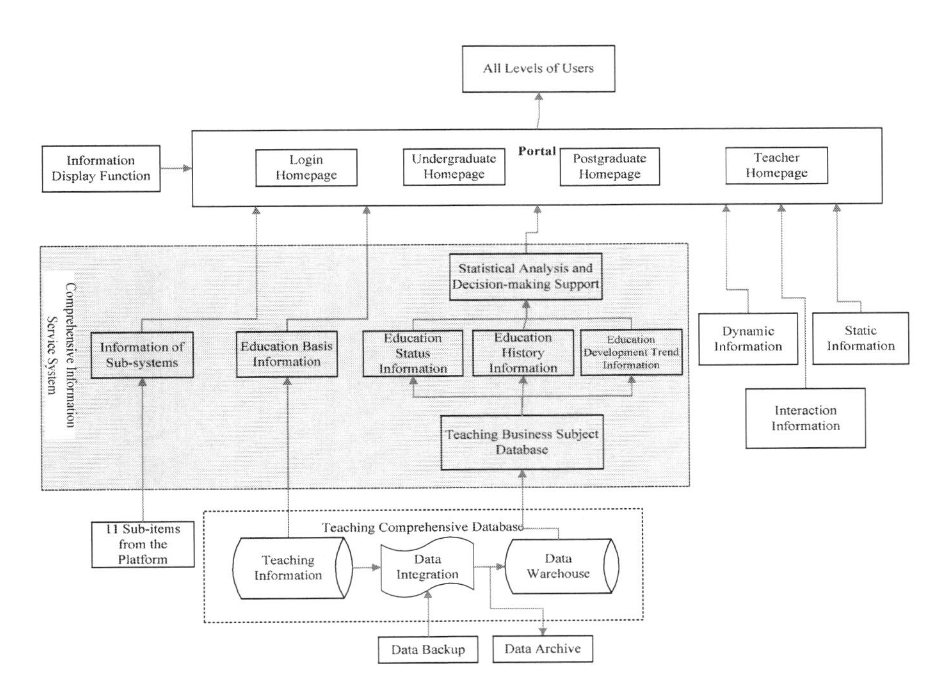

Fig. 415.1 Framework of the information service system

415.4 Information Service Model Construction

Based on information technology including data share and exchange, tree-structure organization, role permission management, information Portal integration and etc., comprehensive information service provides abundant and accurate comprehensive inquiry as well as statistical analysis for universities, departments, schools, teachers and students. These services include data standard release, business subject inquiry, and support for statistical analysis, individual file management and maintenance of user permission.

415.5 Design and Realization of User Function Model

By analyzing the information flow direction of business activities including educational administration, personnel and etc., the comprehensive information service can figure out the relation between internal organization/institution involved in

Table 415.1 User function model

Roles	Role function	Information in resource	Data permission
University leader	Organize and manage enrolment, education, personnel, research and etc	(a) Admission statistic result (b) Education statistical result (c) Teacher and staff statistics	All the university
Admission office	Undergraduate enrolment, employment and management	(a) All admission information (b) Admission statistics.	All the university
Administrative education office	Undergraduate education management	(a) All administrative education information (b) Administrative statistics	All the university
Personnel office	Management of teachers and staff	(a) All personnel information (b) Teachers and staff statistics	All the university
School leader	Education and management of relevant school	(a) Administrative education statistics of school	Relevant school
School administration and education staff	Undergraduate education and management	(a) Administrative education information of school (b) Administrative education statistics	Relevant school

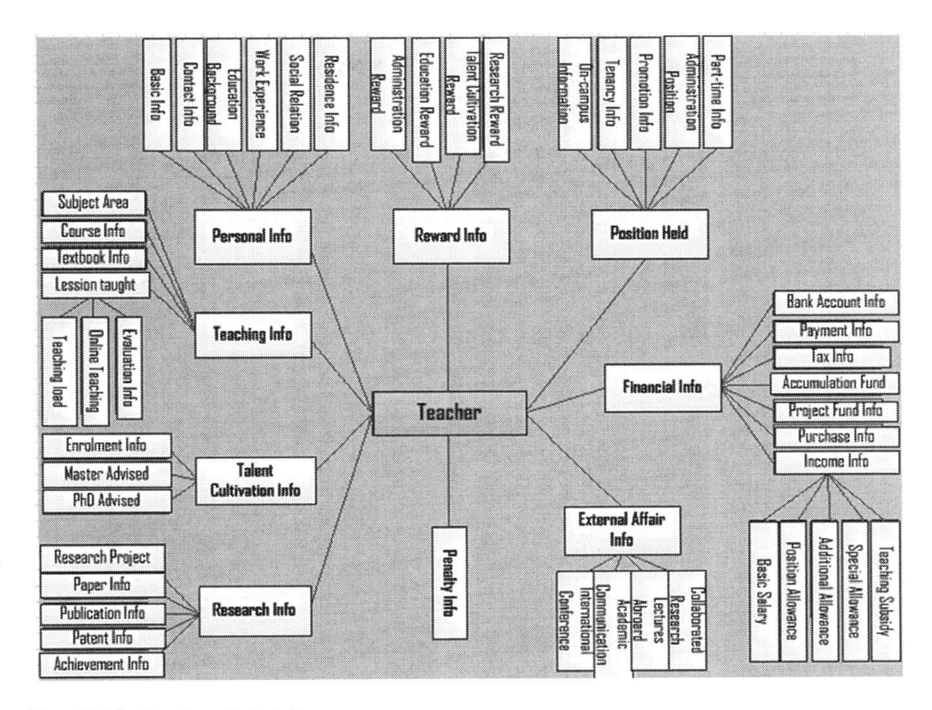

Fig. 415.2 Teacher digital files

management business, a whole set of business inquiry, statistical analysis and role permission model is established and complete control of multi-layer user, multi-level data and multi-business subject can be realized, which improve the security of system and data (Table 415.1).

415.6 Individual File Design and Realization

Based on both the teacher and student subject database, the comprehensive information service provides functions for teachers and students to view and maintain all kinds of personal information in the university. Teachers' individual files, as shown in Fig. 415.2 include personal information, position information, education information, research information, financial information, reward information and etc.

Students' individual files, as shown in Fig. 415.3 include personal information, studentship information, cultivation information, social work, payment information, reward information, penalty information and etc.

Comprehensive information service also provides electronic space for all the teachers and students to save personal photos and upload local files, record events

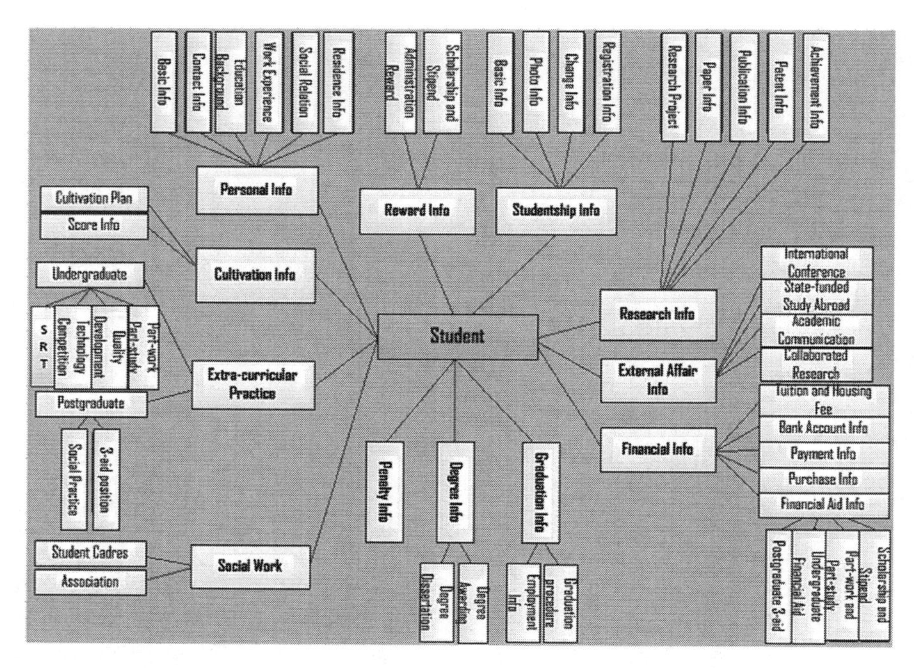

Fig. 415.3 Student digital files

and etc. Meanwhile, publicise teachers' and students' personal information, including personal experience, research information and library record, by integrated with the Portal.

415.7 Conclusions

Talent cultivation is the fundamental task of universities. Digital campus needs to serve such fundamental task and convert the advantage in running schools into the advantage in the improvement of talent cultivation quality with the use of information technology. Ordered organization and centralized management of data would realise the standardisation, integration and authorization of the management of data resource of universities so that the completeness, consistency, orderliness, sharing and manageability can be guaranteed. By organization and management of all kinds of resources in university informationisation, the comprehensive information service enables the users to promptly find out the information resource and service needed, allows managerial staff to manage business in a professional manner, provides perfect environment for online information communication between teachers and students, and provide information for users in the most efficient way so that the expected goal has been achieved.

References

1. Chun Y, Fang Y, Qixin (2011) Exploration and practice of college and university information resource service. Exp Technol Manag 28: 228–230, 243
2. Yang Y, Gang D, Xin S (2005) The Design and Implementation of a service-oriented information service system". J Beijing Univ Technol 31:411–414
3. Chun Y, Fang Y, Qixin L (2012) Design and implementation of personnel-oriented integrated information service system. Paper presented at the 2012 international conference on systems and informatics, 2610–2613
4. Jiang D-x, Liu Q-x, Zheng S-l, Role and activity based digital campus access control model. J Dalian Maritine Univ 36(1):132–134
5. Chun Y, Fang Y, Qixin L (2012) Research and application on university integrated information services. Paper presented at the 2012 international symposium on IT in medicine and education, 323–326
6. Zhang A (2002) Information service patterns in the network environment. J Libr Sci Chin 28:32–34

Chapter 416
Adaptive Tracking Servo Control for Optical Data Storage Systems

Zhizheng Wu, Yang Li, Fei Peng and Mei Liu

Abstract The high precision tracking servo control would play an important role in the next generation near-field optical data storage systems where the desired tracking error should be below 5 nm under various unknown situations. It is proposed in this paper to use an adaptive regulation approach to maintain the tracking error below its desired value, despite unknown track eccentricity and external force disturbance. The experimental evaluation result show the effectiveness of the proposed control approach.

Keywords Adaptive control · Tracking servo · Optical data storage

416.1 Introduction

To accommodate the unprecedented expansion of information, ultra-high density data storage devices are needed for information storage. The next generation near field optical data storage systems would have a storage density of more than 5 TB/in^2 with a tracking error below 5 nm [1]. Due to the extremely high storage density, the tracking servo system is very sensitive to the disturbances such as force disturbance caused by vibration and radial run-out caused by the track eccentricity. One of the major issues associated with the design of a tracking servo controller is the fact that some disturbances have unknown and possibly time varying properties. The traditional PID control system cannot deal with the unknown force disturbance effectively [2]. Repetitive control has been applied for rejecting periodic disturbances. However, the exact knowledge of the period of the external signals is required [3]. Robust control provides the ability to balance

Z. Wu (✉) · Y. Li · F. Peng · M. Liu
Department of Precision Mechanical Engineering, Shanghai University, Shanghai, China
e-mail: zhizhengwu@shu.edu.cn

S. Li et al. (eds.), *Frontier and Future Development of Information Technology in Medicine and Education*, Lecture Notes in Electrical Engineering 269,
DOI: 10.1007/978-94-007-7618-0_416,

disturbance rejection with the model uncertainty. However, the selection of the weighting functions can be time consuming and can result in an overly conservative design if done improperly [4]. It is proposed in this paper to use a Youla parameterized adaptive controller design approach to achieve tracking precision despite unknown track eccentricity or force disturbance. Experimental results illustrate the capability of the proposed adaptive regulation approach to yield the desired tracking performance.

416.2 Adaptive Controller Design

The tracking servo system is needed to read the data from a spiral track. As shown in Fig. 416.1, e is the tracking error which is supposed to be zero, u is the control input, d_1 is the force disturbance and d_2 is the run-out disturbance. The main disturbance of tracking servo system is from run-out caused by eccentricity. The eccentricity is defined by the mismatch of a rotational center with respect to the geometrical center of the data tracks, which can be presented as sinusoidal disturbances to the output y.

Convert the above servo control problem to the generalized regulation problem with a discrete-time linear system model given by:

$$\sum : \begin{cases} x(k+1) = Ax(k) + Bu(k) + Ed(k) \\ y(k) = C_y x(k) + D_y d(k) \\ e(k) = C_e x(k) + D_e d(k) \end{cases} \tag{416.1}$$

where x is the state vector, d represents the unknown track eccentricity and force disturbances The controller basically consists of the interconnection of a fixed block J, and a tuned system Q [5]:

$$J : \begin{cases} \hat{x}(k+1) = (A + LC_y + BK)\hat{x}(k) - Ly(k) + By_Q(k) \\ u(k) = K\hat{x}(k) + y_Q(k) \\ y(k) - \hat{y}(k) = y(k) - C_y\hat{x}(k) \end{cases}$$

$$Q : \begin{cases} x_Q(k+1) = A_Q x_Q(k) + B_Q(y(k) - \hat{y}(k)) \\ y_Q(k) = C_Q x_Q(k) \end{cases}$$

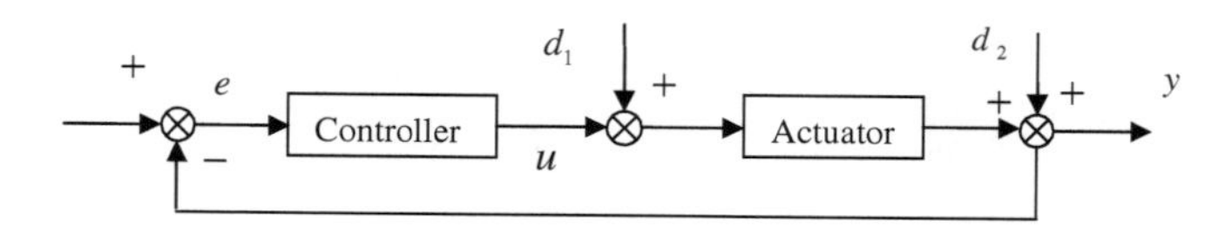

Fig. 416.1 Tracking servo control system

where K is state feedback gain and L is the observer gain. The plant $\sum$ and the block J can be combined into a single block T. The dynamics of the system T can be represented as follows:

$$\begin{bmatrix} x(k+1) \\ \tilde{x}(k+1) \\ e(k) \\ y(k)-\hat{y}(k) \end{bmatrix} = \begin{bmatrix} A+BK & BK & E & B \\ 0 & A+LC_y & -E-LD_y & 0 \\ C_e & 0 & D_e & 0 \\ 0 & -C_y & D_y & 0 \end{bmatrix} \begin{bmatrix} x(k) \\ \tilde{x}(k) \\ d(k) \\ y_Q(k) \end{bmatrix} \tag{416.2}$$

where $\tilde{x} = x(k) - \hat{x}(k)$. Then we have:

$$\begin{bmatrix} e(k) \\ y(k)-\hat{y}(k) \end{bmatrix} = \begin{bmatrix} T_{11} & T_{12} \\ T_{21} & T_{22} \end{bmatrix} \begin{bmatrix} d(k) \\ y_Q(k) \end{bmatrix} \tag{416.3}$$

Let q^{-l} denote the l time step delay operator, and $Q_k = \sum_{i=1}^{n_Q} \theta_i(k-1)q^{1-i}$. The aim of the adaptation is to tune the parameter vector θ so that it converges to the desired parameter vector θ_0 needed to achieve regulation. The performance variable $e(k)$ is then given by:

$$e(k) = T_{11}(q^{-1})d(k) + T_{12}(q^{-1})Q_k F(q^{-1})r(k) \tag{416.4}$$

$F(z)$ is a stable weighted function. Define $r(k) = y(k) - \hat{y}(k)$. Let

$$v_1(k) = T_{12}(q^{-1})F(q^{-1})r(k)$$

$$\phi(k) = [-v_1(k), \ldots, -v_1(k-n_q+1)]^T$$

$$\theta(k) = [\theta_1(k), \ldots, \theta_{n_q}(k)]^T$$

Define $e_2(k) = [T_{12}(q^{-1})Q_k - Q_k T_{12}(q^{-1})]F(q^{-1})r(k)$ and the modified error $\tilde{e}(k) = e(k) - e_2(k)$. The adaptive algorithm is then given as:

$$\begin{aligned} \hat{\theta}(k+1) &= \hat{\theta}(k) + \lambda(k+1)P(k+1)\phi(k+1)\tilde{e}(k+1) \\ P^{-1}(k+1) &= \lambda(k+1)[P^{-1}(k) + \phi(k+1)\phi^T(k+1)] \end{aligned} \tag{416.5}$$

where $\lambda(k)$ is a time varying forgetting factor satisfying $0 < \lambda_{\min} \le \lambda(k) \le \lambda_{\max} < 1$.

416.3 Experimental Result

The proposed adaptive control approach is evaluated on an optical storage servo control system as shown in Fig. 416.2. The optical pick-up head SF-HD850 from Sanyo Corporation and the servo control chipset AM5668 are used to actuate the optical lens. The Polytec OFV552/5000 is used to measure the displacement of the

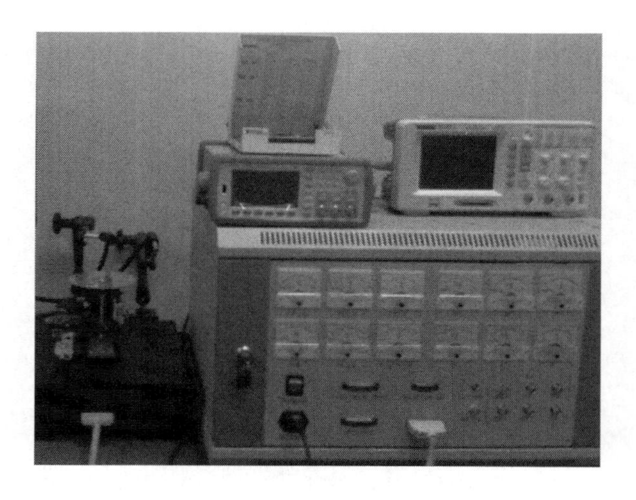

Fig. 416.2 The photo of the experiment system

optical lens in the plane of the tracking movement. The simulated disk eccentricity and force disturbance signals are added to the output of the controller and measurement of the displacement, respectively. The maximum eccentricity is assumed to be 100 μm. The plant model of the tracking servo system is obtained using system identification method as

$$G(s) = \frac{2575.7575}{s^2 + 14.248s + 2575.7575}$$

The experimental result is shown in Fig. 416.3, which illustrates that the tracking error effectively maintains below 4 nm despite the unknown disturbances with the proposed adaptive controller.

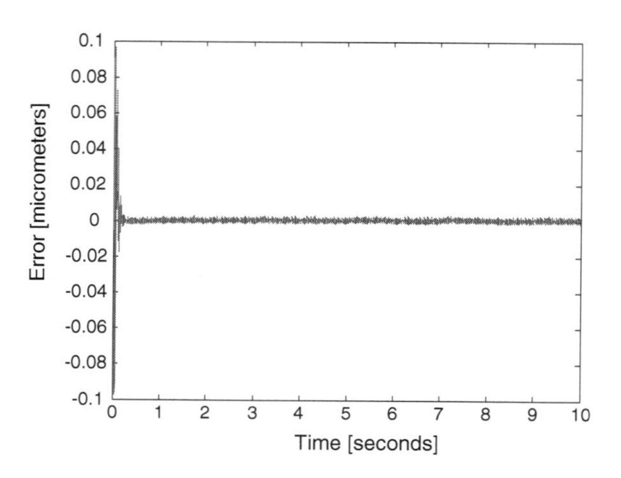

Fig. 416.3 The tracking error based on the adaptive controller

Acknowledgments This work was supported by the National Natural Science Foundation of China (51075254), the Shanghai Pujiang Program (11PJ1404000) and the Innovation Program of Shanghai Municipal Education Commission (11YZ16).

References

1. Park K, Park Y, Park N (2011) Prospect of recording technologies for higher storage performance. IEEE Trans Magn 47(3):539–545
2. Cherubini G, Chung CC, Messner WC (2012) Control methods in data-storage systems. IEEE Trans Control Syst Technol 20(2):296–322
3. Kim K, Lee S, Chung C (2011) A survey of control issues in optical data storage system. In: Proceedings of the 18th IFAC World Congress, pp 854–868
4. Conway R, Choi J, Nagamune R, Horowitz R (2010) Robust track-following controller design in hard disk drives based on parameter dependent Lyapunov functions. IEEE Trans Magn 46(4):1060–1068
5. Wu Z, Ben Amara F (2010) Adaptive regulation in bimodal linear systems. Int J Robust Nonlinear Control 20(1):59–83

Chapter 417
Optimal Focus Servo Control for Optical Data Storage Systems

Zhizheng Wu, Qingxi Jia, Lu Wang and Mei Liu

Abstract In the next generation optical data storage systems, the lens-disk interface gap and the tolerance of the focus error will reduce dramatically. The rotation of the spindle motor could produce repetitive disturbances to the focus servo system due to the misalignment and the skew of the disk, therefore affect the focus precision and cause the lens-disk collision. In this paper, an optimal Q-parameterized controller design approach is proposed and the optimization constraints are formulated in matrix inequalities. The approach is finally evaluated in an optical data storage experimental system.

Keywords Focus servo system · Q-parameterized · Optimal control · Optical data storage

417.1 Introduction

To increase the data storage density for the successive optical disk generations, the depth of focus must be reduced, which leads to a much smaller tolerance for the focusing error. However, the disturbances caused by the misalignment of the spin, the skew of the disk and other vibration forces could reduce the focus control precision and cause the lens-disk collision [1]. Therefore, it is highly desirable to design an effective focus controller which can effectively eliminate all kinds of disturbances and maintain a constant distance between disk and the optical head. Many studies have been conducted to improve the performances of focus servo controller including PID control, robust repetitive control and switching control [2]. However, both PID controller and robust repetitive controller cannot deal with

---

Z. Wu (✉) · Q. Jia · L. Wang · M. Liu
Department of Precision Mechanical Engineering, Shanghai University, Shanghai, China
e-mail: zhizhengwu@shu.edu.cn

S. Li et al. (eds.), *Frontier and Future Development of Information Technology in Medicine and Education*, Lecture Notes in Electrical Engineering 269,
DOI: 10.1007/978-94-007-7618-0_417,

the collision effectively due to the possible big dynamic overshoot in the closed loop system. The switched controller design method has been used in pull-in process [3] and air-gap control [4] in near-field storage system. However the parameters of the controllers and the switch point must be regulated by try and errors in the experiments and the design process is complex. In this paper, a Q-parameterized optimal controller design approach is proposed to eliminate the sinusoidal and random disturbances under an anti-collision constraint. The experiment result shows the effectiveness of the designed controller against various disturbances with a good focus precision.

417.2 Optimal Controller Design

The focus control problem can be formulated as the regulation problem with a discrete-time linear system model given by [5]:

$$\Sigma_P: \begin{cases} \boldsymbol{x}(k+1) = \boldsymbol{A}\boldsymbol{x}(k) + \boldsymbol{B}\boldsymbol{u}(k) + \boldsymbol{D}^x\boldsymbol{d}_r(k) + \boldsymbol{F}^x\boldsymbol{d}_w(k), \\ \boldsymbol{y}(k) = \boldsymbol{C}^y\boldsymbol{x}(k) + \boldsymbol{D}^y\boldsymbol{d}_r(k) + \boldsymbol{F}^y\boldsymbol{d}_w(k), \\ \boldsymbol{e}(k) = \boldsymbol{y}(k), \end{cases} \tag{417.1}$$

where x is the state vector, u is the control input, y is the measurement focus error, e is performance variable to be regulated and δ is the desired flying height, d_r represents the deterministic sinusoidal disturbance and d_r represents the random disturbance. The designed Q-parameterized controller proposed in this paper are constructed by a set of controllers, each controller involve a fixed block J, and a proper stable system Q [5]. The state space representation of the system J and Q are given by:

$$J: \begin{cases} \hat{x}(k+1) = (A + LC^y + BK)\hat{x}(k) - Ly(k) + By_Q(k),\ \hat{x}(0) = \hat{x}_0, \\ u(k) = K\hat{x}(k) + y_Q(k), \\ y(k) - \hat{y}(k) = y(k) - C^y\hat{x}(k). \end{cases} \tag{417.2}$$

$$Q: \begin{cases} x_Q(k+1) = A_Q x_Q(k) + B_Q(y(k) - \hat{y}(k)),\ x_Q(0) = x_Q^0, \\ y_Q(k) = C_Q x_Q(k), \end{cases} \tag{417.3}$$

where $\hat{x}(k)$ is an estimate of the plant state vector $x(k)$, $\hat{y}(k)$ is an estimate of the plant output $y(k)$, K and L are state feedback and observer gains, respectively. Denote $\chi = \begin{bmatrix} x^T & x_Q^T & \tilde{x}^T \end{bmatrix}^T_{1\times N}$, $N = 2n + n_Q$, $\tilde{x}(k) = \hat{x}(k) - x(k)$. Combine formula (417.1, 417.2 and 417.3), then the resulting closed loop system can be represented as:

$$\Sigma^{cl}: \begin{cases} \boldsymbol{\chi}(k+1) = \widehat{\boldsymbol{A}}\boldsymbol{\chi}(k) + \boldsymbol{E}^d\boldsymbol{d}_r(k) + \boldsymbol{E}^w\boldsymbol{d}_w(k), \\ \boldsymbol{e}(k) = \boldsymbol{C}^{ex}\boldsymbol{\chi}(k) + \boldsymbol{D}^y\boldsymbol{d}_r(k) + \boldsymbol{F}^y\boldsymbol{d}_w(k), \end{cases} \tag{417.4}$$

where $\widehat{A} = \begin{bmatrix} A + BK & BC_Q & BK \\ 0 & A_Q & -B_Q C^y \\ 0 & 0 & A + LC^y \end{bmatrix}$, $E^d = \left[(D^x)^T \quad (B_Q D^y)^T \quad - (D^x + LD^y)^T \right]^T$, $E^w = \left[(F^x)^T \quad (B_Q F^y)^T \quad -(F^x + LF^y)^T \right]^T$, $C^{ex} = [C^y \quad 0 \quad 0]$

The optimal Q-parameterized controller needs to eliminate the sinusoidal disturbance d_r and minimize the H_2 norm of the closed loop system with respect to the random disturbance d_w. To achieve these goals, we can exploit the flexibility of Q parameter in the parameterized set of stabilizing controllers for the closed loop system. The regulation against d_r can be presented in the form of interpolation conditions as [5]:

$$A_\theta \theta + B_\theta = 0, \tag{417.5}$$

where $\theta = \left[\theta^1, \ldots, \theta^{n_q}\right]^T$ is the unknown parameter vector in Q, A_θ and B_θ are properly formulated matrices. Furthermore, to achieve the goal of anti-collision performance, the variable should satisfy $|e(k)| \leq |\delta|$. Then the overall multiobjective optimization conditions can be expressed in the following matrix inequalities:

$$\begin{bmatrix} -P + \alpha P & 0 & \left(\widehat{A}\right)^T P \\ 0 & -\frac{\mu}{\kappa} I & \left[E^d \quad E^w\right]^T P \\ P\widehat{A} & P\left[E^d \quad E^w\right] & -P \end{bmatrix} < 0$$

$$\begin{bmatrix} \alpha P & 0 & (C^{ex})^T \\ 0 & \frac{(\beta-\mu)}{\kappa} I & \begin{bmatrix} (D^y)^T \\ (F^y)^T \end{bmatrix} \\ C^{ex} & [D^y \quad F^y] & \beta I \end{bmatrix} > 0$$

$$\begin{bmatrix} -X & X\widehat{A} & 0 \\ \widehat{A}^T X & -X & (C^{ex})^T \\ 0 & C^{ex} & -I \end{bmatrix} < 0$$

$$\begin{bmatrix} X & 0 & XE^w \\ 0 & I & F^y \\ (E^w)^T X & (F^y)^T & S \end{bmatrix} > 0$$

$$A_\theta \theta + B_\theta = 0$$

$$Tr(S) < \gamma^2$$

where $\kappa = \max_{k \geq 0} \left(\|d_r(k)\|^2 + \|d_w(k)\|^2 \right) \neq 0$, $\alpha > 0$ is a preset constant, $P > 0$ $X > 0$ and μ is a positive scalar.

417.3 Experimental Result

The proposed optimal focus controller is evaluated on an optical data storage servo control system as shown in Fig. 417.1. The optical pick-up head SF-HD850 from Sanyo Corporation and the servo control chipset AM5668 are used to actuate the optical lens in the pick-up head. The focus error is obtained based on the astigmatic method using FPGA chipset EPIC20FBGA400 from ALTERA Corporation. The controller algorithm is implemented in the DSP signal processor TMS320C6711 from TI Corporation. A skew disk with 600 μm deflection is used in the experimental evaluation test. An additive voltage signal is added to the output of the controller to simulate various unknown random disturbance. The plant model of the focus servo loop is obtained using the subspace system identification method in Matlab as

$$G(s) = \frac{0.5166s + 567.2}{s^2 + 214.6s + 94790}$$

The standard lead-lag controller commonly used in the DVD system is first applied to the experimental system and results in a steady root mean square (RMS) value of the focus error 88 nm. The experimental result with the proposed optimal controller is shown in Fig. 417.2. After performing several times of the nominal

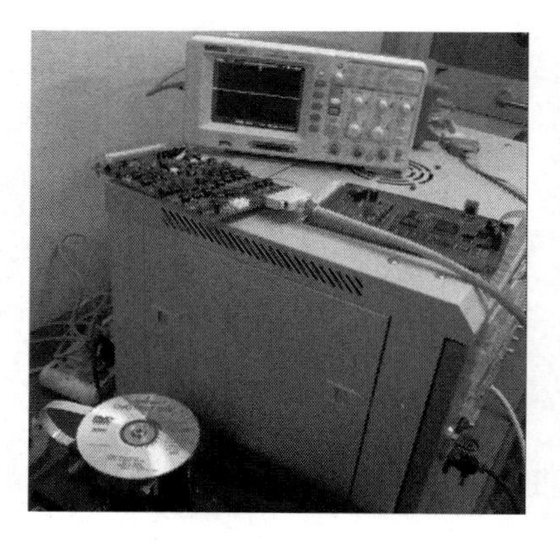

Fig. 417 1 The photo of the experiment system

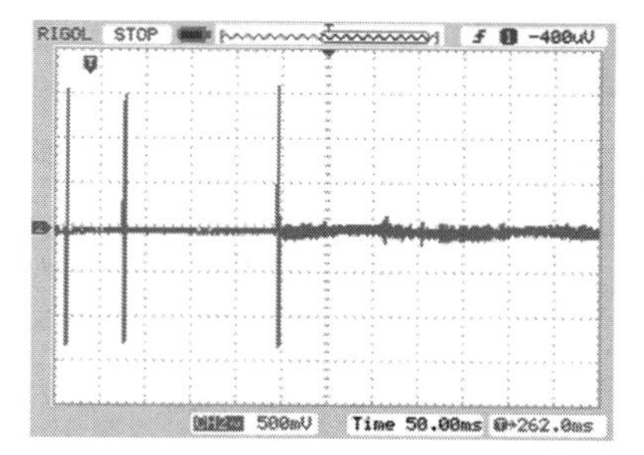

Fig. 417.2 The focusing error based on the optimal servo controller

focus position search with a triangle driving voltage signal, the control loop is then closed with the optimal controller around the focus crossover position. The experimental result illustrates that the final root mean square (RMS) value of the focus error drops to 29 nm, which means the proposed optimal controller is more effective for dealing with the external disturbances.

Acknowledgments This work was supported by the National Natural Science Foundation of China (51075254), the Shanghai Pujiang Program (11PJ1404000) and the Innovation Program of Shanghai Municipal Education Commission (11YZ16).

References

1. Park K, Park Y, Park N (2011) Prospect of recording technologies for higher storage performance. IEEE Trans Magn 47(3):539–545
2. Cherubini G, Chung CC, Messner WC (2012) Control methods in data-storage systems. IEEE Trans Control Syst Technol 20(2):296–322
3. Kwon T, Kim S, Yun H, Kim J (2007) A novel pull-in process using input shaping for solid immersion lens-based near-field recording system. Jpn J Appl Phys 46:1003–1005
4. Kim JG, Kim TH, Choi H, Yoon YJ, Jeong J, Park NC, Yang HS, Park YP (2007) Improved air-gap control for SIL based near-field recording system. IEEE Trans Magn 43:811–813
5. Wu Z, Ben Amara F (2008) Adaptive regulation in bimodal linear systems. Int J Robust Nonlinear Control 18:1115–1141

Chapter 418
Curriculum Design of Algorithms and Data Structures Based on Creative Thinking

Chen Weiwei, Li Zhigang, Chen Weidong, Li Qing, Tang Yanqin, Wu Yongfen and Shi Lei

Abstract Around the cultivation of creative thinking, a Trinity Teaching Content System is proposed, highlighting the cultivation of creative thinking teaching content organization and a new learning method of "read, imitate, change, and research" about "Algorithms and Data Structures" course are introduced. A practice platform establishment is also presented, which is for students' ability training.

Keywords Algorithm · Data structure · Curriculum design · Teaching reformation · Creative thinking

418.1 Overview

In the teaching of "algorithm and data structure" course, in order to deal with the relationship between cultural knowledge, scientific thinking and ability wisdom, we choose the optimal knowledge points as carrier to teach students problem-solving thoughts and algorithm evolution process, to achieve thinking training, ability cultivation and wisdom inspiration.

In the face of students' knowledge structure changing and information technology applications expanding, we need to solve the following three problems.

C. Weiwei (✉) · L. Zhigang · L. Qing · T. Yanqin ·
W. Yongfen · S. Lei
College of Command Information System, PLA University of Science and Technology, Nanjing 210007, China
e-mail: hchcww@263.net

C. Weidong
College of Information System and Management, National University of Defense Technology, Changsha Hunan 410073, China

S. Li et al. (eds.), *Frontier and Future Development of Information Technology in Medicine and Education*, Lecture Notes in Electrical Engineering 269,
DOI: 10.1007/978-94-007-7618-0_418,

- How to further optimize the composition of course content structure to improve students' cognition level and thinking depth.
- How to organize the teaching process in order to integrate thinking training and knowledge teaching to improve students' creative thinking ability.
- How to improve students' learning approach to prominent independent and active learning.

Responding to the above problems, several measures have been made as follows. First, we study the curriculum design approach to embody creative thinking. Second, we make new teaching implementation scheme and new teaching materials including network course. Third, we hold teaching ability competition and different forms of education and teaching practice, such as classroom teaching implementation.

The course has been named excellent course of Communication Bureau of General Staff of PLA in 2011, won first prize in teaching achievement award of Information Bureau of General Staff of PLA. The rest of this paper briefly introduces the details of our work for training students' creative thinking.

418.2 Curriculum Design of Teaching Content and Organization

418.2.1 Teaching Content Reformation

We propose a Trinity Teaching Content System including "data structures, algorithm and inherent computational difficulty of problems" [1]. This system can help students to understand the meaning of optimal algorithm. It can also reflect knowledge coherence and thinking depth.

Specifically, at the problem level, the inherent computational difficulty and NP-hard presence are revealed, to prevent students from attempting to seek algorithms superior to the difficulties inherent. Otherwise the students may do some useless work. At the algorithm level, we want to the students to know what efficient algorithm is, what "good" algorithm is, what "optimal" algorithm is and how to design "good" algorithm by algorithm complexity and evaluation methods. At the data structure level, features of various data structures are described as well as how to properly configure appropriate algorithms to these data structures to obtain processing efficiency. At last algorithms, data structures and program design can be integrated organically. Table 418.1 shows the correlation between the relevant teaching content and thinking training.

Table 418.1 The correlation between teaching content and thinking training

Training levels	Teaching content	Thinking training	Integration
Problem level	Inherent computational difficulty of problems, the relationship between inherent computational difficulty and complexity, P and NP problems	Rational thinking training. Grasp the overall and thoroughness of thinking	Demand as the traction, training students' innovative ability by procedure control (problem analysis, algorithm design, data structure selection and programming)
Algorithm level	The importance of algorithms, recursion, divide and conquer, and balance, greedy method, dynamic programming, backtracking; complexity analysis	Rational thinking training. Grasp the openness and diversity of thinking	
Data structure level	List, tree, graph, hash set, basic operations (search, insert, delete, etc.)	Rational thinking training. Grasp the abstraction, logical and dialectical of thinking	
Program design	Course practice (algorithm programming)	Engineering thinking training. Grasp the serious and compromise of thinking	

418.2.2 Curriculum Teaching Organization

Creative thinking [2] is a psychological process unique to human being. The accomplishments created by human being are all creative thinking externalization and materialization. Humanistic education [3] can be used to stimulate students' creative enthusiasm. We propose innovative education based on shaping innovation environment. We divide the teaching organization into three levels (Fig. 418.1).

The humanistic education focuses on history of algorithm and data structures including historical figures' stories and roadmap to produce technology. It can build innovation environment to improve students' state of mind, to stimulate learning potential and enthusiasm. The method training takes basic knowledge as carrier, is a platform for showing thinking process, models, algorithms, tools and systems. Behavioral experience emphasizes students' practical activities.

418.2.3 Creative Thinking Training Highlighted Curriculum Design

A teaching model of "problem → model → algorithms → evolution" was proposed. The problem is the traction for basic teaching content. It emphases on why do we need this knowledge, what the model features are, what operations needed, how to design algorithm, and how to evolve knowledge to meet different demand. It helps students to think, to study and to explore innovation. For example, Fig. 418.2 shows the procedure that integrates the teaching content, measures and methods together for Kruskal's algorithm teaching.

418.3 Learning Method and Practice System

418.3.1 An Efficient Four Words Learning Method

We propose an efficient four words learning method to help students to build confidence gradually. The four words are "read", "imitate", "change", and "research". This method has a strong operability, so that the students not only grasp the basic knowledge points, but also master methods of learning.

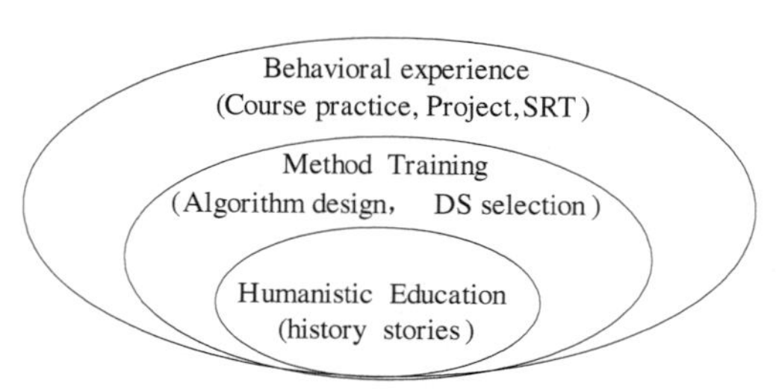

Fig. 418.1 Teaching organization structure chart

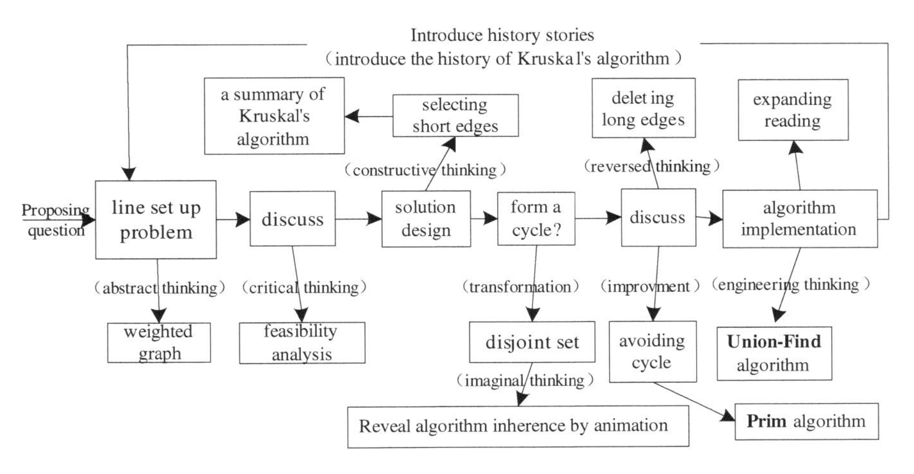

Fig. 418. 2 The teaching process of Kruskal's algorithm

"*Read*" means reading codes. Students can learn other people's algorithm design ideas and description ways by reading other people's codes. It is Enlightenment for learning algorithm design. After that, the students can *imitate* to design algorithms for solving problems by integrating learned knowledge points. When the application scenarios or demand changes, the students can *change* the original algorithms to optimize them. It can help students to comprehend knowledge points. "*Research*" is to make student to study the nature features of problems and to find solutions. It can help student to improve many abilities and their quality.

418.3.2 A Progressive Practice System

Consideration on students' behavior experience is an important part of teaching reformation [4]. A progressive practice system is established for building students' confidence and knowledge pursuit enthusiasm. This system includes "single algorithms—Project—Programming Contest—National Programming Contest".

In "single algorithms" stage, five types of experiments, including case experiments, basic experiments, design experiments, comprehensive experiments, and open experiments, are designed for different levels of students' needs.

The projects take simple realistic problems as carriers. Three students form a group for one project. A project's phase includes "objective analysis → solution design → evaluation → coding → testing, feedback and correction". It also needs document management. The project document includes task division, scheduling, research reports, testing reports and summary.

418.4 Conclusion

After 6 years of construction, "algorithms and data structures" course has acquired many fruits. It is deeply welcomed by the students. A lot of students take this course as their practice field for thinking. It provides a new perspective to look at problems. The most important is that it cultivates students' creative thinking. In our future work, we will enrich our teaching content and cases to pursuit more fruits, based on the results of the existing construction.

Acknowledgments The research is supported by the College Computer Course Reform Project (2-1) of MOE of China.

References

1. Chen W, Wang Q (2010) Data structures and algorithms. Higher Education Press, Beijing
2. Sun Y (2012) Research on mathematics education in the middle school based on the cultivation of creative thinking. Ph.D. thesis, Central China Normal University
3. Zhang C (2011) The Humanities and University Education. Mod Univ Edu, 2:34–37
4. Zhang C (2007) EQO Education is such an education that shows much concern about the fusion of subject and object. J Chin Soc Edu, 8:1–4

Chapter 419
Questionnaire Design and Analysis of Online Teaching and Learning: A Case Study of the Questionnaire of "Education Online" Platform of Beijing University of Technology

Shidong Xu, Shuyi Zhou, Qian Cao, Jin Lei, Xiaoyong Li and Yuhu He

Abstract In this case, "Education Online Platform Application Questionnaire" were sent to teachers and collected by making use of Questionnaire Network System to analysis the role of online teaching, the usage of the platform, the obstacles and incentives of "Education Online", then we can form a valuable reference and make targeted improvements and promotion in technology, design, promotion, application and policy support.

Keywords Education online · Questionnaire · Obstacles · Incentives

By the end of May 2013, our school's "Education Online" (EOL)platform has 23767 student users, 1182 teachers users and 1368 online courses, 682 courses applied by teachers, 1423 classes, The total number of network access is 39,204,891, and 10,200 times of average daily access. And we face a lot of pressure. On the basis of the existing platform, how to facilitate learning, improve curriculum and deepen the network teaching and the construction of digital resources through technical methods, these issues need to be explored and researched.

Therefore, the main purposes of the questionnaire research include to find out how teachers used the EOL platform and theirs satisfaction; to understand the problems found in the teachers' application and collect functionality of the platform needing to improve, such as functional, technical, process; form how to promote the use of online teaching and learning.

S. Xu (✉) · S. Zhou · Q. Cao · J. Lei · X. Li · Y. He
Modern Education Technology Center of Beijing University of Technology, Beijing 100124, China
e-mail: xushidong@bjut.edu.cn

S. Li et al. (eds.), *Frontier and Future Development of Information Technology in Medicine and Education*, Lecture Notes in Electrical Engineering 269,
DOI: 10.1007/978-94-007-7618-0_419,

419.1 The Methods and Processes

Description of research methods, data sampling and questionnaire preparation of the design

1. Online survey research methods Collection and analysis of relevant data using self-compiled questionnaire about EOL platform applications.
2. Data samplingThe subjects of the survey are from teachers of Beijing University of Technology. The network questionnaires are released on the questionnaire and curriculum test platform (http://class.bjut.edu.cn/Questionnaire), and forwarded through the school portal, online education and the Fifth Education Discussion site forward questionnaire. The questionnaire link is sent to teacher users of Education Online through mass-mailing.
3. The design of the questionnaireThis is a real name questionnaire survey. "Expressed deviation" are fixed by 5 persons' test. The answer time is controlled in 9–13 min after adjustment of the amount of questions and the difficulty. The contents of the questionnaire presented showing single page scrolling, and the preamble of the questionnaire explained the purpose and meaning of the investigation activities. The statistical results generated by the system, and respondents can view the statistical results. To prevent personal information leaking, the results filter respondents name and e-mail and other information.

419.2 Questionnaire and Analysis

Describe the contents of the questionnaire and analysis of the results.

419.2.1 Contents of Questionnaire

The questionnaire consisted of objective questions and subjective questions a total of 22 questions. The problem sequentially numbered T1, T2, T3,..., T22. A combination of four dimensions Expand: Basic information of the respondents; the effects of online teaching and learning; usage of the "Education Online" platform; the impediments and incentives of online teaching and learning. Specific preparation is as follows:

Dimension 1 Basic information of the respondents. Measured from the respondents name, gender, age, education, job title, institutes, academic background, the online teaching experience, E-mail, a total of 9 problems, including radio and blank

Table. 419.1 Some example of the impediments and incentives of online teaching and learning

Question	Topic	Options
T20	What hinder teachers in online teaching? (Multiple choice)	Lack of time; lack of technology; lack of computer equipment; lack of incentives; lack of modern educational philosophy and the recognition of online teaching; worry about leakage of teaching and learning materials; worry about online teaching uncontrollable; workload evaluation of teachers in online teaching is not clear; low motivation of students to gain information; other
T22	What incentives and policy support can promote depth development of the network teaching? (Short answer)	

Dimension 2 The effects of online teaching and learning. Measured from whether classroom teaching of university assisted by online teaching or not; whether the demand and pressure from the students access to network information to encourage teachers to carry out the sharing of network teaching or not; cases of online teaching and learning; the effects of online teaching and learning in the school's self-learning courses, a total of 4 small problems

Dimension 3 Usage of the EOL platform. Measured from ever courses on Education Online; whether to continue to use; the satisfaction; which functions are used; what kind of network forms of teaching; the effects of "Education Online" on online teaching; the lack of features and services, a total of 7 small problems

Dimension 4 The impediments and incentives of online teaching and learning. Measured from What factors hinder teachers in online teaching; What incentives support, a total of 2 small problems, part of the example shown in Table 419.1.

419.2.2 Results and Analysis

419.2.2.1 Basic Information of the Respondents

We received a total of 116 valid Teacher Questionnaires. The statistics of T1–T9 (1–9 questions) in Dimension 1 reflect the basic situation of the teachers concerning about online teaching. Among the respondents, the proportion of male teachers is 37.07 % and the proportion of female is 62.93 %. The teachers' ages

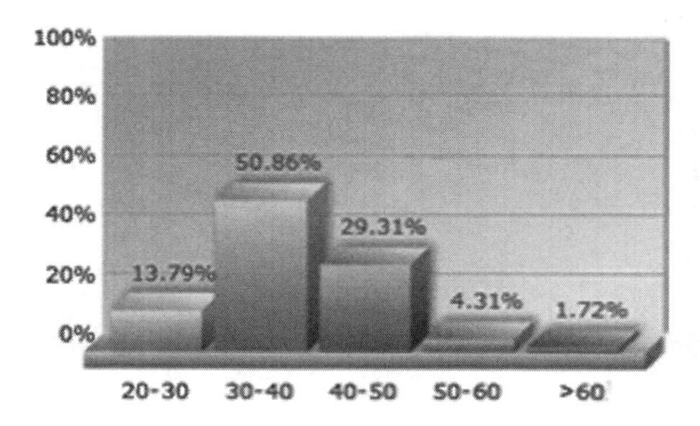

Fig. 419.1 Age chart

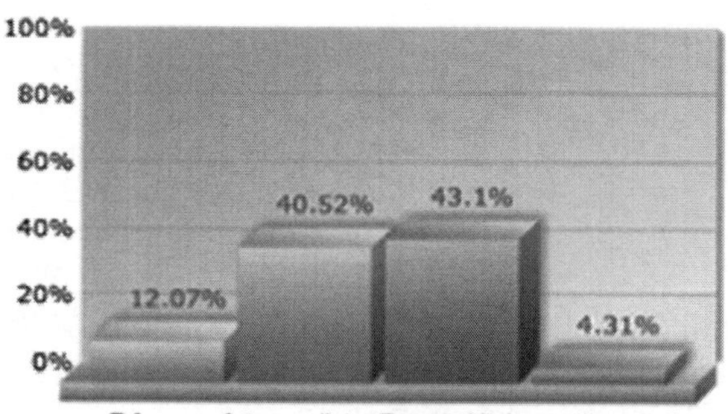

Fig. 419.2 Titles chart

are mostly at the age of 30–50, and the ratio reached 80.17 %, as shown in Fig. 419.1. The proportion of teachers with a master's degree or above is 85.34 %. The proportion of teachers of intermediate and senior vice is 83.62 %, and only 4.31 % are senior teachers, as shown in Fig. 419.2. The teachers from Computer Science, College of Applied Sciences and Electronic Control Institute have higher motivation in Online Teaching. Teachers of science and engineering disciplines accounted for 76.72 %. These data are basically in same with Education Online Teacher user statistics. In general, the teachers of science and engineering disciplines, of intermediate and senior vice, with a master's degree or doctor's degree, at 30–50 years old are the main force to carry out online teaching.

419.2.2.2 The Effects of Online Teaching and Learning

This part of the test checks whether the teachers satisfied with online teaching role, and the answer is yes. 97.41 % of teachers recognized that online teaching could promote classroom instruction, and 95.69 % of teachers recognized that the need of students to gain network learning materials is a contributing factor for teachers in online teaching.

T12 Shares a online teaching case: the visits of "Data structures and algorithms" course BBS on "Education Online" platform is up to more than 120 million times, and the topic posts more than 1800. The retired teacher Moderator "old man" still often returned to the Forum Q & A, and the graduate students for many years often "come back" Q & A and greetings. This course was named "Beijing quality courses". This question gives teachers incentives, and the proportion of teachers is 91.38 %, who believed that "old man" could help students by Forum Q & A, and establish a harmonious relationship between teachers and students. There are 78.45 % of teachers agreed that the love of teaching, perseverance and dedication of "old man" move people and great touch on young teachers to pay attention to teaching. There are 75 % of teachers thinking that IT is not "Midas touch technique", and the teacher is the real magician, and the excellent online teaching needs of teaching technology, design, to operate and adhere to. However, there are 2.59 % of teachers thinking that the "old man" was unwise because delaying the functions of the "research".

T13 explores the effect of online teaching in the school's self-learning courses, and views did not agree. Point 1: independent study based on learning tasks and resources can improve students' independent analysis and exploration capability, suitable for blending learning—the combining form online teaching and classroom teaching. Teachers bring learning tasks and materials in the platform courseware and practice modules; organize and support and monitor the process of learning through BBS activities; close and correct course work in the homework module. Teachers holding this view accounted for 73.28 %. Point 2: Online teaching can only be a supplement to classroom teaching, not suitable for self-learning courses. Teachers holding this view accounted for 23.28 %. According to T13 the majority of teachers agree that the school's self-learning courses are suitable foe blending learning form. It is based on this case, we take the form of online teaching assisting classroom teaching based on Education Online platform, and online teaching is a strong complement to classroom, and the resource of quality courses, audio-visual classroom on platform support students self-learning services.

419.2.2.3 Usage of the EOL Platform

T16 measured to detect teachers' satisfaction with the Education Online platform. There are 66.37 % of teachers very satisfied with the "Education Online", 31.86 % of teachers basically satisfied who made some recommendations. According to T15 there are 85.34 % of teachers who would continue or try to use the EOL platform.

According to T17 the application of teacher on EOL centralized course notification, course description, course outline, courseware, course work and Q & A discussion, while others such as blog and courses introduce ourselves less applied, as shown in Fig. 419.3. It is corresponding to T18 statistics that teachers mainly used courseware, course work, forums, video in online teaching, specific statistics that there are 69.81 % of teachers who used courseware sharing curriculum resources to

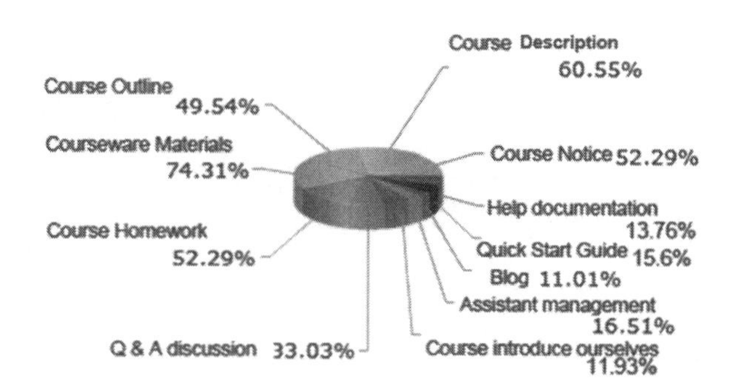

Fig. 419.3 Application of EOL chart

facilitate students to download; 31.86 % of them built curriculum resources and organized discussions on the course forum under the assistant's help; 37.74 % of them sent course work and corrected them on the platform; 23.58 % of them mainly used video teaching mode. To combine with "Education Online" operating data, it also was found that some function modules such as "blog" has lost its meaning, and operation and maintenance energy should be mainly into teachers concern.

According to T19, 90.52 % of teachers think that it's convenient (online teaching is a useful supplement and extension to classroom teaching that share courseware, information, course work and practice); 81.03 % of teachers think that the content is expanded (teachers can organize and send more discipline development information, materials, links to resources and answers to some question that were not introduced in the classroom limited by time, to guide students to think and exchanges); 56.9 % of teachers think that the Interaction are deeper(teachers can organize common learning problems in the forum, to avoid repeated answer common problems, to promote student learning and exchange), shown in Fig. 419.4.

The T21 short answer measurements detect teachers' advices on Education Online features and services, mainly in the course work, courseware copyright protection, browser compatibility, promotion and training. For example the recommendations on course work is to increase the marking function on the download package, the marking document can be uploaded; to increase the rating performance statistics and group management; to make course work republish and secondary upload by students. These proposals are small in the big, very important to optimize the teaching process and improve the quality of teaching that reflects the subject of Educational Technology. We reply these issues one by one by mail, and publish the finishing answers on campus network.

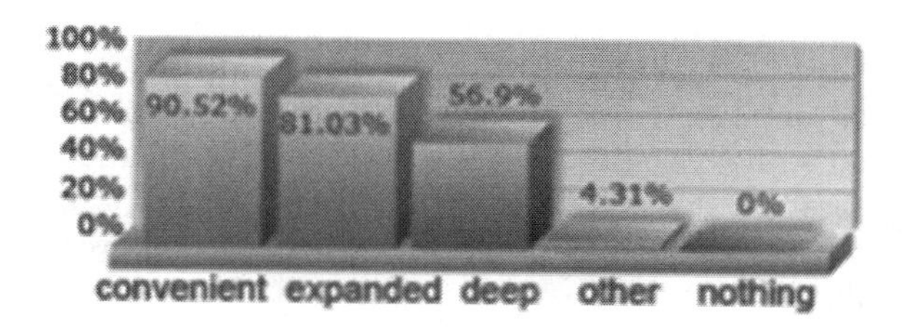

Fig. 419.4 Effect of EOL chart

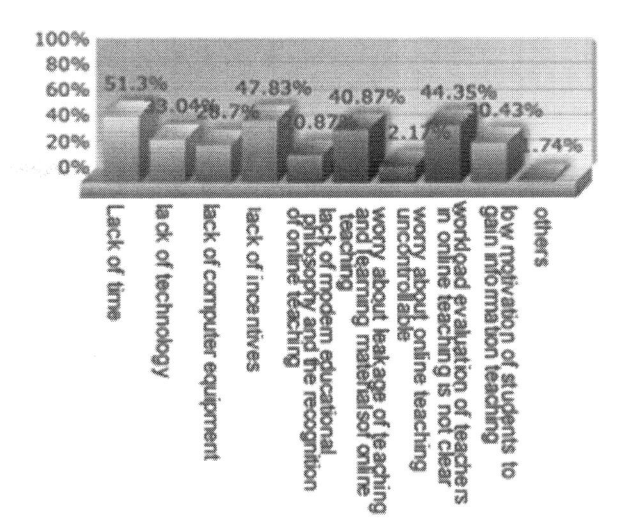

Fig. 419.5 Impediments of online teaching chart

The impediments and incentives of online teaching and learning

T20 multiple-choice test check the online teaching impediments. There are 51.3 % of teachers thinking lack of time; 47.83 % thinking lack of incentives; 44.35 % thinking workload evaluation of teachers in online teaching is not clear; 40.87 % fear of leakage of teaching and learning materials; and some other factors, as shown in Fig. 419.5. The question finds the factors hindering the development of online teaching from the reverse thinking and measures out that the incentives focus on the following aspects: setting the "quality assessment mechanism of online teaching" to reward qualified teachers; equipping assistant to help developing online teaching; setting up "the online teaching outstanding achievement award"; increasing online teaching research projects.

"Lack of time" reflects teachers' competitive pressure difficult to try to put in some effort to engage in online teaching, and teachers want to encourage in this part of the work, and to study out Workload Calculation and coefficients. The issue of copyright protection has restricted network teaching. Actually teachers can solve the problem of copyright protection by converting document formats (such as PDF or swf) or encryption method. Currently, universities' awareness of this part of the work can not form a unified approach. With the increasingly prominent role of online teaching, research and practice related will become the future trend.

419.3 Thinking and Summing

EOL platform is designed to reflect the people-oriented and tailored principle. With the continuous development of Education Online, it integrates of audio-visual classroom and Quality courses resources platform, with function to get expand, basically meeting the needs of teachers, widely recognized. Teachers provide a lot of good advice for it on promotion and application, functional improvement, service, platform integration, incentives and so on. We should summary and improve them, such that the platform is to a certain technical service cycle at the technical level. With the upgrade of the browser, the platform needs to "fix" some code to solve browser compatibility and the editor version.

At the design level, according to the needs of teachers, some modules have little effect, and we could terminate these services. However, some modules need to continually improve, such as course work, forums, courseware to optimize online teaching process.

At the level of the application and promotion, work in these areas has complete, such as help documentation, flash major step animated guide, message boards, supplemented by manual telephone auxiliary, and technical support services. But we still need to synchronously sort out the online teaching mode case and the production of promotional electronic materials, supplemented by small-scale seminars and day-to-day training to promote and deepen the online teaching.

There is no relevant policy support in our school, and teachers carry out teaching through EOL platform with interest and responsibility in our school. In some colleges and universities good policies guide the development of online teaching. Shandong Polytechnic University, for example, adds a "rich curriculum resources" and "online course" building objectives in the "construction quality undergraduate education program of Shandong Polytechnic University" to encourage teaching reform and innovation, and projects 100 courses annually, and organizes projecting, allocation of funds, inspection and acceptance of related teaching and research. Increasing emphasis on curriculum resource's networking and information technology, teachers promote the application in teaching and learning resources, while achieving the educational technology capability. Supported by the small sample size restrictions and some respondents unused EOL, additional the questionnaire having promotional purposes, some of the issues and options set more subjective, which affected the accuracy of the findings. So the findings are for reference only. The analysis and summary is also based on the EOL platform daily data as an important reference drawn.

References

1. Wang H (2007) "People-oriented"— to build a new generation of online education platform. Modern Distance Education, Beijing
2. Zhou S, Zhu X (2008) Design and implementation of the information feedback system based on a new generation of network teaching platform. China Modern Educational Equipment, Beijing
3. Cao Q, Zhou S (2008) Data migration when switching network teaching platform. Modern Educational Technology, Beijing
4. Zhou S, Cao Q, Lei J, Xu S (2008) Adhere to the educational technology research to lead the Educational Technology development. China Modern Educational Equipment, Beijing

Chapter 420 The Application of Telemedicine Technology

Ming-gang Wang, Ying-jun Mao and Wei Li

Abstract Based on the development of telemedicine in the United States and Europe, the article introduces the history and the present situation of telemedicine development. The current telemedicine mainly contains: tele-consultation, tele-diagnose, tele-education, tele-care and tele-medical car, etc. Telemedicine can be applied in homecare, sea medical, emergency treatment and military, etc. The article also discusses some key technology of telemedicine. The technologies used in telemedicine that has gradually transformed from single television monitor or phone remote diagnose to figure, picture and phonic transmission by mobile communication equipment, wired and wireless network. At the same time, monitoring equipment, all kinds of vital-sign monitors and wireless sensors have become smaller and portable. Wearable biomedical instrument is the research focus in the field of telemedicine. Although there are some problems, such as insufficient understanding, high cost, low accuracy and privacy, telemedicine has the advantages of time and space, and effectively solves the problem of irrational allocation of medical resources and imbalance of medical level.

Keywords Telemedicine.homecare · Ele-monitor.technology

Telemedicine is an interdisciplinary high-tech combining modern network technology Communication technology Multimedia technology and medical treatment by telecommunications and information processing technology providing means of information storage and processing transmitting voice images data documents, pictures and even moving color images and other medical activities in long distance space

M. Wang (✉) · Y. Mao · W. Li
The 401st Hospital of PLA, Qingdao, China
e-mail: wmgang@sina.com

S. Li et al. (eds.), *Frontier and Future Development of Information Technology in Medicine and Education*, Lecture Notes in Electrical Engineering 269,
DOI: 10.1007/978-94-007-7618-0_420,

420.1 Introduction

From early 1960s to the mid-1980s, Telemedicine activities are usually known as the first generation of telemedicine. In the early 1960s, the United States National Aeronautics and Space Administration set up Telemedicine test-bed for astronauts in Arizona to provide telemedicine services. The means of communication are satellite and microwave technology, transferring medical information, including electrocardiograms and X-rays. During this period, Canada, Australia and other countries have also initiated telemedicine research. This stage of the development of telemedicine is slow, mainly because information technology is not well developed, the development of telemedicine is limited by the communication conditions.

In the late 1980s. Several higher-valued projects are launched in the globe, representing the second generation of the development of telemedicine. In 1988, United States proposed a concept that telemedicine system should be used as an open distributed system. In 1991, Georgia first built the world's largest and most extensive of distance education and medical networks-education. Which can be do communications activities by wired, wireless and satellite. Later, the U.S. and successfully did telemedicine activities in the Gulf War and Somali peace mission. In 1994, the U.S. Department of Defense established a telemedicine test-bed, launched all kinds of telemedicine projects, the promotion of large-scale telemedicine experiments systems initiated by the European Union further promoted the popularity of telemedicine. A data shows that in 1993 alone, about 2,250 patients in the United States and Canada were treated through the telemedicine system. This phase of telemedicine showed a great application value in military and civil applications.

The U.S. military is starting "Gold Plan III", "man-monitor program" and other research projects. Which is known as the third generation of telemedicine. Gold Plan III will link medical institutions in Hungary, Bosnia and Herzegovina, Germany, Europe and the United States, establishing a telemedicine network. Battlefield telemedicine system developed by the University of Maryland combined field doctor, communications equipment vehicles, satellite communications network, field hospitals and remote medical center together. In this system, soldiers equip with newly developed man-monitor, which is mainly composed by environmental sensors, physiological sensors, GPS locator, wireless phones and other. Once injured, the monitor can measure the soldiers blood pressure and heart rate parameters etc. GPS locator can help doctors to find the injured quickly, and do diagnosis and treatment through the telemedicine system.

From the 1980s, China began to explore telemedicine, after passing qualified acceptance, dozens of hospital websites were formally put into operation in more than twenty provinces including the Chinese Academy of Medical Sciences, Beijing Union Medical College Hospital, Chinese Academy of Medical Sciences Fu Wai Cardiovascular Disease Hospital the hospital, and had done a lot of teleconsultations and tele-educations, which greatly promoted the development of the cause of China's telemedicine. Though telemedicine had achieved initial results, but comparing with the level of developed countries, there is a great gap in the technologies, policies, regulations, applications, which needs continue improvements.

420.2 Application of Telemedicine and Technological Realization

Main applications: remote medical diagnosis system for the purpose of diagnosis, consultation, remote medical consultation system for the purpose of consultation, remote medical education system for the purpose of teaching and training and home care for the purpose of remote beds monitoring system.

420.2.1 Application in Home Monitor

Home monitoring devices which are introduced in the market today, are video interactive combined with video camera, wireless ECG transmission function, wireless auscultation capabilities, broad band cable, satellite communications and digital technology to achieve real-time, two-way high-speed communications, rapid transmission of diagnostic digital clinical images, by using portable wireless detection equipment, passing the patient's physiological parameters to the data center.

As to equipment manufacturers, the majority are US ones. Most of them were built on the existing video conferencing equipment, providing software platforms and network services, such as the United States Vetel company. There are many companies providing a wide variety of monitoring equipment. For example AMD, its remote devices include dozens of subjects of sensor equipments, such as cardiac examination, dental, eye, ear, nose, throat, skin, and ECG, blood pressure, blood oxygen detection, as well as the corresponding camera and endoscopic diagnostic tests, which can directly transmit signal to the care center.

Another is typical video phone. Motion Media Company launched a video telephone instrument, using a standard telephone line PSTN and ISDN or IP telephone service. This monitoring equipment using existing PSTN network to achieve the general information desk, medical education, and it is easy to promote home monitoring mode with less investment. Currently a more outstanding wireless home monitoring is developed by a Canada MARCH company, such series of monitoring devices have the following unique features: achieving the exchange of information with the patients through wireless communication, wireless ECG, auscultation and blood pressure monitoring.

420.2.2 Application in Emergency Treatment

Since the date of birth, Telemedicine is inseparable with Emergency Treatment Medicine. AS human began to fly into space in the 1960s, the NASA had set in telemedicine research, using telemedicine technology to monitor astronauts' physiological functions. As technology continues to improve in all aspects, the scope of application of telemedicine is expanding its role in the field of emergency medicine.

For example, the British Central Cheshire hospital established telemedicine connection by combining the minor trauma medical departments with accident emergency treatment center. This project began in January 1997, with BT cooperation via ISDN for remote PC-based video terminal, and today still got further perfection, mainly used to support nurses practice and telemedicine connection for remote patient care consultation.

Telemedicine technology is introduced to the pre-hospital care of the emergency treatment to in recent years abroad, changing the passive treatment to active treatment, further improving the speed and quality of first aid. The University of Maryland in the United States successful developed a set of ambulance mobile telemedicine system, which can do the real-time transmission of variety of wounded vital signs, voice, images to the emergency center. So that the doctor would have a more comprehensive understanding of the situation of the wounded before arriving, and get ready to do the rescue, if necessary, doctors can also guide the responder to the wounded through the telemedicine system for emergency treatment. Recently they prepared to add GPS to accomplish a dynamic management of all the ambulances and make the full use of the pre-hospital care.

420.2.3 Application in Military

Modern warfare is implemented in a short period of time under high-tech conditions, high-intensity, full range of intense military confrontation, with characteristics of sudden and strong, more serious injuries and complex treatment environment and requiring maneuvers, rapid treatment. The traditional hierarchical ambulance mode can not meet such demand, we must find a more effective treatment approach. Telemedicine has been favored by the national army.

In this regard, the U.S. military is the leading one among them. War wounds treatment research and development before 2010 including the collection, management and delivery of front-line medical data modules, monitoring and diagnosis of physiological sensors and intelligent medicine, telemedicine were proposed in the financial year plan made in 1997. The same content also contains in the development strategy of the 21st century health care system. The U.S. military also set up a special Tele-medicine and Advanced Technology Research Center, TATRC, and actively carry out the research about telemedicine technology and equipment. The U.S. military has been developed Personal the Status Monitor, which combines global satellite positioning system, state of life care and communication functions together to do the wounded precise searching. This device has been successfully used in the Gulf War and the current war in Kosovo rescue missions, greatly improve the survival rate of the soldiers on the battlefield. The U.S. military has recently further developed what is called a "smart jersey injury detection", combining the injured area location, type of injury, injury severity judgment, wireless communication functions. In the shortest possible time, the wounded could get the necessary treatment. "Smart jersey" has now completed the battlefield test, and is equipped by Marines and Special Forces of U.S. begin. Military telemedicine high-tech research center and its cooperation units are also developing a battlefield remote control operation system. With virtual reality, three-dimensional reconstruction and precision machinery technology, the rear experts can control a computer robot to implement remote surgery on the wounded on the battlefield. If combined with microsurgical instruments, can also do microsurgery. The system has been successfully tested on animals. In addition, in recent years, the U.S. military also successfully developed a large number of telemedicine equipments, such as portable field medical assistance, field medical coordinator, trauma care coordinator and trauma modules and portable trauma treatment, storage and transmission of treatment information, the coordination between the various ambulance ladder and auxiliary treatment programs.

Telemedicine applications include almost every aspect of telemedicine technology, such as remote diagnostics, remote consultation, remote monitoring, remote operation, remote consultation.

420.2.4 Telemedicine Education

For medical workers, Telemedicine Education is the latest and most advanced medical information and knowledge to the grass-roots hospitals, the expert experience to the primary health care workers, answer the primary hospital problems encountered in the diagnosis and treatment activities to help grass-roots hospitals and doctors to expand the clinic, standardize the treatment program, obtain the latest medical information and treatment techniques through the telemedicine education system or network platform. In view of this, the telemedicine education is one of the important means to enhance the service level of grass-roots medical staff. For students, telemedicine medical education is to show the students in the medical field a variety of information, knowledge and the ways of medical technology operations by video. The content of education can include the latest developments of the medicine field, medicine dynamic, research results, teaching rounds, surgical demonstration. This form of teaching is more likely to be accepted by the students with interest and passion to learn.

Through satellite communications, computer network and multimedia techniques to create an image of a real-time, interactive simulation classroom environment. The system mainly consists Management Control Center (CMC), multi-point audio and video distribution control unit (MCU) and client software. TCP/IP platform can be extended to IP video telephone network, and on this basis also can establish a point-to-point, point-to-multipoint or multi-point-to-multipoint video conferencing, to meet the needs for long-distance training, technical exchanges, daily meetings and instant message. Such systems can use MPEG-4, JPEG 2000 compression technology, H.263, H.263, H.264, etc. and is compatible with a variety of coding techniques to support multi-resolution options, thus ensuring the quality of audio and video. Using H.323 encoding, H.323 framework based on selection the centralized conferencing systems architecture, and C/S mode as realized mode and MCU multicast to each terminal data to send data in the form of single point on the multi- point data transmission, designed in line with the H.323 standard multi-point video conferencing system. In order to achieve synchronized video and audio, the stereo audio compressed stream can be embedded into the stereoscopic video coding system based on the H.264 standard. In addition, video conferencing systems also involves product maintenance, compatibility, and security issues. Dynamic key, encrypted communication and RSA digital signature are mainly used to ensure video conference security.

420.3 Existing Problems

Telemedicine is an emerging new technology, there are still many problems to be solved in the course of its development.

420.3.1 Doctor-Patient Insufficient Understanding

Remote Consultation provide convenient and efficient health care services for patients, while promoting exchanges and cooperation between the medical staff, but lack the understanding and awareness of the remote consultation for both doctors and patients. On one hand, the medical staff does not know this technology too much, in their view, this is an unproven technology, the effectiveness of this technology is also unknown. They believe a doctor with many years practice with telemedicine experience is a good doctor, and now still can be a good doctor. There are some doctors who are willing to use telemedicine, but have no time to learn how to use it. On the other hand, most patients do not understand the characteristics of this new way of medical services. They are reluctant to try this new technology, resulting in the process of looking for a doctor delaying the best time of treatment, aggravating the condition and bringing serious consequences. Therefore, improving the understanding of both doctors and patients on the remote consultation is very important.

420.3.2 High Cost

The establishment of a telemedicine system hardware cost is very expensive, so as to install and maintain database transmission line. The cost of chat online with experts is not encouraging. Although the cost of the hardware as the development of science and technology will reduce, but the barriers of telemedicine widely used in developing countries still exist. Not to mention other costs. The American scholar Smiths studied telemedicine system used in the United States of Texas, found that the system was used only once a week. She believes that "only 50 times a week is difficult to pay line charges.

420.3.3 Low Accuracy of Telemedicine Diagnosis

It has been reported that the accuracy of telemedicine is lower than the accuracy of the person on-site consultation. Due to the doctor's technology level of the application side and medical condition have a certain gap with the diagnosis side, if lacking the necessary communication, the application physician will easily miss some information which they think is not important in the acquisition process of consultation medical records, resulting case incomplete, affecting the consultation experts to understand, analyze and judge the medical records provided. Secondly, because the staff does not well learn the graphics image reconstruction technology, image blurred, color distortion, deviate from the real data, the transmission of graphic information inaccurate may occur, which will also affect the accuracy of diagnosis.

420.3.4 Privacy

The security of personal data within the system, in particular the leading figure will be reduced. Advanced network technology enables it to become easier to obtain the information of another node from a node, or even modify the data of another node. More security concerns should be given about stealing the patient's privacy by intercepting video or other information. We should take a more comprehensive security policy, such as joint coding, extended personal password, to prevent the patient's medical information, especially highly sensitive information from being exposed.

In addition, the significance of telemedicine in law is yet to be determined. Whether telemedicine is legitimate, whether the doctor should obtain telemedicine license, these are the development of telemedicine need to be resolved.

420.4 Conclusion

Although there are some problems, however, application of telemedicine has changed the traditional medical model. With the advantage of time and space, telemedicine enables remote transmission of medical information, remote monitoring, remote consultation, education and communication, and effectively solves the problem of irrational allocation of medical resources and imbalance of medical level.

References

1. Yasushi S (2011) A remote desktop-based telemedicine system [J]. J Clin Neurosci 18:661–663
2. Wang X,Richard S, Zhou W et al (2003) The Fast development of PAS brings hope for telehomecare in China. In: The 25th Annual international conference of the IEEE engineering in medicine and biology society, Cancun MPxic
3. Maxine LR (1977) Telemedicine: explorations in the use of telecommunications in health care [J]. Soc Sci Med 11:295–296
4. James B, Jane H (2009) Adopting integrated mainstream telecare services [J]. Eurohealth 15:8–10
5. Frederick N, Prathibha V (2011) Are e-health web users looking for different symptom information than callers to triage centers [J]. Telemed e-Health 17:19–25

Chapter 421
A Method of Data Flow Diagram Drawing Based on Word Segmentation Technique

Shuli Yuwen and Kaifei Wang

Abstract The drawing of Data Flow Diagram (DFD) is the key technology in the development of system analysis and design. DFD is not only the key composing part of the logic model in new system, but also the key basis in the system physical designing. According to the author's experience in research and teaching, the paper puts forward a simple method of drawing the DFD based on the word segmentation technology. This method can automatically draw the DFD according to the investigation reports, and this can improve the system analyst's work efficiency.

Keywords Word segmentation technique · Data flow diagram · Substantiality · Data process · Data storage · Data flow

421.1 Introduction

In the course of the system analysis and design, data flow diagram (DFD) is the main tool of describing information system logic model, and it also is an effective communication method between the systems analyst and the users. With a few symbols, DFD easily and comprehensively shows the information condition, which composes the information flowing, processing and storing in the system. Practice has proved that the user can understand the mean of the DFD, as long as the system analyst slightly explains the DFD to the user. At the same time, the DFD is suitable to business investigation for the business people with different levels of management due to DFD's strong levels. Therefore the drawing of the DFD is particularly important in the method of the structured system development. This paper puts forward a simple method of drawing the Data Flow Diagram based

---

S. Yuwen (✉) · K. Wang
School of Management, Hebei University, Hebei, People's Republic of China
e-mail: ywslzxhll@gmail.com

S. Li et al. (eds.), *Frontier and Future Development of Information Technology in Medicine and Education*, Lecture Notes in Electrical Engineering 269,
DOI: 10.1007/978-94-007-7618-0_421,

on the word segmentation technology according to the author's experience in research and teaching, which greatly saves system analyst's conversion time from the investigation report to the DFD.

421.2 Introduction of DFD

Commonly, the DFD consists of four symbols, and we are respectively describing them below:

421.2.1 Substantiality

The substantiality refers to the person or entity outside of the system, and they are the information providers or the users outside of system, which has information transmission relationship with the system. is. Generally, the substantiality exists outside of the system and emerges the persons or the organizations, and it is used to illustrate the data source inputting the system or the data destination and the end users. It is often said with S with serial number.

421.2.2 Data Processing

The data processing id also known as the system function and it is the show and instruction of all the data logic in the system. The data processing is the core of the DFD, and decomposition of the system DFD is based on the decomposition of the data processing. Generally the data processing is said by P with serial number.

421.2.3 Data Storage

The data storage is the long-term or temporary storage data which stored in the system, and it is usually by form of data file, folder, and books and so on. And D is commonly used to represent the data storage with serial number.

421.2.4 Data Flow

The data flow is showing the flowing data and the data flow direction in the system. It is composed of a fixed set of components of data, which can is a data or a group of data, for example, it can be files, documents and so on, at the same time it also can be used to represent the operation of the stored data file. The data flow can flow from one data processing to another data processing, and also can be used between the data processing and the data storage or between the data processing and the substantiality. There may have more data flows between two data processing. Data flow is commonly used to represent by F with serial number.

421.3 Drawing Method of DFD based on the Word Segmentation

Obviously, for the name of the DFD's four components, the substantiality mostly is person or organization, so it is often named by nouns, and the data storage or the data flow mostly are files or documents in the form of existence, so they are also with nouns to name them. Only the data processing is used to indicate the specific data of the system operation, so it is much in the form of a verb. Above all, firstly we can participle the investigation report, and then corroding to the segmentation the system can automatically draw a rough DFD and participle it, finally we can manually adjustment the DFD depending on the needs of the investigation and system. The main idea is as follows:

(1) Analyzing the investigation report, and tagging the report with the part-of-speech by system tool;
(2) picking up the main word from the tagged results, and extracting the nouns and the verbs, then preprocessing these nouns and verbs, such as classifying, sorting, statistical analysis and merging the same or similar the nouns or the verbs according to the user's requirements and so on;
(3) Defining the system's substantiality, the system function and the core data storage, and drawing the top level diagram of the DFD;
(4) Decomposing the system function according to the result of word segmentation, and refining the DFD's hierarchical structure.
(5) Repeating step (4) until the word segmentation results is empty, so then the system DFD is after drawing.

421.4 Case Application

421.4.1 Case Introduction

Depositors will complete a single certificate and sent it with the passbook to the bank clerk. The bank clerk separately handles it according to the two different situations: if it is a deposit, the passbook, the deposit slip and the cash will be sent to the deposit clerk, and the deposit clerk will query the depositor's account and return the depositor the passbook after registration; and if it is a withdrawn, the passbook and the withdrawal slip will be sent to the withdrawal clerk, then the withdrawal clerk will take the cash and return the depositor the passbook with the cash after registration.

421.4.2 Drawing the DFD

421.4.2.1 Results of the Part-of-Speech Tagging and Preprocessing

Table 421.1

421.4.2.2 Drawing the Top DFD

Obviously, the depositor in the nouns list after preprocessing does not belong to the bank clerk or units in the system, so in this case, the depositor is marked as substantiality.

The system's main function is the depositing and withdrawn, so we can name it with them or directly named as system processes.

All above, at the top of the DFD of the case as shown in Fig. 421.1:

Table 421.1 Results of preprocessing

Nouns	Verbs
Depositors	Process
Deposit slip	Deposit
Withdrawal slip	Registration
Cash	Deposit cash
Passbook	Withdrawn
Account	Take cash

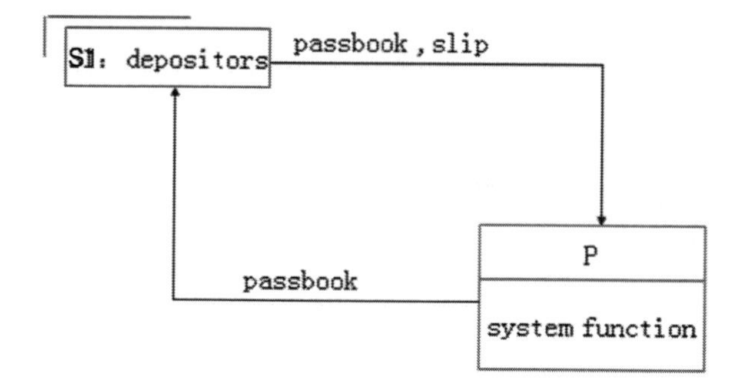

Fig. 421.1 Top DFD

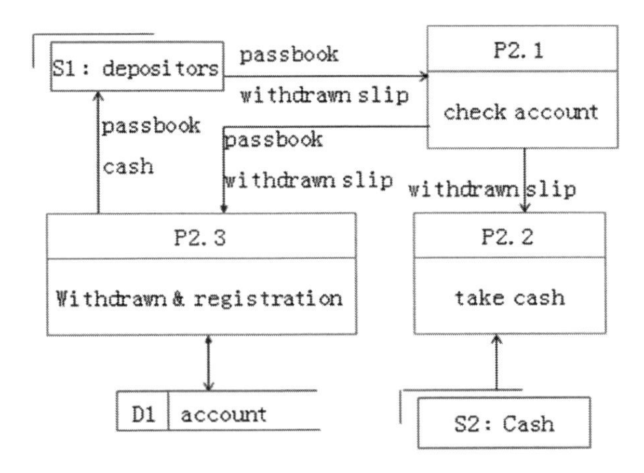

Fig. 421.2 Underlying DFD

421.4.2.3 Underlying DFD

According to the investigation, we can see that the main function of the system can be divided into two handling: deposits and withdrawals processing operations. At the same time, these processing can be discomposed according to each segment verb table, therefore, we can draw the underlying DFD as shown in Fig. 421.2, which is withdrawals.

421.5 Conclusion

The method of the drawing DFD based on the word segmentation technology is the author's teaching achievements of nearly 10 years of the course of the information system analysis and design. This method has proved in practice by more than 20 classes and more than 1000 people in the past 10 years. It has proved that this method is easy to learn and operate, and it also can save the analyst's time and energy on the drawing of the DFD. And this method is accepted by the teachers and students in our school.

At present, a software tool for DFD drawing is developed according to this method, which can automatically draw the rough the DFD due to the investigation report and it need to revise in order to achieve more accurate DFD.

Acknowledgments This research was supported by the Society Science Union of Baoding under Grant 201201054 and 201201118.

References

1. Tiyun H (2009) Management information system 4 th edn. Higher Education Press
2. Huacheng X (2012) Management Information System 6 edn. Tsinghua University Press
3. Yueyang H, Shikun D, Shiyin J, Yuanfang L (2011) Research on the word classification in Chinese word segmenttion. Comput Technol Dev
4. Xiaoxing L, Changxia H (2011) Research on the key technology of WEB text information retrieval. Silicon Valley
5. Chunming Y, Yongguo H (2011) Rapid and automatic keyword extraction algorithm from the field document. Comput Eng Des
6. Jun G, Hao W (2011) Research on the term extraction method based on Chinese text field. Mod Inf Technol
7. Tingting M (2010) Overview of the Chinese automatic word segmentation system. Comput Knowl Technol
8. Tieli S, Yanji L (2009) Research on the Chinese word segmentation technology. Inf Technol

Chapter 422
Chemical Reaction Optimization for Nurse Rostering Problem

Ziran Zheng and Xiaoju Gong

Abstract Chemical reaction optimization (CRO) method is a relative new nature-inspired algorithm. It searches solutions in the problem space by simulating the molecules movement happened during the chemical reaction process. This method has been applied to many problems in recent years. As a NP-hard combinatorial problem, nurse rostering problem (NPR) is a well-known personnel scheduling task whose goal is to create a nurse roster under many hard and soft constraints in a hospital ward. This paper investigates the application of CRO to solve the NRP. We provide the CRO operator under the framework for the rostering problem. The performance of the CRO method is evaluated on several datasets from the first NPR Competition 2010. Experiment results show that this method could obtain good solutions compared to that of genetic algorithm (implemented herein).

Keywords Chemical reaction optimization · Nurse rostering · Timetabling and personnel scheduling · Genetic algorithm

422.1 Introduction

Nurse rostering problem is a kind of personnel scheduling task which could be a difficult. In an hospital ward, managers or head nurses usually design the roster in a period by hand and this leads to a very time-consuming. Since this work often

Z. Zheng (✉)
School of Management Science and Engineering, Shandong Normal University, Jinan, China
e-mail: zzr_nature@163.com

X. Gong (✉)
Provincial Hospital Affliated to Shandong University, Jinan, China
e-mail: happyxiaoju@163.com

S. Li et al. (eds.), *Frontier and Future Development of Information Technology in Medicine and Education*, Lecture Notes in Electrical Engineering 269,
DOI: 10.1007/978-94-007-7618-0_422,

needs the constraints, traditional method cannot obtain the best roster easily. Large amount of methods had been proposed to solve this method. Because this problem is NP-hard, various kinds of combinatorial optimization algorithms are investigate. To solve this problem, various kinds of method are proposed. In literature [1–4], population-based heuristics are provided. Chemical Reaction Optimization is first presented in [5]. It is an new nature-inspired searching technique framework. In this paper, we applied this relative new method to solve the NRP.

In Sect. 432.2, we briefly describe the nurse rostering problem. In Sect. 422.3, we describe the CRO method and the operator we designed. Experiments are presented in Sect. 422.4, and draw the conclusion in the Sect. 422.5.

422.2 Problem Description

The object of the nurse rostering problem is to create a roster dotted with shift types to present the nurse scheduling during a period. In our algorithm, one roster solution uses a multi-dimensional array to represent the solution directly.

Usually two kinds of constraints should be considered, which are hard constraints and soft constraints. The definition of these constraints can be different based on the actual needs or other requirements. Since in this paper we use the dataset from the Nurse Rostering Competition 2010, their constraints are applied here. There are two hard constraints. The first one is the number of nurses needed on a certain day should be defined and any solution must not contradict it. The other one is every nurse could only work one kind of type of shift. Before the searching, the original randomly generated solution is created follow these two and every move during the searching process neither contradict it. The number of soft constraints is much more than that of the hard constraints. The main soft ones are described as follows (Table 422.1):

Given a set of N nurses with each belongs to a working contract and $|N| = 10$; denote D the set of days in a time period with $|D| = 28$; let S be the shift types that contains Night, Early, Late night and Day with the first letter being their abbreviation; we use the C to denote the constraint set and let C1 be the soft constraints stated above for the hard constraints is always met with certain methods during the initial solution generating process. Let X be an solution and the cost function is

Table 422.1 Soft constraints description

Soft constraints	Description
S1	The maximum number of shifts that can be assigned to one nurse
S2	The minimum number of shifts that can be assigned to one nurse
S3	The maximum number of consecutive days on which a nurse works
S4	The minimum number of consecutive days on which a nurse works

$$f(X) = \sum_{i \in N} \sum_{j \in C_1} w_{i,j} f_{i,j} \qquad (422.1)$$

where w is the weight the f is the soft constraint's cost value if the solution contradicts that constraint. We use the direct solution representation for the problem. A candidate solution is represented by an |N| × |D| matrix X where x, i, j corresponds to the shift type assigned for nurse is at day d. If there is no shift assigned to nurse s at day d, then x takes Null.

422.3 Chemical Reaction Optimization for NPR

Chemical Reaction Optimization is a new kind of heuristics to obtain the approximate solutions for an optimization problem. It is as a population-based searching technique as other nature-inspired algorithm like Genetic Algorithm. The algorithm follows the rule that the direction of the chemical reaction—the molecules should evolve toward the stable state. Consider the solutions as molecules, and the process of reaction is the process of searching solution in the space.

Each solution as the molecules in a reaction has its own attributes. It includes the potential energy (PE) which is the fitness value of objective function and kinetic energy (KE) which represents the tolerance of accepting worse solution. There are four kinds of basic reactions which act as the searching movement. Those four are on-wall ineffective collision, decomposition, inter-molecular ineffective collision, and synthesis. These four types of reaction differs in their searching range which means two of them could be considered as the local search and the others two keep the diversity. More detailed description of Chemical Reaction Optimization (CRO) can be found in Ref. [5]. This algorithm has been used in several problems and could obtain very competitive results [6–10].

Although this is a new heuristic, it also needs to design the operator for the independent problem. In our investigation, we provide the operator for the NRP solution.

- On-wall ineffective collision: In this reaction process, the solution simulates the process of molecule colliding to the wall of the container. The solution should change from one to another by just picking a new one in its neighborhood. As for our problem. We randomly choose 4 days, to each of which the operator exchange two nurses' shifts.
- Decomposition: The extent of change in this reaction should be more that the on-wall ineffective one. After this happens, one solution is decomposed to two new solutions. In a roster solution, we just divide one into two by splitting a solution from the mid day. Here we choose the fourteenth day. After the splitting, we randomly created the left two halves to form two new solutions.

Table 422.2 Comparison of two methods

Instance name	CRO best	Avg.	GA best	Avg.
Sprint01	**72**	**73**	75	75
Sprint02	75	75	75	75
Sprint03	69	**69**	69	70
Sprint04	**76**	**75**	80	80
Sprint_late01	**50**	**50**	52	54
Sprint_late02	61	62	60	62
Sprint_late03	**58**	60	59	60
Sprint_late04	57	57	56	57
Sprint_hidden01	**58**	**60**	62	62
Sprint_hidden02	**72**	**75**	76	79
Sprint_hidden03	**93**	**96**	98	98
Sprint_hidden04	89	89	87	88

- Inter-molecular ineffective collision: this movement represents the two molecules' collision and in this process, two old solution changes to two new ones. We randomly choose 4 days from two solutions and exchange each one,
- Synthesis: Make the two molecules into a new one. Firstly we randomly pick a day and two solutions. Then the partly solution before that day and another partly solution after that day form a new one.

Note that there are several operators; parameters like in the first reaction we choose 4 days. In our experiments, we choose them following the try-and-error methods. Nevertheless, for the extent of the solution change should be considered, the parameter is not hard to pick.

422.4 Computational Experiments

We implement the algorithm in C and the simulations are run on a PC with Intel Core 2 duo@ 2.93 GHz and 2 GB RAM. We also implement a Genetic Algorithm to compare the methods. The test dataset is the sprint track of the NRP competition. All the dataset can be found in the official site of the competition.

The main parameters of the CRO are as follows: *Pop Size* = 20, *KE loss Rate* = 0.4, *Mole Coll* = 0.2, *Initial KE* = 100, $\alpha = 50$, $\beta = 5$, *Initial Energy* = 0, and *Iteration Number* = 100000.

We test the some sprint track data both in CRO and a simple Genetic Algorithm in same iterations. The result is presented in Table 422.2. It show that in most of the instances, CRO method obtain better solutions (in bold).

422.5 Conclusion

In this research, we solve the Nurse Rostering Problem using the new heuristics named Chemical Reaction Optimization. Since this method provides a searching framework, the operator for this problem is designed. Experiment results show that it could obtain good results compare to other searching techniques. In this paper, although we have compared it to GA, the algorithm has not reach the best score in other literature. Future directions include improving the algorithm to increase the effectiveness of this method. For example, the operator could use other form of neighbourhood search. Another direction is to make the algorithm more adaptive for solving the problems of various scales.

References

1. Bilgin B, Demeester P, Misir M, Vancroonenburg W, Vanden Berghe G (2011) One hyper-heuristic approach to two timetabling problems in health care. J Heuristics 18(3):401–434
2. Burke E, De Causmaecker P, Berghe G, Van Landeghem H (2004) The state of the art of nurse rostering. J Sched 7(6):441–499
3. Lü Z, Hao JK (2012) Adaptive neighborhood search for nurse rostering. Eur J Oper Res 218(3):865–876
4. Ruibin B, Burke EK, Kendall G, Jingpeng L, McCollum B (2010) A hybrid evolutionary approach to the nurse rostering problem. IEEE Trans Evol Comput 14(4):580–590
5. Lam AYS, Li VOK (2010) Chemical-reaction-inspired metaheuristic for optimization. IEEE Trans Evol Comput 14(3):381–399
6. Xu J, Lam AYS, Li VOK (2011) Stock portfolio selection using chemical reaction optimization. In: Proceedings of the international conference on operations research and Financial engineering. Paris, France
7. Xu J, Lam AYS, Li VOK (2010) Parallel chemical reaction optimization for the quadratic assignment problem. In: Proceedings of the international conference on genetic and evolutionary methods, Las Vegas, NV, USA
8. Xu J, Lam AYS, Li VOK (2010) Chemical reaction optimization for the grid scheduling problem. In: Proceedings of the IEEE international conference on communications, Cape Town, South Africa
9. Xu J, Lam AYS, Li VOK (2011) Chemical reaction optimization for task scheduling in grid computing. IEEE Trans Parallel Distrib Syst 22(10):1624–1631
10. Lam AYS, Xu J, Li VOK (2010) Chemical reaction optimization for population transition in peer-to-peer live streaming. In: Proceedings of the IEEE congress on evolutionary computation.Barcelona, Spain

Chapter 423
Survey of Network Security Situation Awareness and Key Technologies

Zhang Xuan

Abstract Network Security Situation Awareness (NSSA) can significantly improve the monitoring and emergency response capability of the network. It's important to predict the network security trend. In this paper, we described the key technologies of NSSA, and then we discussed the advantages and disadvantages of the various algorithms of network security situation assessment and predict. Finally, we summary the problems of network security situational awareness, and analyzed the future direction of development and trends.

Keywords Network security situation awareness (NSSA) · Network security · Data fusion · Situational prediction

423.1 Introduction

With the rapid development of computer network technology, network openness, sharing and interconnection degree growing computer network has brought more and more convenience. But at the same time, the rapid expansion of network size, complexity and uncertainty increases, network time face serious challenges by the attacks, the threat of unexpected events, availability, security, network security issues have become increasingly prominent. Traditional network security technology functional unit in a separate state, the lack of effective information extraction and information fusion mechanism, unable to establish a link between the network resources, global information about the performance of poor and unable to effectively manage, mass network security information. Network secu-

Z. Xuan (✉)
Teaching Research Department for Basic Causes in Shandong Police College,
Jinan 250014 Shandong, People's Republic of China
e-mail: zx@sdpc.edu.cn

S. Li et al. (eds.), *Frontier and Future Development of Information Technology in Medicine and Education*, Lecture Notes in Electrical Engineering 269,
DOI: 10.1007/978-94-007-7618-0_423,

rity situational awareness techniques have been proposed in this context become the hotspot of the new generation of network security technology and development direction.

423.2 Overview

Network security situational awareness (NSSA) is the complexity of the current network system, borderless, multi-source heterogeneous characteristics, you can integrate all of the available information, the many factors that affect network security such as access to a variety of network equipment operating conditions, network behavior and user behavior, understand, evaluate, display and predict future trends, the precision of the network security situation overall cognitive the safe operation of the network system status evaluation and prediction of the network's security posture.

In 1988, for the first time Endsley explicitly put forward the definition of situational awareness, situational awareness (Situation Awareness, SA) concept refers to the perception of environmental elements within a volume of time and space, the comprehension of their meaning, and the projection of their status in the near future [1], Fig. (423.1).

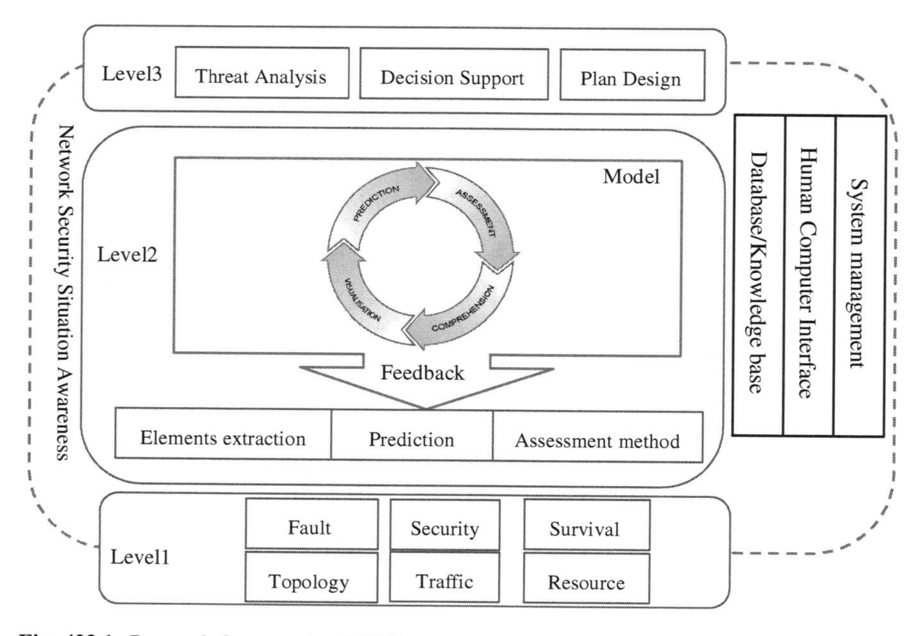

Fig. 423.1 Research framework of NSSA

423.3 The Key Technologies of NSSA

Network security situational awareness is a complex system, has yet to have a strict uniform standards, but researchers are certain consensus of its general framework, network security situational awareness process is divided into three phases: extraction of the elements in the network security situation, understanding of network security situation and prediction of network security situation [2].

423.3.1 NSSA Model

Based on the JDL functional model by Endsley and the situation awareness conceptual model by Bass, later researchers put forward proposals dozens of network security situation awareness model [3], Smart Cycler JDL model, Boyd control loop, waterfall model, Dasarathy model, the Omnibus model, the extended observe, Orient, Decide and Act (OODA) model, perceptual reasoning model [4]. Although each component of different models is not the same, but most of them are built in the JDL and Endsley model.

423.3.2 Extraction of Elements in the Network Security Situation

Extract accurate, comprehensive network security posture elements of network security situational awareness on the basis of the study.

Extract the main source of network security situational factors, including network vulnerability information, network alarm information, the honeypot network data information, net flow traffic information etc. Wang [5] collected network vulnerability information to assess the vulnerability posture of the network; Barford [6] used honey pot network data to assess the trend of network attacks. Gather information from a single point of view, access to the global information flawed, some scholars trying to obtain a full range of network information, such as Wang Juan [7] proposed a network security feature extraction index system, according to the different levels information from different sources and different needs of a variety of situations, refining the four macro two general indicators of the nature of the network, and identified more than twenty-level indicators, extracted through a defined network security index system of network security situation element.

423.3.3 Assessment of Network Security Situation

Network situation assessment in large-scale network environment, level-l integration for various types of network monitoring data, and with the help of a mathematical tool or mathematical model, based on domain knowledge and historical data on the basis of simple processing, through analytical reasoning, the current status of the entire network consisting of various network resources, network operation and user behavior and many other factors make a reasonable explanation.

Fusion Method Based on Logical Relationships Base on the logical relationship between the internal logic of the information, the information integration.

Fusion Method Based on Mathematical Models Comprehensive consideration of the trend factor, structural evaluation function, to create a collection of trend factor R to the momentum space mapping relationship.

Fusion Method Based on Probability and Statistics Probability and statistics-based fusion method, make full use of a priori knowledge of the statistical properties, combined with the uncertainty of information, the establishment of the situation assessment model, then the model evaluation network's security posture,for example Bayesian networks and Hidden Markov Model (HMM).

Fusion Method Based on Rule Reasoning Fusion method of rule-based reasoning, use fuzzy multi-attribute information of uncertainty and logical inference rules to achieve network security situation assessment. D–S evidence combination method and fuzzy logic is the study of hot spots.

423.3.4 Prediction of Network Security Situation

The trend forecast is based on actual data and historical data for the development of network security threats change, the use of scientific theories, methods, and a variety of experience, judgment, knowledge, to predict estimated to analyze changes in a certain period of time possible in the future.

Qualitative forecasting methods System according to people past and present experience, judgment and intuition to predict which human logic judgment, requires only that the direction of system development, status, situation qualitative results. It is suitable for the lack of historical statistics system objects.

Time series analysis According to the historical data of system objects change over time, only consider the variation of the system variables over time, the quantitative prediction of the future performance of the system time. It applies to using simple statistics trend prediction of the object changes with time.

Causal relationship to predict Some causes and consequences of the relationship between system variables to identify several factors that affect a certain result, the mathematical model between cause and effect. Under the direction of changes in the factors variables predict changes in the outcome variables, both forecasting system development to identify specific numerical variation.

423.4 Problems to Be Solved

Network security situational awareness systems are generally deployed in large-scale information systems security center,but there are still difficult issues as follows:

1. Division of labor between the different organizations
2. Deal with the complexity of the network, to shorten the response time
3. Multi-source, multi-point event correlation analysis
4. Reduce the additional network load, system fault tolerance
5. Visualization of the security situation.

423.5 Conclusion

Network security situational awareness technology as a new technology, there is much room for development, and in the course of its development should grasp the following aspects:

1. Real-time situational awareness
2. Trend forecast
3. Unknown attack detection capabilities
4. Adaptive Intrusion response, intelligent decision-making.

References

1. Endsley MR (1988) Design and evaluation for situation awareness enhancement [C]. In: Proceeding of the 32nd human factors society annual meeting.Human Factors and Ergonomics Society, Santa Monica, pp 97–101
2. Zhuo Y (2010) Research of situational awareness based on the network topology and traffic mining [D]. National Defense Science and Technology University
3. Gad A, Farooq M (2002) Data fusion architecture for maritime surveillance. In: Proceedings of the international society on information fusion (ISIF), pp. 448–455. http://www.isif.org/fusion/procecdings/fusion02CD/pdffiles/papers/M4D03.pdf
4. Kadar I (2005) Knowledge representation issues in perceptual reasoning managed situation assessment. In: Proceedings of the FUSION, pp. 13–15. http://ieeexplore.ieee.org

5. Wang L, Singhal A, Jajodia S (2007) Measuring network security using attack graphs[C]. In: Proceedings of the 2007 ACM workshop on quality of protection. ACM Press, New York, pp 49–54
6. Barford P, Chen Y, Goyal A et al (2005) Employing honey nets for network situational awareness [C]. In: Proceedings of the fourth workshop on hot topics in networks. Springer, Berlin, pp 71–102
7. Wang J (2010) Research on Key technology in large-scale network security situation awareness [D]. University of Electronic Science and Technology of China

Chapter 424
Mining ESP Teaching Research Data Using Statistical Analysis Method: Using One-Sample *t* Test as an Example

Yicheng Wang and Mingli Chen

Abstract We demonstrate the usage and effectiveness of a simple statistical analysis method, one-sample *t* test, in mining ESP teaching research data. The statistical analysis software SPSS is used. Our method discovers more information concealed in the data compared to the average or percentage method. Our work also provides some basic survey data for ESP teaching researches, especially for research on local level universities in China. Three issues discovered in data analysis process are discussed: (1) students' behaviors conflict with their anticipations; (2) conflicts exist between course setting and students' practical more imminent issues; and (3) the pros and cons of blackboard writing and multimedia in ESP teaching.

Keywords ESP · One-sample *t* test · Data mining · Questionnaire survey

424.1 Introduction

English for Specific Purposes (ESP) in China's universities has been undergoing a hard time [2]. Researchers did a lot of work aiming to promote the efficiency of ESP teaching. When it comes to data analysis, most researchers use qualitative or very simple quantitative method such as averages or percentages. Such values make little statistical sense, and only limited amount of information is obtained while a large part is left out. Formal data analysis techniques are rarely used in ESP teaching researches [1, 4].

In this paper, we demonstrate the usage and effectiveness of a simple statistical analysis method, namely, one-sample *t* test, in analyzing the questionnaire survey

Y. Wang (✉) · M. Chen
College of Resources and Environment, Qingdao Agricultural University,
Qingdao 266109, People's Republic of China
e-mail: ywangqau@163.com

S. Li et al. (eds.), *Frontier and Future Development of Information Technology in Medicine and Education*, Lecture Notes in Electrical Engineering 269,
DOI: 10.1007/978-94-007-7618-0_424,

data collected from a group of senior undergraduate students with land management major. Results of the tests were interpreted and discussed.

424.2 Data and Results

424.2.1 The Questionnaire

In the questionnaire 23 statements are given, each corresponding to a variable which will be analyzed in the next subsection. Students evaluate each statement and give a score which ranges from 1 to 5, higher score indicating more approval.

v1: Words and phrases should be explained within a context. v2: Words and phrases taught in class are not very related to our major. v3: Words and phrases not related to our major should not be taught in class, although they are new and appear often in reading. v4: Only explain the structure of difficult sentences, no need to translate the whole sentence. v5: English explanation of important specialty concepts should be provided in class. v6: I like the Words of Celebrities before class. v7: Blackboard writing consumes too much time. v8: Using PPT may be better. v9: I would like to see English video clips in class. v10: Video clips should only be related to our major, not to other areas. v11: I would like to make a presentation about what I translated in homeworks. v12: Reading materials should be provided before class. v13: I would like to collect information about a topic which I am interested in. v14: Reading exercise should also be included as homework in addition to translating. v15: Writing exercise should also be included as homework. v16: Only two homework, there should be more. v17: More work should be done in translation homework. v18: Exam can take a variety of forms such as paper writing. v19: I hope my English will be improved by taking this class. v20: This class is expected to improve our capability on all aspects including listening and speaking capabilities. v21: There should be more rollcalls in class. v22: Students who are preparing other exams don't have to come to class. v23: We are busy preparing other exams, teacher should not be too strict on us.

Fifty copies of the questionnaire were distributed, 40 of them were collected back and considered effective answers.

424.2.2 Results

Descriptive statistics for the sample data, including the mean, standard deviation, and standard error, were obtained first. The mean shows the average value of the sample data, while standard deviation indicates the distribution of data. Basically these are the information that descriptive statistics tell us, more importantly, the

Table 424.1 Population means and classification of *t* test results

Population means and categories	Variables
4 (agree)	v1, v5, v6, v8, v9, v12, v13, v18, v19, v20
3 (ok)	v4, v11, v14, v15, v21, v22, v23
2 (disagree)	v2, v3, v7, v10, v16, v17

Note See "424.2.1 the questionnaire" section for the meaning of each variable

mean values are sample means, not population means, and we are not able to statistically judge what the population mean[1] is.

We then did a one-sample *t* test using SPSS. Confidence level was 95 %. Variables were classified into three categories, "agree", "ok", and "disagree", corresponding to, respectively, when null hypothesis "population mean = 4, 3 or 2" was accepted. This classified most variables except variables v1, v10 and v16. For v1, null hypothesis "population mean = 4" was rejected, but "population mean = 4.5" was accepted, v1 was classified into "agree" category. Similarly, for v10 and v16, "population mean = 2" was rejected, but "population mean = 2.5" was accepted, these two variables were classified into "disagree" category (Table 424.1).

424.2.3 Interpretation of Results

424.2.3.1 Category of "Agree"

For variables v5, v9 and v19, null hypothesis "population mean = 4.5" was also accepted. These three variables, together with variable v1, can be considered "strongly agree". This indicates that, on average, students strongly think that: (1) words and phrases should be explained within in a context (v1); (2) specialty concepts and relevant knowledge should be explained adequately in English (v5); (3) Students would love to see English video clips in class (v9); and (4) students hope to improve their English by taking this class (v19).

For variables v6, v12, v13, and v20, only null hypothesis "population mean = 4" was accepted, indicating that, on average, students think that: (1) Words of Celebrities is good (v6); (2) Reading materials should be provided (v12); (3) Students would like to collect English materials which they are interested in (v13); and (4) Students hope to improve their overall English capabilities (v20).

[1] Population mean can be understood as the mean value of scores given by all land management students (or all non-English major students) in China's local level universities.

For variables v8 and v18, "population mean = 3.5" was also accepted, indicating that: (1) students' intendance to see PPT was not strong (v8); and (2) they would accept a variety of forms of the exam, but only to some extent (v18).

424.2.3.2 Category of "Ok"

For variables v4, v14, v15 and v21, null hypothesis "population mean = 2.5" was also accepted, showing an intendance toward "disagree". Specifically, students consider that: (1) It may be ok if difficult sentences are not completely translated, but if they are, it would be better (v4); (2) It may be ok if reading and writing homework are assigned, but if they are not, it would be better (v14, v15); and (3) Teacher can do more roll calls in class but that would not be welcomed (v21).

For variables v11, v22, and v23, null hypothesis "population mean = 3.5" was also accepted, showing an intendance toward "agree". Specifically, students: (1) showed conserved willingness to participate in class activities but they would like to do it if opportunity is provided (v11); (2) will attend this class when they are preparing another exam, but they actually intend not to do so (v22); and (3) would accept a strict teacher, but they would love a teacher who is not that strict (v23).

424.2.3.3 Category of "Disagree"

This category includes six variables. For variables v10 and v16, null hypothesis "population mean = 2" was rejected, and "population mean = 2.5" was accepted. These results indicate that: (1) students think that materials not directly related to their major can also be included in video clips (v10); and (2) students don't want more homework although currently there are only two (v16).

The other four variables indicated a strong "disagree", only "population mean = 2" was accepted. Specifically: (1) students consider that words taught in class are related to their major (v2); (2) they believe that new words are important as long as they appear frequently in reading; (3) to large extent, students accept blackboard writing (v7); and (4) students don't want to do more translation in homework (v17).

424.3 Discussion

424.3.1 Conflicts Between Students' Anticipation and Their Behaviors

Students anticipated that they do well in class but they didn't show a willingness to work hard. This anticipation-behavior conflict may not be unique in ESP class. In our opinion, adequate amount of homework is necessary to put some pressure on students to prompt them to study. Homework may take a variety of forms, though, such as translating product introduction, advertisement, lecture notes, etc. The teacher can encourage students to ask questions, participate in class discussion, and express different opinions to improve class efficiency.

424.3.2 Conflicts Between Class and Imminent Issues

A significant part of students are preparing for other exams such as Graduate Entrance Exam (GEE). Also some students are taking internship in companies. To ensure the internship and future job, students would go to the internship instead of the classroom. One possible solution is to put the class in another semester such as one semester earlier when students have time and energy to study ESP. Another is teaching design [3]. Teaching pattern should be designed from a practical perspective, that is, ESP should aim to improve students' capabilities of using it in practice. Investment negotiations or expos can be simulated in classroom.

424.3.3 Pros and Cons of Blackboard Writing and Multimedia

Students showed acceptance toward blackboard writing, but considering students' strong willingness to learn words and phrases in a context, we suggest that PPT and multimedia are used in a proper way. By "proper" we mean the following. Word font on the PPT slide should be large enough to be easily identified; Words and phrases in a sentence are highlighted; Slides don't go too fast so students can have time to make notes. Also we point out that a video clip should be major-related as possible, and talks in the video is not too fast.

424.4 Concluding Remarks

We have demonstrated the usage and effectiveness of a simple statistical analysis method, one-sample t test, in mining ESP teaching research data. We discussed three issues found in data analysis, and we proposed potential approaches to addressing these issues. These findings provide a basis on which further researches can be carried out and efficient teaching patterns can be designed.

Most ESP researches in China focus on national level universities. Only on some rare occasions were local level universities included but still the data were not analyzed separately from national levels [5]. This survey was carried out in a local level university, that we believe helps to bridge the gap between research need and data deficiency.

Finally, we point out that other data processing and analysis methods, such as principal component analysis, fuzzy evaluation, and cluster analysis, if properly used, can also help in data mining in ESP teaching researches.

References

1. Bao G (2012) A survey on the usage of statistical analysis methods in foreign language teaching researches in China. Foreign Lang World (1):44–51,60
2. Cai J (2010) Some considerations on the orientation of college English teaching in China. Foreign Lang Teach Res 4:306–308
3. Gu Z (2010) A study on the design of ESP teaching. Shanghai Foreign Languages Univ, Master thesis
4. Leong W, Li X (2011) Optimized strategy in English teaching for tourism management major. Tourism Tribune 2:89–94
5. Zhang H (2012) Analysis of the questionnaire on the specialized English of electronic information science. J Wuhan Univ (Nat Sci Ed.) (S2):244–248

Chapter 425
Research on the Impact of Experiential Teaching Mode on the Cultivation of Marketing Talents

Jia Cai and Hui Guan

Abstract Experiential teaching is a brand-new teaching mode and teaching concept. Its unique teaching method plays an important role in cultivating applied talents. This study examines the experiential teaching model which could significantly improve students' knowledge, abilities and qualities through empirical research methods.

Keywords: Marketing talents · Talents cultivation · Experiential teaching

425.1 Marketing Talents' Qualities

The American scholar Ralphl W. Jackson and Rober D. Hisrich have pointed out that there are three special characteristics that only processed by successful markers, which are quality, skill and knowledge. In terms of quality, marketing should have a sense of social responsibility, the determination of the character, honesty and trustworthiness, innovation, adaptability, occupation ethics and professionalism, and so on. In terms of ability, the marketing talents should have the ability to collect process information, language skills, logical thinking ability, communication skills, self-learning ability, management skills, social skills, the ability of market research, marketing planning capability, marketing ability, and so on [2]. In terms of knowledge, marketing in addition to master marketing expertise, also should have knowledge of economics, management, law etc.

J. Cai · H. Guan (✉)
School of Economic Management, Dalian University, Dalian 116622, People's Republic of China
e-mail: gloria366000@163.com

S. Li et al. (eds.), *Frontier and Future Development of Information Technology in Medicine and Education*, Lecture Notes in Electrical Engineering 269,
DOI: 10.1007/978-94-007-7618-0_425,

425.2 Experiential Teaching Content and System

425.2.1 The Connotation of Experiential Teaching

Experiential teaching is a teaching model, in this teaching process, teachers based on students' cognitive characteristics and laws, according to the teaching objectives and content, purposefully create teaching situation or use a variety of teaching methods to stimulate students' senses, inspire students' emotions and then through the guidance of the students, let they personally perceive and comprehend the knowledge, so as to apply the knowledge to the practice [3]. Experiential teaching is a new teaching theory and teaching methods that different from the traditional teaching mode, it is emphasizing the subjectivity of students, students not only conducive to the understanding and mastery of knowledge through personal experience, but also exercise the language skills, communication skills, logical thinking ability, and to develop their own quality.

425.2.2 Experiential Teaching Model

In Bernd H. Schmitt's experience theory, the experience is divided into sensory experience, emotional experience, thinking experience, behavior experience and related experience [4]. The development of the model is based on the experience theory of the Bernd H. Schmitt, constructing the teaching mode of three modules of "sensory emotion", "thinking behavior" and association, let the student to participate, realized "Learning By Doing". The sensory emotional module is implemented through three aspects of multimedia, video data and network platform; the thinking behavior module is achieved by case teaching, seminar-style teaching, simulated teaching, experimental teaching and practice teaching five aspects; the last module "association" through marketing planning season, career planning and entrepreneurial training three aspects to be realized. Therefore, the architecture of experiential teaching mode system is shown in Fig. 425.1.

425.3 The Effect of Experiential Teaching on Students' Knowledge, Ability and Quality

Experiential teaching emphasizes the personal experience of students, in the teaching activities, teachers create a variety of situations; use many teaching methods (case teaching, seminar-style teaching, simulated teaching, experiment teaching, practice teaching, etc.); organize various competitions (marketing planning contest, Challenge Cup entrepreneurship competition, etc.) to enable students to participate in teaching activities, personal experience and perception,

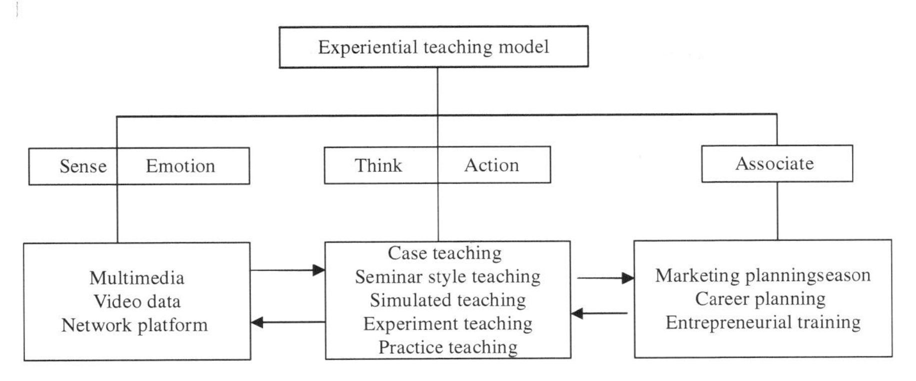

Fig. 425.1 Experiential teaching model system

insight knowledge, thus transforming knowledge into ability. So experience teaching has a great influence on students to acquire knowledge, to improve the capacity and quality.

First, in the sense-emotion experience, teachers make use of sensory teaching methods such as multimedia; video data and network platform to stimulate students' enthusiasm for learning, let students experience the joy of learning, so that they can change from passive learning to active learning. Students will actively participate in teaching activities, not only active classroom atmosphere, but enable students to acquire knowledge in a pleasant state, thus they will be able to better understand and master the knowledge.

Second, in the thinking-action experience, teachers adopt a variety of teaching methods such as case teaching, seminar-style teaching, simulated teaching, experimental teaching and practice teaching to mobilize students' enthusiasm, learning by doing, so students can transform knowledge into ability, thus improve students' ability to process information collected, logical thinking skills, communication skills as well as to enhance the sense of responsibility, teamwork and other qualities.

Finally, in the related experience, by participating in the marketing planning contest, Challenge Cup Entrepreneurship Competition, students can use the theoretical knowledge into practice, while improving the ability of market research, market development and marketing capabilities, marketing planning capability, and management ability, in order to be able to promote students' self-motivation, self-reinforcing, exercise the will of the students, and self-confidence.

In short, experiential teaching plays an important role in students' learning and mastering the professional knowledge, improving the capacity of all aspects and enhancing their own quality.

425.4 Research Design and Data Processing

In order to verify the experiential teaching can cultivate and improve students' knowledge, ability and quality, this study used a questionnaire, conducted a survey on the students of different grades in Dalian University marketing profession, and then by the analysis of the questionnaire's results to verify experience teaching having effect on the students' knowledge, ability and quality.

425.4.1 Questionnaire Design

The items of questionnaire mainly get from the results of interviews with students of all ages on the marketing profession and the number is 20. The questionnaire is divided into three parts: the first part (1–3 questions) is the effect of experiential teaching on students' knowledge; the second part (4–16 questions) is about experiential teaching improves what ability of students; the third part (17–20) is about experiential teaching reinforces what aspects of the quality of students. The questionnaire use Likert-5 scale.

425.4.2 Data Collection

The questionnaire mainly issued in different grades of undergraduate of marketing profession in Dalian University, a total of 150 questionnaires were returned 128 questionnaires, a response rate of 85.33 %, of which 125 valid questionnaires, the effective response rate was 83.33 %.

425.4.3 Data Analysis

425.4.3.1 Factor Analysis

First standardized questionnaire collected data collected, and then making use of SPSS13.0 statistical analysis software analysis the standardized data. Selective principal component analysis, and on maximum variation orthogonal rotation, the retention factor load is greater than the absolute value of 0.5 items, deleting items of cross-factor load, the last remaining 11 items. In accordance with the principle of Eigen values greater than 1 were extracted three factors, the cumulative variance contribution rate is 76.794 %, these factors can illustrate the effect of experiential teaching on students' knowledge, ability and quality in the maximum extent.

Table 425.1 Orthogonal rotation factor loading coefficient

Items				Factors		
No.	Content	Mean	Std.Deviation	1	2	3
X1	Communication skills	4.2160	0.71374	0.797		
X2	Ability to process information	4.2080	0.73282	0.784		
X3	Language skills	4.2480	0.66788	0.776		
X4	Social skills	4.1520	0.69626	0.682		
X5	Logical thinking ability	4.1360	0.73335	0.590		
X6	Exercise will	3.9440	0.78601		0.815	
X7	More honest	3.5120	1.00496		0.765	
X8	Promote self-motivation and self-reinforcing	4.0880	0.68411		0.746	
X9	More responsible	4.0000	0.82305		0.722	
X10	A deeper understanding and memory knowledge	4.2480	0.64328			0.888
X11	Mastery of the knowledge system	4.0560	0.67566			0.712

Through analysis the 11 indicators, the value of Kaiser–Meyer–Olkin(KMO) is 0.899, Bartlett's test of sphericity $\times 2$ value is 1012.682, so common factors exist in the correlation matrix of the population, that the data is suitable for factor analysis.

The factor analysis on these 11 indicators, and using varimax rotated factor of the orthogonal rotation, after five times of rotation after iteration factor load factor as shown in Table 425.1.

As can be seen from the Table 425.1, the first factors including X1, X2, X3, X4 and X5 these five indicators, representing the coordination and communication capabilities, the information collection processing ability, language skills, social skills and logical thinking ability, these indicators reflect the influence of the experience teaching in the students' abilities, and the five indicators load is higher in the first factor; second factors including X6, X7, X8 and X9 these four indicators, representing the exercise of will, more honest, promoting self-motivation and strengthen the sense of responsibility, these indicators reflect the effect of experiential teaching on the students' own quality, these four indicators, and the load is higher in the second factor; third factors including X10 and X11, on behalf of a more profound understanding and memory of knowledge, mastery of the knowledge system, these indicators reflect the experiential teaching's effect on the students' knowledge, and the two indexes load is higher in third factor.

425.4.3.2 Reliability Analysis

The reliability test purpose is to learn more about the 11 indicators and extracted three factors verifying the reliability of effect of experiential teaching on the students' knowledge, ability and quality.

Table 425.2 The total scale and the reliability coefficients of each factor

	Total scale	Ability	Quality	Knowledge
α Coefficient	0.935	0.901	0.870	0.842

United States statistician Hair (the Joseph F. Hair Jr.), Anderson (Jr. Rolph E. Anderson) Tyson (Ronald L. Tathan) and Blackburn (William C. Black,) pointed out that Value greater than 0.7, indicating that the higher reliability of the data, the number of items in the measured foot is less than 6, the value is greater than 0.6 indicates that the data is reliable [5].

The total scale coefficient obtained by the correlation analysis of the three factors is 0.935, then do each time correlation analysis on three factors obtained after each factor coefficients are 0.901, 0.870 and 0.842, so the total scale and the reliability coefficients of each factor are shown in Table 425.2:

From the above Table 425.2 shows: whether total scale's α coefficient or each factor's α coefficient, is greater than 0.7, so the data is reliable, the reliability of the final form of the experience teaching on students' knowledge, ability and quality validation indices can be acceptable.

425.5 Conclusion and Outlook

In this study, through the empirical analysis of the experiential teaching can cultivate and improve the knowledge, ability and quality of students is verified. Empirical evidence shows that, experience teaching allows students a deeper understanding and memory of knowledge and mastery of the entire body of knowledge; the experiential teaching can improve students' communication skills, ability to process information is gathered, language skills, social skills and logical thinking capacity and other aspects of capacity; experience teaching enhance students' own quality, allow students to be more honest, more responsible, exercise the will and promote students' self-motivation and self-reinforcing. Therefore, the results from the study can be seen experience teaching having great influence and effect on cultivate of marketing talents. The advocacy experience teaching mode to cultivate more marketing talents adapt to the development of market economy, the reform is a long way to go.

References

1. Jackson RW, Hisrich RD (2001) Sales management. China Renmin University Press, Beijing
2. Guan H, Wang Y (2007) The contemporary marketing personnel quality measurement scale development. Economist

3. Cui H (2009) Fully carry out experiential teaching to improve the ideological and political theory teaching effectiveness. Qiqihar Teachers Coll
4. Schmitt BH, Yinna L, Jing G, Lijuan L (2004) Experience marketing [M]. Tsinghua University Press, Beijing
5. Xiaoyun H, Cunxiao W (2003) With service companies Customer satisfaction and loyalty. Tsinghua University Press, Beijing

Chapter 426
Lung Segmentation for CT Images Based on Mean Shift and Region Growing

Huang Zhanpeng, Yi Faling and Zhao Jie

Abstract Segmentation of the lungs in chest-computed tomography (CT) is a precursor to most pulmonary image analysis applications. A new lung segmentation based on the 3D CT image series is proposed integrating mean shift smoothing and region growing algorithms together. As medical images are mostly fuzzy, Mean Shift cluster algorithm is used to smooth the CT images. Then some seed points for left and right lung separately are selected by the user, and the growing criterion is calculated automatically by the analyzing the neighboring sub-blocks. Then region growing method is applied to get the final segmentation. Experiments results show the proposed method can efficiently segment the lung region from serial abdominal CT images with little user interaction.

Keywords Lung segmentation · Mean shift · Region growing · CT image serials

426.1 Introduction

Lung disease has been a serious threat to human health, and lung cancer is considered to be one of the most harmful to human health and life currently. In China, lung cancer has been the leading cause of cancer deaths since 1996 and increased at an average annual rate of 4.4 %. Early diagnosis and treatment (EDAT) of lung cancer greatly increases the chances for successful treatment. The research shows that the 5-year survival of patients rose from 14 to 49 % by EDAT [1].

As an important issue in pulmonary image analysis, segmentation has received much attention and many methods have been proposed. Threshold method [2] is a simple and fast method for image segmentation, but failed to effectively remove

H. Zhanpeng (✉) · Y. Faling · Z. Jie
College of Medical Information Engineering, GuangDong Pharmaceutical University, No. 280 Waihuan Road East, Guangzhou 510006, People's Republic of China
e-mail: gdpuhzp@126.com

S. Li et al. (eds.), *Frontier and Future Development of Information Technology in Medicine and Education*, Lecture Notes in Electrical Engineering 269,
DOI: 10.1007/978-94-007-7618-0_426,

the background and tracheobronchial region. In [3], the lung region is extracted by gray-level threshold and a sequence of erosion and dilation operations.

In this paper, a novel segmentation algorithm based on mean shift and region growing is proposed to segment the lung from CT image sequences. Some seed points are chosen from the CT image by the user manually. For reducing noise and preferably keeping the edge of image, and the images are clustered by the mean shift algorithm. Mean shift filtering replaces each pixel's value with the most probable local value, found by a nonparametric probability density estimation method. Then region growing method is used to extract the final area of lung.

426.2 Incorporated with Mean Shift and Region Growing

The mean shift algorithm is a nonparametric clustering technique which does not require prior knowledge of the number of clusters, and does not constrain the shape of the clusters. The method was originally presented for target tracking and classification in 1975 [4]. It was applied to machine vision in [5], which has aroused wide attention. Mean shift is used for robust feature space analysis [6, 7], which is useful to image smoothing and image segmentation.

426.2.1 The Mean Shift Procedure

Kernel density estimation (known as the Parzen window technique in pattern recognition) is the most popular density estimation method. Given n data points xi, $i = 1,\ldots,n$ on a d-dimensional space Rd, the multivariate kernel density estimator obtained with kernel $K(x)$ and bandwidth h is

$$\hat{f}(x) = \frac{1}{nh^d}\sum_{i=1}^{n} K\left(\frac{x - x_i}{h}\right) \tag{426.1}$$

The modes of the density function are located at the zeros of the gradient function. The gradient of the density estimator (426.1) is:

$$\hat{\nabla} f_{h,k}(x) = \frac{2C_{k,d}}{nh^{d+2}}\left[\sum_{i=1}^{n} g\left(\left\|\frac{x - x_i}{h}\right\|^2\right)\right]\left[\frac{\sum_{i=1}^{n} x_i g\left(\left\|\frac{x-x_i}{h}\right\|^2\right)}{\sum_{i=1}^{n} g\left(\left\|\frac{x-x_i}{h}\right\|^2\right)} - x\right] \tag{426.2}$$

where$g(x) = -k'(x)$. The second term

$$m_{h,G}(x) = \frac{\sum_{i=1}^{n} x_i g\left(\left\|\frac{x-x_i}{h}\right\|^2\right)}{\sum_{i=1}^{n} g\left(\left\|\frac{x-x_i}{h}\right\|^2\right)} - x \tag{426.3}$$

is the mean shift. The mean shift vector always points toward the direction of the maximum increase in the density. In practice, we use the sequence of successive location of kernel G from (426.3)

$$y_{j+1} = \frac{\sum_{i=1}^{n} x_i g\left(\left\|\frac{x-x_i}{h}\right\|^2\right)}{\sum_{i=1}^{n} g\left(\left\|\frac{x-x_i}{h}\right\|^2\right)}, j = 1, 2, \ldots \quad (426.4)$$

is the weighted mean at y_j computed with kernel G and y_1 is the centre of the initial position of the kernel. As confirmed in [6], a kernel K that obeys some mild conditions suffices for the convergence of the sequences $\{y_j\}_{j=1,2\ldots}$.

Let x_i and z_i, $i = 1,\ldots,n$, be the input and filtered image pixels. The smoothing algorithm consists of the following steps:

For each $i = 1$ to n

(1) Initialize k = 1 and $y_k = x_i$
(2) Repeat: compute y_{k+1} using the procedures (426.4) until convergence.
(3) Assign $z_i = y_k$

426.2.2 Region Growing Algorithm

Region growing is a procedure that group pixels or sub-regions into larger regions based on predefined criteria for growth. The basic approach is to start with a set of "seed" points and from these grow regions by appending to each seed those neighboring pixels that have predefined properties similar to the seed.

We use an automate method to determine the similarity criteria. In order to reduce the noises of the selected seed points, the sub-blocks with size N*N are used to calculate the similarity criteria. Generally the value of N may set 3 to 5, considering the size of the target region. In our application, the sub-blocks with size 3*3 are chosen as the basic units to compute the homogeneity criterion. For each seed point selected by the users, a seed sub-block is found which the seed point's center in and there are 8 neighboring sub-block with same size. In our approach, homogeneity between seed sub-block and neighboring sub-blocks is calculated as the similarity criteria of region growing. For each seed pint, the stages of the procedure can be outlined in the following way:

(1) Calculate the mean and variance of seed and 8 neighboring sub-blocks by

$$\mu = \frac{1}{n}\sum_{i=1}^{n} f_i \qquad \sigma^2 = \frac{1}{n}\sum_{i=1}^{n} (f_i - \mu)^2 \quad (426.5)$$

where n is the num of pixels in the sub-block.

(2) Compute the weight mean and variance value of seed sub-block and 8 neighboring sub-blocks

$$\overline{\mu} = \frac{\sum_{i=1}^{M} w(i)\mu(i)}{\sum_{i=1}^{M} w(i)} \qquad \overline{\sigma} = \sqrt{\frac{\sum_{i=1}^{M} w(i)\sigma^2(i)}{\sum_{i=1}^{M} w(i)}} \tag{426.6}$$

where M is the num of neighboring sub-blocks considered in algorithm, and M usually is set 9. In the algorithm, the Euclidean Distances between core sub-block and neighborhood sub-blocks are calculated as the weight values $w(i)$.

(3) (3)The consistency criteria for each seed point is the mean of area between $[\overline{u} - 3\overline{\sigma}, \overline{u} + 3\overline{\sigma}]$.

426.3 Result

The lung segmentation algorithm has been implemented using Matlab, and tested in many experiments. The datasets from 64-slice spiral CT were processed.

In our application, we need to segment the lung from CT images. The source image from 64-slice spiral CT is shown in Fig. 426.1a. At the beginning, two seed points are selected by the user for the left and right lung, the image is filtered by mean shift algorithm and the result is shown in Fig. 426.1b. Then region growing are used to extract the lung area, which is shown in Fig. 426.1c. The result shows that the algorithm successfully extracted the lung areas, and the holes in the lung area are the intrapulmonary vessels of the lung, which are useful for future bronchi, pulmonary veins and pulmonary arteries analyzing and 3D visualization. The same image segmented by the traditional region growing method is shown in Fig. 426.1d. Although the traditional region growing method able to basically extract the lung areas, but they are many small holes in the lung area.

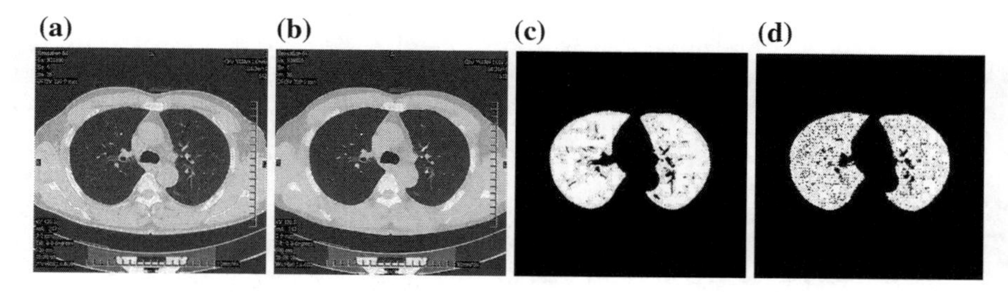

Fig. 426.1 lung segmentation for CT image

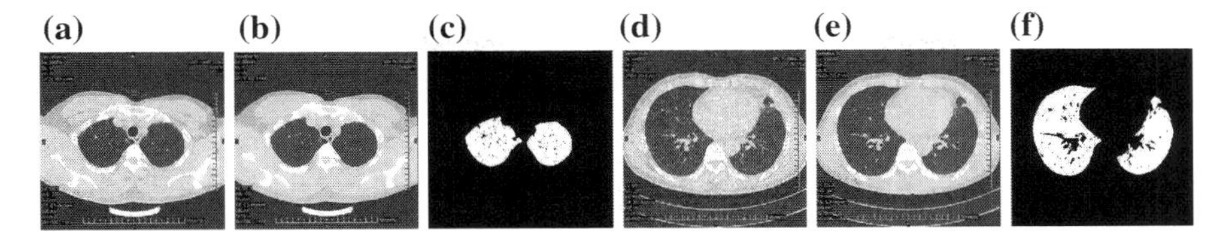

Fig. 426.2 lung segmentation for CT image from same dataset

In Fig. 426.2, two other images from same dataset were processed by the proposed method, and the results are separately shown in Fig. 426.2c and Fig. 426.2f.

References

1. Lin DT, Yan CR, Chen WT (2005) Autonomous detection of pulmonary nodules on CT image with a neural network-based fuzzy system. Comput Med Imag Gr 29(6):447–458
2. Armato SG,Senssakovic WF (2004) Automated lung segmentation for thoracic CT: impact on computer-aided diagnosis. AcadRadio 11(9):1011–1021
3. Hu S, Hoffman EA, Reinhardt JM (2001) Automatic lung segmentation for accurate quantization of volumetric X-Ray CT images. IEEE Trans Med Imag 20:490–8
4. Fukunaga K, Hostetler LD (1975) The estimation of the gradient of a density function with applications in pattern recognition. IEEE Trans on Inf Theory 21(1):32–40
5. Cheng YZ (1995) Mean shift, mode seeking, and clustering [J]. IEEE Trans on Pattern Anal Mach Intell 17(8):790–799
6. Comanicu D, Meer P (2002) Mean shift: a robust approach toward feature space analysis. IEEE Trans Pattern Anal Mach Intell, May 2002
7. Comaniciu D, Ramesh V, Meer P (2000) Real-time tracking of non-rigid objects using mean shift. Proceeding of CVPR 2000

Chapter 427
The Application of Psychological Teaching Combined with Daily Life: The Role of the Internet

Chuanhua Gu

Abstract The mode of psychological teaching combined with daily life emphasizes the connection of psychological teaching with learners' daily life and teachers' instructing learners or students to apply the knowledge of psychology in the process of analyzing the phenomena of psychology in daily life and to learn psychology based on their daily life experiences. It is supported by the relevant psychological research and includes the following basic steps. Firstly, the teacher can collect typical phenomena of psychology from daily life based on the analysis of the teaching goal. Secondly, the teacher can request learners to raise their questions about the phenomena and arouse their interest or motives to explore the phenomena. Thirdly, the teacher can instruct learners to answer the question based on their explorations. Finally, the teacher can direct learners to integrate the extant knowledge with the newly obtained knowledge. In the process the Internet plays an indispensable role. The Internet can be used as the convenient tool of information searching and personalized interactions between learners and between learners and instructors, and it can also be adopted to support online learning and to arouse the learner's interest in learning psychology.

Keywords Psychological teaching combined with daily life · The internet

---

C. Gu (✉)
School of Psychology, Central China Normal University, 152, Luoyu Street, Wuhan 430079, People's Republic of China
e-mail: 502774209@qq.com; guchuanhua_ccnu@sina.cn

C. Gu
Key Laboratory of Adolescent Cyberpsychology and Behavior (CCNU) of Ministry of Education, School of Psychology, Central China Normal University, Wuhan 430079, People's Republic of China

S. Li et al. (eds.), *Frontier and Future Development of Information Technology in Medicine and Education*, Lecture Notes in Electrical Engineering 269,
DOI: 10.1007/978-94-007-7618-0_427,

427.1 Introduction

Psychology has been an important course of general education for undergraduates in normal universities nowadays. Psychology is more associated with the daily life of learners because it aims to understand and investigate the law in mental activities. This lays the foundation for psychological teaching combined with daily life. Nowadays, the prevalent use of the Internet provides great convenience for combining the psychological teaching with the learner's daily life. This paper aims to analyze the possible methods of psychological teaching combined with daily life and the role of the Internet in the process.

427.2 The Significance of Psychological Teaching Combined with Daily Life

The mode of psychological teaching combined with daily life aims to instruct students to obtain psychological knowledge by exploring the behavior or life experiences of people including themselves. In the process of psychological teaching combined with daily life, the instructor should guide the learner to understand or explain their life experiences or typical phenomena and to solve the problem in their daily life based on what they have learned. In other words, the instructor should guide the learner to know how to use the psychological knowledge to explain or understand their life experiences or typical phenomena in daily life. For example, in the process of teaching about perception in general psychology, the learner can raise any question about perception based on the reflection on their own life experiences or typical phenomena about perception, and ask many "whys" about them. What the instructor should do is to instruct the learner with many "whys" to explore independently or cooperate to find the answers to questions, i.e. the possible psychological explanations for their perceptive experiences or typical perceptive phenomena.

We can find mass empirical research supporting the mode of psychological teaching combined with daily life. The study of cognitive process in educational psychology provided enough evidence for psychological teaching combined with daily life. Just as the research results indicated, the level of information processing impacted individual memory, and the deeper the individual processed the learning material, the better the individual learned [1]. The study of problem solving indicated that, successful problem solver could explore the solution with great efforts and passion generally [2]. Psychological teaching combined with the learner's life experience or typical phenomena will arouse the learner's passion for the exploration into the answers to the questions.

Clinchy described ways in which a mode of instruction called connected teaching could be used applied to undergraduate courses in developmental psychology [3]. The mode emphasized thinking over expertise, elicitation and exploration of students' narratives of personal experiences, and respectful consideration of commonsense views of development derived from these experiences. It tried to convince students that they could actively construct, rather than just passively receive, psychological knowledge. It has been proved more useful than the traditional instruction mode for the obtainment of students' knowledge. The mode is also consistent with the learning theory of constructivism [4].

427.2.1 The Role of the Internet in Psychological Teaching Combined with Daily Life

The prevalent use of the Internet provides the convenience for psychological teaching combined with daily life. By the Internet the learner can obtain the timely information that is helpful to their learning. In sum, the Internet is the convenient and fast tool of information searching; it can promote the personalized interaction between learners and between learners and instructors; it can provide the necessary tool and technique for learning, support the online learning of learners, and increase the learner's interest and motivation [5].

Firstly, learners can collect the mental phenomena which are associated with the knowledge that will be learned by the Internet, such as the phenomena about the sense, perception, memory, thinking, competence, temperament, character, and social psychology. Based on the analysis of the phenomena, learners can propose all sorts of psychological questions and try to answer them. On the other hand, the analysis of the phenomena also can help them deepen their understanding into the specific psychological knowledge.

Secondly, learners can obtain all sorts of learning materials by online learning, including all sorts of information the instructor provides for learners to learn specific content, especially all sorts of typical cases and the psychological analysis of them. In fact, learners will obtain learning materials without interrupt, and instructors will control and manage the teaching materials they provide for learners and make teaching process more flexible [6].

What's more, instructors also can collect all sorts of mental phenomena in daily life associated with every topic to inspire students to propose the question and to increase their motivation for learning, and build the teaching material depository or "the depository for life phenomena". Besides, just as some research indicated, because of such functions of the Internet in social interaction as BBS and E-mail, the teacher also can interact with the student to obtain timely teaching materials and feedback about the learning. Both the instructor and the learner can benefit from the Internet [7].

427.3 How to Conduct the Psychological Teaching Combined with Daily Life with the Help of the Internet

Based on the analysis of the process of psychological teaching, the psychological teaching combined with daily life can be divided into the following four steps with the help of the Internet.

427.3.1 Collect Typical Mental Phenomena

At this step, instructors should analyze the teaching goal and learners' daily life, and find the "combining point" of teaching content with the learner's life experience or human's life experience, especially the typical mental phenomena relevant with teaching goal, so that they can encourage learners to analyze the psychological explanation and finally to obtain specific psychological knowledge. In the process the Internet provides much convenience. For instance, by such search engines as Google and Baidu learners can easily find all sorts of psychological phenomena associated with the learning content.

427.3.2 Request the Learner to Analyze the Phenomena and to Propose Questions

The instructor should request learners to explain and analyze the collected typical phenomena, and inspire them to understand the mental activity of human beings. The instructor can instruct learners to use the Internet to search the relevant information about the phenomena analyzed. It is significant for instructors to guide learners to ask "why" for the phenomena, which can help them learn to propose questions and arouse their passion to explore the phenomena.

427.3.3 Request Learners to Answer Questions by Autonomous Exploration

In order to understand the psychological mechanism of the phenomena and answer the question about them, the learner needs to explore independently or by group. In the process, the learner can think about them according to the relevant theory and research. They also can make most use of the Internet to search all sorts of analyses and explanations for typical phenomena, and give their own viewpoints after critical thinking or group discussion.

427.3.4 The Integration of Knowledge

The learner finds the psychological mechanism behind the phenomena of daily life and achieves the aim of teaching. He or she obtains the specific knowledge, skill or attitude, integrates the extant knowledge, skill, or attitude with newly obtained knowledge, skill, or attitude.

This process, in fact, is that of finding knowledge by the Internet under the guidance of teachers, in which the learner's autonomous learning ability, analytic ability, problem solving ability, and creative thinking ability will be strengthened. In the following part, the principal procedures of psychological teaching combined with daily life will be illuminated by the teaching example.

In the teaching of memory, the teacher asks the student to search and collect the typical phenomena about memory that are prevalent in daily learning and life and reflect on his or her own experience about memory such as memory in reading, remembering some names, reviewing lessons before test, and memorizing English words (The first step). Then the teacher encourages the student to explain the phenomena (The second step). Based on this, the teacher asks the student to collect the relevant materials or explanations for them and to understand the natural law behind memory independently or by group (The third step). Finally, the student obtains the expected knowledge and skill about memory, and he or she can use specific knowledge about memory to explain his or her own experience or typical memory phenomena and can apply the knowledge to the improvement of his or her memory. He or she integrates the new knowledge and skill with the extant knowledge and skills about cognition (The fourth step).

In sum, the psychological teaching combined with daily life actually emphasizes the autonomous exploration and finding of learners and the application of psychological knowledge to daily life with the help of the Internet.

The paper is funded by the Central China Normal University Psychology Project for University Special Majors Construction (PSYCHT201214).

References

1. Wang S, Wang A (1992) Cognitive psychology. Beijing Publishing House, Beijing
2. Zhang D (2004) Educational psychology. The People's Education Publishing House, Beijing
3. Clinchy BM (1995) A connected approach to the teaching of developmental psychology. Teaching of Psychology 22(2):100–104
4. Jonassen DH (1992) Objectivism versus constructivism: Do we need a new philosophical paradigm? From ETR & D 39(3):5–14
5. Gu C (2010) Internet-supported creative learning: The application of network in learning. In: Proceedings of the international conference on E-product, E-service and E-entertainment (ICEEE2010) & the international conference on management science and artificial intelligence (MSAI2010), IEEE eXpress Conference Publishing, New York

6. Cummings R, Phillips R, Tilbrook R et al (2005) Middle-out approaches to reform of university teaching and learning: champions striding between the top-down and bottom-up approaches. International review of research in open and distance learning, Available at http://www.irrodl.org/content/v6.1/cummings.html. Cited 03 Nov 2005
7. Chen H (2011) Constructing english teaching environment in new type of college campus at the E-times—A case study of college english teaching reform in Linyi university. Asian Soc Sci 7(8):252–256

Chapter 428
Developing a Pilot Online Learning and Mentorship Website for Nurses

Sue Coffey and Charles Anyinam

Abstract The Ontario Nursing Connection (ONC) was a project funded by the Ontario Ministry of Health and Long-Term Care. It used electronic telecommunication tools via the internet as a vehicle for information exchange and virtual connection for nurses and other healthcare professionals. With a focus on three themes (leadership, mentorship, and interprofessional practice), this innovative website attracted close to 11,000 site visitors in a 12-month pilot period. Registered users (N = 645) who participated in a variety of learning and mentorship opportunities hailed from 29 countries around the world. Enhancements to existing software modules and new programming specific to the design of the project were used to create a rich repository of resources (text-based, audio, audio-visual, and virtual) on a number of topic areas. Additionally, through a virtual mentorship program, the ONC provided real time opportunities for knowledge transfer and support for career mobility. Learning from this project can now be applied to the development of a more permanent portal focusing on these themes and utilizing readily available and easily accessible technology to support continuous learning and professional development for nurses and other healthcare professionals.

Keywords Mentorship · Virtual learning environment · Online mentorship

428.1 Background

In 2007, the Ontario government launched the *Interprofessional, Mentorship, Preceptorship, Leadership and Coaching (IMPLC) Fund* in 2007. The fund, Developed by the Ministry of Health and Long-Term Care as part of *HealthForceOntario,* was

S. Coffey (✉)
University of Ontario Institute of Technology, Oshawa, ON, Canada
e-mail: sue.coffey@uoit.ca

C. Anyinam
George Brown College, Toronto, ON, Canada
e-mail: canyinam@georgebrown.ca

S. Li et al. (eds.), *Frontier and Future Development of Information Technology in Medicine and Education*, Lecture Notes in Electrical Engineering 269,
DOI: 10.1007/978-94-007-7618-0_428,

designed to support the province's health human resources strategy. It was also consistent with the focus on continuous learning as an essential requirement for professional nursing practice in Ontario [1]. Among other things, continuous learning for nurses involves acquisition of knowledge, appreciation of a variety of practice contexts and the pathways to developing career opportunities within them, and personal development [2].

In the spring of 2007, funding was provided by the Ministry of Health and Long-Term Care through the IMPLC Fund to a research team to initiate the Ontario Nursing Connection (ONC). This website was developed as an interactive, open access virtual nursing community. Objectives for this project were centred on learning and mentorship opportunities, and included:

1. Development of a web-based mentorship site serving Ontario nurses across the spectrum of transition to practice
2. Development of resources and supports specifically designed for Internationally Educated Nurses (IENs) and graduates/students of compressed nursing programs
3. Creation of an archived library of resources
4. Provision of both distance and face-to-face opportunities for mentorship with Ontario nurses and collaborative healthcare teams

Through the creation of the ONC website, Ontario nurses, nursing students, and individuals considering nursing as a career were able to explore the possibilities for a career in nursing in this province. Three foundational themes of nursing leadership, mentorship, and interprofessional practice formed the basis for this online professional community. Activities and site features focused broadly on: (a) learning components, (b) mentorship components, (c) profiling nursing in Ontario, and (d) creating a growing archive of resources available to all site users. Usability testing for this website, which was offered in an English-language only format, included both nurses and nursing students. Participants whose first language was English and those who indicated English as a second language took part in robust trials of the navigation of the website to ensure that it was intuitive and experienced positively by site users.

428.2 Website Components

428.2.1 Online Learning

Three modular learning series were developed, focusing on: (a) nursing leadership, (b) mentorship, and (c) interprofessional practice. Each series consisted of tutorials available in text format, synchronized rich media modules, and as podcasts for download. Upon completion of each of the learning series, participants were able to write a quiz based on the learning materials, and earn a certificate of completion.

Within a 12-month period, with very little promotional support, a total of 334 participants registered on the website and completed the various components of the learning activities. An additional 68 registered users viewed an online quiz but elected not to submit their answers in order to receive a certificate of completion.

Best Practice Guideline (BPG) knowledge translation modules were also created as part of online learning opportunities. BPGs are an essential practice tool for bringing best evidence into everyday nursing contexts. However, their lengthy, text-based format creates challenges to easy uptake. Focusing on two relevant Healthy Work Environment BPGs, interactive, online knowledge translation modules were created that included a summary of recommendations; audio, video, and graphic elements; interactive elements; and case studies.

428.2.2 Mentorship Components

Three types of mentorship activities were included in the development of the website. These included group e-mentoring sessions with nurses from around the world, small face-to-face mentoring sessions with Ontario nurses and nursing students, and individual virtual mentoring activities.

Three large group e-mentoring sessions were held. Each was broadcast live via streaming video. Two of the three events focused on nursing mentorship, with in-studio and online audiences and employing a town-hall type format. The third event focused on interprofessional practice, using an expert panel format with an online audience. For all events, members of the online audience engaged in real-time with the studio guests via an online moderator. For all three events, the online audience was comprised of nurses from not only across Ontario and Canada, but also included participants from 28 countries around the world. Each of these events was archived and viewable in streaming video format on the ONC website. Total participation for all three events included 16 panel guests, 28 studio audience members, and an online audience of more than 100 participants.

Three small group face-to-face mentoring sessions also took place, which were audio-recorded and made available on the ONC website. The focus for each event was based on website user requests. Additionally, one-to-one mentoring was also an option available on the ONC website. This took place through informal dialogue via ONC question and answer forums available to all registered users. It also occurred through matched mentor–mentee relationships, with a tally of 72 mentors trained and 77 mentoring matches completed in the 12-month period of operation.

428.2.3 Profiling Nurses in Ontario

Nursing in Ontario was profiled through three web-based components. An interview series featured exceptional Ontario nurses sharing their experiences. Six full-length interviews with exceptional Ontario nurses are available on the ONC website in streaming video format with accompanying transcripts. Two interviews focus on each theme of mentorship, nursing leadership, and interprofessional practice. Additionally, a career paths component of the project provided an alphabetical listing of 27 nursing specialties, with detailed descriptions of the nursing career foci and the preparation required. Rotating photos and quotes from Ontario nurses who are experts in the described practice areas accompany the text description.

428.2.4 Multi-media Resource Archives

A collection of archived resources was made available in multiple formats (streaming video, audio, text-based). Library resources are database searchable and accessible. Packaging for multiple deliverables (high and low bandwidth) was accomplished through the availability of multiple media choices as well as the option to request a DVD containing all rich media components.

428.3 Discussion

In addition to the numbers of participants for each of the components described above, the overall popularity of the ONC website in just 6–12 months is noteworthy. While the original target for site visitors for the pilot period was set at 1,000, during the first 12 months almost 11,000 visitors sought out the ONC website (with a combined total of more than 100,000 page views). Of that number, 645 became registered users, surpassing our initial target of 200.

Mentorship as a key component of education, socialization, and support for healthcare professionals is growing in popularity [3, 4]. However, face-to-face mentorship programs for nurses are limited by the fact that participants must reside in the same geographic location and must take time away from busy lives to create meeting opportunities [5]. They also fail to take into account typical challenges related to work-life balance for busy working healthcare professionals. At the same time, creating learning opportunities for nurses and other healthcare professionals that are easily accessible and relevant to the current healthcare context is imperative [6–8].

This initial project provides solid evidence for ongoing development of virtual mechanisms by which to support nurses, nursing students, and individuals considering a career in nursing or healthcare to connect, learn together, and explore professional possibilities. Within a 12-month period, this pilot online learning and mentorship project showed tremendous uptake, with both the number of site visitors and the number of registered users from around the world far surpassing expectations. Participants were able to engage throughout the process with developing website foci, including the requesting the topics for the live streaming face-to-face mentoring sessions. Feedback from participants was overwhelmingly positive. During usability testing, nurses whose first language was English and nurses for whom English was an additional language expressed equally high satisfaction with the website design and functionality. Both mentor and mentee participants in the online mentorship component expressed satisfaction with the preparation for mentorship learning module and the mentorship experience. Website activity demonstrated a high degree of activity from both new and returning users. Finally, requests for formal use of learning materials posted on the website have been received from multiple health education providers.

Results of this pilot project demonstrated that creating opportunities for nurses and other healthcare professionals both locally and internationally to share and grow professionally was made possible through readily available, easily replicated, internet-based technology. Learning was provided in accessible, visually attractive modules that mirrored user preferences (audio, video, or text-based). Developing a virtual community such as the one described in this pilot creates possibilities for healthcare professionals from around the world to learn from each other, mentor and support each other, and grow together.

Acknowledgments This project was funded by the Ontario Ministry of Health and Long-Term Care through the IMPLC Fund. The authors wish to thank the IT development team at York University for their support of the project.

References

1. College of Nurses of Ontario (2002) Practice standards revised 2002. Author, Toronto
2. Bruce BC, Levin JA (1997) Educational technology: media for inquiry, communication, construction, and expression. J Educ Comput Res 17(1): 79–102 http://alexia.lis.uiuc.edu/~chip/pubs/taxonomy/
3. Tourigny L, Pulich M (2005) A critical examination of formal and informal mentoring among nurses. Health Care Manag 24(1):68–76
4. Beecroft PC, Lacy ML, Kunzman L et al (2006) New graduate nurses' perceptions of mentoring: Six-year programme. J Adv Nurs 55(6):736–747
5. Kalisch BJ, Falzetta L, Cooke J (2005) Group e-mentoring: a new approach to recruitment into nursing. Nurs Outlook 53(4):199–205
6. Axmann M (2001) Effective learning strategies for the online environment: including the lost learner. In: Okamoto T, Hartley R, Kinshuk et al (eds) Advanced learning technology: issues, achievements and challenges. IEEE Comput Soc, Los Alamitos, CA
7. Axmann M (2002) An online mentorship programme for the online educator: patterning for success. In: McNamara S, Stacey E (eds) Untangling the web: establishing learning links. Proceedings ASET Conference 2002. Melbourne, 7–10 July. http://www.aset.org.au/confs/2002/axmann.html
8. Ntshinga WL (2010) World wide web (WWW) Tools enhancing mentorship. In: INTED2010 proceedings, 4th international technology, education and development conference 2010, Valencia, 8–10 March 2010

Chapter 429
Estrogenic and Antiestrogenic Activities of Protocatechic Acid

Fang Hu, Junzhi Wang, Huajun Luo, Ling Zhang, Youcheng Luo, Wenjun Sun, Fan Cheng, Weiqiao Deng, Zhangshuang Deng and Kun Zou

Abstract Study the estrogenic and antiestrogenic effects of protocatechuic acid with the aim of obtaining a safe and effective natural estrogen replacement drugs. Its estrogenic and antiestrogenic effects were evaluated through cell proliferation experiments. The estrogen-receptor (ER) binding abilities of protocatechuic acid were tested by yeast two-hybrid experiment, and their possible binding sites for ERs were performed by computer-aided molecular docking technology. Protocatechuic acid showed significant effects on the proliferation of estrogen-sensitive ER (+) MCF-7 cells in the absence of estrogen, and resulted in antagonistic effects on E_2-induced MCF-7 cell proliferation. However, it could not induce the proliferation of estrogen-negative ER (-) MDA-MB-231 cells. The yeast two-hybrid experiments showed protocatechuic acid had significant but non-selective binding abilities for the two ERs. Protocatechuic acid revealed a double directional adjusting function of estrogenic and antiestrogenic activities, which showed estrogenic agonist activity at low concentration or lack of endogenous estrogen, and the estrogenic antagonistic effect was stimulated at high concentrations or too much endogenous estrogen. Protocatechuic acid had significant binding capacity for ERs. Therefore, protocatechuic acid could be used in the treatment of the estrogen deficiency-related diseases.

Keywords Protocatechuic acid · *Phellinus lonicerinus* (Bond.) · Estrogen · Yeast two-hybrid assay

---

F. Hu (✉) · J. Wang (✉) · H. Luo · L. Zhang · Y. Luo · W. Sun · F. Cheng · Z. Deng · K. Zou
Hubei Key Laboratory of Natural Products Research and Development (China Three Gorges University), College of Chemistry and Life Science, China Three Gorges University, Yichang 443002, People's Republic of China
e-mail: horsedog@163.com

W. Deng
Dalian Institute of Chemical Physics, Chinese Academy of Sciences, Dalian 116023 Liaoning, People's Republic of China

S. Li et al. (eds.), *Frontier and Future Development of Information Technology in Medicine and Education*, Lecture Notes in Electrical Engineering 269,
DOI: 10.1007/978-94-007-7618-0_429,

429.1 Introduction

Protocatechuic acid is a kind of phenolic acids naturally existing in many vegetables, fruits, *Salviae Miltiorrhizae*, *Holly* and other traditional Chinese medicines. It has various pharmacological activities such as antibacterial, anti-platelet aggregation and analgesia. Recently, many studies reported protocatechuic acid showed antitumor effect and can be used as an effective inhibitor of many chemical carcinogens [1].

Protocatechuic acid was isolated from *Phellinus lonicericola* (Bond.) Bond. et sing. *P. lonicericola* is a drug commonly used in Tujia, which had been collected in "Quality Standards of Traditional Chinese Medical Materials in Hubei Province" (2009 Edition) [2]. *P. lonicericola* is one of the best internationally recognized medicinal fungus with anti-cancer effect at present. Studies have shown that *P. lonicericola* have good estrogen-like effect as well as antitumor activity Therefore, we have done estrogen and antiestrogen experiments on original catechins, the composition of *P. lonicericola*, in order to provides the basis for further the development and utilization of *P. lonicericola*.

429.2 Materials and Methods

429.2.1 Materials

Dulbecco's modified Eagle's medium, Leibovitz's L-15 Medium [+] L-Glutamine and Leibovitz's L-15 Medium [+] L-Glutamine [-] Phenol Red were obtained from Gibco BRL (Grand Island, NY, USA.). Fetal bovine serum was purchased from ICN Biomedicals, Inc (Aurora, OH, USA). Streptomycin, 0.25 % trypsin was purchased from Nacalai Tesque Co (Kyoto, Japan). 17β-estradiol was obtained from Calbiochem Co. (Darmstadt, Germany). 3-(4,5-dimethyl-2-thiazolyl)-2, 3-diphenyl-2*H*-tetrazolium bromide (MTT), penicillin, and norit SX-P charcoal were purchased from Wako Pure Chemical Ind., Ltd (Osaka, Japan). Dextran 70T was obtained from Amersham Pharmacia Biotech AB (Uppsala, Sweden). 17β-estradiol assaying ELISA kit was bought from Shanghai Hufeng Biology and Technology Company Limited.

429.2.2 Methods

429.2.2.1 Estrogenic Activities Assay

Estrogen sensitive ER (+) MCF-7 cells were grown in DMEM supplemented with 10 % FBS, penicillin, and streptomycin. The cells were harvested by trypsinization

(0.25 % trypsin) and plated at a concentration of 1.0×10^4 cells/well in DMEM supplemented with 10 % FBS in 96-well tissue culture plates and allowed to attach for 24 h. The culture medium was replaced with phenol red-free DMEM, then protocatechuic acid was added. Dissolution of protocatechuic acid in DMSO was diluted with phenol red-free DMEM, and the final DMSO concentration in culture did not exceed 0.1 %. Estrogen insensitive ER (−) MDA-MB-231 cells were cultured in the same way except the medium (L-15). After 4 days in the incubator with 5 % CO_2 at 37 °C, the proliferation of the cells was measured using the MTT method.

429.2.2.2 Antiestrogenic Activities Assay

Estrogen sensitive ER (+) MCF-7 cells were cultured under the same conditions as estrogenic activity assays. After the culture medium was replaced by phenol red-free DMEM, E_2 (1.0×10^{-9} M) was added to induce the cell proliferation. At the same time, various concentrations of protocatechuic acid were added, respectively. After 4 days in the incubator with 5 % CO_2 at 37 °C, the proliferation of the cells was measured using the MTT method.

429.2.2.3 Yeast Two-Hybrid Assay

The yeast two-hybrid assay was carried out according to the method of Nishikawa [3, 4]. And yeast cells expressing ERs were allowed to grow overnight at 30 °C with shaking in synthetic defined medium lacking tryptophan and leucine. Yeast cells were treated with protocatechuic acid for 4 h at 30 °C, and β-galactosidase activity was determined as follows. The growth of the yeast cells was monitored by measuring the turbidity at 600 nm. The treated yeast cells were collected by centrifugation (8000 *g*, 5 min) and resuspended in 200 mL of Z-buffer (0.1 M sodium phosphate, pH 7.0, 10 mM KCl, and 1 mM $MgSO_4$) containing 1 mg/mL of zymolyase at 37 °C for 15 min. The reaction was started by the addition of 40 μL of 4 mg/mL ONPG as a substrate. When the yellow color appeared (30 min), 100 μL of 1.0 M Na_2CO_3 was added to quench the reaction. The absorbance of solution (150 μL) was measured at 420 nm and 550 nm. β-Galactosidase activity (U) was determined using the following formula:

$$U = 1000 \times 3(A_{420} \times 1.75 \times A_{550})/t \times 0.05 \times A_{600} \quad (429.1)$$

429.2.2.4 Molecular Docking

The atomic coordinates for the structure of ERα and ERβ were downloaded from the Protein Data Bank (PDB Code: 3ERD [3] and 1U3R [6], respectively). The subsequent 3ERD and 1U3R models were subject to the Protein Preparation

Wizard module in Schrödinger [7] as follows: adding hydrogen, assigning partial charges using the OPLS-2001 force field, assigning protonation states. All crystal waters were removed. LigPrep of Schrödinger software suit [7] was used for preparation of ligand. Then molecular docking simulation was performed by Glide (SP mode) [7].

429.2.2.5 Statistical Analysis

Data were processed with the SPSS 13.0 for Windows software package. Values were expressed as mean ± standard deviations (SD). One-way analysis of variance was used for statistical analysis. A value of $p < 0.05$ was considered statistically significant.

429.3 Results

429.3.1 The Effects of Protocatechuic Acid on the Proliferation of MCF-7 Cells

As shown in Tables 429.1 and 429.2. The results indicated protocatechuic acid could significantly induce the proliferation of estrogen-sensitive ER (+) MCF-7 cells in the absence of estrogen. The strongest proliferation appeared at a concentration of 5.0×10^{-6}M ($p < 0.01$), and the proliferative effects declined as continuously increasing the concentration (1.0×10^{-6}-1.0×10^{-7} M). When E_2 (1.0×10^{-9} M) and the different concentrations of protocatechuic acid were treated at the same time, protocatechuic acid could result in antagonistic effects on E_2-induced MCF-7 cell proliferation. The difference was significant when the concentration of protocatechuic acid was 1.0×10^{-7}M compared with the simple use of E_2 ($p < 0.05$). When the concentration of protocatechuic acid increased to 1.0×10^{-5}M, the difference was significant compared with the control group($p < 0.01$).

429.3.2 The Effects of Protocatechuic Acid on the Proliferation of MD-AMB-231 Cells

The in vitro proliferation effects of MD-AMB-231 cells were shown in Table 429.1. Protocatechuic acid could not induce the proliferation of estrogen-negative ER(-) MDA-MB-231 cells.

Table 429.1 The effects of protocatechuic acid on the proliferation of MCF-7 and MD-AMB-231 cells ($\overline{X} \pm S$, n = 6)

Group	Concentration (M)	OD(MCF-7)	Proliferation (% of control)	OD (MD-AMB-231)	Proliferation (% of control)
Control	–	0.316 ± 0.010	–	0.508 ± 0.023	–
E_2	1.0×10^{-9}	0.502 ± 0.023**	159.0 % ± 7.28 %	0.506 ± 0.019	99.61 % ± 3.74 %
Protocatechuic acid	1.0×10^{-5}	0.394 ± 0.055**	124.8 % ± 17.41 %	0.521 ± 0.014	102.56 % ± 2.76 %
	5.0×10^{-6}	0.477 ± 0.013**	150.8 % ± 4.11 %	0.502 ± 0.018	98.82 % ± 3.54 %
	1.0×10^{-6}	0.397 ± 0.044**	125.6 % ± 13.92 %	0.491 ± 0.025	96.65 % ± 4.92 %
	5.0×10^{-7}	0.377 ± 0.010*	119.2 % ± 3.16 %	0.503 ± 0.010	99.02 % ± 1.97 %
	1.0×10^{-7}	0.339 ± 0.009	107.3 % ± 2.85 %	0.491 ± 0.025	96.65 % ± 4.92 %

Asterisks indicate significant difference from the control at $p < 0.05$ (*) or $p < 0.01$ (**)

Table 429.2 The effects of protocatechuic acid on the proliferation of MCF-7 cells in the presence of E_2 ($\overline{X} \pm S$, n = 6)

Group	Concentration	OD	Proliferation (% of E2)
Control	–	0.367 ± 0.025**	–
E2	1.0 × 10¯9 M	0.490 ± 0.022	–
Protocatechuic acid + E2(1.0 × 10-9 M)	1.0 × 10¯5 M	0.384 ± 0.013**	78.37 % ± 2.65 %
	5.0 × 10¯6 M	0.409 ± 0.017**	83.47 % ± 3.47 %
	1.0 × 10¯6 M	0.434 ± 0.013**	88.57 % ± 2.65 %
	5.0 × 10¯7 M	0.455 ± 0.014**	92.86 % ± 2.86 %
	1.0 × 10¯7 M	0.465 ± 0.015*	94.90 % ± 3.06

Asterisks indicate significant difference from the E_2 group at $p < 0.05$ (*) or $p < 0.01$ (**)

429.3.3 Effects of Protocatechuic acid on the Induction of β-Galactosidase Activity in an Yeast Two-Hybrid Assay

The protocatechuic acid induced β-galactosidase activity in a yeast two-hybrid assay results were listed in Table 429.3. The results indicated protocatechuic acid had a significant but non-selective binding abilities for the ERα and ERβ. When the concentration beyond 1.0×10^{-8}M, the difference of ERα and ERβ binding abilities was significant compared with the control group (p < 0.01). All of these indicated protocatechuic acid exerted estrogenic and antiestrogenic effects through binding to ERs.

429.3.4 Docking Study

Docking simulation between protocatechuic acid and estrogenic receptor was performed. The docking results of protocatechuic acid with ERα and ERβ were

Table 429.3 The protocatechuic acid induced β-galactosidase activity in a yeast two-hybrid assay ($\overline{X} \pm S$, n = 6)

Group	Concentration	α-Galactosidase Activity U	β-Galactosidase Activity U
Control	–	129.5 ± 6.5	165.0 ± 17.9
E2	1.0 × 10¯9 M	2126.0 ± 180.2**	1497.5 ± 172.9**
Protocatechuic acid	1.0 × 10¯4 M	675.0 ± 63.7**	1516.2 ± 180.0**
	1.0 × 10¯5 M	405.9 ± 29.8**	1411.1 ± 191.8**
	1.0 × 10¯6 M	322.8 ± 66.5**	787.7 ± 102.1**
	1.0 × 10¯7 M	261.5 ± 36.1**	399.7 ± 11.3**
	1.0 × 10¯8 M	307.1 ± 22.3**	373.1 ± 53.0**

Asterisks indicate significant difference from the control at $p < 0.01$ (**)

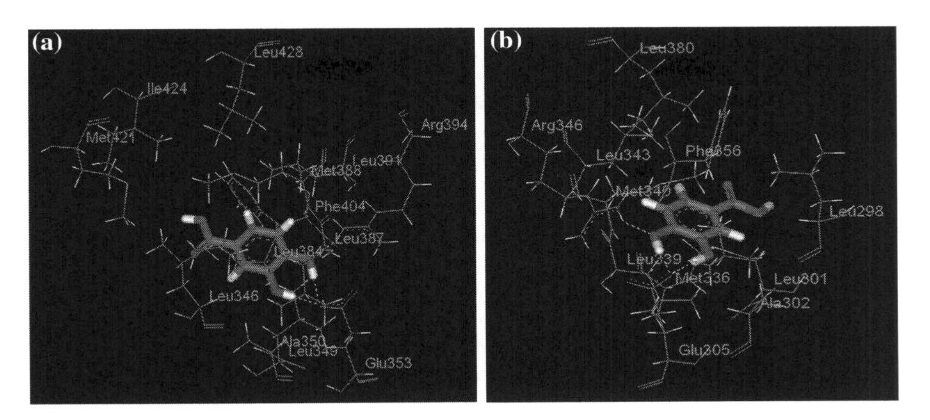

Fig. 429.1 The binding sites of protocatechuic acid-ERα (**a**) and protocatechuic acid-ERβ (**b**)

shown in Fig. 429.1. Gscores of protocatechuic acid-ERα and protocatechuic acid-ERβ docked complexes were −6.46 and −6.67, respectively. The hydrogen bonds are formed between hydroxyl group of protocatechuic acid and the amino acid residues Glu353 and Arg394 of ERα, or Glu305 and Arg346 of ERβ.

429.4 Discussion

Women's quality of life is seriously affected by the deficiency of estrogen. Estrogen replacement therapy (ERT) is a kind of therapeutic method suitable for supplementing menopausal women with E_2 and alleviating their climacteric syndrome. However, the long-term use of estrogen may lead to adverse effects such as breast swelling and venous thrombosis. What's more, estrogen stimulation is also considered to increase the risk of endometrial cancer and breast cancer at present.

In recent years, many efforts were dedicated to finding the safer estrogen replacement drugs. Phytoestrogens are estrogen-like chemicals, which commonly possess estrogenic effects and reduce estrogen deficiency symptoms without any adverse effects [4]. The phytoestrogens could prevent bone loss associated with the menopause and reduce breast cancer risk among pre-menopausal women. The traditional Chinese medicines have been an important source of phytoestrogens [9, 10]. The aim of this work was to find the components' double directional adjusting estrogenic effect from Chinese medicines, overcome the side effects of estrogen and generate the estrogenic effect instead of the estrogen. After screening many traditional Chinese medicines, the extract of the *phellinus lonicerinus* was found the most excellent anti-breast cancer effects and lest toxic to normal cells. Therefore, the component and its estrogenic effect of the *Phellinus Ionicerinus* was furtherly studied with the purpose of obtaining a safe and effective natural estrogen replacement drugs.

Protocatechuic acid was firstly found to possess strong estrogen-like effects and significant research implications in our work. Therefore, the estrogen-related physiological functions of protocatechuic acid should be further studied. Protocatechuic acid exhibited the estrogenic and antiestrogenic double directional adjusting activities through binding to ERs, which showed estrogenic agonist activity at low concentration or lack of endogenous estrogen, and the estrogenic antagonistic effect was stimulated at high concentrations or too much endogenous estrogen. The directional adjusting effects might be associated with its competitively binding to the intracellular ERs with E_2. Protocatechuic acid could also antagonize breast cancer cells growth induced by the high concentrations of estrogen. Consequently, the side effects of estrogen were inhibited, such as blocking estrogen-dependent mammary gland hyperplasia and preventing the breast cancer [11]. Protocatechuic acid is present in many edible and medicinal plants. Protocatechuic acid is a potential cancer chemopreventive product and reported relative safety [6]. Protocatechuic acid might be safer than E_2 when used as estrogen replacement drug, but the in vivo estrogenic effects including the double directional adjusting effects, tissue-selectivities and ERs selectivities were also worthy of further study.

429.5 Conclusion

The estrogenic and antiestrogenic activities of protocatechuic acid were confirmed in this study. The estrogenic agonist activity of protocatechuic acid was generated at low concentration or lack of endogenous estrogen, and the estrogenic antagonistic effect was stimulated at high concentrations or too much endogenous estrogen. Protocatechuic acid had significant binding capacity for ERs. Therefore, protocatechuic acid might be used in the treatment of the estrogen deficiency-related diseases.

References

1. Tanaka T, Kojima T, Kawamori T, et al. (1995) Chemoprevention of digestive organs eareinogenesis by natural produet protocatechuic acid. Cancer 75(6 Suppl): 1433–1439
2. Hubei Food and Drug Administration of China (2009) Quanlity Standard of Chinese Herbal Medicines in Hubei Province Wuhan: Hubei Science and Technology Press 113–114
3. Eguchi K, Ozawa M, Endoh YS, et al. (2003) Validity test for a Yeast Two-Hybrid assay to screen for estrogenic activity, and its application to insecticides and disinfectants for veterinary use. Bull Environ Contam Toxicol 70: 226–232
4. Nishikawa J, Saito K, Goto J et al. (1999) New screening methods for chemicals with hormonal activities using interaction of nuclear hormone receptor with coactivator. Toxicol Appl Pharmacol 154: 76–83
5. Shiau AK, Barstad D, Loria PM et al. (1998) The structural basis of estrogen receptor/ coactivator recognition and the antagonism of this interaction by tamoxifen. Cell 95: 927–937

6. Malamas MS, Manas ES, McDevitt RE et al. Design and synthesis of aryl diphenolic azoles as potent andselective estrogen receptor-beta ligands. J. Med. Chem 47: 5021–5040
7. Schrödinger LLC (2010), New York, NY www.schrodinger.com
8. Eden JA (2012) Phytoestrogens for menopausal symptoms: a review. Maturitas. 72:157–159
9. Hsiao WL, Lium L, (2010) The role of traditional Chinese herbal medicines in cancer therapy–from TCM theory tomechanistic insights. Planta Med 76: 1118–1131
10. Man S, Gao W, Wei C et al. (2012) Anticancer drugs from traditional toxic Chinese medicines. Phytother Res 26: 1449–1165
11. Prins GS, Korach KS (2008) The role of estrogens and estrogen receptors in normal prostate growth and disease. Steroids 73: 233–244
12. Takuji T, Takahiro T, Mayu T (2011) Potential cancer chemopreventive activity of protocatechuic acid 3: 27–33

Chapter 430
A Study on Learning Style Preferences of Chinese Medical Students

Yuemin Ding, Jianxiang Liu and Xiong Zhang

Abstract With the fast development of China, today's medical students in China are very diverse in education backgrounds, experiences, culture, and learning styles. There are four major sensory modes of learning: visual (V), auditory (A), reading-writing (R), or kinesthetic (K). To determine whether a particular teaching method might satisfy the requirement of students, a learning preference survey with the VARK questionnaire was given to our second-year medical students of Zhejiang University City College School of Medicine. As a result, 98 of 133 students (74 %) returned the completed questionnaire. Only 14.3 % of the students preferred a single mode of information presentation. In contrast, most students (85.7 %) preferred multiple modes of information presentation. The current result suggests that medical instructors in China should be aware of the student's individual preferences in order to make the educational experience more productive and enjoyable.

Keywords Learning styles · Medical education · Preference · Physiology

430.1 Introduction

With the fast development of China, today's medical students in China are very diverse in education backgrounds, experiences, culture, and learning styles. This diversity presents a challenge for instructors to meet the educational needs of all students. It is reported that when instruction is adapted to student learning styles, student motivation and performance improves [1]. Thus, knowing the different

Y. Ding (✉) · J. Liu · X. Zhang
School of Medicine, Zhejiang University City College, Hangzhou 310015, People's Republic of China
e-mail: dingyuemin@zucc.edu.cn

S. Li et al. (eds.), *Frontier and Future Development of Information Technology in Medicine and Education*, Lecture Notes in Electrical Engineering 269,
DOI: 10.1007/978-94-007-7618-0_430,

learning styles among the medical students is important for designing curriculum and developing appropriate teaching approaches to promote student learning [2].

Learning styles are the effective and efficient ways that one used in the learning process [3]. Specifically, the students' preferred mode of learning in terms of the sensory modality is the characterization of learning styles. There are four major sensory modes of learning: visual (V), aural (A), reading-writing (R), and kinesthetic (K), which is called the VARK instrument. Although students can use all of these sensory modes of learning, one mode is often dominant and preferred. Briefly, visual students learn through seeing pictures, animations and other image-rich teaching tools. Auditory students learn by listening to lectures. Reading-writing students learn through interaction with textual materials, whereas kinesthetic students learn through touching and experiences.

Physiology is the discipline focusing on the biological manifestations of the normal body. Traditionally, the learning of physiology at medical schools has relied heavily on classroom lectures. More recently, with changes to the medical curricula globally, it is increasingly being taught in a number of different ways, ranging from web-based distance learning, problem based learning, experiment based learning and a combination of many processes. A current trend on physiology education is to highlight ways in which the teaching of physiology can be successfully integrated into both traditional and web-based learning orientated curricula.

The advantage of web-based support of instruction by making all teaching materials, including visual, aural and reading-writing materials, available 24 h per day, 7 days per week, may meet the needs of different students with various learning styles and help instructor to develop appropriate teaching approaches.

Since we introduced the Blackboard learning system as the web-based support platform in the course of physiology, we were interested in knowing the preferred learning styles of our medical students in the course of physiology so that we could develop appropriate teaching approaches. To achieve this goal, we designed a descriptive study. The rational for this descriptive study was to help us design a lesson plan that addressed all students and to identify areas for further research.

430.2 Methods

430.2.1 Design

The VARK questionnaire was designed to investigate the preferences of students for particular modes of information presentation and was administered to our second-year medical students to determine their preferred modes. The questionnaire was included with the class packet for the physiology course, and 98 of the 133 students (74 %) returned the completed questionnaire. The questionnaire was administered on the Blackboard platform so that it can be completed online. The analysis of the questionnaire was completely managed on this virtual learning environment.

430.2.2 Procedures

The questionnaire was administered at the end of our medical physiology class at Zhejiang University City College, School of Medicine. The class consisted of 133 s-year medical students.

430.2.3 Data Analysis

Analysis for the VARK component was performed online, at the VARK home page. The number of students who preferred each mode of learning was divided by the total number of responses to determine the percentage of students in each category.

430.3 Results

The data shown in Table 430.1 indicate that more than 80 % of the total 98 students preferred visual modes (video and/or animation) and traditional reading-writing modes of teaching information presentation (blackboard and/or handouts). The kinesthetic mode (learning from experiments) was preferred by 76.5 % of the students. Only 64.3 % preferred auditory mode (sound record). In the present study, 14.3 % of the students preferred a single mode (either unimodal V, unimodal A, unimodal R or unimodal K) of information presentation, while the majority of students (85.7 %) preferred multiple modes (multimodal) of information presentation.

Taking unimodal and multimodal together for consideration as 100 %, 16 students preferred two modes (bimodal, 16.3 %), 19 students preferred three modes (trimodal, 19.4 %), and 49 students preferred four modes (quadmodal,

Table 430.1 Overall learning preferences of 98 medical students

Learning preferences	Number of students	Percentage(%)
Visual (V): Video and/or Animation	79	80.6
Aural (A): Sound record	63	64.3
Reading-Writing (R): Blackboard and/or Handouts	82	83.7
Kinesthetic (K): experiments	75	76.5

Fig. 430.1 Overall learning mode preferences of medical students

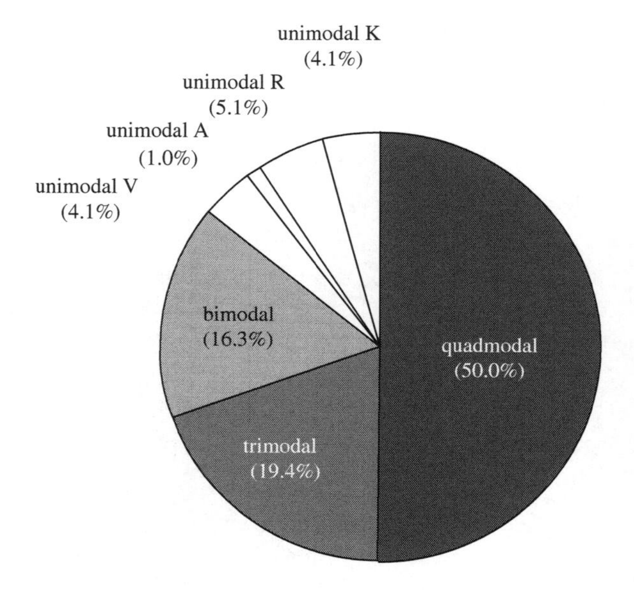

50.0 %). The percentage distribution of single mode preference was as follows: unimodal V (4.1 %), unimodal A (1.0 %), unimodal R (5.1 %) and unimodal K (4.1 %). Fig. 430.1 presents the percentages of students who preferred single, two, three, or four modes of information presentation.

Be consistent with the above results, when asked about the traditional classroom lectures, 96.6 % of the students preferred Powerpoint (PPT) slides show, which may include amount of teaching approaches related to different sensory modes, such as pictures, animations, flashes, videos, etc. Of the students who preferred PPT presentation, some students preferred the combination of PPT and blackboard drawing (48.2 %), some students preferred the combination of PPT and discussion (29 %), and some students preferred PPT alone (19.4 %), only (3.4 %) of them preferred blackboard drawing or discussion alone.

430.4 Discussion

To determine the preferred learning styles of our medical students in the course of physiology, in the present study, we administered the designed questionnaire to our second-year medical students. Ninety-eight of the 133 students (74 %) returned the completed questionnaire. Only 14.3 % of the students preferred a single mode of information presentation. Most students (85.7 %) preferred multiple modes of information presentation.

When analyzing the learning modes, 80.6 % of the medical students preferred visual modes of teaching information presentation. These students preferred information to arrive in the form of graphs, charts, videos and animations. They were sensitive to changing spatial arrangements. Similarly, 83.7 % of the students preferred reading-writing modes of teaching information presentation. They preferred receiving information by printed or written words. The kinesthetic mode was preferred by 76.5 % of the students. These students were satisfied by manipulating models, role playing [4] and experiments. Only 64.3 % preferred auditory mode. Auditory students are reached through discussion during peer instruction [5], collaborative testing, debate, games, and answering questions. When a blend of visual, auditory, reading-writing, and kinesthetic activities was provided, most students learned more effectively. To meet the need of each individual student, teaching approaches were suggested to be multi-sensory and the integrated teaching strategies become extremely important.

The Blackboard learning system has been introduced in the teaching of physiology from the spring of 2009. It enable us to load a vast array of learning materials to make sure each student can find the kind of materials that best suit his/her learning style. This feature helps students to become strategic learners by stressing the relations between educational contents and curriculum objectives. The use of such varied multimedia materials also facilitates the learning of abstract concepts, which are particularly prominent in Physiology course.

In conclusion, Chinese medical students have different learning styles. The medical instructors should be aware of the student's individual preferences to develop appropriate teaching approaches and make the educational experience more productive and enjoyable. Use of web-based multimedia materials facilitates both instructors and students in teaching and learning process in Chinese medical schools.

References

1. Smith AR Jr, Cavanaugh C, Jones J et al (2006) Influence of learning style on instructional multimedia effects on graduate student cognitive and psychomotor performance. J Allied Health 35:182–203
2. Tanner K, Allen D (2004) Approaches to biology teaching and learning: learning styles and the problem of instructional selection–engaging all students in science courses. Cell Biol Educ 3:197–201
3. Andrusyszyn MA, Cragg CE, Humbert J (2001) Nurse practitioner preferences for distance education methods related to learning style, course content, and achievement. J Nurs Educ 40:163–170
4. Kuipers JC, Clemens DL (1998) Do i dare? using role-play as a teaching strategy. J Psychosoc Nurs Ment Health Serv 36:12–17
5. Cortright RN, Collins HL, Rodenbaugh DW et al (2003) Student retention of course content is improved by collaborative-group testing. Adv Physiol Educ 27:102–108

Chapter 431
Design and Implementation of the Virtual Experiment System

Liyan Chen, Qingqi Hong, Beizhan Wang and Qingqiang Wu

Abstract Firstly, this paper introduced the features of virtual lab and showed advantages during teaching. Then it mainly discussed the combination of VRML and Java, including realizing dynamic client interface with Java Applet technology and communicating between HTTP protocol tunnel and backstage servlet, which is supposed to bring interaction and individuation education come true. Finally, this paper described the constructing idea and system structure of the virtual experiment system.

Keywords: Virtual experiment system · VRML · Java

431.1 Introduction

The traditional engineering course teaching adopts the model of teachers' explaining and demonstration as well as students' listening and practice after class. To a certain extent, this kind of teaching model neglects students' principal role in teaching activities, not reflecting the course synthesis and practice of teaching characteristics. This not only has a bad effect on students to develop their autonomy independence, but also teachers can not consider students' actual understanding during explanation. Besides, for the equipment hardware, it is replaced quickly and has a lot of wear and tear, some experiment also cannot be finished in laboratory. These existing problems restrict engineering course to foster students' practice ability. The presenting of 3D virtual reality technology provides the breakthrough point for practical teaching reform, resolves the contradiction between teaching and learning, achieving a multiplying effect. And it can provide

L. Chen · Q. Hong (✉) · B. Wang · Q. Wu
Department of the Software, Xiamen University, Xiamen, China
e-mail: hongqq@gmail.com

S. Li et al. (eds.), *Frontier and Future Development of Information Technology in Medicine and Education*, Lecture Notes in Electrical Engineering 269,
DOI: 10.1007/978-94-007-7618-0_431,

students the vivid, lifelike learning environment, and students can become a participator of the virtual environment, playing a role in the virtual environment, which has a positive effect on breaking through the emphasis focal point and difficulties of teaching as well as fostering students' skills.

431.2 VRML and Java

431.2.1 VRML Technology

VRML is a kind of language used to establish a model of the real world or a colorful world made by people. As in international standard, it is the main kind of program language based on the "www" net building, which is defined by ISO, the kind of MIME is x-world or x-VRML. The most important thing is that it has no relationship with the operating system. Otherwise, because of the birth of VRML 2.0, its ability of describing the dynamic condition gets better, and the interaction of the internet evolved too. The use of VRML will bring a revolutionary change.

431.2.1.1 Integrating JAVA and VRML

To supply a gap of full programming language functionality's absence, VRML provides Script node defining an interface between VRML world and a script written in a regular programming language such as Java. Additional, VRML also provides another API for programming language interaction: the External Authoring Interface (EAI). Script node is typically used to program the behavior in a scene such as signifying a change or user action, receiving events from other nodes, and effecting change somewhere else in the scene by sending events. Relative to uncomplicated Script node, EAI, designed to allow external application to access nodes in a VRML world using the existing VRML event model, covers all forms of access to a VRML world from external applications. Taking complexity of CVES into consideration; we emphasize on EA1 mechanism to enhance programming capability.

431.3 Advantages of Virtual Experiment System

Compared with the traditional laboratory, the virtual lab embodies its advantages on courses extension, knowledge learning and experiment exploring.

431.3.1 Courses Extension

As the new technology's rapid development, the former experiment material and teaching method cannot meet students' requirement, so courses need to be extended urgently. The 3D virtual reality educational system makes a breakthrough in teaching material category and expanding educational content, and pays attention to the integration of new technology and new knowledge, that ensuring the integrity and contemporary of courses content and advancing with the times in courses.

For the construction of teaching resources, the 3D virtual reality educational system breaks the current situation of paper nature resource as main body, presents stereoscopic all-around content of teaching and learning, and develops the resource system that consists of virtual resource as characteristics, network resource as main body and E-textbooks as assistant. According to the character of courses content, a large number of text resources, video tutorials, electronic resources, network resources and video cases are developed. These resources formation not only create and provide conditions for the realization of network education, research study and self-learning, but also provide guarantee for the constructing of courses teaching mode.

For the teaching mode, students can be self-learning by teachers' assigning through network platform, and ask their interesting questions and feedback learning proposals. Teachers can analyze proposals from students and learning process data to determine the degree-of-difficulty of classroom teaching contents, and also to judge the type of teaching contents: for theoretical knowledge, explanation teaching is primarily adopted; for practical skill, demonstration method is primarily used, and to arrange relevant experimental teaching task. After class, students can make group activity of experimental project through virtual laboratory, making virtual simulation training according to experiment guide to obtain basic experiment skills, and present problem and suggestion of experiment operation. According to feedback from students, teachers can give students necessary guidance and make experiment preparation for students' handing.

431.3.1.1 Knowledge Learning

Knowledge learning means that students use virtual reality system to learn all kinds of knowledge. It has two aspects in application field: one is reproduction of natural phenomenon or changing process which cannot be observed in real life, to provide students vivid, lifelike and perceptual learning materials, to help students solve difficulties during study. For example, text, picture, sound and animation can be mixed together through VRML technology when introducing principles of computer components, to show computer's components for students with 3D, and students can also assemble computer in the virtual three-dimensional space.

Another application of the 3D virtual reality technology in knowledge learning is to make the abstract concept visual and intuitive, which is convenient for students to understand.

431.3.1.2 Experiment Exploring

The practical teaching is the most important process in computer course, and with the appearance and development of VRML technology, it provides us the effective way for practical teaching. We can use the 3D virtual reality technology to build different kinds of virtual laboratory, to provide students vivid, lifelike experimental situation and convenient, natural experimental method, to better help students understand knowledge and enhance memory, and to provide effective technical support for improving teaching quality.

Network virtual lab can provide students an online participation and the interactive experiment environment. Using 3D and VR technology can realize the requirement of immersion and interaction of virtual reality. For experiment content, considering the design cost and the selection of detail experimental content, it can be designed as a simple 3D virtual reality technology, which doesn't need special helmets, data gloves, sensing device and so on, users only need mouse operation.

In the laboratory, students can freely simulate different kinds of experiments freely. Through test in the virtual laboratory, it can be not only reduced the experiment time, but also be obtained the intuitive and real effect. Meanwhile, students can also make a team through the virtual platform, and work together to complete a virtual experimental project.

The 3D virtual reality technology not only can perform experiment, but also can make virtual operation for different questions from students and supposed model in the teaching, and can visually observe questions or the final result of supposed model. Students can also study and explore, thus stimulates their interest during study and foster their creative ability. But using the virtual experiment in teaching process cannot replace the real experiment operation completely, and the virtual experiment should be combined with the real experiment in operation, so as to improve experiment effect.

431.4 Construction of Virtual Laboratory

Construction of virtual laboratory is the integrated application of multiple technologies, and the system architecture mainly includes two aspects: model construction and the realization of interaction.

431.4.1 Model Construction of Virtual Laboratory

Scene modeling and different kinds of equipments that are required by experiment process are needed to be constructed firstly. Three dimensional virtual scene modules are built to be based to a real scene, in order to construct a virtual experiment environment with reality sense, so the field survey of laboratory environment is needed before modeling the virtual scene,. And it is complicated to build complex 3D models of equipment through VRML language, moreover, the modeling method of VRML is short of visualization. However, 3DSMAX is widely used in 3D virtual scene because of its powerful modeling function and format output function for VRML file. And modeling method should be selected according to the feature of model during building process. Simple models will directly use simple geometry patch-based texture method of VRML, and complex scene will use the 3DSMAX modeling which will be converted to VRML file format for output. Of course, a lot of work on modeling in virtual laboratory make a high requirement for software's efficiency, so Canoma can be adopted, which is a high efficient software in the modeling process.

Making use of it, 3D model can be built directly by one or several pictures without modeling. Because of using real pictures to create 3D model, the effect is very real, and Canoma also can make VRML file for network. In order to show the characteristic of equipment, sometimes Flash technology is adopted to realize the reality of equipment, and to provide some basic interaction.

431.4.1.1 Realization of Experiment System's Interaction

Interaction is the important issue of virtual experiment system. When users browsing the scene, the main input equipment is mouse, at this time the detector actually is checking different actions of mouse by users, for example, pointing, clicking, dragging and so on, accordingly the virtual scene will make feedback. The detector used for monitoring action is touch-type monitor. Describing this kind of monitor's nodes include touch sensor node, plane sensor node, sphere-sensor node and cylinder sensor node. Another is to judge the close degree of some object between users and scenes, to make the object response accordingly, and forming the interaction between users and virtual objects. After adding all equipments into scenes successfully, users can freely pick up their required equipment to make experiment, so the interface of selecting equipment apparatus for users is needed to provide. And the selection button for users is involved in the prototype equipment apparatus. Because of users' requiring interaction with system and system's needing communicating with backend database according to users' selection, so the Java Applet can be adopted. Utilizing the Java Applet technology to achieve dynamic client interface can realize the interaction and individuation education through the communication between HTTP protocol tunnel and backstage server Servlet. Applet has good and transparent network transmission performance. Figure 431. 1 shows the process of browser's database access through applet.

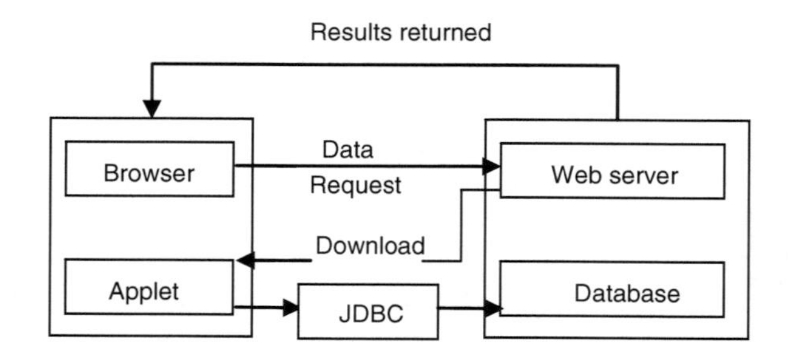

Fig. 431.1 Process of browser's database access through JDBC

431.5 Conclusion

Importing the virtual reality technology into education with the characteristic of scene-teaching and powerful interaction is the necessary trend of new education technology development, also is the one of best ways to realize the virtual reality technology itself-value.

VRML technology as a new science and technology is related to many different science domains. The technology potential of this field is huge and the application prospect is also wide. In teaching field, the VRML technology is especially suitable for engineering courses with powerful practice. Compared with the traditional education model, with a more lively teaching method coordinating student's autonomous learning, it can stimulate students' interest, and guide students to be in learning state step-by-step through the application of the VRML technology.

Although at the present time currently the VRML technology has been applied in computer teaching, there are still some unsolved theory problems and unconquered technical difficulties. For example, display equipment can not receive good quality and lifelike images, in addition, the real-time and the generated speed of images are required to be improved in complex condition. As the rapid development of the VRML technology, it will make greater development in education application in future.

References

1. Hannafin MJ, Land SM (1997) The foundations and assumptions of technology-enhances, student-centered learning environments. Instructional science 25(3):167–202
2. Saliah HH, Villardier L, Assogba B (2000) Resource management strategies for remote virtual laboratory experimentation. In: Proceedings of the 30th annual frontiers in education conference, Kansas City, USA
3. Xuan Z (2009) The virtual reality technology applied in the experimental teaching. J Yiyang Vocat Tech Coll 6:64–66

Chapter 432
Application of Simulation Software in Mobile Communication Course

Fangni Chen and Zhongpeng Wang

Abstract Mobile Communication is an important course for the communication engineering specialty. According to the current 3G (the third generation) era background in China, mobile communication technology develops rapidly and it has a lag in experimental teaching. Exploring a teaching system for combining theory with practice is very important. Therefore, we propose the reform of curriculum content and experimental methods by using the simulation software which is called WCDMA simulation system. It helps to design and analyze the mobile system in computer instead of building the very expensive hardware system in the lab. The experimental teaching software helps to improve the students' learning interest and achieves satisfactory teaching effect.

Keywords Simulation · Software · Mobile communication · WCDMA

432.1 Introduction

With the rapid development of mobile communication and the popularization of application in the current society, it has penetrated into every aspect of people's life. As a major course of communication engineering, Mobile communication course is based on several basic courses such as "circuit principles", "electronic technology", "high frequency circuits", "signal and system", "communication principles". It is a comprehensive course which includes a wide range of knowledge, such as mobile communication coding and modulation, mobile networking technology, GSM mobile communication network, the third generation mobile communication network and so on.

F. Chen (✉) · Z. Wang
Zhejiang University of Science and Technology, Hanzhou, Zhejiang, China
e-mail: cfnini@163.com

S. Li et al. (eds.), *Frontier and Future Development of Information Technology in Medicine and Education*, Lecture Notes in Electrical Engineering 269,
DOI: 10.1007/978-94-007-7618-0_432,

After the release of 3G licenses in China, the third generation mobile communication is in its rapid development. Under the background of 3G, the innovation of mobile communication technology and the development of market make communication enterprises put forward higher requirements for communication students.

432.2 Teaching Problems in Mobile Communication Course

However, the present teaching situation of mobile communication course cannot adapt to the coming of the 3G era. There are four main problems in the process of teaching:

(1) Existing textbook of mobile communication course can hardly keep up with the pace of the development of mobile technology. Thus it causes a lag of knowledge which the student are learning and it will influence the students' work ability in the future.
(2) Generally the mobile communication curriculum only discusses the theory and its algorithm, but seldom involves the application environment and objects. It causes a severe separation with the industry requirements.
(3) Being restricted by the experiment equipment, the comprehensive experiment is difficult to open, which leads the students' lack of global view of the mobile communication system.

Facing with these problems, the preferred solution is to build a good teaching system which can combine the theory and practice together, and can strengthen the practical engineering skills and communication occupation accomplishment.

432.3 Simulation Software

The experiment is the important part of mobile communication teaching. Giving the grim students' employment situation, most employers welcome the students who have both a solid theoretical foundation and strong practical ability. Therefore, the practice teaching plays an important role to cultivate and improve students' comprehensive quality and creative ability. However, some experimental contents are very difficult to open because of the expensive cost of the laboratory hardware. In order to let the students further understand the basic principle of mobile communication systems, we can use the simulation software to carry on the experimental contents instead of hardware implementation.

Specifically, experimental realization of mobile communication can use three different levels of experimental methods, namely, the principle level, the simulation level and the engineering level. Here we focus on the second and third level. In these three levels, considering the development of communication industry, simulation experiments of engineering level are most important. It can further promote students' learning interest; improve their professional ability and occupation quality. We applied WCDMA simulation software in our mobile communication course. The software simulates a virtual communication building, let the student goes into the control room to see and learn the WCDMA hardware. This simulation experiment of engineering level effectively improves the students' interest in learning, and achieved satisfactory teaching effect.

The WCDMA system simulation software we are using is supplied by Shenzhen Xunfang Communication Technology Company. The software is based on the WCDMA hardware equipment produced by Huawei Company. It take the configuration of the hardware as a typical example, vividly shows the physical structure of RNC (radio network controller) and base station equipment Node B. Meanwhile, students can complete the operations of system backstage management, data configuration, alarm management, dynamic data management, signaling message tracking and so on. Through WCDMA system simulation software, students can carry out the following 5 categories of experiment:

1. Global configuration experiment of WCDMA RNC equipment.
2. IU_CS interface configuration experiment of WCDMA RNC equipment.
3. IU_PS interface configuration experiment of WCDMA RNC equipment.
4. Iub interface and the wireless side configuration experiment of WCDMA RNC equipment.
5. Configuration experiment of WCDMA Node B equipment.

432.4 The Application of WCDMA Simulation Software

The wireless network controller RNC and base station equipment Node B together constitute the mobile access network UTRAN. The function of RNC is radio resource management including system information broadcasting, switching, cell resource allocation etc. Node B is the wireless signal transceiving equipment serving one cell or multiple cells. Node B exchange the data with RNC through the standard Iub interface, and communicate with UE (the user equipment) through the Uu interface. It mainly completes the processing of Uu interface protocol and Iub interface protocol.

Figure 432.1 shows the communication building and the control room which are simulated in the software. Students can "go into" the building and the control room. Figure 432.2 shows the RNC equipment rack and Node B equipment. By moving the mouse to each single board on the RNC, it will display the description and function of this single board. Students can study the knowledge about RNC equipment on their own. Also we can see the video of Node B installation by

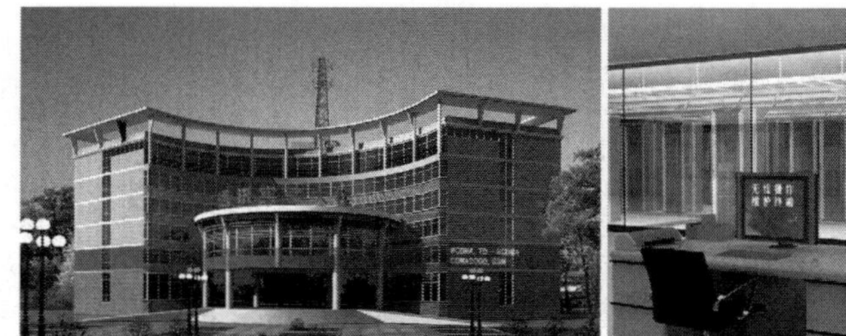

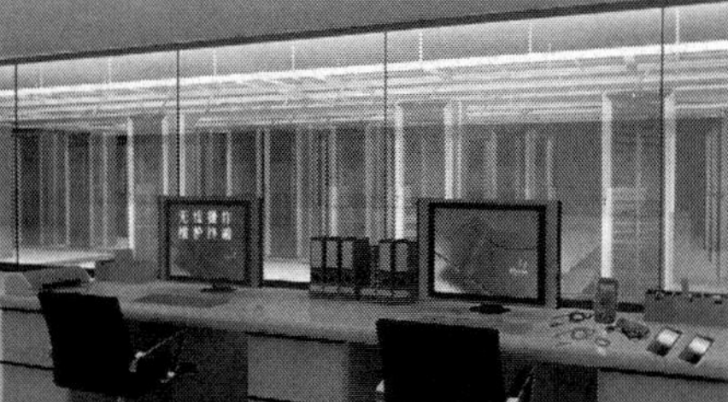

Fig. 432.1 The communication building and the control room

clicking the mouse on the Node B equipment. These figures and video made a strong impression on the students and help them to understand the structure and function of the real hardware equipment of WCDMA system.

Next we will take the basic data configuration of the Node B experiment as an example to introduce the application of the software.

After logging in the WCDMA simulation system, we can choose the operation and maintenance interface of Node B equipment. The configuration of Node B includes steps as follows:

(1) Configure Node B basic information.
(2) Configure Node B equipment information.
(3) Configure Node B panel information and radio unit.
(4) Configure the Ethernet port information.
(5) Configure IUBCP data.
(6) Configure IPPATH data.
(7) Configure OMCH data.
(8) Configure IP routing data.
(9) Configure wireless data.

The configuring page of step 3 are shown in Fig. 432.3 as an example.

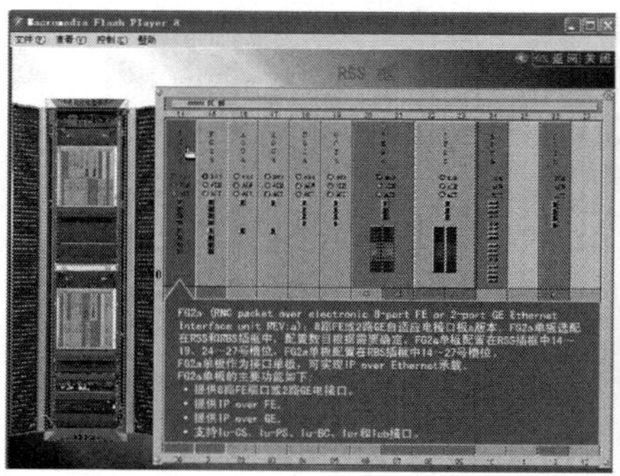

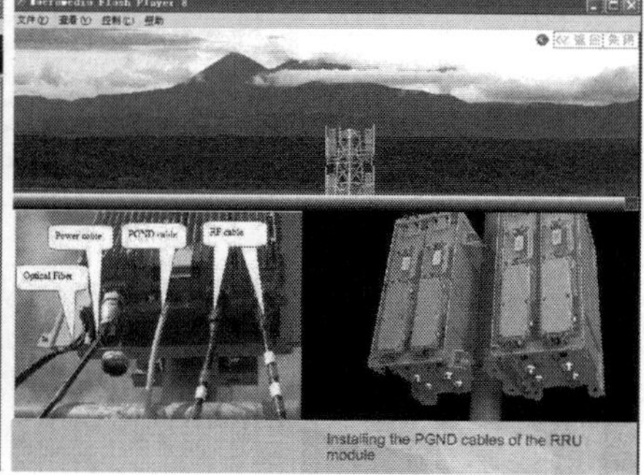

Fig. 432.2 RNC equipment rack and Node B equipment

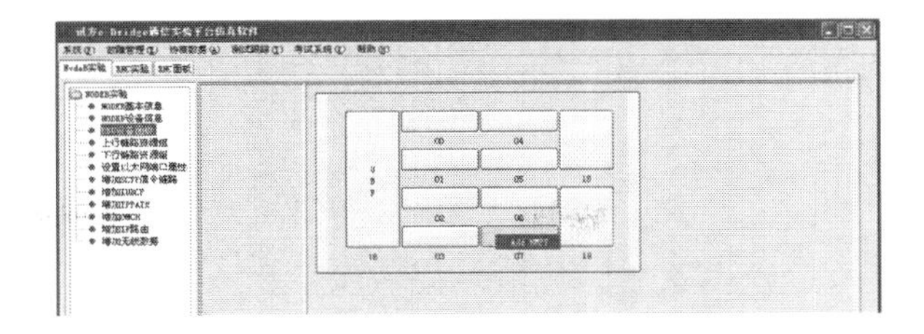

Fig. 432.3 Configure Node B panel information

When the configuration is finished, students can check the configuration result by dial simulation through the software. If the configuration is perfect, the dial will success; otherwise, the dial will fail.

432.5 Conclusions

WCDMA system simulation software can simulate the WCDMA network hardware much more rapidly, effectively and accurately. Through the experiments of equipment configuration and maintenance, it helps to save the investment and improve students' learning initiative. All these advantages make it an effective tool of practical teaching of mobile communication course.

References

1. Chen Y (2011) Teaching reform of mobile communication under the model of instruction of BTEC in Britain. Nat Sci Teach 12:107–108
2. Dai CQ, Ran HX, Bao NH (2012) Mobile communication experimental teaching reform and platform construction. Exp Technol Manage 29(2):144–145
3. WCDMA simulation system experiment book (2011) Shenzhen Xunfang Communication Technology Company
4. WCDMA DBS3900 hardware structure (2012) HUAWEI Technologies CO., LTD
5. WCDMA BSC6800 hardware structure (2012) HUAWEI Technologies CO., LTD

Chapter 433
Study on the Effect of Astragalus Polysaccharide on Function of Erythrocyte in Tumor Model Mice

Chen-Feng Ji, Yu-bin Ji and Zheng Xiang

Abstract To study the effect of astragalus polysaccharide on function of erythrocyte in tumor model mice. S_{180} mice were made as tumor model mice and treated with APS by i.p. for 7 days, and then the erythrocytes were collected. Band 3 and GPA content were determined by SDS-PAGE, test kits were used to measure phospholipids, cholesterol and sialic acid contents, DPH dye was used to determine membrane fluidity. Erythrocytes were labeled by rat anti-mouse CR1 antibody and FITC-conjugated goat anti-mouse antibody, flow cytometry was used to determine the number of CR1, then the DTER and RBC-C3bRR was determined by microscope. The results showed that Astragalus polysaccharide increased phospholipids content and decreased cholesterol content of erythrocyte membrane in tumor model mice, and increased both Band 3 and GPA contents and sialic acid content, also it improved erythrocyte membrane fluidity. Asparagus polysaccharide even increased CR1 number and activity of erythrocyte in tumor model mice. These results indicate Astragalus polysaccharide can adjust the abnormality of erythrocyte and improve its function.

Keywords Astragalus polysaccharide · Erythrocyte · Function · Tumor

C.-F. Ji (✉) · Y. Ji · Z. Xiang
Engineering Research Center of Natural Anticancer Drugs, Ministry of Education, Harbin University of Commerce, Harbin 150076, China
e-mail: smilejcf001@sina.com

C.-F. Ji · Y. Ji · Z. Xiang
Center of Research on Life Science and Environmental Science, Harbin University of Commerce, Harbin 150076, China

S. Li et al. (eds.), *Frontier and Future Development of Information Technology in Medicine and Education*, Lecture Notes in Electrical Engineering 269,
DOI: 10.1007/978-94-007-7618-0_433,

433.1 Introduction

Astragalus polysaccharides (APS) has a good role in immune regulation and anti-tumor effect [1]. Modern research indicates red blood cells act as one of immune cells and are involved in the development and progression of tumors, so it plays an important role in the anti-tumor immune response. It has been reported that many of polysaccharides could promote and regulate erythrocyte immune function. In this study, we studied the effect of astragalus polysaccharide on membrane structure and components of erythrocyte in tumor model mice.

433.2 Materials and Methods

433.2.1 Animals and Administration

Mice were divided into three groups with 10 mice in each group: Normal, tumor control group and APS treated group. The drug was given to mice 0.2 mL once a day for 7 days.

433.2.2 Preparation of the Erythrocyte Suspension and Membrane

Fresh blood was drawn and washed with PBS for 5 min at 1500 r/min. Erythrocyte residue was drawn and diluted with PBS. Erythrocytes were hemolysised in Tris–HCl, and the protein was separated by centrifuge (12000 × g, 15 min, 4 °C). The content of protein in the membrane was quantified by kit.

433.2.2.1 The Content of Phospholipids, Cholesterol, GPA, Band and SA in erythrocyte membrane

Membrane solution was drawn and added into 3 mL mixed solution of chloroform and methanol, then was centrifuged at 3000 r/min for 5 min, and the low layer was drawn. The content of phospholipids and cholesterol was determined with kits.

The SDS-PAGE was applied to separate the protein. The gel was dyed by PAS For GPA analysis and dyed by CBB R250 for Band 3 analysis.

The content of SA was determined on spectrophotometer depending on a purple compound formed by oxidated SA and 5-Methylresorcinol.

433.2.3 The fluidity of Erythrocyte Membrane

DPH probe solution was added to cell suspension, and incubated for 30 min at 25 °C and then centrifuged at 3000 r/min for 10 min twice and then diluted into PBS. It was measured by fluorescence spectrophotometer.

433.2.4 The Number and Activity of CR1 on Erythrocyte

4 μL rat-anti-mouse CD35 antibody was added to erythrocyte suspension, and then incubated for 30 min at room temperature, rinsed with PBS and centrifuged at 1500 r/min for 5 min. The supernatant was discarded, and 100 μL FITC-goat-anti-rat antibody was added and incubated for 30 min, rinsed with PBS and centrifuged for 5 min at 1500 r/min, diluted into PBS and tested by flow cytometer.

RBC-C3bRR and DTER were measured with protocols developed by Guo Feng.

433.2.5 Statistical Processing

Data were processed using SPSS 15.0, with results for the various groups expressed in the form $\bar{x} \pm s$. Variance test was used to compare the samples.

433.3 Results

433.3.1 Effect of Astragalus Polysaccharide on the Content of Phospholipids, Cholesterol, Band 3, GPA and SA on Erythrocyte Membrane in S180 Mice

The results showed the content of phospholipids in S180 mice was remarkably low and cholesterol in S180 mice was higher than that in normal mice, and APS could increase phospholipids content and decrease cholesterol content remarkably compared with control group ($P < 0.05$). And the band 3 and GPA content in S180 mice was lower than that in normal mice, and APS could increase both proteins content remarkably compared with control group ($P < 0.05$). The content of SA in S180 mice was lower than that in normal mice, and APS could increase the content remarkably compared with control group ($P < 0.01$). As shown in Table 433.1.

Table 433.1 Effects of APS on content of PL, Ch, Band 3, GPA and SA on erythrocyte membrane

Group	PL (mmol/L)	Ch (mmol/L)	Band 3(%)	GPA (%)	SA (mmol/L)
Normal	1.72 ± 0.03**	1.38 ± 0.05**	23.12 ± 2.93**	84.07 ± 3.08*	1.09 ± 0.10**
Control	1.32 ± 0.05	1.55 ± 0.15	14.55 ± 2.55	73.19 ± 5.88	0.67 ± 0.04
APS	1.49 ± 0.06*	1.49 ± 0.10*	17.43 ± 1.95*	80.59 ± 4.35*	0.90 ± 0.08**

*$P < 0.05$, **$P < 0.01$ versus control group

433.3.2 *Effect of Astragalus Polysaccharide on Fluidity of Erythrocyte Membrane in S180 Mice*

The results showed the erythrocyte membrane fluidity in S180 mice was remarkably low compared with that in normal mice ($P < 0.01$), and APS could improve membrane fluidity remarkably compared with control group ($P < 0.05$). As shown in Table 433.2.

433.3.3 *Effect of APS on the Number and Activity of CR1 on Erythrocyte*

The results showed the number of CR1 in S180 mice was remarkably low compared with that in normal mice ($P < 0.01$), and APS could increase CR1 number remarkably compared with control group ($P < 0.05$). As shown in Table 433.3.

The results also showed the RBC-C3bRR and DTER in S180 mice was remarkably low compared with that in normal mice ($P < 0.01$), and APS could increase RBC-C3bRR and DTER remarkably compared with control group ($P < 0.05$). As shown in Table 433.3.

Table 433.2 Effects of APS on erythrocyte membrane fluidity

Group	Dose (mg/kg)	*P*	η	LFU
Normal	–	0.13 ± 0.02**	0.83 ± 0.10**	20.13 ± 2.15**
Control	–	0.18 ± 0.03	0.96 ± 0.10	11.30 ± 1.04
APS	50	0.16 ± 0.03*	0.90 ± 0.07*	14.46 ± 1.17*

*$P < 0.05$, **$P < 0.01$ versus control group

Table 433.3 Effects of APS on the number and activity of CR1

Group	Dose (mg/kg)	MFI	DTER (%)	RBC-C3bRR (%)
Normal	–	17.10 ± 0.53**	36.51 ± 0.81**	20.1 ± 1.5**
Control	–	14.67 ± 0.31	17.38 ± 0.68	11.4 ± 0.5
APS	50	15.60 ± 0.67*	20.51 ± 1.21*	14.6 ± 0.9*

*$P < 0.05$, **$P < 0.01$ versus control group

433.4 Discussion

Cell membrane is framed by liquid lipid bilayer and mainly composed of phospholipids and cholesterol. Phospholipids array as bi-molecular layer and bond with protein by non-covalent bond, which constitute the main structure of the cell membrane. When the body is in a pathological state, the structure and function of cell membranes change, and the change of membrane lipid fluidity is obvious [2, 3]. The results showed Astragalus polysaccharides restored membrane structure and components, and improved membrane fluidity and function. It increased band 3 protein and glycophorin A content on erythrocyte membrane, increased phospholipids content and decreased cholesterol content, increased sialic acid content, adjusted membrane fluidity.

The erythrocyte complement receptor 1 (CR1, CD 35), or the C3b/C4b receptor is an important material basis for erythrocyte immunology. It has been shown that erythrocytes facilitate the phagocytosis of CIC by phagocytes through the adhesion of CR1 on their membrane, thus enhancing the capacity of the organism to eliminate CIC [4, 5]. Some drugs can help to enhance the immunity of the erythrocytes of patients mainly because they can increase the natural capacity of CR1 to adhere to tumor cells. The main mechanism is that the drugs can affect the structure and activity of CR1 either by directly increasing the activity and the number of CR1, or by strengthening the antigenicity of the tumor cells and activating the complements, or through the erythrocyte glycoprotein receptors adhering to glycoprotein immunity-enhancers and thus affecting membrane structure. The results showed Astragalus polysaccharides increased CR1 number, increased RBC-C3bRR and DTER, which indicated it could enhance the regulation of erythrocyte CR1 on immunological reaction.

In conclusion, Astragalus polysaccharides can effectively regulate red blood cell function and immune response, which may provide a scientific basis for the comprehensive developments and utilizations of Astragalus.

References

1. He WJ, Yuan ZJ, He XS (2012) Research progress on pharmacological effects of Astraglus polysaccharide. Chin J Biochem Pharm 33:692–694
2. Brad SK, James DH, James RS et al (2009) Changes in Band 3 oligomeric state precede cell membrane phospholipid loss during blood bank storage of red blood cells. Transfusion 49(7):1435–1442
3. Angel HH, Marina CR, Abel LR (2006) Alterations in erythrocyte membrane protein composition in advanced non-small cell lung cancer. Blood Cells Mol Dis 36:355–363
4. Liu D, Niu ZX (2009) The structure, genetic polymorphisms, expression and biological functions of complement receptor type 1 (CR1/CD35). Immunopharmacol Immunotoxicol 31:524–535
5. Seregin SS, Aldhamen YA, Appledorn DM (2009) CR1/2 is an important suppressor of Adenovirus-induced innate immune responses and is required for induction of neutralizing antibodies. Gene Ther 16:1245–1459

Chapter 434
Anti-Diabetes Components in Leaves of Yacon

Zheng Xiang, Chen-Feng Ji, De-Qiang Dou and Kuo Gai

Abstract The inhibitory effect of four new compounds (smallanthaditerpenic acids A–D) previously isolated from leaves of *Smallanthus sonchifolius* (yacon) on α-glucosidase were examined and their IC_{50} were determined to be 0.48, 0.59, 1.00, and 1.17 mg/mL respectively. In addition, a rapid, reliable HPLC method for the analysis of smallanthaditerpenic acids A and C in yacon leaves was established, and the variation in their contents in leaves from plants cultivated in different places and collected at different times of the year were compared. The established analytical method for determining smallanthaditerpenic acids A and C presented good results and could be used as a method for the quality control of *S. sonchifolius* leaves.

Keywords *Smallanthus sonchifolius* · Smallanthaditerpenic acid · Diabetes · HPLC

434.1 Introduction

Yacon, *Smallanthus sonchifolius* (Peoepp. & Endl.) H. Robinson (family Asteraceae), an indigenous plant of the Andes, was introduced into China via Japan in the early 1990s. It has been reported that its leaf extract has potential

Z. Xiang · C.-F. Ji · D.-Q. Dou (✉)
Engineering Research Center of Natural Anticancer Drugs, Ministry of Education, Harbin University of Commerce, Harbin 150076, China
e-mail: doudeqiang2003@yahoo.com.cn

Z. Xiang · C.-F. Ji · D.-Q. Dou
Center of Research on Life Science and Environmental Science, Harbin University of Commerce, Harbin 150076, China

D.-Q. Dou · K. Gai
College of Pharmacy, Liaoning University of Traditional Chinese Medicine, Dalian 116600, China

S. Li et al. (eds.), *Frontier and Future Development of Information Technology in Medicine and Education*, Lecture Notes in Electrical Engineering 269,
DOI: 10.1007/978-94-007-7618-0_434,

antidiabetic effects [1]. Chemical investigations of yacon have revealed that its leaves contain monoterpenes, sesquiterpenes and diterpenes, which have a physiological role in the pest-resistant and antimicrobial activities of the plant [2–4].

Previously, kaurene derivatives, pentacosaol, cannabiside D, platanionoside B, octadecatrienoic acid and smallanthaditerpenic acids A, B, C and D (Fig. 434.1) have been isolated from leaves of yacon cultivated in China [5–7]. In continuation of this work, we found that smallanthaditerpenic acids (SA) A, B, C and D possessed stronger inhibitory activity of α-glucosidase than that of caffeic acid, which had been regarded as the major component possessing this property [8]. An HPLC method has also been developed and validated for the quantification of SAs A and C in yacon and used to study the variation of these compounds in leaves collected from plants cultivated at different places and collected at different times of the year.

434.2 Results and Discussion

The inhibitory effect of SA A∼D on α-glucosidase was determined, which indicated that they possess strong inhibitory activity (Table 434.1). In this experiment, acarbose was used as the positive control. Its maximum inhibition ratio (70 %) was found at a concentration of 1.25 mg/mL, whereas the inhibitory effects of SA A, B, C and D were stronger (Table 434.1).

Because of this strong inhibitory activity of the SAs on α-glucosidase, a HPLC method for determination of their contents in yacon leaves was established. Separation conditions were optimized in order to achieve satisfactory resolution. Full details are presented in the Experimental section. Because of the low contents of SA B and D, only SA A and C were determined.

The HPLC method was validated as follows. The calibration curves (correlation coefficient) for SA A and C were $y = 2961.5x - 72.475$, ($r^2 = 0.9996$, n = 6, 0.01 − 0.2 mg/mL); $y = 2962.3x + 34.26$, ($r^2 = 0.9998$, n = 6, 0.05 − 1.0 mg/mL). The limits of quantification of SAs A and C were determined to be 0.02 and 0.04 μg, respectively. The limits of detection, defined as the lowest sample concentration, were 0.005 μg (SA A) and 0.01 μg (SA C), which were determined

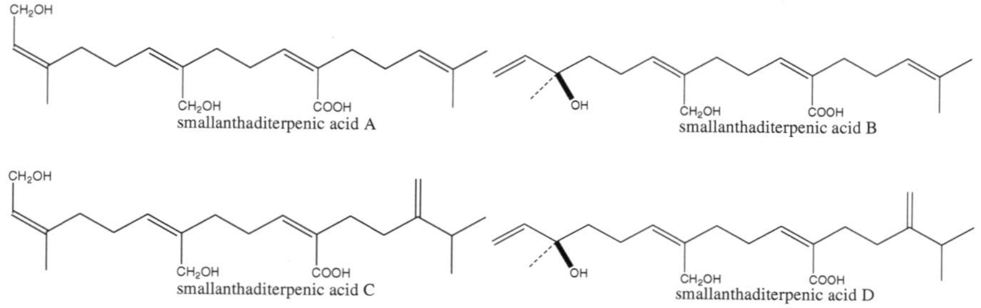

Fig. 434.1 Chemical structures of smallanthaditerpenic acids A–D

Table 434.1 Inhibitory activity of α-glucosidase of smallanthaditerpenic acids

Substance	IC_{50} (mg/mL)	IC_{50} (μM)
Smallanthaditerpenic acid A	0.48	1.43
Smallanthaditerpenic acid B	0.59	1.76
Smallanthaditerpenic acid C	1.00	2.86
Smallanthaditerpenic acid D	1.17	3.34

with a signal-to-noise ratio (S/N) of 3. The variation coefficients of SA A and C were 0.16 and 0.18 % for the intra-day assays.

The accuracy of the method was examined by performing recovery experiments according to the method of standard additions. SA A and C stock solutions were added before the extraction at different concentration levels to half of the analyzed amounts in yacon leaves (500 mg). Samples were prepared in triplicate at each level. Mean recoveries of SA A and C were 97.4 % (RSD % = 2.5), 99.6 % (RSD % = 1.7), respectively, which presented good accuracy for the analysis.

The SA A and C contents of yacon leaf extracts from plants cultivated at different places were evaluated by HPLC (Table 434.2). The leaves collected from Anshan (China) had the highest content of SAs A and C, whereas the leaves from Japan had the lowest content of SAs A and C. The leaves obtained from these various places were not collected at the same time of the year, and it seemed that there was no regularity in the content changes of the evaluated compounds in yacon leaves based on these different places of collection. Therefore, yacon leaves were collected at different times of the year from Yunnan, a main production area of yacon in China, to compare the content changes of SAs A and C. The results (Table 434.3) indicated that the younger leaves had the highest contents of SA A and SA C; these decreased with increases in growing time.

Table 434.2 Content of smallanthaditerpenic acids in yacon leaves cultivated at different places (Mean±SD, μg/g)

Sample productions	SA A	SA C
1 Anshan (China)	382.6 ± 3.2	519.3 ± 4.9
2 Dalian (China)	65.1 ± 0.6	304.7 ± 3.0
3 Yunnan (China)	129.3 + 1.2	386.3 ± 3.8
4 Japan	46.3 + 0.57	139.0 ± 1.4
5 Japan	46.0 + 0.54	138.5 ± 1.5
6 Korea	89.3 ± 1.16	224.4 ± 2.6
7 Peru	46.9 ± 0.52	266.0 ± 2.7
8 Peru	47.3 ± 0.51	265.9 ± 2.8

Table 434.3 Content of smallanthaditerpenic acids A, C in yacon leaves from Yunnan at different harvest times (Mean±SD, μg/g)

Harvest times	SA A	SA C
25th, June	129.3 ± 1.3	386.9 ± 3.9
25th, July	142.6 ± 1.5	292.9 ± 3.0
25th, August	100.1 ± 1.0	307.0 ± 3.0
25th, September	88.6 ± 0.79	220.4 ± 2.1
25th, October	60.5 ± 0.65	258.6 ± 2.7
25th, November	52.6 ± 0.61	230.6 ± 2.5

434.3 Experimental

Plant material S. sonchifolius leaves were collected from Dalian, Anshan, and Yunnan (China). The leaves cultivated in Korea were purchased by Professor Young-Ho Kim in Korea, and those from Japan and Peru were obtained from its tea products. The leaves were identified by Professor Kang Tingguo, University of Traditional Chinese Medicine. A voucher specimen (No. 20081205) has been deposited at the Pharmacognosy Laboratory, Liaoning University of TCM.

Chemicals α-Glucosidase (EC 3.2.1.20) and PNPG (4-nitrophenol-α-D-glucopyranoside, CAS: 3767-28-0) were purchased from Sigma-Aldrich (New Jersey, USA). Reduced glutathione was obtained from Xinjingke Chemical Co. (Beijing, China). Acarbose was purchased from Bayer Healthcare Company Ltd. Organic solvents for HPLC analyses were purchased from Kermel Chemical Co. (Tianjin, China) and filtered through 0.45 μm organic membranes prior to use. Water was purified using Mill-Q-plus filter systems (Millipore, Bedford, MA, USA). SAs A, B, C and D were isolated and identified in our laboratory from *S. sonchifolius*. All other reagents were of either analytical or HPLC grade.

Inhibitory activity of α-glucosidase Smallanthaditerpenic acids A, B, C and D were dissolved in DMSO, and the final concentrations of the stock solutions were 75.03, 83.16, 167.32, and 199.83 mg/mL, respectively. Inhibitory activities of all fractions were monitored according to the reported method [9]. Reduced glutathione solution (25 mL containing 1 mg/mL), 35 μL α-glucosidase solution (0.8U/mL), 10 μL smallanthaditerpenic acid standard solution and 860 μL potassium phosphate buffer (67 mmol/L, pH 6.8) were added to the tubes, which were then incubated at 37 °C for 10 min. PNPG (70 μL of a 50 mmol/L solution) was added as substrate and incubated at 37 °C. After 20 min, 5 mL Na_2CO_3 solution (0.1 mol/L) was added to stop the reaction. Absorbance was measured at 400 nm by a UV–vis spectrophotometer (UV-2100, Unique Co. China) at room temp. All SAs were dissolved in DMSO, which had no inhibitory activity on α-glucosidase at a concentration of 1 % (v/v).

Preparation of standard solutions for HPLC analysis SAs A, C, caffeic acid and chlorogenic acid were dissolved in methanol to produce stock solutions containing 73.36, 167.0, 96.25, and 101.0 μg/mL, respectively.

Preparation of samples for smallanthaditerpenic acids content analysis Dry, powdered yacon leaves (approx.1 g, accurately weighed) were extracted by refluxing with a mixture of KOH (0.5 g) and 70 % EtOH (50 mL) for 2 h, twice. The mixture was diluted with water (100 mL) and filtered. The filtrate was extracted thoroughly with 3 × 100 mL of light petroleum. The aqueous phase was then acidified with dilute HCl (pH = 4) and extracted with 3 × 100 mL of light petroleum. The light petroleum extract was dried over anhydrous magnesium sulfate. After filtration, the remaining solvent was evaporated to dryness using a rotary evaporator, the residue dissolved in methanol, and made up to 5 mL in a volumetric flask with methanol. The sample solution was filtered through 0.45 μm organic membranes prior to use.

HPLC Determination was achieved using analytical HPLC with an Agilent 1100 series HPLC system with pump (Agilent model G1314A VWD), and an Agilent reverse-phase Eclipse XDB-C_{18} column (4.6 × 150 mm, 5 μm particle size) protected by a pre-column from the same company, and thermostated at 30 °C.

References

1. Aybar MJ, Sanchez RAN, Grau A et al (2001) Hypoglycemic effect of the water extract of *Smallanthus sonchifolius* (yacon) leaves in normal and diabetic rats. J Ethnopharmacol 74:125–132
2. Kakuta H, Seki T, Hashidoko Y et al (1992) Ent-kaurenoic acid and its related compounds from glandular trichome exudate and leaf extract of *Polymnia sonchifolia*. Biosci Biotechnol Biochem 56:1562–1564
3. Lin F, Hasegawa M, Kodama O (2003) Purification and identification of antimicrobial sesquiterpene lactones from yacon (*Smallanthus sonchifolius*) leaves. Biosci Biotechnol Biochem 67:2154–2159
4. Consolacion Y, Ragasa AB, Alimboyoguen SU et al (2008) A bioactive diterpene from *Smallanthus sonchifolius*. Nat Prod Commun 3:1663–1666
5. Qiu YK, Kang TG, Dou DQ (2008) Three novel compounds from the leaves of *Smallanthus sonchifolius*. J Asian Nat Prod Res 10:1109–1115
6. Xiang Z, Gai K, Dou DQ et al (2009) New compounds from the leaves of *Smallanthus sonchifolius*. Nat Prod Commun 4:1201–1204
7. Dou DQ, Tian F, Qiu YK (2008) Structure elucidation and complete NMR spectral assignments of four new diterpenoids from *Smallanthus sonchifolius*. Magn Reson Chem 46:775–779
8. Sumio T, Kikuo I, Akira Y (2006) The constituents relate to anti-oxidative and α-glucosidase inhibitory activities in Yacon aerial part extract. Yakugaku Zasshi 126:665–669
9. Xiang Z, Dou DQ (2009) Effects of arctigenin on α-glucosidase activity. Zhong Guo Xian Dai Zhong Yao 11:28–29

Chapter 435
Nitric Oxide Donor Regulated mRNA Expressions of LTC4 Synthesis Enzymes in Hepatic Ischemia Reperfusion Injury Rats

FF Hong, CS He, GL Tu, FX Guo, XB Chen and SL Yang

Abstract Cysteinyl LTs were associated with hepatic ischemia and reperfusion (I/R) injury. LTC4 synthesis enzymes including leukotriene C4 synthase (LTC_4S), microsomal glutathione S-transferase (mGST) 2 and mGST3 can all conjugate LTA4 and reduced glutathione (GSH) to form LTC4, which involved hepatic ischemia–reperfusion (I/R) injury. This experiment was designed to further investigate the effects of V-PYRRO/NO (a selective liver nitric oxide donor)on the gene expressions of LTC4 synthesis enzymes during hepatic I/R. Adult male SD rats were divided into 3 groups: sham group (Control), I/R group and V-PYRRO/NO + I/R groups. Liver subjected to 1 h of partial hepatic ischemia followed by 5 h of reperfusion, saline or V-PYRRO/NO (1.06 μmol/kg/h) was administered intravenously through all the experimental periods. The mRNA levels of LTC4 synthesis enzymes in rat liver tissue were examined by RT-PCR. We observed that hepatic mRNA expressions of LTC4S and mGST3 were lower whereas mGST2 mRNA levels were higher in V-PYRRO/NO +I/R group than those in I/R group. Compared with control, only mGST3 mRNA was significantly declined in V-PYRRO/NO +I/R groups. These results suggest that NO donor V-PYRRO/NO can downregulate the mRNA expressions of LTC_4S and mGST3 but upregulate mGST2 mRNA expressions during hepatic I/R injury.

Keywords NO donor · Microsomal glutathione S-transferase · Ischemia reperfusion injury · Liver

F. Hong · F. Guo · X. Chen · S. Yang (✉)
Department of Physiology, College of Medicine, Nanchang University, Nanchang 330031, China
e-mail: yangshulong@yahoo.cn

F. Hong · G. Tu
Department of Experimental Teaching, Nanchang University, Nanchang 330031, China

C. He
Health Supervision Station of Jinggangshan, Jinggangshan 343600 Jiangxi, China

S. Li et al. (eds.), *Frontier and Future Development of Information Technology in Medicine and Education*, Lecture Notes in Electrical Engineering 269,
DOI: 10.1007/978-94-007-7618-0_435,

435.1 Introduction

Hepatic injury secondary to warm ischemia and reperfusion (I/R) is an important clinical issue. It has been implicated in the pathogenesis of a variety of clinical conditions including trauma, thermal injury, hypovolemic and endotoxin shock, reconstructive vascular surgery, liver transplantation, and liver resectional surgery. Hepatic I/R injuries occur during transplantation, liver resection for tumor, and circulatory shock [1].

The cysteinyl leukotriene (LT)s mediate a wide variety of biologic responses including enhanced vascular permeability, smooth muscle contraction, mucus hypersecretion, bronchial hyperreactivity [2]. Our previous studies showed cysteinyl LTs were associated with hepatic I/R injury [1, 3–5]. It is known that LTC4 synthesis enzymes including leukotriene C4 synthase (LTC_4S), microsomal glutathione S-transferase (mGST) 2 and mGST3 can conjugate LTA4 and reduced glutathione to form LTC4, which is the first committed synthesis step of the cysteiny LTs, LTC4, LTD4, and LTE4 [3–5].

Nowadays the relationship between Cysteinyl LTs and NO has been shown [3, 6–8]. Larfars et al. first demonstrated that the cysteinyl LTs LTC4 and LTD4, as well as LTB4, activate NO release from human PMN by surface receptor, G-protein and [Ca2 +]i-dependent mechanisms [6].The addition of NO via the infusion of sodium nitroprusside (SNP,0.05 mM, 1 mM) reduced the effect of leukotriene D4 on portal flow, bile flow and bile acid secretion whereas the leukotriene D4 effects on hepatic glucose output remained unaffected. Correlation coefficient between decrease in portal flow and reduction of bile flow by infusing leukotriene D4 was higher than that while in the presence of SNP [7].LTB4 decreased hepatocyte NO synthesis in a concentration-dependent manner when the cells were stimulated with a combination of cytokines or IL-1 alone [8].Reduced synthesis of NO_{2-} was associated with reduced iNOS mRNA levels suggesting that the induction of iNOS was inhibited. These findings demonstrate that eicosanoids can regulate hepatocyte NO synthesis in vitro. In addition, our recent reports have indicated that NO donor, sodium nitroprusside (SNP) regulated LTC4 generation during rat liver I/R injury. But, up to now, the effects of the selective liver nitric oxide donor, V-PYRRO/NO, on the mRNA expressions of LTC4 synthesis enzymes during hepatic I/R in rats have not been fully clear. Thus, the present experiment was explored to further explore whether V-PYRRO/NO, a selective liver nitric oxide donor can influence the mRNA expressions of LTC4 synthesis enzymes during hepatic I/R in rats.

435.2 Materials and Methods

435.2.1 Materials

Male Sprague–Dawley rats, weight 230–250 g, were obtained from the Experimental animal Center, Nanchang University (Nanchang, China). V-PYR-RO/NO was purchased from Cayman Chemical (Michigan, USA). TRIzol Reagent and MmuLV reverse transcriptase were from GIBCO BRL (Gaithersburg, MD), reduced glutathione and *Taq* DNA polymerase were from Sangon (Shanghai, China). cDNA probes for rat mGST2, mGST3, LTC4S were synthesized by Sangon (Shanghai, China). All other chemicals were of the highest purity commercially available.

435.2.2 Animal Model of Hepatic Ischemia and Reperfusion Injury

The rats were housed and treated in accordance with the Guidelines for the Care and Use of the Experimental Animals Center of Nanchang University (Nanchang, China). The study was approved by the local animal ethics committee. Animals were fasted for 12 h but allowed to drink water prior to the operation and randomized into five groups: I/R group, animals were anesthetized with pentobarbital 50 mg/kg intraperitoneally, the external jugular vein catheter was created using a polyethylene tube of 0.9 mm inner diameter (Becton–Dickinson Medical Devices, Suzhou, China) and subjected to midline laparotomy, the liver was exposed, and the left lateral and median lobes were rendered ischemic by clamping the hepatic arterial and portal venous blood supply using a microaneurysm clamp. Following 60 min of hepatic ischemia (or sham), livers were reperfused for 5 h by removing the clamp and the peritoneal cavity was sutured closed for 5 h. Saline solution (3 mL/Kg/min) was intravenously injected by external jugular vein at 15 min before the start of ischemia through 5 h reperfusion. Sham group (Control), surgeries were performed on anesthetized rat in which hepatic blood flow was not occluded. V-PYRRO/NO (1.06μmol/kg/h) + I/R groups, surgeries were performed on anesthetized rat as I/R group, and V-PYRRO/NO (1.06μmol/kg/h) was intravenously injected by external jugular vein at 15 min before the start of ischemia through 5 h reperfusion respectively. Following 5 h of reperfusion, Serum was collected from each animal for NO2- determinations, livers were removed, medium lobe fixed in 10 % Formalin for immunohistochemistry, left lobule snap frozen in liquid nitrogen and then stored at −80 °C for RNA determinations and western blotting analysis.

435.2.3 Reverse Transcriptase Polymerase Chain Reaction

The mRNA expressions of mGST2,mGST3 and LTC4S were performed as described in our previous report [3–5]. Briefly, total RNA was isolated from whole liver tissue using TRIzol Reagent according to the manufacturer's instructions and quantified by measurement of ultraviolet absorption at 260 nm. 1 μg of total RNA from each sample was reverse-transcribed to synthesize the single-stranded cDNA using an antisense specific primer and 200 units of MmuLV reverse transcriptase (Gibco BRL). Sequences of PCR primers for rat β-actin, mGST2,mGST3 and LTC4S were derived from published sequences [3, 5] (see Table 435.1). Aliquots of the synthesized cDNA (1.5 μl) were amplified with proper cycle using each primer and 1.5 U of *Taq* DNA polymerase in a Mastercycler gradient (Eppendorf, Germany). The reactants were cycled at 95 °C for 45 s, 55.8 °C/58 °C for 45 s, and 72 °C for 45 s. The PCR products were separated by electrophoresis using 1.5 % ethidium bromide-stained agarose gel and visualized by ultraviolet trans-illumination. The intensity of each band was measured by a Bio-Imaging Analyzer (Bio-Rad) and quantified using Quantity One version 4.2.2 software (Bio-Rad). Using amplification of β-actin as a control, the degree of expression of the mRNA of these products was compared.

435.2.4 Statistical Analysis

Data are expressed as means ± S.D. Kruskal–Wallis test was used to compare the three groups. The Student t test was used for the comparison of two groups. $P < 0.05$ was considered to be significant.

Table 435.1 Oligonucleotide primer used for the analysis of LTC4-S, mGST2, mGST3 and β-ACTIN genes by RT-PCR

Genes	Sense and antisense	PCR product (bp)	PCR cycles	Annealing temperature (°C)
LTC4-S	5′-CGAGTACTTTCCGCTGTTC-3′ 5′-TAGTGTGCCAGGGAGGAAG-3′	237	35	55.8
mGST2	5′-TGCAGTCTCCCTTCTGTGTG-3′ 5′-CAGGAATCTGCTTGCTACCC-3′	367	30	58
mGST3	5′-GGAATATGGATTCGTGCTTCTC-3′ 5′-GGGTACACCTCCAATGTGTTCT-3′	189	30	58
β-actin	5′-TGACGGGGTCACCCACACTGTGCCCATCTA-3′ 5′-CTAGAAGCATTTGCGGTGGACGATGGAGGG-3′	660	25	58

435.3 Results

435.3.1 RT-PCR Analysis of Hepatic mRNA Expression of LTC4 Synthesis Enzymes (LTC4S, mGST2 and mGST3) in Control, I/R and V-PYRRO/NO + I/R Groups Rats

A representative of hepatic mRNA expressions of LTC4S, mGST2 and mGST3 was shown in Fig. 435.1a, b displayed densitometric analysis of PCR products of LTC4 synthesis enzymes in the control, I/R and V-PYRRO/NO (1.06 μmol/kg/h) + I/R groups rats. Compared with I/R group, the mRNA expression of LTC4S in liver tissue was significantly decreased after 5 h reperfusion in V-PYRRO/NO (1.06 μmol/kg/h) + I/R groups ($P < 0.05$). However, V-PYRRO/NO (1.06 μmol/kg/h) increased mGST2 mRNA but decreased mGST3 mRNA level when compared to I/R group ($P < 0.05$). Compared with control, mGST3 mRNA was significantly decreased and no change of mGST2 mRNA presented in V-PYRRO/NO (1.06 μmol/kg/h) + I/R groups ($P > 0.05$).

435.4 Discussion

LTs are ubiquitous mediators of a wide variety of physiologic and immunologic effects in liver function and disease [9–11]. A growing body of evidences implicates LTs in the pathogenesis of the hepatic I/R injury [12–14]. The committed step in cysteinyl LTs (LTC4, LTD4 and LTE4) biosynthesis is catalyzed by LTC4S, mGST2 and mGST3 [15, 16]. LPS was shown to down-regulate cysteinyl LT release and LTC4 synthase gene expression in mononuclear phagocytes by an NF-κB-mediated mechanism [17]. Research over the past 20 years has identified endogenous NO as a key messenger molecule in the cardiovascular, nervous and immune systems [18]. The relationship between Cysteinyl LTs and NO has been shown [6–8].Here we used a rat model of hepatic ischemia 60 min and 5 h reperfusion to prove whether the selective liver nitric oxide donor V-PYRRO/NO could regulate the gene expression of LTC4 synthesis enzymes in I/R injury rats.

Previous study demonstrated that LTC4S mRNA was detected in whole liver, hepatocytes, and sinusoidal endothelial cells, but not in Kupffer cells [19]. There were no significant changes in the mRNA expression of LTC4-S in liver tissues during I/R injury in rats [13]. We have recently indicated that SNP regulated the mRNA expressions of LTC4 synthesis enzymes during hepatic I/R injury [5]. In this study we further found that just like SNP, V-PYRRO/NO (1.06 μmol/kg/h) reversed completely up-regulation of LTC4S gene expression in hepatic I/R rats. However, V-PYRRO/NO upregulated mGST2 mRNA levels but down-regulated mGST3 mRNA levels during hepatic I/R injury in rats. Even compared with

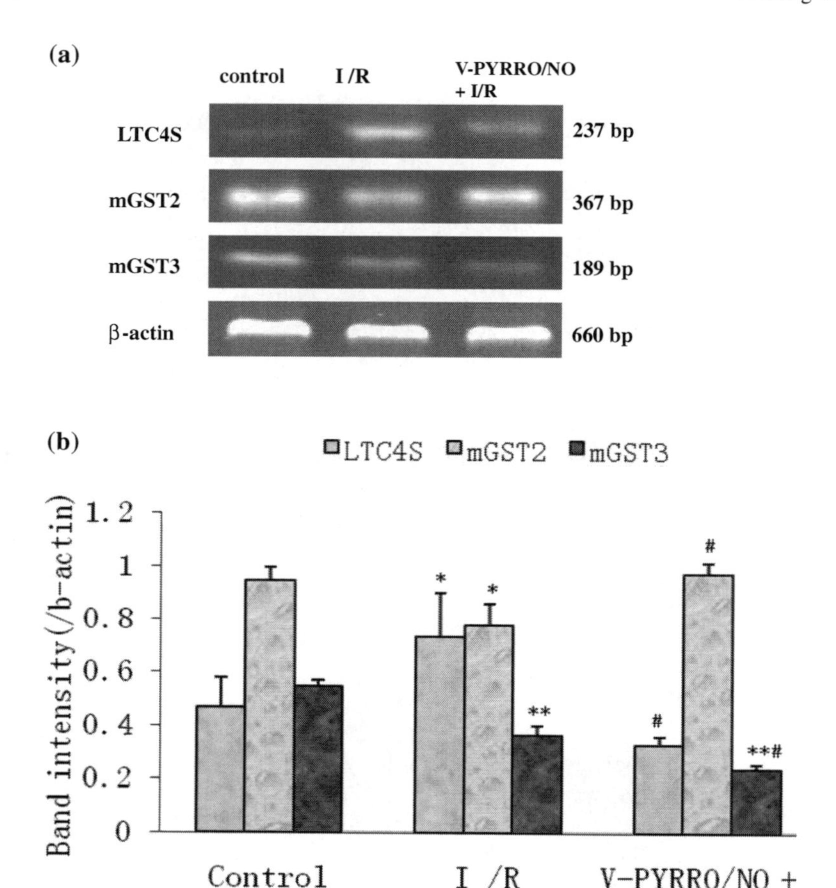

Fig. 435.1 Hepatic mRNA expression of LTC_4S, mGST2 and mGST3 in the control, I/R and V-PYRRO/NO (1.06 μmol/kg/h) +I/R groups rats. **a** A representative of hepatic mRNA expression of LTC_4S, mGST2 and mGST3 in the control, I/R and V-PYRRO/NO (1.06 μmol/kg/h) + I/R groups rats. Single-stranded cDNA synthesized from total RNA (1 μg) was used for PCR amplification with specific primers with optimal cycles for LTC_4S, mGST2, mGST3 and β-Actin. The PCR products were electrophoresed on 1.5 % agarose gel. **b** Densitometric analysis of PCR products of LTC_4S, mGST2 and mGST3 in the control, I/R and V-PYRRO/NO (1.06 μmol/kg/h) + I/R groups rats. The intensity of each band was normalized to that of the corresponding band of β-Actin and calculated as the ratio to the value in the control. Values represent the mean ± S.D ($n = 3$). Compared with Control, *Indicates $P < 0.05$, ** Indicates $P < 0.01$; Compared with I/R, # Indicates $P < 0.05$

control, V-PYRRO/NO (1.06 μmol/kg/h) also down-regulated mGST3 mRNA but didn't affect the mGST2 mRNA expressions. Thus, V-PYRRO/NO, the selective liver nitric oxide donor appeared to be a dual influence on the regulation of the mRNA expressions of mGST2 and mGST3.

435.5 Conclusions

Our findings demonstrate that a selective liver nitric oxide donor V-PYRRO/NO down-regulated the mRNA expression of LTC_4S, but appeared to be a dual influences on the regulation of the mRNA expressions of mGST2 and mGST3.

Acknowledgments This work was supported by National Natural Science Foundation of China (No. 81260504) and Educational Commission of Jiangxi Province of China (No. GJJ12073) and Health Department of Jiangxi Province of China (No. 20123175, 2012A131 and 20132018).

References

1. Hong FF, Yang SL (2012) Ischemic preconditioning decreased leukotriene C4 formation by depressing leukotriene C4 synthase expression and activity during hepatic I/R injury in rats. J Surg Res 178(2):1015–1021
2. Samuelsson B et al (1987) Leukotrienes and lipoxins: structures, biosynthesis, and biological effects. Science 237(4819):1171–1176
3. Yang SL, Lou YJ (2007) Sodium nitroprusside decreased leukotriene C4 generation by inhibiting leukotriene C4 synthase expression and activity in hepatic ischemia-reperfusion injured rats. Biochem Pharmacol 73(5):724–735
4. Yang SL et al (2007) Increased leukotriene c4 synthesis accompanied enhanced leukotriene c4 synthase expression and activities of ischemia-reperfusion-injured liver in rats. J Surg Res 140(1):36–44
5. Yang SL et al (2007) Sodium nitroprusside regulates mRNA expressions of LTC4 synthesis enzymes in hepatic ischemia/reperfusion injury rats via NF-kappaB signaling pathway. Pharmacology 80(1):11–20
6. Larfars G, Lantoine F, Devynck MA, Palmblad J, Gyllenhammar H (1999) Activation of nitric oxide release and oxidative metabolism by leukotrienes B4, C4, and D4 in human polymorphonuclear leukocytes. Blood 93(4):1399–1405
7. Beckh K et al (1997) Effects of nitric oxide on leukotriene D4 decreased bile secretion in the perfused rat liver. Life Sci 61(19):1947–1952
8. Harbrecht BG et al (1996) PGE2 and LTB4 inhibit cytokine-stimulated nitric oxide synthase type 2 expression in isolated rat hepatocytes. Prostaglandins 52(2):103–116
9. Sjolinder M et al (2000) Aberrant expression of active leukotriene C(4) synthase in CD16(+) neutrophils from patients with chronic myeloid leukemia. Blood 95(4):1456–1464
10. Gonzalez J et al (1992) Leukotriene C4 detection as an early graft function marker in liver transplantation. Transplant Proc 24(1):135–136
11. Gonzalez J et al (1992) Role of leukotrienes B4 and C4 in liver allograft rejection. Transpl Int 5(Suppl 1):S659–S660
12. Wettstein M, Haussinger D (1994) Effect of hypoxia on nitric oxide formation and leukotriene metabolism in the perfused rat liver. Zentralbl Chir 119(5):328–333
13. Takamatsu Y et al (2004) Role of leukotrienes on hepatic ischemia/reperfusion injury in rats. J Surg Res 119(1):14–20
14. Okboy N et al (1992) The effect of iloprost and NDGA in ischemia reperfusion injury in rat liver. Prostaglandins Leukot Essent Fatty Acids 47(4):291–295
15. Jakobsson PJ, Mancini JA, Ford-Hutchinson AW (1996) Identification and characterization of a novel human microsomal glutathione S-transferase with leukotriene C4 synthase activity and significant sequence identity to 5-lipoxygenase-activating protein and leukotriene C4 synthase. J Biol Chem 271(36):22203–22210

16. Jakobsson PJ et al (1997) Identification and characterization of a novel microsomal enzyme with glutathione-dependent transferase and peroxidase activities. J Biol Chem 272(36):22934–22939
17. Serio KJ et al (2003) Lipopolysaccharide down-regulates the leukotriene C4 synthase gene in the monocyte-like cell line, THP-1. J Immunol 170(4):2121–2128
18. Megson LL (2000) Nitric oxide donor drugs. Drugs Future 25:701–715
19. Shimada K et al (1998) Expression and regulation of leukotriene-synthesis enzymes in rat liver cells. Hepatology 28(5):1275–1281

Chapter 436
An Optimal In Vitro Model for Evaluating Anaphylactoid Mediator Release Induced by Herbal Medicine Injection

Zheng Xiang, Chen-Feng Ji, De-Qiang Dou and Hang Xiao

Abstract The Xue-Sai-Tong injection, a traditional Chinese medicine injection with total saponins extracted from Sanqi Ginseng, was used to treat coronary artery disease. Adverse drug reaction of the injection occurred frequently in recent years. This study was to establish an in vitro model for assaying the mediator release from the degranulation of mast cell and RBL-2H3 cells stimulated by herbal medicine injection. Mediators released from mast cells and RBL-2H3 cells caused by Xue-Sai-Tong injections were assayed by the method of fluorospectrophotometry, ELISA and spectrophotometry respectively. It revealed that histamine release induced by XST injection could not be assayed accurately by the method of fluorospectrophotometry owing to the existence of saponin and unknown components in the injection. Rat peritoneal mast cells was also not an optimal cell model for determining histamine and β-hexosaminidase release due to the higher spontaneous release rate of allergic mediator. So, ELISA could be the suitable method to evaluate the histamine release from RBL-2H3 cells, and this method could also be utilized in evaluating degranulation of herbal medicine injection.

Keywords RBL-2H3 · Degranulation · Saponin · Herbal medicine injection

Z. Xiang · C.-F. Ji · D.-Q. Dou
Engineering Research Center of Natural Anticancer Drugs, Ministry of Education, Harbin University of Commerce, Harbin 150076, China

Z. Xiang · C.-F. Ji · D.-Q. Dou
Center of Research on Life Science and Environmental Science, Harbin University of Commerce, Harbin 150076, China

D.-Q. Dou (✉) · H. Xiao
College of Pharmacy, Liaoning University of Traditional Chinese Medicine, Dalian 116600, China
e-mail: doudeqiang2003@yahoo.com.cn

S. Li et al. (eds.), *Frontier and Future Development of Information Technology in Medicine and Education*, Lecture Notes in Electrical Engineering 269,
DOI: 10.1007/978-94-007-7618-0_436,

436.1 Introduction

Herbal medicine injections are widely used in China and other countries. The complicated ingredients are the outstanding characteristic of the injections, which make their quality difficult to be controlled. Thus adverse drug reactions (ADRs) of herbal injections occurred frequently [1, 2]. In recent years, more and more reports indicated that the ADRs of herbal injections are serious and China's SFDA had noticed to stop the production of 7 kinds of herbal injections in 2006.

Sanqi ginseng, the roots of *Panax notoginseng* (Burk.) F. H. Chen, is an important ancient herbal medicine widely used for more than two thousands years to treat atherosclerosis and cerebral infarction [3]. Sanqi ginsenosides with the purity of over 80 % are the active components of Xue-Sai-Tong (XST) injections generally used as anti-coronary medicine [4–7]. Clinically XST injection was reported to possess acute anaphylactic and hemolytic ADR. Hemolysis is one of saponins' properties and can lead to hemolytic ADR of injections. Prediagnostic methods for the hemolysis of injections containing saponins were established by authors in the previous research [8]. Anaphylactoid reaction is another major ADR of herbal injections. Histamine and β-hexosaminidase are the main mediator in mast cell and granulocyte released by the direct stimulate of the drug at high concentration [9].

Mast cells play a crucial role in the development of anaphylaxis, but degranulation research of mast cell is often hampered by difficulties originating from the isolation and primary culture of cells [10–12]. So, the continuous cell line of rat basophilic leukemia, RBL-2H3, was considered a useful tool to take the place of mast cell for in vitro work, as a great number of cells can be obtained rapidly.

In a continuing study, an optimal in vitro model for evaluating anaphylactoid reaction of Xue-Sai-Tong injection was established for the first time.

436.2 Materials and Methods

436.2.1 Chemicals and Reagent

RBL-2H3 cells were from the American Type Culture Collection. Fetal bovine serum was purchased from GIBCO Invitrogen. Histamine assay kit was purchase from IBL International GMBH. Histamine phosphate was purchased from the National Institute for the Control of Pharmaceutical and Biological Products. Compound 48/80, 4-nitrophenyl N-acetyl-β-D-glucosaminide, *O*-phthalaldehyde (OPT), percoll solution, trypan and toluidine were purchased from Sigma-Aldrich, Co., Xue-Sai-Tong injection was purchased from Kunming Pharmaceutical CO., LTD. (09LJ12). All other chemical reagents were purchased from Kermel Chemical Co.. Multimode microplate reader was purchased from Tecan Group Ltd..

436.2.2 Cell Culture

RBL-2H3 cells were cultured in DMEM supplemented with 10 % fetal bovine serum and 100 U ml^{-1} penicillinstreptomycin at 5 % CO_2 and 37 °C. Cells were subcultured using trypsin when reaching 80 % confluency.

436.2.3 Histamine and *β*-hexosaminidase assays of RBL-2H3 cells

100 μL of RBL-2H3 cell suspension were plated at 5 × 10^5 cells/mL in 96-well plates for 24 h. Then, the medium was removed and washed twice with PBS. 200 μL XST injection or compound 48/80 (positive drug) solutions of different concentrations were incubated at 37 °C for 30 min with the cells in wells, then the contents of histamine and *β*-hexosaminidase in the supernatant were determined.

The histamine release assay of RBL-2H3 induced by sample solutions were assayed either using a histamine ELISA kit or by using a reported fluorometric assay. To 50 μL of supernatant from each well or histamine phosphate standard solution (in 0.1 N HCl), 50 μL of 0.4 N NaOH and 10 μL of 0.1 % OPT were added. The supernatant was then incubated at room temperature for 10 min. The reaction was stopped by addition of 50 μL of 0.1 N HCl. The concentration of the fluorescent product of the reaction was measured using a fluorescence microplate reader set at: $\lambda_{ex} = 349$ nm and $\lambda_{em} = 448$ nm, respectively. 100 % release of histamine in the cell was caused by Triton X-100 (0.1 %, v/v). The release rate was determined as follows: Release rate (%) = $(C_{eg}-C_{nc})/(C_{100\ \%}-C_{nc})$, where C_{eg} and C_{nc} represent the content of experimental group and negative control group, respectively.

β-Hexosaminidase release assay was obtained as the published method [13]. 50 μL of supernatant was added into a 96-well plate which contained 50 μL of substrate (4-nitrophenyl N-acetyl-*β*-D-glucosaminide, 1 M) and incubated for 1.5 h at 37 °C. The reaction was stopped by adding 200 μL Na_2CO_3–$NaHCO_3$ buffer (1 M) to each well and the formed *p*-nitrophenolate was measured spectrophotometrically at a wavelength of 405 nm. The release rate was determined as follows: Release rate (%) = $(OD_{eg}-OD_{nc})/(OD_{100\ \%}-OD_{nc})$, where OD_{eg} and OD_{nc} represent the absorbance of experimental group and negative control group, respectively.

436.2.4 Histamine and β-hexosaminidase Assays of Rat Peritoneal Mast Cells

Rat peritoneal mast cells (RPMC) were obtained as the reported method [13] with minor modification. Male Wistar rats (200–300 g) were killed in atmosphere saturated with CO_2. 15 ml BSS was injected i.p. and the abdomen was gently massaged for 2 min. The crude cell suspension was aspirated following a midline incision and centrifuged for 5 min (4 °C, 1000 rpm). Cells were washed three times with BSS. The crude cells were purified using a percoll/BSS density gradient. After centrifugation for 15 min (4 °C, 2500 rpm), RPMC whose viability and purity were more than 95 % were separated and resuspended in BSS (5×10^5 cells/mL).

100 μL of RPMC were added into tubes containing 200 μL of sample solution with different concentrations. The test tube were centrifuged for 10 min (4 °C,1000 rpm) after incubated at 37 °C for 30 min. Then, 50 μL of the supernatant was used to assay the release rate of histamine and β-hexosaminidase by the method of ELISA and spectrophotometry above, respectively.

436.3 Results and Discussion

436.3.1 Histamine Analysis of RBL-2H3 Cells by Fluorospectrophotometry

The wavelength of excitation and emission of histamine were determined to be 349 nm and 448 nm by fluorescence microplate reader respectively. Standard curve of histamine was constructed, and the equation as follows: $y = 0.3812x + 7.4503$ ($R^2 = 0.9999$), in which x is the fluorescence intensity and y is the concentration of histamine. Histamine release of RBL-2H3 cells stimulated by sample solutions was determined as above method. The results indicated that fluorescence intensity of histamine in the experimental group raised as the sample solutions' concentrations increased, but the intensity was almost the same with that of the sample solution itself (Blank group). One reason for this phenomenon could be the interference of unknown components in the injection and another probably reason was the hydroxyls in the saponin molecules which could induce aldol condensation with OPT. So, fluorospectrophotometry is not a suitable method to assay the histamine release of cells stimulated by XST injection.

436.3.2 Histamine and β-hexosaminidase Assays

The results of degranulation of RPMC indicated that the RPMC could be direct stimulated by compound 48/80 (1000 μ/mL) to release allergic mediators (histamine and β-hexosaminidase), and the release rates of histamine and β-hexosaminidase were 96.2 ± 4.4 and 82.3 ± 6.9 %, respectively. But, there were no differences in release rate of allergic mediators between the negative control group and experimental group. So, RPMC was also not an optimal cell model for evaluating the sensibilization of herbal medicine injection or other drugs with degranulation slightly due to its obvious spontaneous release rate of histamine and β-hexosaminidase.

In order to find a sensitive indicator to appreciate the degranulation of RBL-2H3 cells by herbal medicine injection, histamine and β-hexosaminidase release from the cells were assay by the method of ELISA and spectrophotometry as above at the same time, respectively. Mediators release from RBL-2H3 cells stimulated by Xue-Sai-Tong injection and compound 48/80 were evaluated. It showed a similar tendency that the rate of histamine release was higher than that of β-hexosaminidase release stimulated by the injection or compound 48/80 at the same concentration. It was deemed that histamine was more sensitive than β-hexosaminidase in evaluating degranulation of RBL-2H3 cells.

In this study, degranulation of RBL-2H3 and RPMC stimulated by XST injection were assayed in vitro. Histamine is more sensitive than β-hexosaminidase in evaluating the degranulation of cells. ELISA was the suitable method to assay the histamine release from RBL-2H3 cells. An optimal model for evaluating anaphylactoid reaction of XST injection was established. This model could also be utilized in evaluating degranulation of herbal medicine injection.

References

1. Xu XH (2006) Severe adverse effects of Puerarin injection in 18 cases. Shanghai J TCM 40:71–72
2. Yi D, He Y, Zhou YL (2009) Analysis of 26 adverse drug reactions cases of Ginkgo leaf injection. Chin J Pharm 6:411–414
3. Wang N, Wan JB, Li MY et al (2008) Advances in studies on *Panax notoginseng* against atherosclerosis. Zhong Cao Yao 5:787–791
4. Dou DQ, Zhang YW, Zhang L et al (2001) The inhibitory effects of ginsenosides on protein tyrosine activation induced by hypoxia/reoxygenation in cultured human umbilical vein endothelial cells. Planta Med 67:19–23
5. Yao XH, Li XJ (2001) *Panax notoginseng* saponins injection in treatment of cerebral infarction with a multicenter study. Zhong Guo Xin Yao Yu Lin Chuang Za Zhi 20:257–260
6. Yu JL, Dou DQ, Chen XH et al (2005) Protopanaxatriol-type ginsenosides differentially modulate type 1 and type 2 cytokines production from murine splenocytes. Planta Med 71:202–207
7. Qiu YK, Dou DQ, Cai LP et al (2009) Dammarane-type saponins from *Panax quinquefolium* and their inhibition activity on human breast cancer MCF-7 cells. Fitoterapia 80:219–222
8. Dou DQ, Xiang Z, Yang G et al (2011) Prediagnostic methods for the hemolysis of herbal medicine injection. J Ethnopharmacol 138:445–450
9. Sun DR, Qi P (2003). adverse drug reaction. People's Medical Publishing House, Beijing
10. Coutts SM, Nehring RE, Jariwala NU (1980) Purification of rat peritoneal mast cells: occupation of IgE-receptors by IgE prevents loss of the receptors. J Immunol 124:2309–2315
11. Horigome K, Bullock ED, Johnson EM (1994) Effects of nerve growth factor on rat peritoneal mast cells. Survival promotion and immediate-early gene induction. J Biol Chem 269:2695–2702
12. Saito H, Kato A, Matsumoto K et al (2006) Culture of human mast cells from peripheral blood progenitors. Nat Protoc 1:2178–2183
13. Egle P, Carsten E, Helen S et al (2009) RBL-2H3 cells are an imprecise model for mast cell mediator release. Inflamm Res 58:611–618

Chapter 437
Change Towards Creative Society: A Developed Knowledge Model for IT in Learning

M. Yu, C. Zhou and W. Xing

Abstract The Information Technology (IT) has brought a "learning revolution" and the change towards the "Creative Society". It drives this paper to understand roles of IT in learning by a knowledge creation approach. So we develop a knowledge creation model where we can link the relationships between creativity, knowledge and learning process, where we can also deeply understand IT as stimuli of "explicit—collective knowledge" in the dynamic process of knowledge creation. So a case of using Web 2.0 for supporting PBL learning environment at Aalborg University (AAU), Denmark will be introduced. Therefore, this study contributes to implications of better pedagogical design for building creative learning environment and better use of IT in education in future.

Keywords Creativity · Knowledge creation · IT · Learning

M. Yu (✉)
College of Humanities and Social Science, China Medical University, Shenyang 110001 Liaoning, China
e-mail: yumiaocmu@163.com

C. Zhou
Department of Learning and Philosophy, Aalborg University, Sohngaardsholmsvej 2, Aalborg 9000, Denmark
e-mail: chunfang@learning.aau.dk

W. Xing
College of Sciences, Northeastern University, Shenyang 110004 Liaoning, China
e-mail: awxing@mail.neu.edu.cn

S. Li et al. (eds.), *Frontier and Future Development of Information Technology in Medicine and Education*, Lecture Notes in Electrical Engineering 269,
DOI: 10.1007/978-94-007-7618-0_437,

437.1 Change Towards Creative Society: "Learning Revolution" Brought by IT

In the 1980s, there was much talk about the transition from "Industrial Society" to the "Information Society". No longer would natural resources and manufacturing be the driving forces in our economies and societies. Information was the new king. However, in the 1990s, people began to talk about the "Knowledge Society". We began to realize that information itself would not bring about important change. Rather, the key was how people transformed information into knowledge and managed that knowledge. The shift in focus from "information" to "knowledge" is an improvement that leads to a conception of "Creative Society" formulated. This conception means in the future, success will be based not on how much we know, but on our ability to think and act creatively [1].

The Information technology (IT) has accentuated the need for creative thinking in all aspects of our lives, and has also provided tools that can help us improve and reinvent ourselves [1]. IT makes possible asynchronous learning, or learning characterized by a time lag between the delivery of instruction and its reception by learners [2]. The educators must make sure that students' creativity is nourished and developed. To achieve this goal will require a deep understanding of relationships between creativity, knowledge and roles of IT in learning. Accordingly, in this paper, we will focus on a question: how can we understand roles of IT in achieving new knowledge and developing creativity in learning process? By answering this question, this paper will implicate for a better pedagogical design for creativity and the better uses of IT in education in future.

437.2 A Knowledge Creation Approach to IT in Learning

437.2.1 A Model of Knowledge Creation

Recently, knowledge creation has been discussed as a social process that means new ideas and innovations emerge between rather than within people [3]. The studies on tacit knowledge and explicit knowledge indicate learning happens in the transformation between the two kinds of knowledge [4]. The knowledge-creation approach conceptualizes learning and knowledge advancement as collaborative processes for developing shared objects of activity [3]. Therefore, the interactions between tacit knowlege and explict knowlege and between individual knowledge and collective knowledge have been emphasized by, for example, Baumard's model [5] (Fig. 437.1).

As the Fig. 437.1 shows, there are four types of knowlege in Baumard's Model for understanding knowlege creation. First, knowledge which is explicit and individual provides techniques that allow us to counter nets and traps. Second, through collective and explicit knowledge we achieve profound knowledge of a

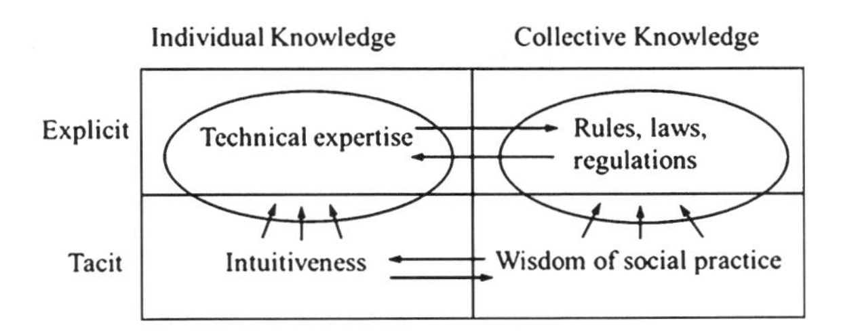

Fig. 437.1 Baumard's model for understanding knowledge creation

terrain, the environment, rules, and laws. Third, knowledge which is tacit and collective is of the unspoken, invisible structure of a practice. Lastly, knowledge can be tacit and individual; where tacit expertise is complemented by "hard" technical knowledge—a sort of inimitable technical skills. Therefore, the fundamental hypothesis in Baumard's model is that learning happens in the complex conversions between different types and levels of knowledge [6].

Although there are other models of knowledge creation, such as the one developed by Nonaka and Takeuchi [7], Baumard's model is focused on here because it provides spaces of developing this model for further understanding of IT as a stimuli for knowledge creation in learning, as what will be illustrated in the below.

437.2.2 IT As Stimuli for Knowledge Creation in Learning

437.2.2.1 A Developed Model for Linking Creativity, Learning and IT

The knowledge creation approach to learning indicates that creativity is imbedded in learning process; since creativity has been generally defined as developing new and useful ideas that means creativity may offer students opportunities to shape new knowledge [8]. So in collaborative settings, learning and creativity go hand in hand. This drives us to develop Baumard's model that regards creatvity could be a "spiral" growing from the junction of the four types of knowledge. In the educational environment, IT could be a stimulator for the growing the "spiral" of creativity in process of achieving new knowledge (Fig. 437.2).

In the developed model in Fig. 437.2, we think that creativity in the learning process is dynamic but not linear, and contains uninterrupted knowledge conversations between different knowledge types. The concept of back burnering an idea is essential in the process of individual reflection and common engagement in collaborative learning settings. In order to stimulate the "spiral" of creativity that grows from such a process, IT should be emphasized here because it helps students communicate more effectively when learning collaboratively in groups. The internet provides the common platform to individual students for sharing new knowledge. IT therefore could be one stimuli of "explicit—collective knowledge" and could facilitate the learning loop as well as creativity development (Fig. 437.2).

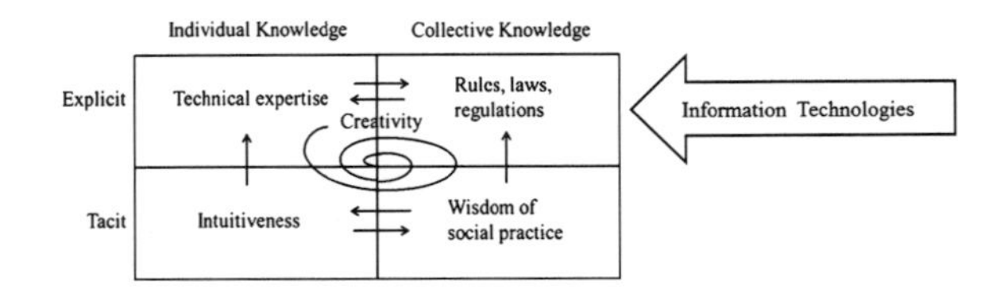

Fig. 437.2 A developed model for understanding IT as stimuli for creativity

437.2.2.2 A Case of Using Web2.0 at Aalborg University, Denmark

Aalborg University (AAU) in Denmark has a tradition of Problem-Based Learning (PBL) since 1974. Students at AAU are required to complete in each semester approximately 50 % coursework and 50 % project work in groups. The IT has brought the new elements to AAU. In order to support students learning activities, Web2.0 has been introduced to their online learning environment, which is called "Ekademia" (Ecademy) (Fig. 437.3) [9].

When 180 undergraduate students began their education within Humanistic Informatics in September 2007, they were met with Ekademia as a new educational online environment supplementing the existing system (Lotus Quickr). Quickr acted as a more traditional VLE segmented into semesters and course-pages with schedules and announcements, whereas the Humanistic Informatics faculty intended Ekademia to be more social and interactional. The faculty therefore chose to base Ekademia on the open source software Elgg, because the system reflects a social networking or e-portfolio metaphor, and contains a number of web 2.0 features such as blogs, personal profiles, podcasting, widgets, RSS-integration and tagging [9]. Therefore, Ekademia provides platforms for both individual and group learning that are basic conditions of building a creative learning environment.

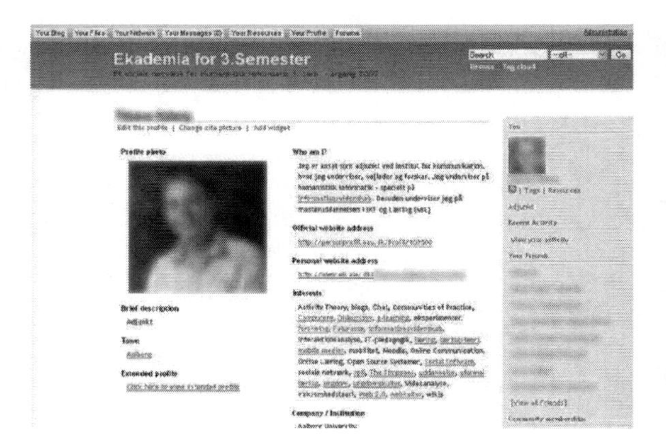

Fig. 437.3 An example of a profile page of Ekademia (pictures and names are deliberately blurred)

437.3 Implications for Future Pedagogical Design

The knowledge creation approach to learning indicates the implications of better pedagogical design for building creative learning environment and better use of IT in education in future.

First, instead of a centralized-control model, we should take a more entrepreneurial approach to learning. Students should become more active and independent learners, with the teacher serving as consultant, not chief executive.

Second, instead of dividing up curriculum into separate disciplines, we should focus on themes and project that cut across the disciplines, taking advantage of the rich connects among different domains of knowledge.

Third, instead of letting students learn "what they should learn", we should focus more on "strategies for learning to become better learners". The education environment must prepare students with the new skills and ideas that are needed for living and working in a creative society [1].

References

1. Resnick M (2002) Rethinking learning in the digital age. In: Kirkman G (ed) The global information technology report: readiness for the networked word. Oxford University Press, Oxford
2. Tinio L (2003) ICT in education. http://139.179.20.111/egitim/eprimer-edu.pdf. Accessed 30 May 2012
3. Paavola S, Lipponen L, Hakkarainen K (2004) Models of innovative knowledge communities and three metaphors of learning. Rev Educ Res 74:557–576
4. Koskinen U, Pihlanto P, Vanharanta H (2003) Tacit knowledge acquisition and sharing in a project work context. Int J Proj Manage 21:281–290
5. Baumard P (1999) Tacit knowledge in organizations. Sage Publications, London
6. Zhou C, Kolmos A, Nielsen D (2012) A Problem and Project-Based Learning (PBL) approach to motivate group creativity in engineering education. Int J Eng Educ 28(1):3–16
7. Nonaka I, Takeuchi H (1995) The knowledge-creating company: how Japanese companies create the dynamic of innovation. Oxford University Press, New York
8. Craft A (2005) Creativity in schools: tensions and dilemmas. Routledge, New York
9. Ryberg T, Dirckinck-Holmfeld L, Jones C (2010) Caterin to the needs of the 'digital natives' or educating the 'net generation'? In: Lee MJW, Hershey CM (ed) Web 2.0-based e-learning: applying social information for tertiary teaching. IGI Global, Hershey

Chapter 438
TCM Standard Composition and Component Library: Sample Management System

Erwei Liu, Yan Huo, Zhongxin Liu, Lifeng Han, Tao Wang and Xiumei Gao

Abstract This paper introduces a sample management system for Traditional Chinese Medicine (TCM) standard composition and component library, including the general framework, module division, functions of each part and main interfaces of the system. The system is user-friendly and easy to master, which will play an important promoting role in realizing TCM research information delivery and standardization.

Keywords TCM composition · Sample · Management system

E. Liu · L. Han
TCM Institute of Tianjin University of Traditional Chinese Medicine, Yuquan Road 88, Nankai, Tianjin 300193, China
e-mail: Liuwei628@hotmail.com

L. Han
e-mail: hanlifeng1@sohu.com

Y. Huo
Tianjin University of Traditional Chinese Medicine, Yuquan Road 88, Nankai, Tianjin 300193, China
e-mail: hyqqshuizi@163.com

Z. Liu
School of IT and Science of Nankai University, Weijin Road 93, Nankai, Tianjin 300071, China
e-mail: lzhx@nankai.edu.cn

T. Wang · X. Gao (✉)
Tianjin TCM Chemistry and Analysis Key Laboratory, Yuquan Road 88, Nankai, Tianjin 300193, China
e-mail: gaoxiumei1984@hotmail.com

T. Wang
e-mail: wangt@263.com

S. Li et al. (eds.), *Frontier and Future Development of Information Technology in Medicine and Education*, Lecture Notes in Electrical Engineering 269,
DOI: 10.1007/978-94-007-7618-0_438,

438.1 Introduction

Traditional Chinese Medicine (TCM) is a treasure of China for many years and an immortal legend during the development of human civilization. Along with the economic globalization, the development and modernization of traditional Chinese medicine is facing new opportunities and challenges [1]. The basic tasks for technology to promote the modernization of traditional Chinese medicine are *inheritance, development, innovation and internationalization* [2] since the beginning of the *Eleventh Five-Year Plan*. Promoting the internationalization of traditional Chinese medicine in China is the need of social progress and the development of the times.

At present, the researches on modernization of traditional Chinese medicine mostly focuses on application of modern science and technology to illustrate the scientific connotation of traditional Chinese medicine and reflection of the idea of *Chinese learning as the fundamental structure, Western learning as the application* [3]. Natural pharmaceutical chemistry always focuses on extraction of the active ingredients, separation, sample preparation, repeated testing, and finally developing drugs and other products with special efficacy. If we can clearly describe the pharmacodynamic material basis of traditional Chinese medicine and be well aware of the effective chemical components possibly extracted or separated from natural plants or medicinal materials, we will be able to avoid safety stability and other problems caused by the complexity of traditional Chinese medicine, which is of great significance for the researches on modernization of traditional Chinese medicine. Composition TCM development on this basis is an important direction of modernization for traditional Chinese medicine, and a lot of achievements have been made over many years of hard work [4–8].

The basis of TCM modernization research is the researches on pharmacodynamic material basis of TCM. By combining with the latest research achievements of natural pharmaceutical chemistry to make standard component preparation and systematic plant-chemical separation, we can get a series of TCM standard composition/component samples with stabilized preparation, controllable quality and repeatability. Recently, computer information revolution, as the pilot of the new technological revolution, has developed quickly into all areas of life. Introduction of advanced computer technology into TCM research will promote the modernization of traditional Chinese medicine. Currently, Tianjin University of Traditional Chinese Medicine has done a lot for TCM component separation and standardization. The staff of this university has formed more than 18,000 TCM standard components and more than 8,000 compounds, with the information corresponding to each standard composition/component, including preparation, structure, representation, etc. In order to effectively manage these huge data, we have designed and developed the TCM Standard Composition and Component Library—Sample Management System of Tianjin University of Traditional Chinese Medicine. With this system, we can effectively manage and mine these data and combine with Chinese herbs and prescriptions to establish the standard library of samples (Chinese herbs, standard composition, chemical components and prescriptions) through computer management, with the information including sample codes, descriptions and sample properties (physical and chemical properties, to be detailed). This system specifies the composition standard of all the samples, makes actual storage, requisition and discarding processes of the prepared samples, and has realized the actual sample informationization. The application of this system plays an important role in promoting the standardization and modernization of TCM researches in our university.

Compared with other similar management systems, TCM Standard Composition and Component Library—Sample Management System has the following major innovations:

(1) The freezers, sample holders and sample boxes used in the visual sample database management are consistent with the material objects. The sample management operations of this system are the same with the actual situation, which is easy for us to use.
(2) The Processed sample management for the out/storage process of this system focus on the continuity of business, and performs in a different way from the usual functional management. It will encourage the members to co-operate and improve their work efficiency.
(3) This system has flexible allocation of management rights. The functional limitations and data limitations for users are managed separately which makes it flexible to control. Users with the same functional limitations can operate separately through different departments or businesses group.

438.2 General Framework of the System

The TCM Standard Composition/Component Library—Sample Management System of Tianjin University of Traditional Chinese Medicine is developed by using Java language, making full use of modern network communication technology, in which good information communication and data sharing has been realized. The software adopts the B/S structure system, which reduces the requirements for the clients, and it is easy for remote login and remote control. The system's database is managed by ORACLE 10G, to ensure the security and reliability of data storing. The currently popular J2EE + EXT + iBATIS + STRUTS2 technical architecture is adopted by this system.

The main functions of this system include system privileges, basic information, sample information and inventory management, as shown in Fig. 438.1 The functions of each part of the system are as follows:

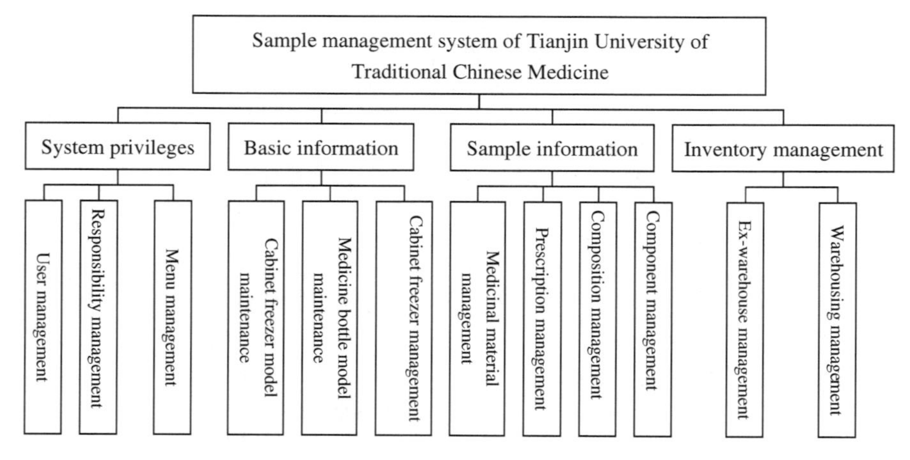

Fig. 438.1 System framework

(1) System privileges:

This part realizes system privilege setting, user creating, modifying and deleting and other functions. The system users are divided into different responsibilities, such as system administrator, basic library administrator and sample administrator. One set of menus shall be set corresponding to each responsibility and each set of menus shall set up its own functions, and the system can select different functions to make each set of menus for each responsibility.

(2) Basic information:

The system administrator is responsible for maintenance of the serial number, model, state and number of available shelves of the cabinet freezer.

Cabinet freezer model maintenance: maintain the models of cabinet freezers existing or introduced later, for example, cabinet freezers can be classified as 5-layer and 7-layer cabinet freezers, which is easy for cabinet freezer management.

Medicine box maintenance: maintain the models of medicine boxes existing or introduced later, for example, medicine boxes can be classified as 3 × 3, 9-grid boxes and 4 × 4, 16-grid boxes, which is easy for cabinet freezer management.

The cabinet freezer management page consists of two parts, hierarchical tree and the corresponding graphical interface. When clicking each node in the hierarchical tree, a corresponding graph will show up. When clicking a medicine bottle graph at the box node, the basic information of this sample will show up. The system administrator can add, modify and delete information at the nodes of each hierarchy. When adding new cabinet freezers, the freezers are numbered according to certain rules; cabinet freezer models show up in the form of a drop-down selection box, and the contents are the information entered at cabinet freezer model maintenance. Similarly, when adding new medicine boxes, this method is also adopted for easy operation and reducing the complexity in information entry.

(3) Sample information:

In order to facilitate sample information sharing, ordinary users can add samples into the sample library, while visitors can view the information, but have no right of modification.

The basic information of sample is classified into four categories, medicinal materials, compositions, components and prescriptions. Ordinary users shall enter the basic information of samples into the system after sample experiments. On the sample information list page, users can enter query conditions to make combination queries for the appropriate information, which will be displaced in the list. If the information is found incomplete, the users can fill out a requisition application, continue to make researches on the sample, and complete the information by creating, deleting and modifying after research. Before filling out the requisition application, the users can view the existing inventory information to determine whether to extract the sample again.

The basic information on the pages of medicinal material, composition, component and prescription adding shall be filled in according to the actual need.

(4) Inventory management:

Warehousing management: the inventory administrator can record sample provider, warehousing time, sample information and storing location. Once ordinary users finish sample research, the sample shall be stored in a cabinet freezer, and inventory administrator shall put the sample at the corresponding location and enter the sample information into the system for easy later queries.

Ex-warehouse management: Inventory administrator can check the inventory quantity and view the details of the inventory. If the inventory quantities and the actual quantities in system are different, the administrator can adjust the inventory quantities in the system and fill in the names of the adjusted samples, reasons and quantities, to ensure the correctness of the system.

438.3 Workflow and Main Interfaces of the System

The personnel using this system mainly include basic library administrator, sample administrator and ordinary viewing users, and these three types of personnel cooperate together to realize TCM standard composition/component sample library management and maintenance. The workflow of the system is shown in Fig. 438.2.

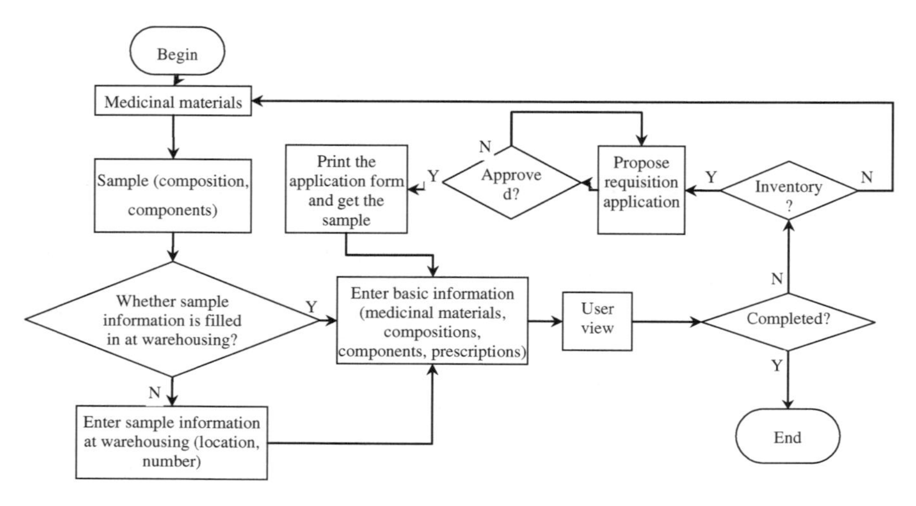

Fig. 438.2

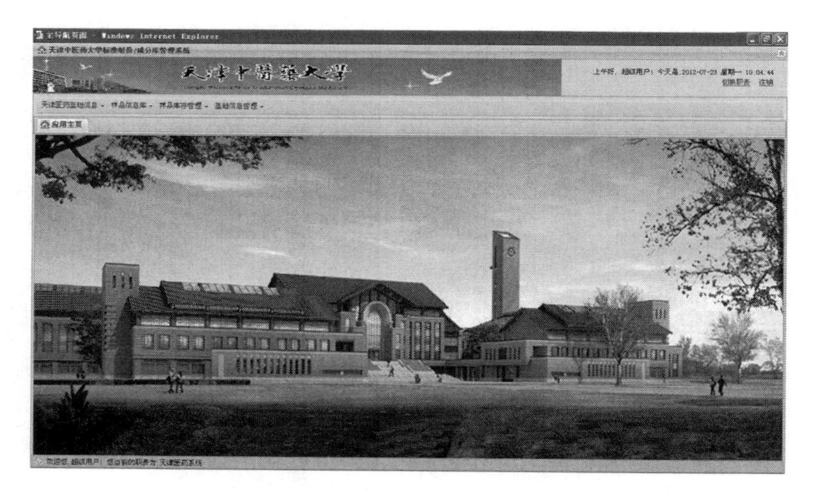

Fig. 438.3 Main interface of the system

438.3.1 Main Interfaces

When users with different rights log in, the home page displayed may be different. The home page for the administrators is demonstrated as shown in Fig. 438.3.

Users can switch over their rights according to their needs, so as to complete different functions with corresponding role.

438.3.2 Basic Information Management

Basic information management is the basis of this system, including various basic information of the system, cabinet freezer, medicine box and bottle maintenance information, medicinal material, prescription, composition and component maintenance information, etc. In basic information, cabinet freezer, medicine box and bottle maintenance information adopts graphic management, which is easy for use and maintenance. The following Figs. 438.4 and 438.5 show the interfaces for cabinet and medicine bottle maintenance.

438.3.3 Sample Information Management Interface

Sample information library is mainly used to achieve the purpose of sample information sharing. Administrators add samples into the sample information library. The normal users can view the information, but have no rights to add, modify and delete, and users can enter query conditions to main combination queries to appropriate information, which is displayed in the list as shown in Fig. 438.6.

438.3.4 Sample Inventory Management

This part includes sample warehousing list, sample ex-warehouse list and proofreading management. The users can make corresponding queries, make sample inventory management. When sample quantity in the system is different from the

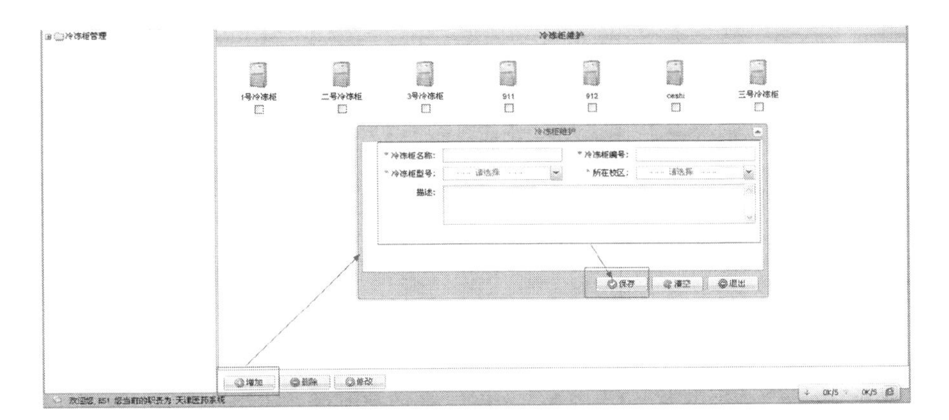

Fig. 438.4 Cabinet freezer management interface

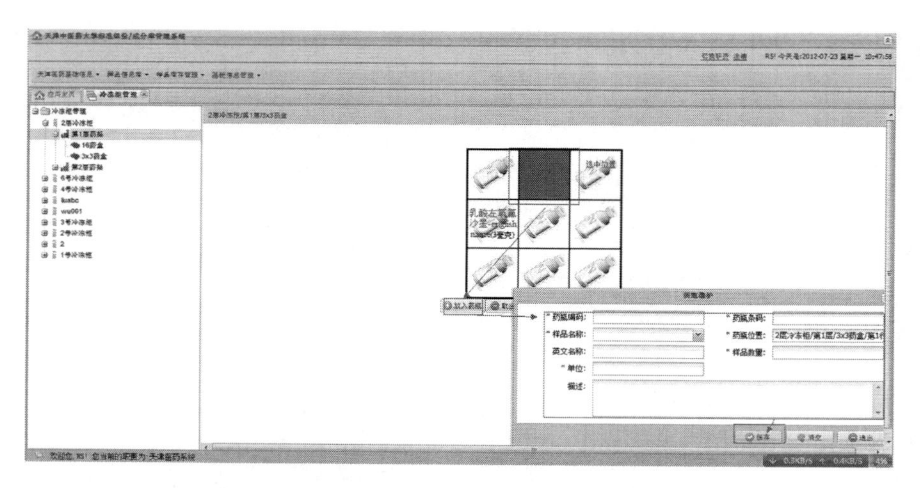

Fig. 438.5 Medicine bottle maintenance interface

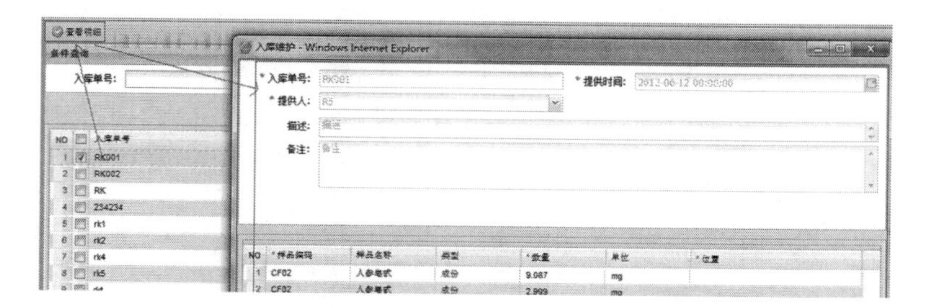

Fig. 438.6 Sample information homepage

Fig. 438.7 Inventory sample information view

actual sample quantity, they can make sample quantity maintenance in the system. Fig. 438.7 shows an interface for inventory sample information view.

438.4 System Operation Effects

This TCM standard composition/component sample library management system started trial operation in the beginning of 2012 and started formal operation in July 2012, and had been working stably for nearly half a year. Currently, in system operation, researchers, project directors and research supervisors can be online simultaneously and realize sample use application, approval by research supervisors and other functions according to the corresponding account rights. It is guaranteed that the researchers can get samples as soon as possible, the research supervisors can make overall arrangements of sample use, and the project directors can make statistics on sample use, which is easy for project fund use and management. Application of this system has avoided the cumbersome procedure that samples are obtained after the application form is signed by the leaders. The paperless office work and processing is also realized via this system, and this system plays a very active role in promoting TCM standard management and improving research efficiency in our university.

438.5 Conclusion

The modernization of research methods is an inevitable trend of TCM research in China. We have fully exploited the scientific connotation of traditional Chinese medicine. Adopting modern technology to make scientific management of TCM under the guidance of TCM theory, we have designed this TCM standard composition/component sample library management system. This paper mainly introduces the general framework, module division, functions of each part and main interfaces of the system. The system is user-friendly and easy to use, which plays an important promoting role in realizing TCM research informationization and standardization.

References

1. Liang X, Xu Q, Xue X, Zhang F, Xiao Y (2006) Composition TCM system research. World Sci Technol 8(3):1–7
2. Zou J (2006) Blow the advance horn for comprehensive development of traditional Chinese medicine—medium and long-term technological task prospect for modernization of traditional Chinese medicine in China. World Sci Technol 8(1):1–2
3. Luo G, Wang Y, Liang Q et al (2010) Systems biology. Science Press, Beijing
4. Cui X, Zhang G (2009) Composition TCM and TCM modernization. Lishizhen Med Mater Med Res 20(5):1290–1291
5. Ji W, Chen L, Gu J et al (2008) Multi-component TCM compound group release synchronism evaluation methodology. Acta Pharmaceutica Sinica 43(6):647

6. Liu D, Yu D, Sun E, Jia X (2012) Construction of TCM composition and composition biopharmaceutics classification system. J Chin Materia Medica 37(19):2997–3000
7. Zhang G, Luo R, Wang Y (2007) TCM pharmacodynamic composition theory and TCM composition science. Chin Herb Med 30(2):125–126
8. Zhang JW, Chen LB, Yang M et al (2008) Novel theory and methods for chemomic multi-component release/dissolution kinetics of traditional Chinese medicines. Chin J Nat Med 6:48

Chapter 439
The Teaching Method of Interrogation in Traditional Chinese Diagnostics

Jingjing Fu, Haixia Yan and He Jiancheng Ding Jie

Abstract Interrogation is one of the fundamental skills that must be mastered by students of traditional Chinese medicine (TCM). This paper aims to improve the teaching quality by investigating the effective approaches in TCM diagnostics teaching through several aspects, including the combination of classroom teaching and clinical practice; application of appropriate heuristic teaching, clinical training and intensive training in practice and internship; the adoption of standardization, and the exploration of the possible applications of an interrogation training software.

Keywords TCM diagnostics · Interrogation · Teaching method

Interrogation plays a vital role in traditional Chinese medicine (TCM) clinical diagnosis. According to "Essential Recipes for Emergent Use Worth A Thousand Gold" (*Qian Jin Yao Fang*), written by Sun Simiao in the Tang Dynasty, "it is accurate to ask before diagnosis." Zhang Jiebin explained in detail the interrogation content and its significance in differentiating between symptoms and signs, while in Jing Yue's complete work, he proposed that interrogation is the key to diagnosis and the first step that must be taken in clinical practice. Therefore, interrogation is one of the fundamental skills that must be mastered by TCM students [1].

Fu Jingjing and Yan Haixia are the parallel first authors of this chapter.

J. Fu (✉) · H. Yan · H. J. D. Jie
Shanghai University of Traditional Chinese Medicine, No. 1200 Cailun Road, Shanghai, People's Republic of China
e-mail: fujj_tcm@163.com

H. Yan
e-mail: hjy2012ok@163.com

S. Li et al. (eds.), *Frontier and Future Development of Information Technology in Medicine and Education*, Lecture Notes in Electrical Engineering 269,
DOI: 10.1007/978-94-007-7618-0_439,

The current teaching content related to interrogation in TCM diagnostics is the traditional classroom teaching, in which only the theories and techniques pertaining to various interrogation methods are being taught, and the specific interrogation skills of the students are not developed. Many students feel nervous when facing patients in clinical practice, because they often have no opportunities to ask patients or if they do, they have insufficient interrogations skills to help them gather the information they need form the patients. All of these directly affect the writing of medical records and the accurate diagnosis of diseases. Training and improving the interrogation skills of TCM students requires urgent attention that must be solved in the current revolution of TCM diagnostics teaching. With years of teaching experience, we, the teaching and research section, propose some suggestions in this work to improve future teaching methods of interrogation in TCM diagnostics.

439.1 The Close Combination of Classroom Teaching and Clinical Practice

The process of interrogation refers to the communication between doctors and patients. The effective communication between patients and doctors plays an indispensable role in diagnosis and in the mental healing of patients, by increasing their compliance with the treatment. Communication also improves the clinical skills and confidence of the doctors as well as the satisfaction of patients. Appropriate teaching of interpersonal communication skills during interrogation helps students understand the benefits of good communication skills and of improving the interrogation efficiency, enabling them to apply such skills in their respective practices and internships.

Furthermore, through classroom teaching students can learn how to perform the step-by-step interrogation process, depending on the actual situation of each patient; here, role play is used to simulate clinical interrogation, while teachers can guide and correct the students on site.

439.2 Appropriate Heuristic Teaching

During heuristic teaching, various teaching methods are required based on teaching aims, teaching content, level of knowledge and the ability of students to learn laws, thus inspiring students to learn and cultivate their abilities. In turn, such methods enable them to actively learn; to master the methods of logical reasoning, generalization and summarization; to learn by analogy; and to develop the abilities of independently analyzing and solving problems. Take a simple interrogation procedure to determine pain as example; this is a case wherein heuristic teaching can be employed. Here, students are required to read and discuss the case before explaining the content. Below is a sample dialogue between a doctor and his patient.

Doctor	*What hurts you?*
Patient	*It hurts here* (pointing to the right rib, i.e., the location of pain, with his hand)
Doctor	*What causes it?*
Patient	*Three years ago, I felt pain in the right rib. After examination, it was said to be cholecystitis, and then I underwent transfusion and injection. Later, I felt better. Sometimes, I took anti-inflammatory agents. Recently, I felt pain again, and the anti-inflammatory medicines I used to take do not work anymore*
Doctor	*How long have you been in such situation?* (Past medical history, the onset and diagnosis of current disease)
Patient	*Almost one week* (pain time)
Doctor	*Continuously or in short bursts?*
Patient	*In short bursts* (the law of pain onset)
Doctor	*Is it serious?*
Patient	*Yes* (the degree of pain)
Doctor	*What do you feel when eating?*
Patient	*I have no appetite and I always feel bloated* (accompanying symptoms)
Doctor	*Let me have a look at your tongue* (white and greasy coating on the tongue)
Doctor	*Let me feel your pulse* (taut pulse)

...

Raise Question 1: What should the doctor focus on when asking about the pain? Students try to summarize the related content to answer the question. Later, teachers introduce the content of the interrogation of pain with case and discussion, and then explain what needs attention during the interrogation.

Raise Question 2: What is the chief complaint in the case and what needs to be improved in the way by which the doctor is performing the interrogation? In this way, the content of the chief complaint can be reviewed, and clinical summarization training can be provided to the students, enabling them to apply their improved interrogation skills in actual clinical practice.

439.3 Intensive Training in Clinical Practice and Internship

In our school, freshmen students are arranged to clinically practice in the primary period of the first year, which is a perfect opportunity to train their clinical skills. Clinical teaching gives students the opportunities to see, observe, and practice.

This period also helps the teachers to immediately identify the insufficiency of a student's skills, facilitating correction that, in turn, augments the shortcomings of theoretical teaching. In turn, this encourages students and gives them self-confidence as they prepare for their future clinical practice.

By the end of the first two periods of the first academic year, students are expected to have completed the courses of Basic Theories of TCM, Traditional Chinese Diagnostics, Traditional Chinese Pharmacology, and Traditional Medical Formulae. During practice, students can interrogate patients face-to-face under the guidance of teachers, allowing them to gradually gain familiarity with the process and develop their interrogation skills. In this process, the teachers also alternately explain some knowledge points of Basic Theories of TCM, Traditional Chinese Pharmacology, and Traditional Medical Formulae, thus consolidating their theoretical knowledge. This helps the students apply what they have learned, activate their learning experience, and enhance their professional ideology.

439.4 The Adoption of Standardization in Treating Patients

Currently, different Chinese medicine colleges are limited by the lack of practice base, guidance teachers and teaching time, thereby leading to the shortened practice in actual teaching. Thus, clinical teaching cannot be carried out. Standardization is widely applied in overseas medical schools in developing the clinical skills of students; the same is also applied in some local schools [2]. Accordingly, this method can be learned to train simulated patients who master correct specifications of the operation. As a training platform, standardization can be used in Chinese medicine teaching practice, thus, improving the clinical techniques of the students, including interrogation.

Due to the long training period of standardization in treating patients, its application is limited. In some cases, local Chinese medicine colleges choose to replace the simulated patients with teachers, helping the teachers determine the learning situation related to interrogation content and the utilization of interrogation skills in a timely manner. This way, they can find and solve problems, as well as help students gain mastery of the interrogation skills in actual situations. This method is easy to conduct and can also be learned in our proposed teaching method.

439.5 The Development of an Interrogation Training Software

A kind of interrogation training software, which can simulate human–computer dialogues, can also be developed with the help of existing artificial intelligence technologies. Related attempts have been carried out. TCM interrogation content can be programmed, with the computer simulating as the "patients" and the students acting as "doctors." Students draw from their knowledge base to interrogate the "patient," while the computers answers accordingly. Through such a dialogue, the "doctor" evaluates the symptoms based on the information. Finally, the computer makes an evaluation of the data, and the goal of the training is achieved.

With years of teaching experience and the combination of various teaching methods, our teaching and research section has perfected a teaching method to improve interrogation skills, which is applicable for college students. The proposed method enables students to grasp and master the basic skills of interrogation in theoretical learning, thus enriching their classroom learning of TCM diagnostics.

Acknowledgment Funded by the Shanghai University of Traditional Chinese Medicine English Course Construction Project (a subproject of the 085 Projects, under Project No. P3040907), the Shanghai University of Traditional Chinese Medicine Postgraduate Courses Construction Project (Project No. K130211), and the 13th Course Construction Project of the Shanghai University of Traditional Chinese Medicine (Project No.).

References

1. Li M, Xu R (2003) The theoretical basis and clinical application of interrogation. J Chin Med 21(10):1772–1773
2. Li Y, Shufen Y, Sui S et al (2008) The present situation and tendency of standardization patients in chinese medical education. Chin Higher Med Educ 3:97–98

Chapter 440
Designing on system of Quality Monitoring on Instruction Actualizing

Zhang Yan

Abstract Oriented towards system of quality Supervision on instruction actualizing, confirm the framework of system, Provide the whole design of system, select the supporting platform of system development and B/S processing mode, partition system into four sub-system, initial stages supervision, on-line supervision, phases supervision and end supervision, Study the value index system and value mode.

Keywords Instruction quality · Monitoring · Index · E-R

440.1 Introduction

The realization of the teaching process quality monitoring is carried out through the teaching examination at some various stage and quality analysis after the end of the teaching process, Specific mode of operation including interim teaching order examination, the lesson plans examination, papers checks, statistical analysis of student achievement at the end of the period and the students' evaluation to teaching. In the conditions of the university digital and network construction with a certain scale, the operation mode is slower, One outstanding problem is that monitor may be easy to become a mere formality, cannot truly reflect the teaching actual situation, also can't timely feedback on teaching effect. Teaching quality monitoring system is designed based on making full use of the network conditions, can solve the above problems, and can play a significant role in improve the quality of teaching.

Z. Yan (✉)
Teaching Department of Computer and Mathematical Foundation of Shenyang Normal University, 110034 Huanghe North Street 253, Huanggu, Shenyang, Liaoning, China
e-mail: Zhangyan_synu@126.com

S. Li et al. (eds.), *Frontier and Future Development of Information Technology in Medicine and Education*, Lecture Notes in Electrical Engineering 269,
DOI: 10.1007/978-94-007-7618-0_440,

440.2 The Design on Overall Structure of the System

440.2.1 System Design Ideas

Design thinking is to establish an instruction running information monitoring platform in a network environment, set different access and the using interface for all kinds of personnel at all levels, determine and load the raw data into the database by the school teaching management departments, departments staffs in charge of the teaching, students, teachers, auxiliary teaching staff, the superintendent and so on, obtain results of analysis and evaluation by using the corresponding evaluation system, which play a guiding role for adjusting teaching schedule, teaching instrument maintenance, the direction of the teaching management work and so on. The whole system processing mode choice browser/server mode, constitute a system with presentation layer, application logic layer and data server.

440.2.2 Division of Subsystem

Through the analysis of the whole system, combined with the arrangement and characteristics of school work, the best way of division of subsystem is according to the time characteristics of the monitoring. Each subsystem is described as following.

The main function of early monitoring subsystem is to summary and evaluate and make statistical analysis to record of teaching programs, curricula, educational calendar, teaching materials, expected student achievement, teaching and research activities plans, teaching equipment, conduct inspection before the commencement of the teaching process. The purpose of early monitoring subsystem is to clear indicators that should be completed in the teaching process, to guide the teaching work in a planned and targeted way, step by step to complete.

The main function of real-time monitoring subsystem is usually specific to each link of teaching process to conduct a comprehensive monitoring, can involve all of the teachers, students, classrooms, laboratories and experimental instruments and equipment, etc. The purpose of real-time monitoring is to ensure the correct implementation of the teaching plan, the completion of teaching tasks and teaching purpose.

The main function of stage monitoring subsystem is to implement monitoring every period and make evaluation according to the rules and norms in advance. Stage monitoring is usually aimed at all kinds of teaching activities, can involve teaching research activity, theme activities, teachers' lesson plans and completion status, etc. It is necessary to make statistics and analysis on stage monitoring data periodically, compare the analysis results with the original teaching plan, find the problem in time and urge the relevant departments or the teacher to correct.

The main function of final stage monitoring subsystem is to make the last evaluation on teaching quality after teaching process, In particular, to make statistics and analysis through the test paper composition, overall results of student, student evaluation information on teachers and courses, etc. The purpose of final stage monitoring is to master students' cognitive ability and level of development status and trend, further defined the direction of teaching and adjust teaching plan, make the whole teaching quality steadily rising.

440.3 Establishment Database and Evaluation Model of Monitoring Target

440.3.1 Design Information Database

Information database is the collection of data tables established in accordance with the monitoring topics and tasks. In the database design stage, can start from the local E-R (entity-relation) figure, and then through E-R to get the integration, then to obtain a global conceptual model. Finally, the E-R diagram is converted to a logical model of the database, complete the design and establishment of related data tables in database. Here is the design of each data table in teaching operation information database:

- Lecture table includes lecture number, course number, teacher number, classroom number, the number of student number, weeks, starting plan time, ending plan time, notes, etc.
- Curriculum table includes course number, course name, hours, credit, types, teaching plans, teaching outline, teaching calendar, etc.
- Teacher table includes teacher number, name of teacher, the subordinate departments, job title, professional, academic, etc.
- Classroom table includes classroom number, name of the classroom, number of teaching equipment, number of laboratory equipment, etc.
- Teaching operation information table includes lecture number, course number, teacher number, classroom number, starting time, ending time, students attendance number, late students number, sick leave students number, lesson plan, interaction between teachers and students, the teaching schedule, the practice teaching, total number of devices, using device number, teaching evaluation personnel, etc.

440.3.2 Set up Evaluation Index System and Evaluation Model

The evaluation model system can adopt efficiency index in the index system. The system including two levels with primary indicators and secondary indicators, the first level indicators include teaching status, teaching plan formulation, teaching plan implementation, daily teaching management and teaching effects, etc. Teaching status includes secondary indicators such as leadership attention, stable teacher team, stable management team, complete teaching file. Teaching program formulation and implementation includes secondary indicators such as teaching planning, the implementation of teaching plans and teaching activities. Daily teaching management includes secondary indicators such as secondary indicators including teaching operation, teaching awards, teaching accidents punishment. The teaching effect includes secondary indicators such as the evaluation of teaching, student achievement and the quality of papers, etc. Evaluation model includes three links:

1. The determination of index weight

Considering the main purpose of this system is for quality control, timely found the factors that teaching quality cannot meet the requirements of teaching, so can use relatively simple expert method to determine the weight of each index. In particular, can get by formula (1), where n represents the number of experts, w_{ij} is weights j expert given to i index.

$$w_i = n^{-1} \sum_{j=1}^{n} wij \tag{440.1}$$

2. The determination of index assessment value

For qualitative indexes, fuzzy theory can be applied to the determination of index assessment value. Specific approach is:

- Determine the comment set $V = \{v_1,v_2,v_3,v_4,v_5\}$ = {Excellent, good, general, poor, bad}, the experts team members review certain qualitative index f_i respectively, obtain the single factor evaluation vector $X_i = \{x_{i1},x_{i2},\ldots,x_{ik},\ldots,x_{i5}\}$,$x_{ik}$ is membership degree of f_i to evaluation V_k.
- According to maximum membership principle, get the comments V^* to f_i, $V^* = \{v_i|\max(x_{ik}),1 \leq k \leq 5\}$
- Quantify the evaluation V^*, set numerical collection $Y = \{9,7,5,3,1\}$ corresponding with comments set V = s{Excellent, good, general, poor, bad}, $y_i = \{y_i| v_i,1 \leq i\leq5\}$, y_i is the assessment value of f_i.

To the quantitative indicators, can directly take its original value, its statistical value y_i is the assessment value of f_i.

3. Comprehensive evaluation

- The index system of this system contains both the qualitative indicators also contains the quantitative indicators, comprehensive evaluation can do according to the all levels index from inside to outside. Specific approach is:
- Standardize the indicators. For qualitative indicators, can get r_i by formula $r_i = (y_i - 1)/(9 - 1)$, r_i is the assessment value of index f_i. For quantitative indicators, can get r_i by formula $r_i = (y_i-\max)/(\max-\min)$, the max and min express upper and lower critical value of f_i, r_i is the assessment value of f_i.

- When integrated each layer indicators, can adopt the method of weighted sum to get evaluation result of the layer index.
- In order to guarantee the intelligent monitoring, system can obtain the target quality level according to the result of comprehensive evaluation, such as excellent, good, qualified and unqualified.

440.4 Conclusion

In order to achieve the quality control of teaching process, needs to arouse the enthusiasm of all participants in the process of teaching, make the system able to get the information through various channels, take advantage of network, database, and mathematical modeling techniques to finish all kinds of information integrating, loading, extract, analysis and information feedback in time, so as to strengthen the effective guidance of teaching work, and effectively promote the improvement of teaching quality in colleges and universities.

References

1. Liu H (2007) Research and practice of construction of normal universities teaching quality monitoring index system. Liaoning Educ Res 8:62–63
2. Gui G, Chang Q, Huang J (2007) Problems and countermeasures of teaching quality monitoring system of Newly-built local undergraduate colleges. China High Educ Res 7:50–51
3. Xiao W (2007) Guarantee and monitoring of internal teaching quality in colleges and universities. Educ Occup 10:36–38
4. Qiu J, Zhang Y (2006) Research on management information system of university evaluation. Inf J 25(1):115–121
5. Lin Q (2003) Decision analysis. Beijing University of posts and telecommunications publishing house, Beijing
6. Zhang Y, Li A (2008) The structure of Supervision on Instruction Quality. J Shenyang Normal Univ (Nat Sci Edn) 26(2):251–253
7. Zhang Y, Li A (2008) Reformation on prsentiment system of university students score. J Shenyang Normal Univ (Nat Sci Edn) 26(2):225–228

Chapter 441
Comparisons of Diagnosis for Occult Fractures with Nuclear Magnetic Resonance Imaging and Computerized Tomography

Ying Li, Huo-Yan Wu, Zhi-Qiang Jiang and Zhang-Song Ou

Abstract Objective-To study comparisons of diagnosis for occult fractures with nuclear magnetic resonance imaging and computerized tomography. Methods-Seventy six cases of patients with bone fracture including 45 males and 31 females were recruited in this study. And the data of X-ray, nuclear magnetic resonance Imaging (MRI) and computerized tomography (CT) were collected. Results-CT examination revealed 61 cases of patients with occult fractures and the accuracy rate was 80.26 %. MRI examination revealed 70 cases of patients with occult fractures and the accuracy rate of diagnosis was 92.11 %. There was no statistically significant difference between two methods in accuracy rates of fractures around the knee and recessive traumatic fracture ($P > 0.05$). For vertebral fractures and recessive bone fracture, the diagnosis rate of CT were 72.22 and 73.68 %, respectively the diagnosis rate of MRI were 91.67 and 94.74 %, respectively, there was statistically significant difference($P < 0.05$). Conclusion-While both computerized tomography and MRI can easily detect the bone fractures that are not recognized from X-ray film and whose clinical signs and symptoms are not clear, MRI can easily detect the occult fractures that are not shown by x-ray film and computerized tomography imaging and it can clarify many types of injuries and thus has high value and clinical applications.

Keywords Nuclear magnetic resonance imaging · Computerized tomography · Occult fractures

---

Y. Li (✉) · H.-Y. Wu · Z.-Q. Jiang · Z.-S. Ou
Department of Orthopaedics, Guangdong Province Integrative Medicine Hospital, Guangdong 528200 Foshan, People's Republic of China
e-mail: gdszxy@163.com

S. Li et al. (eds.), *Frontier and Future Development of Information Technology in Medicine and Education*, Lecture Notes in Electrical Engineering 269,
DOI: 10.1007/978-94-007-7618-0_441,

441.1 Introduction

Occult fractures are mainly caused by violent injuries. For this type of bone fracture, x-ray examination is usually negative. The reason for their negativity with x-ray examination is due to the impalpability of bone fracture lines that is not adequate to cause relocation of the bone fracture ends and the bone morphology still remain intact [1, 2]. While nuclear magnetic resonance Imaging (MRI) technology and the technology of three-dimensional reconstruction by computerized tomography (CT) have played important roles in early diagnosis and early treatment of bone fracture, there are certain differences in the accuracy in diagnosis between two technologies. In this study, we restrictively reviewed the imaging data of 76 cases of patients with occult fractures, aiming to evaluate the values in diagnosis of recessive bone fracture with NMRI and computerized tomography.

441.2 Methods

441.2.1 General Information

Seventy six (76) cases of patients with bone fracture including 45 males and 31 females were recruited in this study. All patients were admitted to this hospital with knee-joint pain or with pain in the lumbar region and backache after trauma. Based on their case histories in combination with results of relevant examinations, those patients with highly susceptive bone fractures or whose possible existence of recessive bone fracture cannot be eliminated were further examined with MRI and computerized tomography. Among these patients, 40 cases were diagnosed with knee-joint recessive bone fracture and 36 cases of patients were diagnosed with vertebral recessive bone fracture. According to the classification of recessive bone fracture, there were 38 cases of patients with recessive traumatic bone fracture with a total 51 sites and 25 cases of patients with recessive bone fracture inside the bones with a total of 38 sites. There are 13 cases of patients with both types of bone fractures.

441.2.2 Diagnostic Criteria

(1) Patients with clear acute injury case history and with such relevant symptoms as local pain or movement disorder; (2) Routine X-ray examination did not reveal noticeable bone fracture lines; (3) Cortical bone and TIWI line- or spot-like weak signals within bone marrow cavity can be seen in MRI imaging, T2W1 displayed high signals or high signals surrounding the low line-like signals but no abnormal

bone morphology was seen; (4) Cortical bone or broken trabecular bone were seen in computerized tomography imaging but no abnormal bone morphology was seen.

441.2.3 Examination Methods

Examination with computerized tomography: A 16-layer computerized tomography was used for performance of isotropic scanning at the patient's injury sites with 5-mm collimation, 5-mm section thickness, 120 kVp, 70 mAs, pitch of 1, and a 512 × 512 matrix, and axial, sagittal and coronal reconstructions were obtained.

Examination with MRI: The Siemens Avanto 1.5T scanner was used to obtain MRI. The SE series T1W1 and T2W1 were used for performance of cross-section scanning, vertical plane scanning, and coronal plane scanning. The lipid inhibition series T2W1 was used for performance of vertical plane scanning and coronal plane scanning. Fast spin echo (FSE) series and spectral presaturation inversion recovery (SPIR) series were used for performance of vertical plane scanning, coronal plane scanning and axial scanning. The scanning parameters included T1W1 TR300–450 ms, TE 10–17 ms, T2W1 TR 3200–4000 ms, TE100–150 ms; Parameters for BWI/SPIR series included TR 2600–3000 ms, TE 10–15 ms, the layer thick was 4 mm, distance between layers was 0.4 mm, field of vision was 150 ram and matrix was 512 × 512.

441.2.4 Imaging Evaluation

All the imaging pictures were cooperatively and completely evaluated by two senior radiologists and two senior orthopedists. When their evaluations were in agreement with each other, the diagnosis was made. The evaluation parameters included the distributions of bone fracture, bone morphology, imaging signals and the scope, and the status of bone injury and soft bone injury.

441.2.5 Statistical Analysis

Statistical analysis of the data was performed with SPSS 16.0 software. The calculated data were texted with X^2 test. The $P < 0.05$ was considered to be statistically significant.

441.3 Results

441.3.1 Comparisons of the Accuracy in Diagnosis of Occult Fractures Between MRI and Three-Dimensional Reconstruction by Computerized Tomography

X-ray anterioposterior and lateral films of 76 cases of patients revealed cortical bone and trabecular bone continuity and no contorted bone breaking and no abnormally brightening lines. CT examination revealed 61 cases of patients with occult fractures and the accuracy rate was 80.26 %. The CT imaging pictures displayed sharp edges and clear bone fracture lines without dislocation of the broken ends. Increased local trabecular bone intensity was seen in a few imaging pictures but the arrangement of trabecular bone was disorder. Swollen soft bone tissues surrounding the injured bone and joint effusion were seen in a part of the imaging pictures. MRI examination revealed 70 cases of patients with occult fractures and the accuracy rate of diagnosis was 92.11 %. The MRI displayed that the bone fracture lines in T1W1 series showed line-like signals or irregular sheet-like low signal whereas in T2W1 series and the lipid inhibition series, the bone fracture lines showed low signal and there were high spot-like signal of oedema imaging surrounding the low line-like signals but the boundary lines were not clear.

CT examination diagnosed 35 cases of patients with bone fracture around the knee-joints and the accuracy rate was 87.5 %. MRI revealed 35 cases of patients with bone fracture around the knee-joints and the accuracy rate was 95 %. Comparing the results with two methods, there was no statistically significant difference ($P > 0.05$). CT examination diagnosed 26 cases of patient with vertebral bone fracture and the accuracy rate was 77.22 %. MRI examination diagnosed 32 cases of patients with vertebral bone fracture and the accuracy rate was

Table 441.1 Comparison of accuracy rates with computerized tomography and MRI examinations in diagnosis of patients with bone fracture around knee-joints

	N	Bone fracture around knee-joints		Accuracy rates
		+	–	
CT	40	35	5	87.5 %
MRI	40	38	2	95 %

Table 441.2 Comparison of accuracy rates with computerized tomography and MRI examinations in diagnosis of patients with vertebral bone fracture

	N	Vertebral bone fracture		Accuracy rates
		+	–	
CT	36	26	10	72.22 %
MRI	36	33	3	91.67 %

91.67 %. Comparing the results with two methods, there was a statistically significant difference ($P < 0.05$) (Tables 441.1 and 441.2).

441.3.2 Comparison of the Diagnostic Accuracy Rates in Classification of Bone Fractures

The accuracy rate in diagnosis of recessive trauma bone fracture with computerized tomography examination was 94.12 % in comparison with the 90.20 % accuracy rate with MRI examination, there is no statistically significant difference between two methods. However, the accuracy rate of MRI examination in diagnosis of recessive bone fracture inside the bone reached as high as 94.74 % in comparing with the 73.68 % of the accuracy rate with computerized tomography examination. There was a statistically significant difference between two methods ($P < 0.05$) (Table 441.3 and 441.4).

441.4 Discussion

Injuries to bones and joints frequently occur. The routine X-ray examination for bone fractures after trauma usually obtains satisfactory diagnostic results and the bone fractures can be treated in time. However, for the structurally complex, overlapping joints in four limps of body, pelvis, vertebral body and their accessory tissues, there are limitations with routine X-ray examination. In particularly, the occult fractures are not effectively detected by routine X-ray examination. Thus, clinically, occult fractures are hardly to be diagnosed or missed diagnosed or

Table 441.3 Comparison of accuracy rates with computerized tomography and MRI examinations in diagnosis of patients with recessive trauma bone fracture

	The number of fracture	Recessive trauma bone fracture		Accuracy rates
		+	–	
CT	51	48	3	94.12 %
MRI	51	46	5	90.20 %

Table 441.4 Comparison of accuracy rates with computerized tomography and MRI examinations in diagnosis of patients with recessive bone fracture

	The number of fracture	Recessive bone fracture		Accuracy rates
		+	–	
CT	38	28	10	73.68 %
MRI	38	36	2	94.74 %

misdiagnosed, and thus miss the treatment opportunity [6, 9]. Vellet et al. [12] found that among the patients with the recessive osteochondrous bone fracture and the associated recessive cortical bone fracture due to cortex compression, 67 % of the cases of patients developed seriously osteochondrous complications during a short period of 6–12 month follow up visit. The reason for this is due to the impalpability of bone fracture lines and the overlapping coverage of these bone fracture lines by the bone structure; no dislocation of the bone fracture ends and no abnormal bone morphology. A part of bone fracture is trabecular bone fracture which is not involved in cortex. Thus, paying attention to recognizing the occult fractures is of importance for early diagnosis and early treatment for occult fractures.

The development and availability of computerized tomography and MRI technologies have substantially improved the diagnosis of occult fractures. While X-ray imaging allows observation of the swollen soft tissues, it hardly displays clearly the joint effusion. CT examination can show clearly the anatomy relationships. Full use of the software treatment technology after CT imaging and the CT values is of significance for decisive diagnosis of bone fracture, the vacuum within the joints, hematocete and fatty tissues. Computerized tomography can also show bone fracture and whether it is involved in the nearby joints, whether or not the surrounding tissues are damaged, whether or not there is hematoma and the degree of their involvement. Thus, computerized tomography examination has certain advantages over X-ray examination. It not only has a faster scanning speed but also has higher density and special resolution. Furthermore, through the reconstruction technologies such as MPR, CPR, SSD, and 3D, computerized tomography can show more clearly and stereoscopically the morphology and location of bone fractures [11]. Imerci et al. [5] pointed before conservative treatment of patients, especially in cases of possible cervical spine and pelvic region fractures, CT should be requested, even if the radiography is normal.

MRI has the advantages of forming imaging at any angles and having higher resolution toward soft tissues. It can show clearly the abnormal signals of the bone continuity breaking, bone marrow blooding and oedema. On one hand, it can eliminate the influence of the X-ray's overlapping shade, overcome the disadvantage of uneasily recognizing the bone fracture due to the limitation of patient's body position; On the other hand, it has high resolution toward soft tissue and can perform multi-layer and multi-series scanning, can recognize the local bleeding and oedema within bone marrow cavity caused by trabecular bone breaking and can also show clearly the bone fracture lines formed by intertwining the broken trabecular bone [4, 7]. Hakkarinen et al. [3] believed that although 64-slice CT was helpful in the diagnosis of occult hip fracture, but one should not completely exclude the diagnosis based on a negative 64-slice CT scan in a patient with persistent, localized hip pain who cannot bear weight. Sankey et al. [10] illustrated the high incidence of fractures which were not apparent on plain radiographs, and showed that MRI was useful when diagnosing other pathology such as malignancy, which may not be apparent on plain films. Oka et al. [8] believed that MRI played an un-replaceable role in diagnosis of recessive bone fracture and in making the decision for treatment scheme for bone fracture. Thus, MRI is considered as the best method for early diagnosis of recessive bone fracture.

Comparing with MRI, computerized tomography has limitations in resolution toward soft tissues and cross-section scanning. It has a lower sensitivity in diagnosis for bone fracture underneath cortical bone and for a part of the occult fractures whose bone fracture lines are arranged horizontally. This disadvantage has been confirmed by this study. In present study, we found that there was no statistically significant difference in accuracy rate in diagnosis of the bone fracture around the knee-joints and the traumatic recessive fracture between computerized tomography and MRI. The reason is that the bone fracture around the knee-joints and the traumatic recessive fracture are mainly cortex bone fracture and they can be shown relatively clearly by both computerized tomography and MRI. However, for the vertebral bone fracture and the recessive osteochondrous bone fracture, the accuracy rates of diagnosis with computerized tomography were 72.22 and 73.68 %, respectively, in comparison to accuracy rates of 91.67 and 94.74 %, respectively, with MRI. There are statistically significant differences in both rates between two methods ($p < 0.05$). Its reason is that the vertebral bone fracture and the recessive osteochondrous bone fracture are mainly the local bleeding and oedema within the bone marrow cavity. While MRI is not as good as computerized tomography in showing the bone fracture lines, MRI most clearly shows noticeable comparison of T1W1 with the bone morrow-containing normal bone tissues and is highly sensitive to bone marrow oedema after trauma. Furthermore, because it has the advantages of good resolution toward the soft tissue density, multi-layer and multi-series imaging, MRI can show clearly the status of soft tissues around the bone fractures, which further confirm bone fractures.

441.5 Conclusions

In summary, with the popularization of computerized tomography and MRI in diagnosis of trauma and increasing attentions toward the diagnosis of recessive bone fracture, minimization and prevention of the complications caused by occult fractures, such as long-term pain and movement disorder, osteochondrous injury, and degenerated joint diseases, is of clinical importance and significance. While both computerized tomography and MRI can easily detect the bone fractures that are not recognized from X-ray film and whose clinical signs and symptoms are not clear, MRI is highly sensitive to bone marrow bleeding and oedema and has the advantages of having better resolution toward the soft tissues and is capable of forming multi-layer and multi-series imaging. MRI can easily detect the occult fractures that are not shown by x-ray film and computerized tomography imaging and it can clarify many types of injuries and thus has high value and clinical applications.

References

1. Ahn JM, El-Khoury GY (2007) Occult fractures of extremities. Radiol Clin North Am 45(3):561–579, ix
2. Gumina S, Carbone S, Postacchini F (2009) Occult fractures of the greater tuberosity of the humerus. Int Orthop 33(1):171–174
3. Hakkarinen DK, Banh KV, Hendey GW (2012) Magnetic resonance imaging identifies occult hip fractures missed by 64-slice computed tomography. J Emerg Med 43(2):303–307
4. Hayter CL, Gold SL, Potter HG (2013) Magnetic resonance imaging of the wrist: bone and cartilage injury. J Magn Reson Imaging 37(5):1005–1019
5. Imerci A, Canbek U, Kaya A et al (2013) Distribution of occult fractures detected in emergency orthopedic patient trauma with computerized tomography. Ulus Travma Acil Cerrahi Derg 19(2):157–163
6. Kim KC, Ha YC, Kim TY et al (2010) Initially missed occult fractures of the proximal femur in elderly patients: implications for need of operation and their morbidity. Arch Orthop Trauma Surg 130(7):915–920
7. Nachtrab O, Cassar-Pullicino VN, Lalam R et al (2012) Role of MRI in hip fractures, including stress fractures, occult fractures, avulsion fractures. Eur J Radiol 81(12):3813–3823
8. Oka M, Monu JU (2004) Prevalence and patterns of occult hip fractures and mimics revealed by MRI. AJR Am J Roentgenol 182(2):283–288
9. Rennie WJ, Finlay DB (2003) Posttraumatic cystlike defects of the scaphoid: late sign of occult microfracture and useful indicator of delayed union. AJR Am J Roentgenol 180(3): 655–658
10. Sankey RA, Turner J, Lee J et al (2009) The use of MRI to detect occult fractures of the proximal femur: a study of 102 consecutive cases over a ten-year period. J Bone Joint Surg Br 91(8):1064–1068
11. Stevenson JD, Morley D, Srivastava S, et al (2012) Early CT for suspected occult scaphoid fractures. J Hand Surg Eur vol 37(5):447–451
12. Vellet AD, Marks PH, Fowler PJ et al (1991) Occult posttraumatic osteochondral lesions of the knee: prevalence, classification, and short-term sequelae evaluated with MR imaging. Radiology 178(1):271–276

Chapter 442
Identifying Questions Written in Thai from Social Media Group Communication

Chadchadaporn Pukkaew and Kanchana Kanchanasut

Abstract To encourage greater student participation and more efficient instruction, we propose a method for classifying text questions communicated through a social media channel used as an informal complement to academic coursework. Specifically, we implement a system that uses basic regular expressions (BRE) to extract and organize Thai questions posted in class-related Facebook groups. Test data is used to identify the most effective identifiers and to evaluate the system as a whole, in a practical academic context.

Keywords Thai question classification · Pattern matching · Regular expression · Text classification · Information retrieval and filtering · Facebook group

442.1 Background

As described by Nguyen [1] and Pagram and Pagram [2], teachers in Thailand are traditionally respected and considered authoritative. As a result, Thai students may not feel as comfortable asking questions and/or voicing their opinions as western students. Recently, we have found that social networks, used as informal complements to the classroom, present a less forbidding channel of communication between students and teachers. Given the popularity of Facebook among college students, we see a significant opportunity to overcome traditional barriers to course-related communication, via Facebook-style groups and group-supportive

C. Pukkaew (✉) · K. Kanchanasut
Asian Institute of Technology, 58 Moo 9, Km. 42, Paholyothin Highway, Klong Luang, Pathumthani 12120, Thailand
e-mail: chadchadaporn.pukkaew@ait.ac.th

S. Li et al. (eds.), *Frontier and Future Development of Information Technology in Medicine and Education,* Lecture Notes in Electrical Engineering 269,
DOI: 10.1007/978-94-007-7618-0_442,

communication functions. We also see an opportunity for instructors to monitor and address a larger number of student questions than would be possible under traditional communication channels.

Formal and systematic use of Facebook in instructional settings remains rare and the potential to strike a more productive balance between fun and serious work in education is relatively unexplored [3, 4]. Students' primary motive for using Facebook is social presence, including the real-time presence provided by Facebook's messaging functions [5]. A typical student spends 10–60 min/day using Facebook to keep in touch with friends, even in the face of known risks to privacy and security [4].

In Thailand, Socialbakers [6], May) reported that there are approximately 18 million Facebook users. Of these, the largest age group is 18–24, comprising a total of 6 million, or 33 % of Thai Facebook users, followed by the next largest age group, 25–34. This concentration of young adult users presents a massive opportunity for Facebook as an educational channel, complementing either traditional or distance learning in both formal and informal contexts.

442.2 Related Work on Question Classification

A number of techniques for question classification have been successfully applied to question answering systems. Most notable are those involving natural language processing (NLP), machine learning, and support vector machines (SVM) [7–12].

Thai question answering systems have been proposed by several researchers. Jitkrittum et al. [13] implemented an open-domain question answering system using Thai Wikipedia as a knowledge base. Specifically, they harvested the information provided in the "infoboxes" of Thai Wikipedia articles and restructured it according to the resource description framework (RDF). Kongthon et al. [14] implemented a semantically enabled question answering system, focused on Thailand tourism information. Question answering systems for farmers have also been proposed, by Suktarachan et al. [15]. Their study focused on query analysis and annotation, relying on the semantic model of "what" and "how" queries, lexical inference identification, and semantic roles, to find the best answer.

Our approach differs from the above in three respects. First, we want to use Facebook as a casual communication channel among students and instructors, and thereby reduce the sense of formality and authority that traditionally hampers such communication. Second, we want to provide Facebook as a complementary channel through which students can post questions, ask for explanations, and share opinions about class sessions with both instructors and peers. Third, we want to identify and extract questions relevant to a given course so that the instructor can more easily manage answers and explanations.

442.3 Proposed Approach

As an informal complement in education, this approach is a very first solution for identifying questions written in Thai communicated through a social media channel. Thai is a highly ambiguous, non-inflectional language. Most Thai words are built by compounding two or more words, without affixations of nouns and verbs, tenses of verbs, ablaut, umlaut, and long-short vowel alternations.

Close relatives and friends always use informal Thai when speaking amongst themselves. This informal language, which has long been distinct from the formal, written language established under Old Thai, has undergone a number of sound alterations throughout history. As a result, the informal text messaging of Thai teenagers differs significantly from conventional written Thai (e.g., เปล่า (plāo[1]) to ปาว)pāo), อะไร (arai) to อาราย) ārāi), เหรอ(roē) to หรอ(rø), and ไม่เสร็จ(mai set) to ม่ายเสด)māi sēt)).

442.3.1 *Regular Expression*

Basic Regular Expressions (BREs) provide a computational method for locating character sub-strings using a context-independent syntax [16–18]. Our approach uses a single BREs to locate Thai question keywords in Facebook group posting.

442.3.2 *Thai Question Keywords*

Basic Thai Question Keywords (BThQkeywords) Some of our question keywords are taken directly from the LEX*i*TRON[2] dictionary, which also provides synonyms and related words. We omitted LEX*i*TRON keywords that could be used in either questions or statements such as หรือ) reū—meaning "or"), ยังไง) yang-ngai—meaning "how"), and ไง)ngai—meaning "how"). Because Thai is a non-inflectional language, however, these omitted keywords could be included in combination with words used to end a yes–no question (e.g., roē) and the gendered particle used after a vocative or at the end of a question, as in, for example, คะ)kha—for women) and ครับ (krub—for man). In these cases, the combined pattern could be treated reliably as a question indicator, as in ยังไงเหรอ(yang-ngai roē), ไงเหรอ) ngai roē), ยังไงคะ (yang-ngai kha), ยังไงครับ (yang-ngai krub), หรือคะ (reū kha), and หรือครับ (reū krub). In all, our BThQkeywords includes 51 Thai question keywords from the dictionary (including the question mark '?').

---

[1] The pronunciation of Thai words were quoted from http://dict.longdo.com/index.php

[2] LEX*i*TRON Thai-English Dictionary. Available at: http://lexitron.nectec.or.th

Additional Thai Question Keywords (AThQkeywords) Besides the question keywords drawn from the dictionary, certain words used in conversation were added. These words were identified through observation of two sources of data: (1) the frequently ask questions (FAQ) and question and answer (Q&A) sections of several Thai websites covering a number of topics, and (2) 31 Facebook groups covering a range of topics and mostly populated by college instructors and students. The former resource had 2,000 messages containing nearly equal numbers of questions and non-question messages. The latter resource had a total of 3,450 messages with a relatively small proportion of questions. Tests were performed using the BThQkeywords search pattern on these datasets, revealing that some questions were identified as non-questions (False Negative: FN), and some non-questions were identified as questions (False Positive: FP). We also found that some question keywords with the same meaning, but different spellings, had been used by students. For instance, a number of teenagers typed the word เหรอ (roē) as หรอ(rø), ไหม (mai) as มั๊ย(māi), and ทำอย่างไร (tham yāngrai—meaning "how") as ทำไง) tham ngai). In addition, negative words such as ไม่ได้ (mai dāi—meaning "not") and ไม่ใช่ (mai chai— meaning "not") were combined to the word เหรอ (roē) to make them interrogative (e.g., ไม่ได้เหรอ (mai dāi roē), ไม่ได้หรอ (mai dāi rø), ไม่ใช่เหรอ (mai chai roē), and ไม่ใช่หรอ (mai chai rø)). Some forms of questions that anticipate an answer were also added to the search pattern. For example, the word ขอถาม (khø thām—meaning "ask for"), ขอคำแนะนำ (khø khamnaenam—meaning "ask for suggestion"), and รบกวนถาม (ropkūan thām—meaning "disturb someone by asking a question"). To select these 160 additional Thai question keywords, we used the AThQkeywords search pattern illustrated in Fig. 442.1.

It should be noted that two keywords, ฤ (reu) and ฤา (reu), were omitted because they are strongly associated with poetic expression, and do not appear in regular conversation. In all, the 212 Thai question keywords we targeted are expressed in the pattern listed in Fig. 442.2.

442.3.3 Thai Question Identification Process

The process of identifying questions written in Thai are illustrated in Fig. 442.3.

First, FAQ and Q&A messages were taken and stored in a database while Facebook group resources (e.g., basic user and group information) were

```
$ptn="(ใคร(คะ|ครับ|เหรอ|หรอ|หนอ))|((ยัง|ยาง)*(ไง|งัย|งาย)(เหรอ|หรอ|คะ|ครับ|คับ))|
    ((ไหม|หรือ|เหรอ|หรอ)(คะ|ครับ|คับ))|((ไม่|ม่าย)(ใช่|ช่าย|ได้|ด้าย)(หรือ|เหรอ|หรอ))|
    (ด้วย(หรือ|เหรอ|หรอ))|((ทำ|ทาม)(ไม|มาย|ไง|งัย|งาย))|((มั้ย|เหรอ|หรอ)(คะ|ครับ|คับ)*)|
    (อยาก(ทราบ|รู้|ถาม))|((ขอ|เรียน|สอบ)*ถามว่า)|((ขอ|เรียน)ถาม)|((อย่าง|อะ|อา)(รัย|ราย))|
    (หรือ(เปล่า|ป่าว|ไม่)(คะ|ครับ|คับ)*)|((รบกวน)*ขอ(ความรู้|คำแนะนำ|ความคิดเห็น|ปรึกษา))|
    (ขอ(เรียน|คำ)*ปรึกษา)|(มี(ความเห็น|คำแนะนำ)(ว่า)*(ยังไง|อย่างไร))|(ช่วย(แนะนำ|ชี้แนะ))|(ขอคำชี้แนะ)";
```

Fig. 442.1 The 160 AThQkeywords search pattern

กี่, เมื่อใด, ขณะใด, เมื่อไร, ตอนไหน, เมื่อไหร่, คราวไหน, ครั้งไหน, เพียงใด, แค่ไหน, เพียงไร, ไฉน, ฉันใด, ทำไม, เพราะเหตุใด,
อย่างใด, อย่างไร, เช่นใด, เช่นไร, กระไร, เพราะเหตุไร, เพื่ออะไร, ด้วยเหตุใด, เพราะอะไร, เท่าไร, กี่มากน้อย, เท่าไหน, เท่าไหร่,
เท่าใด, เพราะเหตุอะไร, เหตุใด, เหตุไฉน, เวลาใด, คราใด, ครั้งไร, ไหน, สิ่งไร, หรือไร, หรือไง, หรือไม่, หรือเปล่า, หรือยัง, เหตุไร,
ที่ไหน, ที่ใด, แห่งไหน, แห่งใด, อะไร, ประการใด, อย่างไรบ้าง, อย่างไรเล่า, ใครคะ, ใครครับ, ใครเหรอ, ใครหรอ, ใครหนอ, ไงเหรอ,
ไงหรอ, ไงคะ, ไงครับ, ไงคับ, งัยเหรอ, งัยหรอ, งัยคะ, งัยครับ, งัยคับ, งายเหรอ, งายหรอ, งายคะ, งายครับ, งายคับ, ยังไงเหรอ,
ยังไงหรอ, ยังไงคะ, ยังไงครับ, ยังไงคับ, ยังงัยเหรอ, ยังงัยหรอ, ยังงัยคะ, ยังงัยครับ, ยังงัยคับ, ยังงายเหรอ, ยังงายหรอ, ยังงายคะ,
ยังงายครับ, ยังงายคับ, ยางไงเหรอ, ยางไงหรอ, ยางไงคะ, ยางไงครับ, ยางไงคับ, ยางงัยเหรอ, ยางงัยหรอ, ยางงัยคะ, ยางงัยครับ,
ยางงัยคับ, ยางงายเหรอ, ยางงายหรอ, ยางงายคะ, ยางงายครับ, ยางงายคับ, ไหมคะ, ไหมครับ, ไหมคับ, หรือคะ, หรือครับ, หรือคับ,
เหรอคะ, เหรอครับ, เหรอคับ, หรอคะ, หรอครับ, หรอคับ, ไม่ใช่หรือ, ไม่ใช่เหรอ, ไม่ใช่หรอ, ไม่ช่ายหรือ, ไม่ช่ายเหรอ, ไม่ช่ายหรอ,
ไม่ได้หรือ, ไม่ได้เหรอ, ไม่ได้หรอ, ไม่ด้ายหรือ, ไม่ด้ายเหรอ, ไม่ด้ายหรอ, ม่ายใช่หรือ, ม่ายใช่เหรอ, ม่ายใช่หรอ, ม่ายช่ายหรือ,
ม่ายช่ายเหรอ, ม่ายช่ายหรอ, ม่ายได้หรือ, ม่ายได้เหรอ, ม่ายได้หรอ, ม่ายด้ายหรือ, ม่ายด้ายเหรอ, ม่ายด้ายหรอ, ด้วยหรือ, ด้วยเหรอ,
ด้วยหรอ, ทำไม, ทำมาย, ทำไง, ทำงัย, ทำงาย, ทามไม, ทามมาย, ทามไง, ทามงัย, ทามงาย, มั้ย, เหรอ, หรอ, มั้ยคะ, มั้ยครับ, มั้ย
คับ, เหรอคะ, เหรอครับ, เหรอคับ, หรอคะ, หรอครับ, หรอคับ, อยากทราบ, อยากรู้, อยากถาม, ถามว่า, ขอถามว่า, เรียนถามว่า,
สอบถามว่า, ขอถามว่า, เรียนถาม, อย่างรัย, อย่างราย, อะรัย, อะราย, อารัย, อาราย, หรือเปล่า, หรือป่าว, หรือไม่, หรือเปล่าคะ, หรือ
เปล่าครับ, หรือเปล่าคับ, หรือป่าวคะ, หรือป่าวครับ, หรือป่าวคับ, หรือไม่คะ, หรือไม่ครับ, หรือไม่คับ, ขอความรู้, ขอคำแนะนำ, ขอ
ความคิดเห็น, ขอปรึกษา, รบกวนขอความรู้, รบกวนขอคำแนะนำ, รบกวนขอความคิดเห็น, รบกวนขอปรึกษา, ขอปรึกษา, ขอเรียน
ปรึกษา, ขอคำปรึกษา, มีความเห็นยังไง, มีความเห็นอย่างไร, มีคำแนะนำยังไง, มีคำแนะนำอย่างไร, มีความเห็นว่ายังไง, มีความเห็นว่า
อย่างไร, มีคำแนะนำว่ายังไง, มีคำแนะนำว่าอย่างไร, ช่วยแนะนำ, ช่วยชี้แนะ, ขอคำชี้แนะ, ?

Fig. 442.2 The 212 Thai question keywords

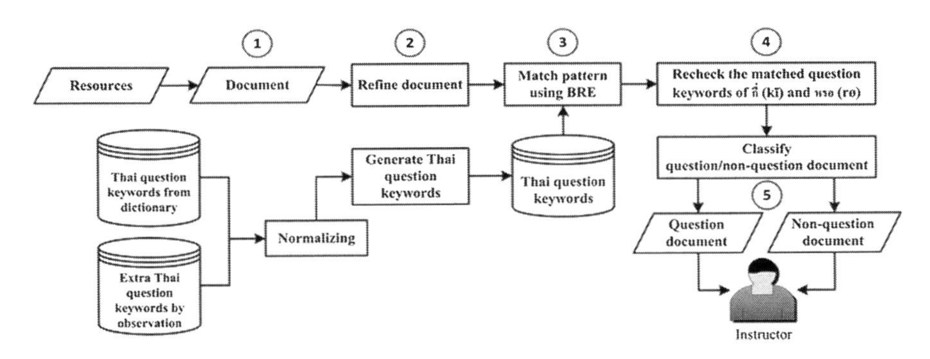

Fig. 442.3 Logical view of Thai question classification process

extracted using the Facebook API (http://developers.facebook.com/). Two applications, based on the same Thai question identification scheme were then used to process the messages from both resources.
Second, a filter was applied to remove irrelevant messages and contents, including emails, URLs, and emoticons.
Third, the question identifier, based on the search pattern described in Sect. 442.3.2, was used to classify documents as questions or non-questions.
Fourth, questions were rescanned for the question keywords กี่ (kī—meaning "how much" or "how many") and หรอ (rø) to increase precision.
Finally, the classified documents were presented to the instructor.

442.4 Experiments and Discussion

The following sections discuss the results of our question identification process when used on test data.

442.4.1 Results for the FAQ and Q&A Datasets

The collected 2,000 datasets were divided into 10 volumes of varying size so that performance with different volumes of data could be compared. The efficiency of the identifiers was measured using three ratings: precision, recall, and F1-measure.

Performance of BThQkeywords Search Pattern Identifier Results indicated an average precision of 95.20 % and an increase in recall scores as dataset size increased. F1-measures increased slightly and then leveled off after 800 documents.

Performance of AThQkeywords Search Pattern Identifier Results indicated an average precision of 95.94 % and an increase in recall scores as dataset size increased. Again, F1-measures increased slightly and then leveled off after 800 documents.

Comparison of Identifiers' Performance on FAQ and Q&A Content Although AThQkeywords generally outperformed BThQkeywords, the AThQ-keywords identifier was more stable overall, as it uses both dictionary and spoken language question keywords to identify less formal questions from the dataset. Note that the FAQ and Q&A datasets used more formal language, and so had fewer typo and spelling errors (Fig. 442.4).

442.4.2 Results of the 31 Facebook Groups Dataset

As above, the collected 3,450 datasets were divided into 12 volumes of varying sizes and the precision, recall, and F1-measure of the identifiers were measured.

Performance of BThQkeywords Search Pattern Identifier of Facebook Groups Results indicated an average precision of 81.24 % and an increase in recall

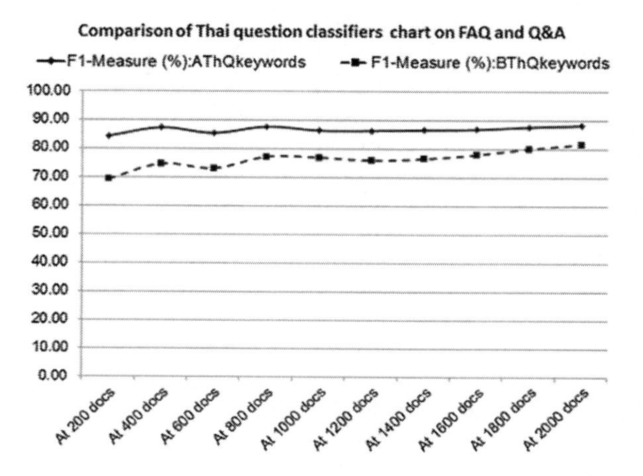

Fig. 442.4 Thai question identifier performance chart on FAQ and Q&A datasets

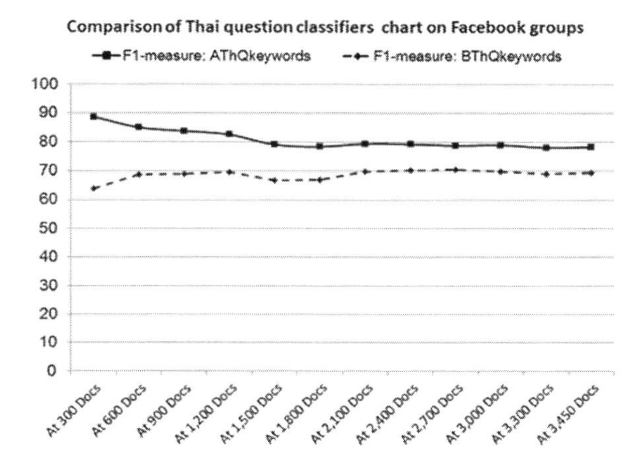

Fig. 442.5 Thai question identifier performances chart on facebook group dataset

scores as dataset size increased. F1-measures increased slightly and then leveled off after 2,100 documents.

Performance of AThQkeywords Search Pattern Identifier of Facebook Groups Results indicated an average precision of 83.04 % and an increase in recall scores as dataset size increased. F1-measures increased slightly and then leveled off after 1,500 documents.

Comparison of Identifiers' Performance on Facebook Groups The AThQkeywords identifier generally outperformed the BThQkeywords identifier. Note that, compared to the FAQ and Q&A content, these datasets contained less formal use of the language, as well as more typos and spelling errors (Fig. 442.5).

Performance of AThQkeywords Identifier on Facebook Groups Used as Informal Communication Channels in Education In the Facebook groups dataset, nine of the 31 groups processed were for different courses taught by four separate instructors. The messages extracted from these nine Facebook groups were taken only from the last 3 months of two semesters in 2012. The first instructor had a total of 419 posts in his Facebook groups, the second instructor 94 posts, the third 39 posts, and the fourth 78 posts. On these, the AThQkeywords identifier showed 94.19 % precision, 76.42 % recall, and 84.38 % F1-measure.

Note that some non-questions were misidentified as questions, due to occasional use of keywords in non-question contexts. Likewise, questions may have been misidentified as non-questions, due to typos or unanticipated abbreviations. It should be noted that the present identification scheme does not include question keywords transliterated from regional dialectical question words.

When using Facebook groups as an informal educational communications channel, especially in Asia, we suggest that an instructor set up a Facebook group for the given course, with the explicit purpose of encouraging informal communications. To keep usage of the Facebook group focused, s/he can post guidelines for politeness and topicality while also making clear that messages need not be limited to course material.

442.5 Conclusion and Future Work

In this paper, we presented a BRE-based system for identifying Thai questions among text posts to course-related SNS groups. Question keywords were drawn from the LEX*i*TRON dictionary and observational data to form a single search pattern covering 212 keywords in total. We performed experiments on 2,000 datasets taken from the FAQ and Q&A sections of various websites and on 3,450 datasets taken from 31 different Facebook groups, all of which were used as informal communication channels by instructors, college students, and/or other communities. Based on these experiments, we found that the AThQkeywords identifier generally outperforms the BThQkeywords identifier.

We believe our approach can be applied to non-inflectional languages besides Thai. In future work, we want to extend question classification into subtopics, so that inquiries can be properly summarized for instructors. We would also like to apply our approach to domain ontologies, knowledge acquisition, and information extraction.

Acknowledgments The author wishes to acknowledge the Office of the Higher Education Commission, Thailand, for a support grant under the Strategic Scholarships for Frontier Research Network program for a Joint Ph.D. Program; and Rajamangala University of Technology Lanna for the partial support given to her during her study at the Asian Institute of Technology (AIT), Thailand. In addition, the author would like to express their greatest appreciation to Dr. Choochart Haruechaiyasak for his valuable suggestions during the planning as well as Professor Dr. Sumanta Guha for his valuable comments of this study.

References

1. Nguyen T (2008) Thailand: cultural background for ESL/EFL teachers. [online] Available at: http://www.hmongstudies.org/ThaiCulture.pdf. Accessed 25 October 2012
2. Pagram P, Pagram J (2006) Issue in e-learning: a Thai case study. Electron J Inf Syst Dev Ctries 26(6):1–8
3. Green T, Bailey B (2010) Academic uses of facebook: endless possibilities or endless perils? J TechTrends 54(3):20–22
4. Hew KF (2011) Students' and teachers' use of facebook. Comput Hum Behav 27(2):662–676
5. Cheung CMK, Chiu P, Lee MKO (2011) Online social networks: why do students use facebook? Comput Hum Behav 27(4):1337–1343
6. Socialbakers (2013) Check facebook. [online] Available at: http://www.checkfacebook.com/. Accessed 19 May 2013
7. Hacioglu K, Ward W (2003) Question classification with support vector machines and error correcting codes. In: Proceedings of the 2003 conference of the North American chapter of the association for computational linguistics on human language technology: companion volume of the proceedings of HLT-NAACL 2003–short papers, vol 2. Canada, pp 28–30
8. Harabagiu SM, Maiorano SJ, Paşca MA (2003) Open-domain textual question answering techniques. Nat Lang Eng 9(3):231–267
9. Li X, Roth D (2002) Learning question classifiers. In: Proceeding of the 19th international conference on computational linguistics, vol 1. Stroudsburg, PA, USA: Association for Computational Linguistics, pp 1–7

10. Moschitti A (2003) Answer filtering via text categorization in question answering systems. In: Proceeding of the 15th IEEE international conference on tools with artificial intelligence, IEEE, pp 241–248
11. Saquete E, Martınez-Barco P, Munoz R, Vicedo JL (2004). Splitting complex temporal questions for question answering systems. In: The 42nd annual meeting on association for computational linguistics, Association for computational linguistics, pp 566–574
12. Suzuki J, Taira H, Sasaki Y, Maeda E (2003) Question classification using HDAG kernel. In: Proceedings of the ACL 2003 workshop on multilingual summarization and question answering, July 11, 2003, Sapporo, Japan, pp 61–68
13. Jitkrittum W, Haruechaiyasak C, Theeramunkong T (2009) QAST: question answering system for ThaiWikipedia. In: Proceeding of the 2009 workshop on knowledge and reasoning for answering questions, ACL-IJCNLP 2009, pp 11–14
14. Kongthon A, Kongyoung S, Haruechaiyasak C, Palingoon P (2011) A semantic based question answering system for Thailand tourism information. In: Proceeding of the KRAQ11 workshop, pp 38–42
15. Suktarachan M, Rattanamanee P, Kawtrakul A (2009). The development of a question-answering services system for the farmer through SMS: query analysis. In: Proceeding of the 2009 workshop on knowledge and reasoning for answering questions, ACL-IJCNPL 2009, pp 3–10
16. Cox R (2007) Regular expression matching can be simple and fast. [online] Available at: http://swtch.com/ ~ rsc/regexp/regexp1.html. Accessed 30 April 2012
17. The IEEE and the Open Group (2004). Chapter 9 regular expressions. [online] Available at: http://pubs.opengroup.org/onlinepubs/009695399/basedefs/xbd_chap09.html. Accessed 30 April 2012
18. Thompson K (1968) Programming techniques: regular expression search algorithm. Commun ACM 11(6):419–422
19. Arpavate W, Cheevasart S, Dejasvanong C (2011) Communication Behavior on facebook of students at Rajamangala University of Technology Phra NaKhon. Rajamangala University of Technology Phra NaKhon, Bangkok

Chapter 443
A Programming Related Courses' E-learning Platform Based on Online Judge

Xiaonan Fang, Huaxiang Zhang and Yunchen Sun

Abstract Coding practice is the most efficient way in learning of programming related courses. In this paper, we propose a programming related courses' E-learning platform based on online judge. This platform is designed according to B/S structure, and page optimization techniques such as Gzip are applied to boost the access speed. Teaching achievements prove that the platform can markedly improve the learning effect of programming related courses.

Keywords ACM-ICPC · Online judge · E-learning · Program design

443.1 Introduction

In programming courses at colleges and universities, the effective method to improve students' programming capability is long-term and a lot of coding practices. This also requires teachers must evaluate the code submitted by the students timely and accurately. Since the artificial evaluation of students' code is time consuming and does not guarantee the accuracy, the teaching results are always not satisfactory.

X. Fang (✉) · H. Zhang · Y. Sun
School of Information Science and Engineering, Shandong Normal University, Jinan, China
e-mail: franknan@126.com

H. Zhang
e-mail: huaxzhang@163.com

Y. Sun
e-mail: sunyunchen@gmail.com

X. Fang · H. Zhang · Y. Sun
Shandong Provincial Key Laboratory for Novel Distributed Computer Software Technology, Jinan, China

S. Li et al. (eds.), *Frontier and Future Development of Information Technology in Medicine and Education*, Lecture Notes in Electrical Engineering 269,
DOI: 10.1007/978-94-007-7618-0_443, © Springer Science+Business Media Dordrecht 2014

Online judge (OJ) system can automatically evaluate programs submitted by the students based on pre-set condition and give feedback to them in a timely manner, make the teacher only need to add and maintain database, without having to care about the evaluation process, so teachers can grasp of students' ability of learning and programming more timely and accurately.

In recent years, some of the teachers and ACM-ICPC coaches began to try to use the online judge system in the teaching and practice of programming courses in university, and have achieved good results. Wen-xin L and Wei G described Poj [1] in their paper, which has been widely used in programming design courses in marking exercise and online test [2]. Kosowski et al. designed SPOJ—a contest and online judge system and applied it to the process of course teaching [3]. Jutge.org is a free access online programming judge developed by Petit et al. Both students and teachers can get help in this system, especially, the authors offer some case studies in this paper [4]. Based on POJ (PKU Judge Online) [1] Luo et al. developed a system called Programming Grid (PG) and it has served for computer-aided education in programming teaching. Practices in computing course prove that PG is useful [5]. Wang et al. presents a practice teaching model of data structure course based on Online Judge. This paper introduces the methods and contents of this model [6].

In this paper, we propose a programming related courses' E-learning platform based on online judge of Shandong Normal University [7]. This system is designed for courses based on program design including Introduction to Computing, C (or Java, C++) programming, Data Structure and Algorithms Design etc. We select classic B/S structure for this platform, and use optimization techniques such as Gzip to improve the access speed. Practices verify that the platform can efficiently improve the teaching effect of programming related courses.

The rest of the paper is organized as follows. First we introduce the Online Judge system in Sect. 443.2. Then the design of the platform and system application is shown in Sects. 443.3 and 443.4. Finally, we conclude in Sect. 443.5.

443.2 Online Judge System

Online judge system was originally used to automatically judge and rank in International Collegiate Programming Contest (ACM-ICPC) [8]. Nowadays it is extensively used for university students' programming training, selection of the team member of the programming contest, the teaching and experimental process in the programming related courses around the world.

443.3 System Design

As a programming related courses' E-learning platform, use in practical teaching process is more important. Therefore, in addition to complete the basic functionality of OJ system, we add capability that can support and manage different programming languages. The platform should also be used to categorize questions, and support online job submission and examination.

443.3.1 System Structure

The main structure of the platform is based on classic B/S framework, and the elements are shown in Fig. 443.1:

In Fig. 443.1, the browsers are the part that the user can directly contact. The web server can handle requests from the browser, realize the user operation, obtain the needed information through exchanging data with the database server and judge server, then returns the result to browsers. The database server is used to store all the data of the system. The judge server is utilized to evaluate the code submitted by the user, then returns the results to web server.

443.3.2 Page Compression

Because performing the program on the server and transporting information from server to the browser consumes a lot of time, and the servers always located within the education network of schools, non-education network access may be very slow, it is necessary to compress the pages of the platform.

In HTTP 1.1 protocol (rfc2616), it is allowed to transfer data using compression algorithms. In the process of the request, the browser can be set supported decompression algorithms in Accept-encoding of the head file, the server gets the decompression algorithm that the browser supports, then use the corresponding compression algorithm compresses, to reduce transmission slowness caused by bandwidth reasons. Most of the current browsers support two compression algorithms, Gzip and Deflate, respectively. As Gzip's compression rates higher, we choose it as the compression algorithm of system pages. Table 443.1 compares some important OJ system files' size before and after compressing using Gzip algorithm.

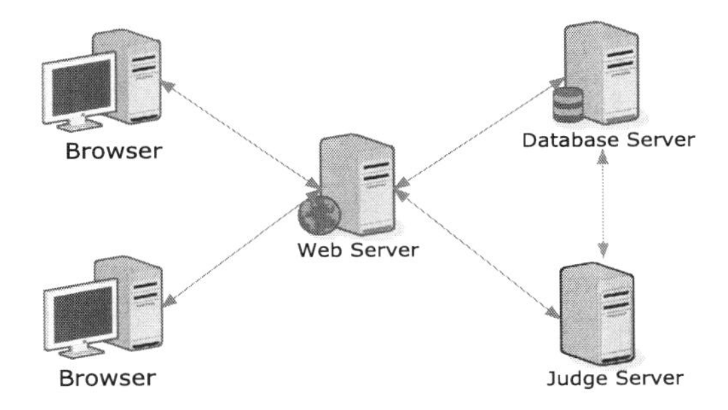

Fig. 443.1 System structure

Table 443.1 Comparison of some important OJ system pages' size

Page name	Before/after compression/ compression ratio	Description
Default.aspx	6.46 KB/2.89 KB/44.74 %	Home page of OJ system
ProblemSet.aspx	33.76 KB/6.36 KB/18.84 %	First page of the list of questions (100 questions)
Problem.aspx	7.02 KB/2.60 KB/37.04 %	The first question page (A + B problem)
Ranklist.aspx	16.80 KB/4.09 KB/24.35 %	First page of the user ranking list (50)

We can see from the table that Gzip's compression rate is satisfactory, especially in the case of these are a large number of similar content or similar format on a single page, the compression rate is particularly high. So if the CPU usage of the web server is not high, subsequently opening the page compression is very useful for faster access.

443.4 System Applications

As shown in Fig. 443.2, the platform's menu items are consisted of online judge module, online training module, online contest module, and user panel module. After register and login users can choose a programming course or ACM-ICPC problem to practice.

Since the E-learning platform has been implemented, more and more teachers have begun to select our platform as an E-learning environment, and about 1200 students have used this platform for program design learning. In 2012, our university received the gold medal of the ACM-ICPC Shandong province contest, and the bronze medal of the ACM-ICPC Asian regional contest.

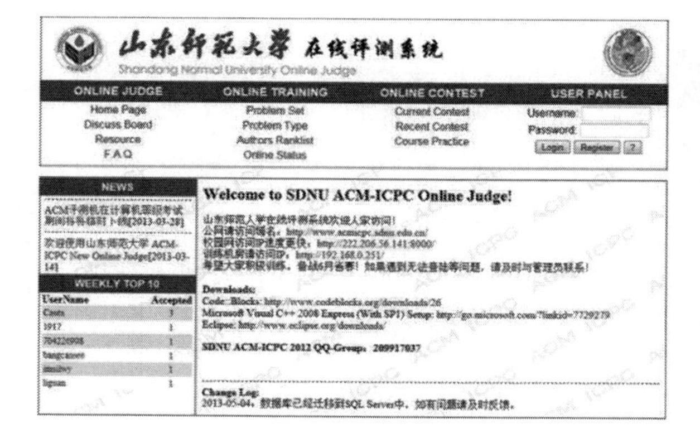

Fig. 443.2 Main interface of the platform

443.5 Conclusion

Facts prove that the E-learning platform can greatly reduce the teachers' time spent on checking the correctness of the student code, algorithm performance, plagiarism, homework completion and accuracy of statistical work, make teachers have more time to communicate with students, answering questions and give reasonable evaluation result, fully mobilize students' learning interest and motivation. In our future work, we will focus on further improving the execution efficiency of the OJ system and adding new programming languages to the platform.

Acknowledgments This research is supported by the National Science Foundation of China (No.61170145), the Specialized Research Fund for the Doctoral Program of Higher Education of China (20113704110001), the Science and Technology Projects of Shandong Province, China (ZR2010FM021, 2008B0026 and 2010G0020115) and the Teaching Reform Projects of Shandong Normal University (2012).

References

1. POJ. POJ[EB/OL]. http://poj.org/
2. Li W, Wei G (2005) Peking University online judge and its applications. J Changchun Post and Telecommun Inst, S2
3. Kosowski A, Małafiejski M, Noiński T (2008) Application of an online judge & contester system in academic tuition. Advances in web based learning–ICWL 2007. Springer, Berlin, pp 343–354
4. Petit J, Giménez O, Roura S (2012) Jutge. Org: an educational programming judge. In: Proceedings of the 43rd ACM technical symposium on computer science education. ACM, pp 445–450
5. Luo Y, Wang X, Zhang Z (2008) Programming grid: a computer-aided education system for programming courses based on online judge. In: Proceedings of the 1st ACM summit on computing education in China on first ACM summit on computing education in China. ACM, p 10
6. Wang T, Luo Y, Zuo K (2010) The research in practice teaching of data structure based on online judge. Comput Educ 10:028
7. SDNUOJ. SDNUOJ[EB/OL]. http://www.acmicpc.sdnu.edu.cn/
8. Skiena SS, Revilla MA, Revila MA (2003) Programming challenges: the programming contest training manual. Springer, Heidelberg

Chapter 444
Leading and Guiding Role of Supervisors in Graduate Education Administration

Huaqiang Zhang, Xinsheng Wang and Hannan Fang

Abstract Education administration is a quality supervision and security system in the process of graduate education. It is important both in innovation and development of graduate education and improvement of academic dissertations. The practice ability for innovation is a basic standard of the education quality. Supervisors play a leading position and guiding role during the period. The reason is that the level of dissertation, the realization of innovation and the formation of ideal faith for graduates are highly related to their supervisors' academic ability and character. A new education mode can benefit resources integration, group wisdom playing and improve the education quality.

Keywords Graduate · Administration · Supervisor · Cultivate quality · Education mode

444.1 Introduction

Graduate education is involved in many fields such as admission, cultivation, student status, discipline, degree, supervision, morality, employment and so on. Strengthening system construction, improving educational administration and awareness of services are basis for doing a good job of graduate management. As a quality supervision and security system in the process of graduate cultivation, education management plays a significant role in innovation and development of graduate education and improvement of academic dissertations. Faced with the difference between academic and practical graduate cultivation models, graduate education administration should make normative documents which cater to

H. Zhang (✉) · X. Wang · H. Fang
Harbin Institute of Technology, Wenhua Xi Road 2, Weihai 264209, China
e-mail: zhq@hit.edu.cn

S. Li et al. (eds.), *Frontier and Future Development of Information Technology in Medicine and Education*, Lecture Notes in Electrical Engineering 269,
DOI: 10.1007/978-94-007-7618-0_444,

development of colleges and insist on tracking management which means tasks being shared, inspected, supervised, feedback and adjusted as well as human-oriented management and service conception. The leading and guiding role of supervisors in graduate education can give a full play of their potential in teaching.

444.2 Connotations of Graduate Educational Management

Cultivation scale and quality are not only important mark of improving educational levels, but also the motivation sources of promoting academic development. The aim of graduate education is to cultivate high-quality talents who are equipped with a solid foundation of theories and professional knowledge as well as creative ability to do research. Cultivation of specialized knowledge during graduate period is the extension of professional knowledge instead of time continuing of undergraduate education period. It requires that graduates should be equipped with broad knowledge reserves and active thinking skills to integrate and overlap disciplines [1]. Supervisors are the disseminators of knowledge and practitioners of cultures because of their knowledge structures and educational conceptions.

The essence of graduate education is to cultivate versatile talents with studying and creative ability by finishing disciplines, participating in science and technology innovation activities, taking specific projects. The guidance and influence of supervisors are lying in imparting professional knowledge, inheritance of national culture, the guidance of the scientific research subject and academic achievements enhancement, throughout the process of graduate cultivation. Supervisors' own value orientations, academic accomplishments, personalities affect the academic style and level of graduate constantly.

444.3 Instruction Models of Supervisors

Moral education is preliminary because it is infiltrated into professional education [2]. Communication between graduates and teachers, schools, enterprises, social is involved in classroom teaching, graduation projects studying and innovation practice process. Cultivating creative talents who adapt to socialist modernization construction should start from the cultivation of noble moral sentiments and solid professional knowledge. Teachers' team construction is the key to improve quality of graduate education.

444.3.1 Quality of Supervisors

Supervisors' own quality is embodied in professional quality and moral quality. The so-called professional qualities advocate scientific spirit of seeking truth from facts. It requires that the supervisors should have high academic level, rich teaching experience, active scientific thinking and gain recognition from graduates and peers. The so-called moral qualities require dedicated spirit of responsibility and education. It is embodied in the noble professional ethics, strong sense of responsibility and mission, effective organization and coordination ability.

Supervisors should have rich teaching experience, high academic level and certain influence so that they can guide the graduates in correctly selecting scientific projects, confirming research methods and refining innovation means. Teachers should focus on discipline development and maintain research direction so that they can keep pace with time and lay a foundation for subject selection.

At present, graduate tutors not only bear teaching tasks, but also a lot of scientific researches. Without scientific research projects, there is no platform for tutors to cultivate practices skills. However, too many scientific research tasks will take more time, therefore supervisors should ensure plenty of energies to guide them. Graduates have higher learning and management ability, but it needs an adaptive process to transfer from undergraduates to graduates. As graduates, they are faced with many problems such as busy courses learning, less chance to meet teachers and to take part in the sciences researches maybe they will feel troubled and confused. So the supervisors should usually concern them, especially in the mental health and the changing of thinks.

444.3.2 Professional Guidance of Supervisors

Supervisors are leaders in graduates learning. Supervisors should give timely guidance on learning methods. They should create science and technology practice opportunities by reforming innovation education and actively building face-to-face platform. It is important that exploring the connotation of academic graduate and applied graduate classification cultivate. Improving science and technology practice and training quality of graduates [3, 4].

With the enlargement of graduate education scale, the supervisors should expand their research scope and refine new research subjects because their research topics may not meet the requirements of multiple graduates. Supervisors should make reasonable assessments of subjects such as research depths, innovative points and so on.

Graduates will encounter all sorts of problems in research process, some are even beyond the research field of tutor which requires teachers to keep pace with time, raise their academic accomplishments, widen new knowledge and consult the couples.

Accumulation of knowledge is important because there are no creative achievements without substantive research. Cultivating graduates' ability to find and solve problems independently. At present, the graduate education is mostly single-teacher training mode. Improving the cultivation of single mode has become more and more important. The training mode with dual supervisors is worthy of extension. This form includes many ways such as campus–campus model, college–college model, college-enterprise joint cultivation model, etc. [5]. Exploring dual-supervisor training mode which is beneficial to widening the graduate's field of vision will promote the all-round development of graduate education.

Teachers and students are friends in "Tutor taking responsibility system" [6], because the difference between graduates is inevitable. Therefore, teachers should equally treat every graduate, respect the equal relationship between teachers and graduates.

444.4 Conclusions

Supervisors play a great role in graduate education. Tutors' spirits of enterprising, responsibility and dedication are three major pillars of graduates' growth. The combination of theory and practice promotes the discipline intersection and integration of knowledge. Dual-supervisor cultivation model will integrate scientific research resources among mentors and cultivate innovative graduate with high quality. Tutor system will give graduates correct guidance according to individual differences and aptitudes so that graduates can form the correct outlook on life and values, self correction in learning and research activities and become a pillar of the community talent.

References

1. Geng J (2009) An analysis of graduate education management's influence and role [J]. Graduates Forum 10:124–126
2. Zhang H, Wang X, Fang H (2012) Position and role of supervisors in graduate education administration. J Harbin Inst Technol (Soc Sci Edn) 14(Supplement 2):19–21
3. Niu G, Zhang H (2011) Characteristics of professional degree and professional degree graduate education quality [J]. J Grad Stud Educ Res 4:81–85
4. Zheng X, Li W (2012) Some thinking on reform of the professional degree postgraduate education. Degree Grad Educ 4:15–19
5. Zeng F, Cao M, Tang Y (2008) The construction of multi-tutor cultivation model. Wuhan Inst Technol (society & science) 21(2):264–267
6. Diao C (2010) Modern society calls for mentors [J]. Degree Grad Educ 11:22–23

Chapter 445
Development of Dental Materials Network Course Based on Student-Centered Learning

Shibao Li, Xinyi Zhao, Lihui Tang and Xu Gong

Abstract Network course is a sum of subjects that related to teaching content and activities through network. Student-centered learning is a modern learning methodology comparing to the traditional teacher-centered learning, it is an active learning of students in the state of dominant position. Dental Materials is an important course for dental school students. The course covers typical aspects of dental materials science such as basic science for dental materials and clinical dental materials. According to the basic characteristics of network course and independent learning, we have designed and developed Dental Materials network course based on student-centered learning. The practice shows that the network courses based on student-centered learning has built an open, and real-time space where teachers guide students and students study independently. At the same time, a variety of teaching methods and medium are coexistent and interactive. Dental Materials network course has promoted innovation capacity of students favorably. It's a good way to improve teaching and learning quality of dental materials.

Keywords Network course · Student-centered learning · Dental materials · Design and development

445.1 Introduction

As the development of modern information technology in the education, e-learning becomes more and more important in the teaching profession field. Network course, is an necessary component of the network educational resources, which is the main way to promote innovation in education, to share high quality teaching resources,

S. Li · X. Zhao (✉) · L. Tang · X. Gong
Department of Dental Materials, School of Stomatology, The Fourth Military Medical University, 145# Changle West Road, Xi'an 710032 Shaanxi, China
e-mail: zhaoxinyi@fmmu.edu.cn

S. Li et al. (eds.), *Frontier and Future Development of Information Technology in Medicine and Education*, Lecture Notes in Electrical Engineering 269,
DOI: 10.1007/978-94-007-7618-0_445,

and comprehensively improve the quality of education [1, 2]. But some colleges and universities have reported dropout rates over 60 % in e-learning courses [3–5]. Recently, developments in education have emphasized student-centered learning over teacher-centered learning. Student-centered learning is based on a constructivist theory of learning whereby each individual students constructs their own understanding based on their prior knowledge and current learning experiences. By student-centered learning, the learners can use and actively control their cognition, motivation and behavior to study online course [6, 7]. Dental Materials is an important course for dental school students, the course covers typical aspects of dental materials science such as basic science for dental materials, clinical dental materials, laboratory and related dental materials. The success or failure of many forms of dental treatment depends upon the right selection of materials, possessing adequate properties, as well as careful manipulation of these materials [8, 9]. By studying dental materials course, students can grasp the fundamental knowledge about the capabilities and limitations of various dental materials. This knowledge will be of prime importance for all clinical courses and dental treatment that require the use of dental materials. There are some big challenges for students to learn dental materials by traditional teaching methods.

According to the network course characteristics and the requirements of learners independent study, how educators build dental materials network course based on student-centered learning and implement the best teaching effect of online course are important issues currently.

445.2 Design of Dental Materials Network Course Based on Student-Centered Learning

445.2.1 The Concept of Student-Centered Learning

Student-centered also called autonomous learning or flexible learning relates to the change in focus in the classroom from the teacher to the student. This is based on a constructivist theory of learning whereby each individual student constructs their own understanding based on their prior knowledge and current learning experiences. Student-centered learning is a modern learning comparing to the traditional teacher-centered learning. Student-centered learning takes students as the learning subject and students learn more independently. Students learn objectives by independent analysis, exploring, practice, question, creating and some other ways. In this learning model, students can select learning content, determine learning method, design learning time, monitor learning process, and evaluate learning result by themselves. Student-centered learning reflects the initiative, autonomy, and consciousness of students as the main body of learning, it enables students to regulate their psychology and behavior in a planned fashion according to their own learning goals.

Table 445.1 Student-centered and teacher-centered continuum

Student-centered learning	Teacher-centered learning
High level of student choice	Low level of student choice
Student active	Student passive
Power primarily with the student	Power is primarily with teacher

Learning is often presented in this dualism of either student-centered learning or teacher-centered learning. In the reality of practice the situation is less black and white. A more useful presentation of student-centered learning is to see these terms as either end of a continuum, using the three concepts regularly used to describe student-centered learning (see Table 445.1).

445.2.2 Network Course Design Based on Student-Centered Learning

Student-centered learning refers to integrated learning activities of student independently obtaining knowledge and using knowledge to solve problems under the guidance of teachers. According to the characteristics and composition of network course and the requirements of student-centered learning, we have built and designed the network course. There are different interfaces (i.e. web pages) for students and teachers, for example, when a student logs in the network course, the web page include nine modules, i.e. teaching tips, real-time learning, discussion, works, questions, testing (including self-testing, examination, and score) notes, learning log, and related resources. When a teacher logs in the network course, the web page include 10 modules, i.e. teaching tips, real-time teaching, discussion, works assignment, answering questions, exam marking, notes, teaching log, related resources, and e-classroom configuration.

445.3 Development of Dental Materials Network Course Based on Student-Centered Learning

445.3.1 Learning Content Design and Preparation

According to characteristics of the curriculum and requirements of learning objectives, we provide students with content-rich learning resources and system-perfect knowledge structure. The purpose of the Dental Materials course is to provide a thorough understanding of the fundamental nature and behavior of dental materials. The course content will include study of the composition, properties,

Table 445.2 The modules of dental materials network course

Module 1 Curriculum planning	Module 2 Resources preparation	Module 3 Curriculum configuration	Module 4 Teaching and learning	Module 5 Evaluation and analysis
Curriculum information	Raw materials	Teaching tips	Real-time teaching	Teacher's log
Chapter structure	Textbook	Web textbook	Discussion	Resources statistics
Knowledge points	Exam questions	E-teaching plans	Works assigning	BBS statistics
E-classroom style	–	Teaching lectures	Works marking	Works analysis
E-class homepage	–	Related resources	Questions answering	Exam analysis
–	–	–	Exam organization	Questions analysis

application, and manipulation of metal, ceramic and polymeric dental materials. The characteristics of dental materials are content complex, abstract, systematic poor, and application strong. The "composition-structure-performance-manipulation" relationship of material is the mainline of the course. The teachers should grasp the mainline when organize course content, choose the most suitable activities to achieve the objectives. As a whole structure of the course website, Dental Materials network course composes of five modules including curriculum planning, resources preparation, curriculum configuration, teaching and learning, evaluation and analysis as shown in Table 445.2. For example, when we dealt with raw materials management in module 2 resource preparation, we prepared enough resources, i.e. audio segment 50, animation 26, video section 62, pictures and images 364, literatures and references 217, and exam questions 620. When we dealt with teaching lectures in model 3 curriculum configuration, we recorded teachers' teaching lectures more than 40 h.

In order to facilitate student learning, according to the mainline of "composition-structure-performance-manipulation" relationship of materials, we integrated learning content into five knowledge modules in each chapter including introduction, chapter study, something about material, knowledge expo and video download. Thus, course content is more efficiently and integrated mainline is much clear. A wealth of supporting information related to the course is displayed, content rich learning resources and system-perfect knowledge structure are provided.

445.3.2 Online Teaching and Learning

In student-centered learning method, teachers should establish a student-centered concept, change students' role, use modern educational thoughts to guide students learning, thinking and creating in the process of independent study. We have established teachers guidance modules and teacher–student communication space (i.e. BBS). Each chapter also has a study guide, test guide and other guidance modules to help students self-learning. At the same time, online exchange community is established, students can consult to teachers online, teachers can guide students learning online. Teachers and students also can communicate by emails.

445.3.3 Evaluation and Analysis

In order to test the learning effect, in the network course, each knowledge unit or each chapter is designed with self-testing and formative exam module. Online exercises and testing module provide different types of exercises and test questions for students, along with suggested answers to help students understanding their own grasp of the content. By this way, students can assess their learning effect and get further guidance to develop further study plan.

445.4 Practice Results

The developed Dental Materials network course has been used successfully for dental school students for 3 years. During the past 3 years, the students have learnt two chapters via network course independently, and learnt other chapters via traditional course and network course. We have had formative six examinations online. Students have raised 124 questions by BBS system. The practice shows that the network courses based on student-centered learning has built an open, multi-level, and real-time space where teachers guide students and students study independently. At same time, a variety of teaching methods and medium are coexistent and interactive.

445.5 Summary

Teaching and learning by network course, the teachers have changed their roles from simple knowledge transmitter and classroom management into a provider of educational resources and navigator of student learning. Dental Materials network course has promoted innovation capacity of students favorably. It’s a good way to improve teaching and learning quality of dental materials.

References

1. Xie Y (2005) Development and application of network course. Electronic Industry Press, Beijing
2. Renata B, Jana M (2012) E-learning as a motivation in teaching physics. Proc Soc Behav Sci 64:328–331
3. Levy Y (2007) Comparing dropout and persistence in e-learning course. Comput Educ 48:185–204
4. Sun P, Tsai R, Finger G et al (2008) What drives a successful e-learning? An empirical investigation of the critical factors influencing learner satisfaction. Comput Educ 50:1183–1202
5. Nichols A, Levy Y (2009). Empirical assessment of college student-athletes' persistence in e-learning courses: A case study of a U.S. National Association of Intercollegiate Athletics (NAIA) institution. Internet and Higher Education, pp 1214–25
6. Lindahl B, Dagborn K, Nilsson M (2009) A student-centered clinical educational unit-description of a reflective learning model. Nurse Educ Pract 9:5–12
7. Wang H (2011) Development and implementation of engineering materials and thermal processing network course based on autonomous learning. Proc Eng 15:127–131
8. Noort R (2002) Introduction to dental materials (Second edition). Mosby Ltd, London
9. Sakaguchi R, Powers J (2012) Craig's restorative dental materials (Thirteenth edition). Elsevier Mosby, Philadelphia

Chapter 446
Research and Practice of Practical Teaching Model Based on the Learning Interest

Tao Gao, Bo Long, Pingan Du and Yefei Li

Abstract In this research, the practical teaching model based on the learning interest has been investigated. Taking the course 'CAD/CAE/CAM' into consideration, a practical teaching platform based on the differences of students' learning interest has been built, and then the experimental course and the learning process have been designed. And a good teaching effect is achieved in practice.

Keywords Interested differences · Computer-aided design · Computer-aided engineering · Computer-aided manufacturing · Practical teaching platform

446.1 Introduction

The undergraduate education is a critical period for students to learn the basic knowledge and to know the overall quality, so it is in the basis and guiding position in the personnel training system of the research-oriented university [1]. How to do in the undergraduate education of the research-oriented university is an important issue of Chinese universities converting to world-class university with 'Features, Research-oriented, and Opening up-style'. Raising the students' learning interest and teaching students according to their aptitude are one of the most important parts for achieving the goal of the undergraduate education of the research-oriented university.

Many world-class universities treat the organic combination of social needs and personal interests as an important basis for building innovative training model [2, 3].Comparing with the similar foreign universities, the most obvious difference of China's university is whether to put the interest of the students in the first place.

T. Gao (✉) · B. Long · P. Du · Y. Li
School of Mechanical, Electronic, and Industrial Engineering, University of Electronic Science and Technology of China, Chengdu 611731 Sichuan, China
e-mail: gaotao@uestc.edu.cn

S. Li et al. (eds.), *Frontier and Future Development of Information Technology in Medicine and Education*, Lecture Notes in Electrical Engineering 269,
DOI: 10.1007/978-94-007-7618-0_446,

In recent years, China's universities also do a lot of attempts on training model based on the students' interest, such as recruiting students by the large classification of subjects, turning professional in college, dual-degree, double major and minor professional. But the effect is not obvious enough. Mainly performances are that the concept of education cannot adapt to development needs of the social and economic, the incentives cannot mobilize the enthusiasm of the teaching reform, and the teaching environment and conditions cannot meet the demand for personnel training based on students' interests. Therefore, the concepts of education must be changed, the students' subject choices and personal expression must be emphasized, the investment in teaching software and hardware must be increased, and the needs of different learning interest students must be meted. In this research, a practical teaching model based on the students learning interest has been designed and practiced.

446.2 Design and Practice of Practical Teaching Platform Based on the Students' Interest

446.2.1 Overall Design Ideas

There are significant differences of student interest in learning something. The students' interest should be taken into account while designing the practical teaching platform. In order to improve its function and optimize its performance, the practical teaching platform needs to be sustained secondary development, and the cycle of 'test-assessment-retest' needs to be repeated. Its overall design concept is shown in Fig. 446.1.

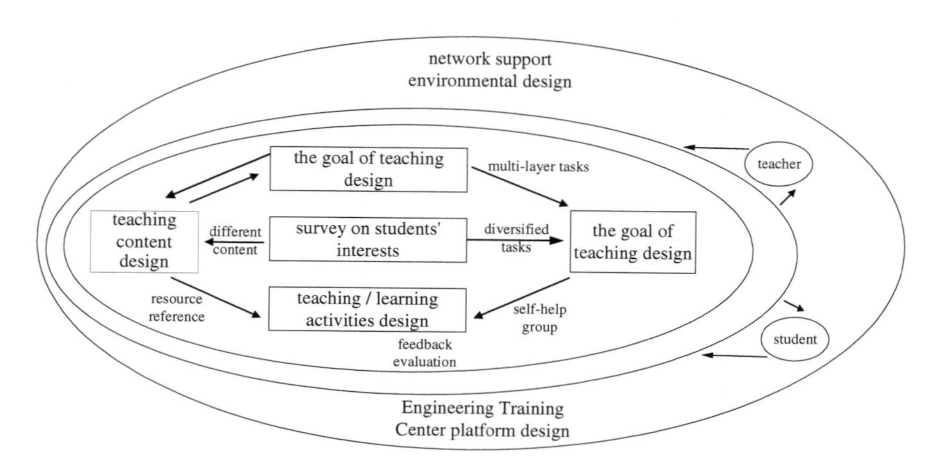

Fig. 446.1 The overall design ideas of the practical teaching platform

446.2.2 Teaching Experimental Design

The course 'CAD/CAE/CAM' involves in computer graphics, numerical control technology, finite element method, computer simulation and integrated technology of computer information, and covers the entire process from product design and analysis to numerical control programming. Because this course requires the higher level of practice and there are significant differences in the students' interest and focus point, the teaching experiments of this course have been taken into consideration in this research. The hierarchical experimental teaching system has been proposed [4, 5]. It is based on theoretical teaching, and plays the important role in obtaining the innovative consciousness and innovation capability. The teaching experiments consist of cognitive practice, basic experiment, selected experiment and innovative experiment. In the cognitive practice, students are organized and arranged to visit these research and development departments of the advanced enterprises. The cognitive practice can help the students to understand the application of CAD, CAE, CAM technology in the large-scale manufacturing enterprises, and help them to increase the intuitive understanding to the technology in industrial applications and to arouse students' enthusiasm for learning. The basic experiment consists of establishing the three-dimensional model of the bracket and the coffee pot, analyzing the structural beams, the sheet round hole and the coupling with finite element software, using the Mastercam to automatic program for 2D milling and using the Mastercam to numerical control program for 3D the milling surface machining. According to the latest developments in machinery industry, the basic experiment will be revised annually. The aim is to consolidate the theoretical knowledge and to master the methods and skill of the basic operation. The selected experiment is more difficult than the basic experiment. It is consisted of the design of the assembly modeling, the static analysis for gear, three-dimensional bearing analysis for the thin-walled cylindrical, the dynamic analysis and the thermal analysis. The experiments combine with the cutting-edge dynamic of scientific research, the research projects and the social application. It requires the students to select the experimental subjects with their interests. The purpose is to train the research thinking of the students. The teachers use the sub-topics within the capability of the undergraduate as the innovative experiment. The students can select the innovative experiment with their own ability and interest.

446.2.3 Teaching Platform Design

The design of the Practical teaching platform based on the learning interest is consisted of the design of the teachers' platform and the design of the students' platform. Each section contains multiple functional modules. The system structure is shown in Fig. 446.2.

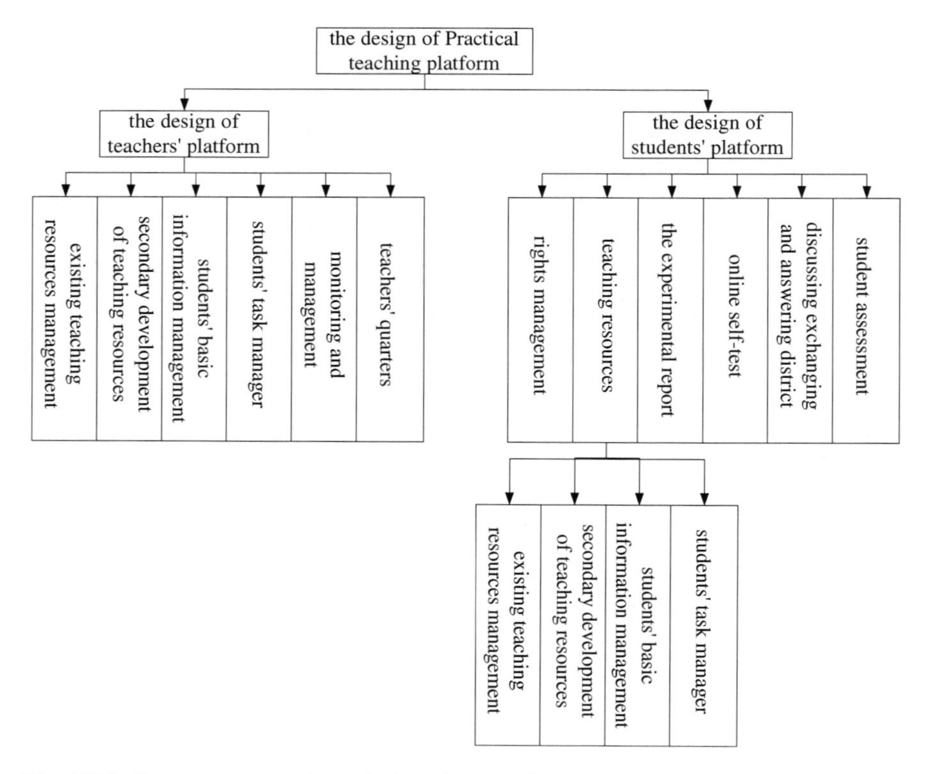

Fig. 446.2 System structure of practical teaching platform

The design of teachers' platform is consisted of six modules, which is designed for teachers to have the permissions to operation. The works of teachers have four main aspects: information dissemination, information management, 'teachers' quarters' and the secondary development of the teaching content of practical experiments.

The information dissemination includes publishing practical experiment content, self-test questions and learning tasks. Their formation managements include students' basic information management, student task management and monitoring management. The 'teachers' quarters' is a personal web page which is designed for the teachers. The teachers can publish the courseware, send and receive operations, browse students' Message and answer the problems of the students in the 'teachers' quarters'. It makes the combination of the classroom teaching and online teaching, the curricular learning and extra-curricular learning come true. And the Interactive teaching mechanism is established. According to the news of the machinery industry, teachers develop some typical practical teaching experiment. The secondary development of the teaching content of practical experiments can meet the different needs of students.

The main works of the students are accessing the teaching resources, submitting the experimental reports and completing the online self-test, discussing and exchanging between the teachers and students, and evaluating the practical teaching platform. The teaching resources include the latest industry information, academic lectures, links to related sites and sub-level practical experiments. Through evaluating the practical teaching platform, teachers can understand the inadequacies of the work and correct the platform.

446.2.4 The Learning Process Design

The learning process has been designed as follows.

(1) After the students log in the platform, they have to accomplish all the basic experiments independently and submit appropriate lab report. The teachers audit the report. After passing the audit, the students can participate in the post-test module test. The students who pass the test (test scores between 80 and 100) can select the selected experiment with their interests.
(2) After entering the selected experiment, the students can take the research individually or group work discussion, and select and complete the experiments, the number of experiments required to achieve the provisions of the college. And then, the students have to submit appropriate lab report. After passing the audit, the students can participate in the post-test module test. The students who pass the test (test scores between 60 and 100) can select the innovative experiment with their interests.
(3) After entering the innovative experiment, the students can take the group work discussion, select at least one innovative experiment. And then, the group has to submit the report. After passing the audit, the students can participate in the post-test module test. The students who pass the test (test scores between 60 and 100) can obtain the credits of this course.

In practical experiment learning of the three levels, the students whose test scores failed must continue to participate in the experimental study, they can also enter the experimental study of a lower level. Before passing the current experiment, they are not allowed to enter the higher level experiment. The students who pass the test scores can enter all level experimental learning.

446.2.5 The Results Achieved

The course group of the 'CAD/CAE/CAM' of Mechanical and Electronic Engineering of UESTC purposed the practical teaching model, and it greatly changed the concept of teacher education and achieved good teaching results.

On the one hand the students change from passive learning to active learning and change from emulate verify to actively explore. The knowledge structure of the students are strengthened and improved in the sub-level experiment. Hands-on capability has been improved. The ability to combine theory and practice of .students and the research capacity on accessing to information, analyzing problems and solving problem is cultivated. On the other hand, students accumulate knowledge, train capacity and exercise thinking in the discussion. Taking more than 360 of the 12 classes of 08 and 09 undergraduate students of Mechanical and Electronic Engineering for example, through the learning and training of the hierarchy of practical teaching experiment based on each student interested, the students' overall quality is significantly improved. Each student has the innovation consciousness and ability of research universities required in the direction of their interest. And experts and students praise it. Specific circumstances visible to the following page: http://222.197.165.195/wlxt/ncourse/cadcaecam/web/cad/jxxg/thpj.html.

446.3 Conclusions

The interest in learning is the internal driving force for the students. In the experimental teaching process of the course 'CAD/CAE/CAM', the practical teaching platform has been developed for students with different learning interest. It provides the multi-level and wide-ranging practical teaching experiment, and it provides multiple choice and wide stage for students. It makes a good teaching and achieves the objectives of undergraduate education for the research-oriented universities.

References

1. Wang J, Zhang W, Wang H (2005) Create research undergraduate teaching system to enhance the quality of teaching. Tsinghua J Educ 26(4):1–4
2. Yu X, Zhang H, Jing Z (2009) Research of personalized talent cultivation model and teaching methods. China Univ Teach 2:34–36
3. Heacox D (2004) Differentiated instruction-help every student to be successful (trans: Yang X). Chinese Light Industry Press, Beijing
4. Gao T, Du P (2010) Discussion on teaching method of "CAD/CAE/CAM technology. Exp Sci Technol 8(1):88–90
5. Du P, Gao T, Li Y (2010) Teaching and practice of "CAD/CAE/CAM technology. Exp Sci Technol

Chapter 447
Developing and Applying Video Clip and Computer Simulation to Improve Student Performance in Medical Imaging Technologist Education

Lisha Jiang, Houfu Deng and Luyi Zhou

Abstract It is generally agreed that practice section is a mandatory part for effective medical imaging technologist education. In order to improve student performance in practice section in medical imaging technologist education, video clips and a computer simulation system were developed and applied. Student performance was evaluated and compared between two classes, one with the application of the video clips and computer simulation system, the other without. The students scored 4.5 points higher in the 4 three-hour practice sections because of the help of video clips and computer simulation. Statistical analysis using independent samples *t*-tests indicated that the difference was statistically significant. However, there was no significant difference between the scores in other aspects of student performance, including multiple-choice question sections and Q & A section in the term exam. It was concluded that in medical imaging technologist education, video clips and computer simulations that focus on practical procedures improved student performance in practice section.

Keywords Video clip · Computer simulation · Mathematical model · Medical imaging technologist · Nuclear medicine

447.1 Introduction

It is generally agreed that practice section is a mandatory part for effective medical imaging technologist education. While we are seeing a rapid expansion of full-time residential students in the discipline of medical imaging technologist education,

L. Jiang · H. Deng · L. Zhou (✉)
Department of Nuclear Medicine, West China Hospital, Sichuan University Sichuan University, Chengdu 610041 Sichuang, China
e-mail: zhouluyi@scu.edu.cn

S. Li et al. (eds.), *Frontier and Future Development of Information Technology in Medicine and Education*, Lecture Notes in Electrical Engineering 269,
DOI: 10.1007/978-94-007-7618-0_447,

we developed and applied video clips and computer simulations to improve student performance and help more effective use of limited practice hour and practice facilities.

447.2 Materials and Methods

447.2.1 Course Description

The compulsory course, named "basic nuclear physics and nuclear medicine instrument", is offered to medical imaging technologist student who, after graduation, is expected to be a capable medical imaging technologist in clinical departments of radiology, nuclear medicine, and ultrasound. It is also an elective course for students from related disciplines such as medical physics. Apart from several introductory lecture on basic nuclear physics, the course offers lectures and 4 three-hour practice sections in nuclear medicine instrumentation—fundamental theory and practical application of mechanical and electrical devices used in nuclear medicine technology including gamma cameras, single photon emission computed tomography (SPECT) and positron emission tomography (PET). Instrumentation includes theory, acquisition, processing, and quality control procedures.

447.2.2 Video Clips

Video clips were used to motivate and increase the interest of the students to learn nuclear medicine instruments and their applications (Fig. 447.1).

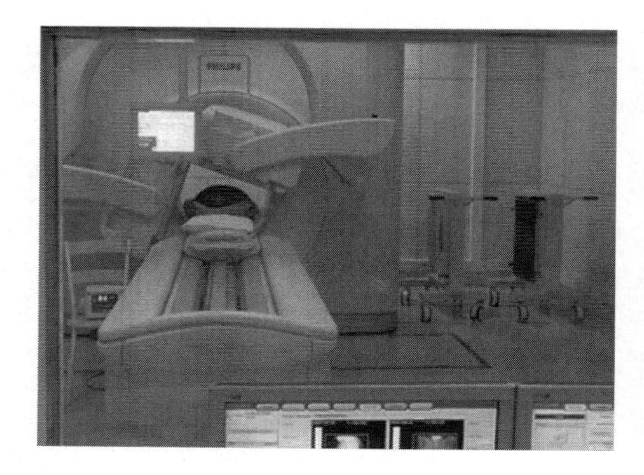

Fig. 447.1 Screenshot of a video clip on gated cardiac SPECT acquisition

Video clips were recorded and edited to demonstrate topics that are difficult to show with static images or text such as a procedure that has multiple steps. The students will learn how nuclear medicine procedures (acquisition and processing) are conducted and the general rules of conducting a procedure. Video clips included content in the following- selecting instrument and imaging data acquisition parameters for a procedure, positioning the patient and obtaining images, recognizing artifacts on static, dynamic, gated and SPECT images that are due to instrumentation malfunction.

447.2.3 Computer Simulation

Computer simulation focused on nuclear medicine image acquisition. A nuclear medicine planar image acquisition simulation system was developed using MATLAB 7.0 (The Mathworks, Inc.), which can simulates the performance of a gamma camera under various conditions such as intrinsic resolution, matrix size, collimators, acquisition duration, etc. This simulation system is a further development and application of our previous mathematical model [1]. Using that mathematical model, we were able to generate realistic images with artificial lesions of changeable location, shape, size and lesion/background ratio from previously acquired images. To simulate the performance of gamma camera, variables and parameters were augmented, modified, and/or fine tuned.

Figure 447.2 demonstrates a example of such changes in order to simulate static image acquisition of a gamma camera with an open acquisition duration. This type of acquisition is difficult and highly skilled because in the acquisition the technologist has to judge the quality of the image in term of lesion detectability and noise level. Once started, the acquisition will run continuously until the technologist decide that the quality is adequate to make diagnosis. In Fig. 447.2a, an image with lesion is generate using the mathematical model. In Fig. 447.2b, a low pass filter is applied to remove the noise from the image. In Fig. 447.2c, the image pixel counts are normalized in accordance with the elapsed acquisition time and randomized with Poisson distribution, and the image is displayed to students. In Fig. 447.2d, steps in Fig. 447.2c is repeated, with a longer elapsed acquisition time. Note that in Fig. 447.2c, because the pixel counts are low and noise level high, the lesion is hardly visible and the acquisition should continue. But in Fig. 447.2d, the pixel counts are adequate and the lesion is visible and the acquisition could be terminated. In actual nuclear medicine image acquisition, nuclear radiation is inevitable, but this simulation system make it possible for students to practice the acquisition procedures as many times as they like without worry about radiation hazard.

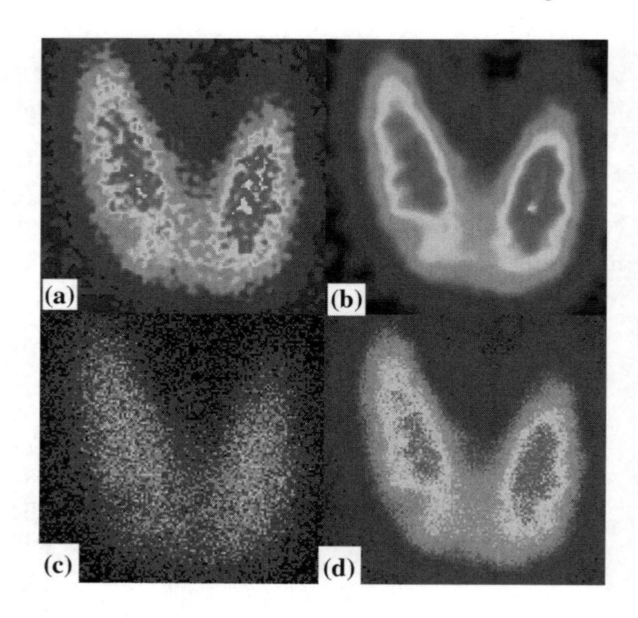

Fig. 447.2 Steps in the simulation of gamma camera static acquisition (detailed in the paragraph)

447.2.4 Application and Student Performance Evaluation

During the academic term of year 2012, the video clips and computer simulation system were used in a class of 48 medical imaging technology students. The student performance was compared with the performance of another class of 40 medical imaging technology students who had the same course content and lecture instructors, and practice instructors, except the above mentioned video clips and computer simulation system, in the year 2011. The student performance included the average score of 4 three-hour practice sections, score of term exam, score of each section in the term exam, and the term final score which was derived from the practice sections, term exam, class presentation and homework. The term exam questions were drawn from the same test bank used for the medical imaging technology students. And the term exam were composed of a single-choice question section, a multiple-choice question section and a Q & A section. Scores were compared using independent samples *t* test at 95 % confidence level, with SPSS for Windows 11.0 (SPSS Inc.) The goal was to determine if the application of the video clips and computer simulation system produced any significant difference in student performance between the two classes.

447.3 Results

Student performance was evaluated by comparing the scores between the two classes. As is evident from Table 447.1, the students scored 4.5 points higher in practice sections after using the video clips and computer simulation. Statistical

Table 447.1 Comparison of student performance in year 2011 and 2012

Item	Years	Mean	Std. deviation	*T*	P value (two tailed)
Practice	2011	82.48	9.64	−2.319	0.023[1]
	2012	87.00	8.44		
Term exam	2011	80.98	8.58	−0.864	0.390
	2012	82.64	9.44		
Term final	2011	83.66	5.42	−1.010	0.315
	2012	84.87	5.85		
Single-choice	2011	42.65	4.65	0.647	0.519
	2012	42.02	4.41		
Multiple-choice	2011	29.25	5.30	−1.938	0.056
	2012	31.50	5.57		
Q & A	2011	9.07	1.30	−0.128	0.898
	2012	9.11	1.59		

[1] Statistically significant at 95 % confidence level

analysis using independent samples *t*-tests indicates that the difference is statistically significant. However, there is no significant difference between the scores in other aspects.

447.4 Discussion

Studies demonstrated that virtual experimentation provided by interactive computer simulations has a positive impact on students' evolving skills, attitudes and conceptual understanding [2, 3]. When it comes to medical imaging technologist education, the current study indicated that video clips and computer simulations that focus on practical nuclear medicine procedures improved student performance in practice section. In the meantime, they have the follow benefits-overcoming the need for multiple sets of specialized and expensive equipment (e.g. SPECT), and enabling students to perform sophisticated procedures which otherwise requires high levels of technical skill, and maintaining radiation safety.

References

1. Zhou LY, Li L, Kuang AR et al (2003) Developing and application of a mathematical model to generate realistic images with artificial lesions from acquired images. J Nucl Med 44(5S):274P–274P
2. Zacharia ZC, Anderson OR (2003) The effects of an interactive computer-based simulations prior to performing a laboratory inquiry-based experiments on students' conceptual understanding of physics. Am J Phys 71(6):618–629
3. de Jong T (2006) Computer simulations-technological advances in inquiry learning. Science 312(5773):532–533

Chapter 448
Research on the Quality of Life of Patients with Depression Based on Psychotherapy

Zhou Xiaoqiu

Abstract The impact of psychotherapy on the quality of life of patients with depression has been explored. The 102 cases of patients with depression receiving radiotherapy or chemotherapy during treatment with the music, a measured assessment of the quality of life of the indicators of quality of life questionnaire (QLQ-C45) before and after the intervention. Insomnia score was statistically significant ($P < 0.06$) before and after the intervention. Application of psychotherapy can improve sleep; improve patients' quality of life.

Keywords Psychotherapy · Patients with depression · Quality of life

448.1 Introduction

Psychotherapy as a method of psychological intervention clinical application in various fields will help ease the patient tense psychological pressure, lower blood pressure. Studies have shown that psychotherapy on patients rebuild the emotional activities, motivate thinking, increased interest in the surrounding, to motivate behaviours, improve retreat tend to have a positive effect. Especially in the field of patients with depression treatment, because patients with depression patient anxiety, depressive disorder incidence of up to 47–49 %. Patients with depression is a treatment and recovery a long illness, it will make the patient is subjected to the pain of the different stages of treatment and quality of life have also been varying degrees of impact. In recent years, the quality of life of patients with depression there is a growing trend, on this basis; we explore the application of psychotherapy on the quality of life of patients with depression.

Z. Xiaoqiu (✉)
University Hospital, Beihua University, 132013 Jilin, China
e-mail: zhouxiaoqiu@126.com

S. Li et al. (eds.), *Frontier and Future Development of Information Technology in Medicine and Education*, Lecture Notes in Electrical Engineering 269,
DOI: 10.1007/978-94-007-7618-0_448,

448.2 Materials and Methods

Clinical data 2004 January 2007—April sick patients, diagnosed with patients with depression, and more than a primary school education, no previous history of mental illness and disturbance of consciousness, Karnofsky Functioning Scale (Karnof-sky performance status, KPS) score\ 60. Into the group of patients with a total of 38 cases, of which 15 cases of nasopharyngeal carcinoma, lung patients with depression in 11 cases, six cases of breast patients with depression after six cases of liver patients with depression; youngest 19 years old, maximum 76 years, an average of 45.56 years.

448.2.1 Rating Scale

Patients with depression quality of life scale (Quality of Life Questionnaire-Core 30 QLQ-C30), a total of 30 projects, functional subscale physical functioning (PF), role function (RF), cognitive function (CF), emotional function (EF), social function (SF), 3 symptom subscales (fatigue, pain, nausea, vomiting), an overall health subscale (GH) and a single measurement projects (difficulty breathing constitute, insomnia, lack of appetite, constipation, diarrheal, financial difficulties). The Functioning Scale the PF, RF and GH higher the score, the better quality of life; CF, EF, SF and symptom scale and individual measurements project the higher the score, the worse the quality of life. The questionnaire was comparable with that in different countries and regions, its reliability and validity and sensitivity has been validated in a number of countries, successfully used in the clinical studies of patients with depression. Questionnaire by the researchers under the unified guidance language.

448.2.2 Cartesian Functioning Scale

KPS into 10 grades, according to the assessment of the functional status of patients given the range of 0 to 100 points, the higher the score, the better physical function. Up to 100 points, followed by 90, 80, 70 points, which means that researchers different assessment of the patient's physical condition from high to low. 100 indicating normal, with 10 indicating critically ill dying, with 0 representing death. Space environment to a certain extent affect the patient's therapeutic effect, and should therefore be avoided noisy interference environment. We choose a single area of 26 m^2, and from the wards, offices at some distance from a dedicated treatment room; built-in with living flowers and murals with health education, information, and as warm as possible, so that the patient is relaxed, natural and comfortable environment.

448.2.3 Methods Selection

The principles of the "symptomatic soundtrack", based on the patient's level of cultural enrichment, music appreciation and hobby selections. Nervousness, irritability patients election relaxation, quiet music, such as the "Palace Moon" "cold duck swimming" mysterious circle "; dizziness, weakness, fatigue, physical decline the patients selected cheerful kind of music, such as" Clouds Chasing the Moon "Red Beans Love" Minuet "; upset, palpitations, chest tightness patients choose the soft, beautiful, lyrical music, such as" Spring Song "" Gorillas in the Mist "; the depression patients election cheerful kind of music, such as" step by step" "radiant," "Swan Lake Waltz". Based on content classification in compiling the music CD, each music CD playback time of 30 min.

448.2.4 Interfere with the Preparation and Methods

Before the intervention, the patient emptying urine, lying in bed, eyes closed, in a natural state of relaxation. Music player, stereo space surround playback, and in order to avoid the interference of others, each time only one person, per day, each time 30 min, 5 times a week for 4 weeks for an intervention treatment. All patients studied before and after the intervention test of the quality of life; 1st measurement time after the patient is admitted to the acoustic space around the player, in order to avoid the interference of others, each time only one person, once a day, each time for 30 min per week 5 for 4 weeks for an intervention treatment. All the patients studied in the test of the quality of life before and after the intervention; 1st measurement time of patients admitted to hospital after receiving radiation therapy and chemotherapy before intervention. 2nd measurement time 2 d after the end of the intervention applied again QLQ-C30 quality of life assessment situation.

Table 448.1 the intervention QLQ-C30 in function subscale scores

Time	Number of cases	Physical function	Role and function	Cognitive function	Emotional function	social function
Before intervention	38	7.81 ± 1.44	3.65 ± 0.73	3.52 ± 1.63	7.76 ± 2.47	5.24 ± 2.15
After intervention	38	7.77 ± 1.45	3.64 ± 0.62	3.54 ± 1.29	7.80 ± 2.22	5.25 ± 1.86
i		0.175	0.465	−0.865	−1.499	−0.634
p		0.862	0.645	0.394	0.144	0.531

Table 448.2 QLQ-C30 score of six individual measurement items

Time	Number of cases	Difficulty breathing	Insomnia	Lack of appetite	Constipation	Diarrhea	Economic difficulties
Before intervention	38	1.65 ± 0.86	2.11 ± 0.98	1.67 ± 1.02	1.87 ± 1.03	1.11 ± 0.30	3.02 ± 1.15
After intervention	38	1.63 ± 0.79	1.51 ± 0.62	1.70 ± 1.06	2.21 ± 0.76	1.21 ± 0.42	3.05 ± 1.12
t		1.099	2.516	−0.229	−1.871	−1.680	−1.648
p		0.280	0.017	0.820	0.071	0.103	0.110

Table 448.3 QLQ-C30 symptom subscale and overall health subscale score

Time	Cases	Fatigue	Pain	Nausea and vomiting	Overal health
Before intervention	38	5.05 ± 2.69	3.25 ± 1.93	2.89 ± 1.305	9.21 ± 2.21
After intervention	38	5.06 ± 2.59	3.13 ± 1.86	2.88 ± 0.987	9.23 ± 1.95
t		−0.205	1.928	1.222	−0.316
p		0.839	0.190	0.231	0.754

448.3 Statistical Results

SPSS 10.0 statistical package for statistical analysis using the t test was used to compare the before and after intervention quality of life (Tables 448.1, 448.2 and 448.3).

Shown in the table, after the intervention the insomnia score is lower than before the intervention ($P < 0.05$), other quality of life and overall health evaluation before the intervention were not statistically significant ($P > 0.05$).

448.4 Conclusion

According to foreign Derogates (1983) reported that 47 % of patients with depression have significant psychological stress response or psychological disorders. As Hang said, fear of patients with depression is global, because patients with depression means extreme suffering and death. Due to the incidence of patients with depression usually does not cause people's attention, so many patients are diagnosed in the late often accompanied by other symptoms, such as pain, insomnia, indigestion, and most patients; and the long duration of treatment, the patient need to face treatment the emergence of side effects, such as chemotherapy, nausea, vomiting, constipation, fatigue, mouth ulcers, these factors could materially and adversely affect the patient's overall quality of life. This study is based patients with depression psychological and disease characteristics, the implementation of the principle of mainly symptomatic soundtrack. When people get sick, the rhythm of the body is in an abnormal state, choose the appropriate music, harmony through music audio, allows the body to a variety of vibration frequency coordination of activities, to the benefit of the patient back to health. The results of this study show that psychotherapy has a good effect to improve the quality of sleep in patients with patients with depression, statistically significant ($P < 0.05$) before and after the intervention. Due to the application of nature music easily beat the promotion of sound waves of sleep, the sleep center of the brain gradually relaxed, and goes to sleep. Johnson and abroad personalized music for insomnia in elderly women (age > 70 years) is similar to the findings, both of which can improve the patient's quality of sleep. On the positive side, the music as a wonderful sound waves, the role of the human brain, people feel the life force from the natural world, in order to stimulate the love of life; the other hand, it can enrich people's imagination, people with good ideas and vision for the future. For patients with depression, to arouse their courageous battle with patients with depression, recognizing the value of self-existence, face reality, cherish every second of life, actively cooperate with treatment, improve treatment compliance, you can improve the patient's quality of life.

References

1. Min Lu, Xu Hefen, Xia Yuanyuan (1999) Patients with depression with anxiety and depression survey. Chin Ment Health J 13 (3): 187
2. Zhang H (2000) Chen Rong Fang tumor, nursing. Tianjin Science and Technology Press, Tianjin, p 261
3. Wang J, Cuijun N, Chen Z (2008) Patients with depression quality of life and related factors. Chin J Clin Psychol 8 (1):23–26
4. Huang Yao ball, (2004),Wang Kai ovarian patients with depression quality of life survey and analysis. J Nurs 19 (10):938
5. Olschewski M, Schulgen G, Schumacher M et al (1994) Quality of life assessment in clinical patients with depression research. Br J Patients depression 70(1):1–5
6. Hang X, Butow PN, Mciscr B et al (1999) Att-itudes and information needs of Chinese migrant patients with depression and their relatives. Aust NZ J Med 29:207–213

Chapter 449
On Systematic Tracking of Common Problems Experienced by Students

Sylvia Encheva

Abstract Evaluation processes in higher education have been addressed by both educators and computer scientists. While the first group is occupied mainly with the learning side of the problem the latter one is concentrating on approaches that can extract the most useful information from previously collected data applying statistical methods. Results obtained from evaluation of students knowledge can also be analyzed with non-probabilistic methods. They appear to be very helpful for locating those places where improvements have to be made.

Keywords Knowledge · Visualization · Dependencies

449.1 Introduction

Evaluation processes in higher education are in need for improvement. Web-based tests are used in nearly all subjects and learners expect immediate responces. While such demands are no longer a technological problem it is still necessary to work out reliable methods for pattern recognition in educational data. Both educators and computer scientists are occupied with providing solutions to that. While the first group is occupied mainly with the learning side of the problem the latter one is concentrating on approaches that can extract the most useful information from previously collected data applying statistical methods. In this work we consider a non-probabilistic approach.

Applications for computational diagnostics are presented in [1]. Learning and instruction processes are discussed in [2]. Test results in [3] are discussed in terms of option fixation, the base-rate fallacy, response criteria, and alternative

S. Encheva (✉)
Stord/Haugesund University College, Bjørnsong. 45 5528 Haugesund, Norway
e-mail: sbe@hsh.no

S. Li et al. (eds.), *Frontier and Future Development of Information Technology in Medicine and Education*, Lecture Notes in Electrical Engineering 269,
DOI: 10.1007/978-94-007-7618-0_449, © Springer Science+Business Media Dordrecht 2014

plausibility. Two answers were generated for each question: a small answer consisting of their favorite alternative, and a large answer consisting of all alternatives except for their least favorite one.

449.2 Preliminaries

A closure system on a finite set M is a set F of subsets of M such that

(1) $M \in F$ and
(2) $C, C^1 \in F \Rightarrow C \cap C^1 \in F$

A closure system on set M is convex geometry if it satisfies the following properties:

- The empty set is closed
- For every closed set $M_1 \neq M$ there exists $m \notin M_1$ such that $M_1 + m$ is a closed set.

Convex geometries are closure systems which satisfy anti-exchange property, and they are known as dual of antimatroids.

A lattice is a partially ordered set, closed under least upper and greatest lower bounds. The least upper bound of x and y is called the join of x and y, and is sometimes written as $x + y$; the greatest lower bound is called the meet and is sometimes written as $x\dot{y}$, [4, 5].

The set of closed sets of a convex geometry, form a lattice when ordered by set inclusion. Such lattices are precisely the meet- distributive lattices. A lattice L is meet-distributive if for each $y \in L$, if $x \in L$ is the meet of (all the) elements covered by y, then the interval [x, y] is a boolean algebra.

Antimatroids are dual to convex geometries, [6, 7]. Antimatroids have been used to generalize a greedy algorithm for optimally solving single-processor scheduling problems, [8] to model the ordering of events in discrete event simulation systems, [9] as well as to model progress towards a goal in artificial intelligence planning problems, [10].

A number of theorists have noted that people tend to be overconfident when they make decisions [11, 12]. In [11] it is shown that students writing the SAT Reasoning Test omit answers in which they have low confidence in order to avoid the penalty for errors.

449.3 Different Paths

Suppose a Web-based test contains five questions. A stem is followed by a correct answer (c), incorrect answer (w), partially correct answer (p), or it is left without any response.

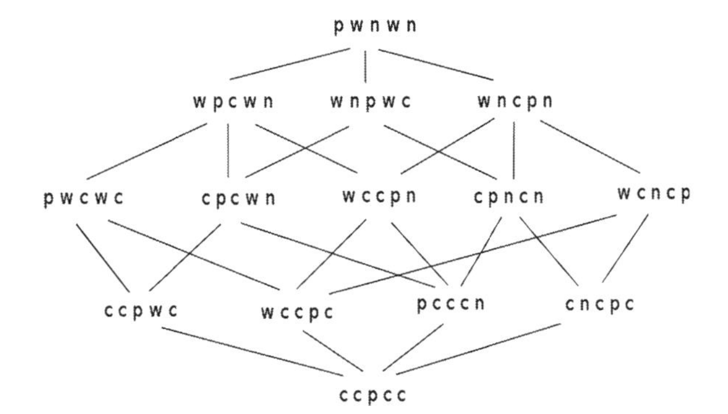

Fig. 449.1 A lattice with two wrong answers as a start

Closure system theory is applied for summarizing students' responses in Figs. 449.1, 449.2, and 449.3. It is of a particular interest to figer out when a wrong answer or an ommited one is follwed by a correct answer when a test is taken repeatedly. Each path contains sets where only one elements is changed on the next step. This provides an opportunity to see the effect of provided help and learning materials. Thus future changes are responding to real data.

In Fig. 449.1 we begin with a case where there is no correct answer in the first response.

In Fig. 449.2 we begin with a case where three wrong ansers are included in the first response.

In Fig. 449.3 we begin with a case where four wrong ansers are included in the first response.

This approach can be applied to provide personalized assitence to each learner. At the same time one can search for patterns of problems experienced by different groups of learners and later on incorporate appropriate changes into the system. There is clearly a need for research exploring other ways in which students might regulate accuracy on university examinations, [3].

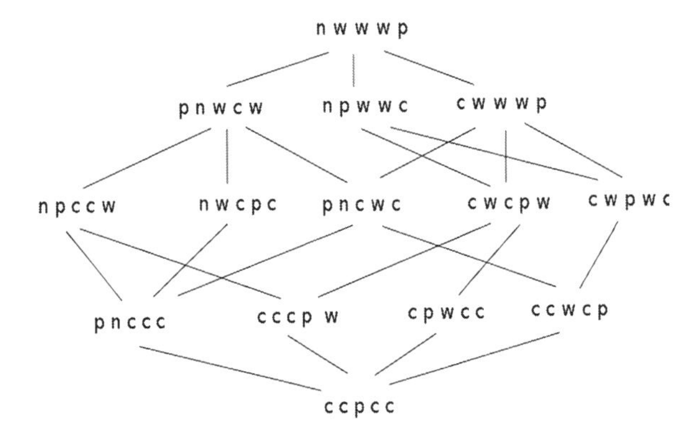

Fig. 449.2 A lattice with three wrong answers

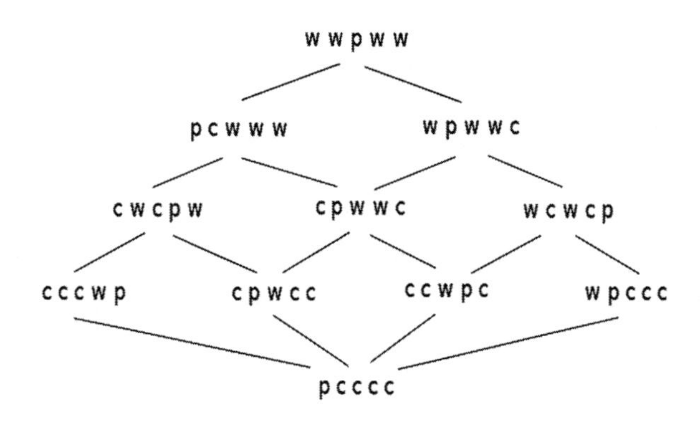

Fig. 449.3 A lattice with four wrong answers

449.4 Conclusion

Students' knowledge are difficult to assess. Methods originating from statistics employed in evaluations derive good conclusions about group achievements in a particular setting but do not provide indication of what what would happen if certain changes are introduced. The presented approach exploits some concepts of convex geometries. The removal process allowing elimination of one problem at a time while preserving the rest unchanged has been applied repeatedly.

References

1. Dummer P, Ifenthaler D (2010) Automated knowledge visualization and assessment. Comput Based Diagn Syst Anal Knowl 2:77–115
2. Ifenthaler D (2010) Learning and instruction in the digital age. In Spector JM, Ifenthaler D, IsaÃ-as P, Kinshuk, and Sampson DG (eds) Learning and instruction in the digital age: making a difference through cognitive approaches, technology-facilitated collaboration and assessment, and personalized communications, Springer, New York, pp. 3–11
3. Higham P (2013) Regulating accuracy on university tests with the plurality option. Learn Instr 24:26–36
4. Carpineto C, Romano G (2004) Concept data analysis: theory and applications. John Wiley & Sons, Ltd
5. Davey BA, Priestley HA (2005) Introduction to lattices and order. Cambridge University Press, Cambridge
6. Edelman PH, Jamison RE (1985) The theory of convex geometries. Geom Dedicata 19:247–270
7. Gruber P, Wills J (1993) Handbook of convex geometry. Elsevier, Amsterdam
8. Boyd EA, Faigle U (1990) An algorithmic characterization of antimatroids. Discrete Appl Mathe 28(3):197–205
9. Glasserman P, Yao DD (1994) Monotone structure in discrete event systems, Wiley series in probability and statistics. Wiley, New York
10. Parmar A (2003) Some mathematical structures underlying efficient planning, AAAI spring symposium on logical formalization of commonsense reasoning
11. Higham PA (2007) No Special K! A signal detection framework for the strategic regulation of memory accuracy. J Exp Psychol Gen 136:1–22
12. Sieck WR, Merkle EC, Van Zandt T (2007) Option fixation: a cognitive contributor to overconfidence. Organ Behav Hum Decis Process 103:68–83

Chapter 450
Research on Nerve Electrophysiology of Chronic Pharyngitis Based on Automobile Exhaust Pollution

Chunxin Dong

Abstract The clinical characteristics of the study in patients with chronic pharyngitis, peripheral neuropathy and nerve electrophysiological testing analysis. The method detected 80 cases of patients with chronic pharyngitis median nerve, nerve, perennial motor nerve conduction velocity (MCV) and F-wave, tibiae nerve, median nerve, ulnas nerve sensory nerve conduction velocity (SCV) and F-wave and 78 cases of healthy people without drinking hobby as control. 80 patients with chronic pharyngitis MCV decreased abnormal rate of 65.6 %, SCV decline, abnormal rate of 81.8 %. Significant difference compared with the control group ($P < 0.01$), the SCV involvement more MCV. Detection of neurons physiological abnormalities is earlier than clinical symptoms. The electrical nerve is detecting early diagnosis of chronic pharyngitis and guide treatment.

Keywords Chronic pharyngiti · Electrophysiology · Peripheral neuropathy · Automobile exhaust pollution

450.1 Introduction

As people socialize frequently and social pressures increase, the population of alcohol dependence has continued to increase. The incidence of chronic pharyngitis is gradually increasing trend. Chronic pharyngitis insidious on set manifestation. Involving the central and peripheral nervous system, the highest incidence of peripheral neuropathy, and more for the initial performance. Nerve electrophysiological testing can accurately reflect the early lesions of peripheral nerves, and provide a basis for the timely diagnosis and treatment. August 2001–June

C. Dong (✉)
Environmental and Biological Engineering College, Jilin Institute of Chemical Technology, 132013 Jilin, China
e-mail: dongchx@126.com

S. Li et al. (eds.), *Frontier and Future Development of Information Technology in Medicine and Education*, Lecture Notes in Electrical Engineering 269,
DOI: 10.1007/978-94-007-7618-0_450, © Springer Science+Business Media Dordrecht 2014

2005, 80 cases of patients with chronic pharyngitis, the clinical features of peripheral neuropathy and nerve electrophysiological testing analysis. The results reported below.

450.2 Materials and Methods

Mental disease classification schemes and diagnostic criteria based on the Chinese Medical Association Psychiatric Association developed in 1995 to confirm the diagnosis of chronic pharyngitis 80 patients were set in the observation group. 78 males, 2 females, age 32–65 years, mean 46.5 years. History of drinking five to 35 years, an average of 20 years, each meal daily drinking, drinking in high spirits. The amount of daily drink liquor (200–800) ml, average daily drinking is about as 250 ml, more than a brief history of alcoholics. Clinical manifestations of upper limb parentheses 46 cases, 58 cases of lower limb parentheses, numbness, lower limbs step on the cotton-like feeling, shoes do not know who, vibratory sensation subsided. Twelve cases of muscle weakness and diminished tendon reflexes, muscle atrophy eight cases. Sleep disorders, near thing memory loss, and decreased attention in 30 cases. Limb tremor in 36 cases. Ataxia in 3 cases. Admission delirium or drowsiness consciousness disorder patients. Jaundice in 12 cases. The chest of spider veins and facial telangiectasia 16 cases. Control group, 78 cases no drinking hobby healthy persons, 75 cases were male and 3 females, aged 29–64 years, mean 40.6 years, no nervous system diseases and signs.

450.2.1 Rating Scale

Cancer patients quality of life scale (Quality of Life Questionnaire-Core 30 QLQ-C30), a total of 30 projects, functional subscale physical functioning (PF), role function (RF), cognitive function (CF), emotional function (EF), social function (SF), 3 symptom subscales (fatigue, pain, nausea, vomiting), an overall health subscale (GH) and a single measurement projects (difficulty breathing constitute, insomnia, lack of appetite, constipation, diarrheal, financial difficulties). The Functioning Scale the PF, RF and GH higher the score, the better quality of life; CF, EF, SF and symptom scale and individual measurements project the higher the score, the worse the quality of life. The questionnaire was comparable with that in different countries and regions, its reliability and validity and sensitivity has been validated in a number of countries, successfully used in the clinical studies of cancer patients. Questionnaire by the researchers under the unified guidance language (Fig. 450.1).

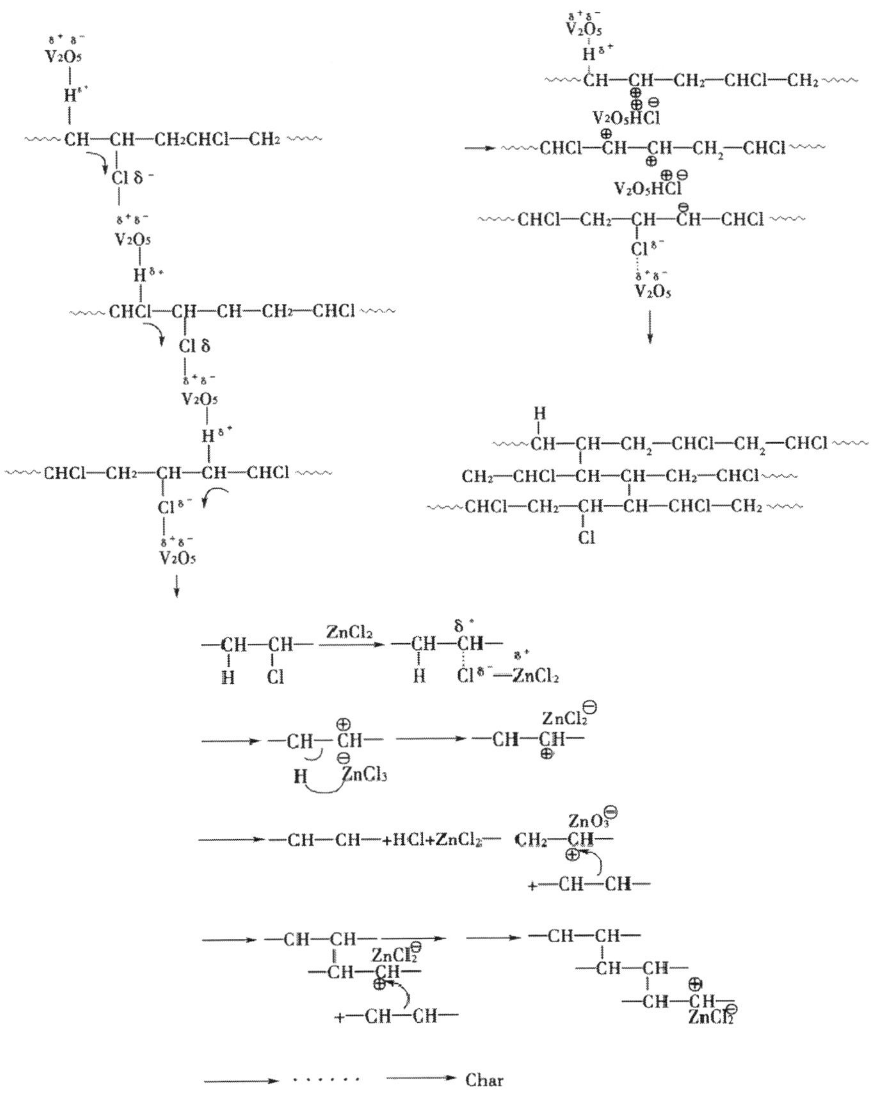

Fig. 450.1 Wine suppression mechanism model

450.2.2 Cartesian Functioning Scale

KPS into 10 grades, according to the assessment of the functional status of patients given the range of 0–100 points, the higher the score, the better physical function. Up to 100 points, followed by 90 points, 80 points, 70 points, which means that researchers different assessment of the patient's physical condition from high to

Table 450.1 Observation group and control group MCV, SCV determination (x ± s) Unit m/s

Groups	Cases	Median nerve	Ulnar nerve	Peroneal nerve	Tibial nerve	Median nerve	Ulnar nerve
Observation group	80	43.69 ± 6.68	46.36 ± 5.64	38.65 ± 6.82	34.56 ± 6.72	42.56 ± 7.82	38.55 ± 8.92
Control group	78	58.89 ± 6.10	56.62 ± 4.69	53.35 ± 5.98	46.56 ± 5.68	72.56 ± 6.58	56.52 ± 7.63
t		14.92	12.42	14.39	12.11	26.06	13.59
p		<0.01	<0.01	<0.01	<0.01	<0.01	<0.01

Table 450.2 Case group compared with the control group F wave (x ± s) in m/s

Seized nerve	Observation items	Observation group	Observation group	t	p
Observation	F Wave velocity (m/s)	62.21 ± 3.25	64.65 ± 3.01	17.99	<0.001
Median nerve	F Wave velocity (m/s)	53.28 ± 2.98	56.06 ± 2.9	18.26	<0.001
Tibial nerve	F Wave latency (m/s)	25.78 ± 1.16	23.62 ± 1.80	79.07	<0.001
Wave velocity	F Wave latency (m/s)	40.88 ± 1.24	38.86 ± 1.98	50.65	<0.001

low. 100 indicating normal, with 10 indicating critically ill dying, with 0 representing death. Space environment to a certain extent affect the patient's therapeutic effect, and should therefore be avoided noisy interference environment. We choose a single area of 26 m^2, and from the wards, offices at some distance from a dedicated treatment room; built-in with living flowers and murals with health education, information, and as warm as possible, so that the patient is relaxed, natural and comfortable environment.

450.3 Statistical Results

SPSS 10.0 statistical package for statistical analysis using the t test was used to compare the before and after intervention quality of life Tables 450.1 and 450.2.

450.4 Conclusion

According to foreign Derogates (1983) reported that 47 % of cancer patients have significant psychological stress response or psychological disorders. As Hang said, fear of cancer is global, because cancer means extreme suffering and death. Due to the incidence of cancer usually does not cause people's attention, so many patients are diagnosed in the late often accompanied by other symptoms, such as pain, insomnia, indigestion, and most patients; and the long duration of treatment, the patient need to face treatment the emergence of side effects, such as chemotherapy, nausea, vomiting, constipation, fatigue, mouth ulcers, these factors could materially and adversely affect the patient's overall quality of life. This study is based cancer patients psychological and disease characteristics, the implementation of the principle of mainly symptomatic soundtrack. When people get sick, the rhythm of the body is in an abnormal state, choose the appropriate music, harmony through music audio, allows the body to a variety of vibration frequency coordination of activities, to the benefit of the patient back to health. The results of this study show that music therapy has a good effect to improve the quality of sleep in patients with cancer, statistically significant ($P < 0.05$) before and after the intervention. Due to the application of nature music easily beat the promotion of sound waves of sleep, the sleep center of the brain gradually relaxed, and goes to sleep. Johnson and abroad personalized music for insomnia in elderly women (age >70 years) is similar to the findings, both of which can improve the patient's quality of sleep. On the positive side, the music as a wonderful sound waves, the role of the human brain, people feel the life force from the natural world, in order to stimulate the love of life; the other hand, it can enrich people's imagination, people with good ideas and vision for the future. For cancer patients, to arouse their courageous battle with cancer, recognizing the value of self-existence, face reality, cherish every second of life, actively cooperate with treatment, improve treatment compliance, you can improve the patient's quality of life.

References

1. Min L, Xu H, Xia Y (1999) Cancer patients with anxiety and depression survey. Chin Mental Health J 13(3):187
2. Zhang H, Chen R, Fang T (2000) Nursing. Tianjin Science and Technology Press, Tianjin, p 261
3. Wang J, Nan C, Chen Z et al (2000) Cancer patients quality of life and related factors. Chin J Clin Psychol 8(1):23–26
4. Huang Yb, Wang K (2004) Ovarian cancer quality of life survey and analysis. J Nurs 19(10):938
5. Olschewski M, Schulgen G, Schumacher M et al (1994) Quality of life assessment in clinical cancer research. Br J Cancer 70(1):1–5

Chapter 451
The Status and Challenge of Information Technology in Medical Education

Jun Li, Ming Zhao and Guang Zhao

Abstract Information technology (IT) has been greatly developed over the past decades. The developed IT becomes an important component in our life, which will affect the teaching and learning process. There are both big challenges and huge potential in the use of IT in education. With some unique characteristics in medical education, using IT as a tool can affect the medical curriculum and profession. This article presents the status and challenge of IT in medical education. First, the rapid development of IT used in general education is described, which is compared with the status of IT in medical education. Then, the challenge of IT facing teachers and students is discussed. Lastly, the promise of IT in medical education is provided. Both China and other countries need to develop new IT in medical education.

Keywords Status · Challenge · Information technology · Medical education

451.1 Introduction

After information technology (IT) was developed, it has been widely used to improve education for decades. The developed IT has important implications in modernization of education. One implication in the education reform is that the learning organizations need to foster originality and innovation for professional development by incorporating research findings of IT into the classroom. The other implication is in the transformation of education from the teacher-centered to the student-centered learning system. It is necessary for teachers to use new IT to create an ideal learning environment by using new IT. On the other hand, using new IT may bring challenges to teachers and students because there are many

J. Li (✉) · M. Zhao · G. Zhao
School of Chemical Biology and Pharmaceutical Sciences, Capital Medical University, Beijing 100069, China
e-mail: lijun88@ccmu.edu.cn

S. Li et al. (eds.), *Frontier and Future Development of Information Technology in Medicine and Education*, Lecture Notes in Electrical Engineering 269,
DOI: 10.1007/978-94-007-7618-0_451,

changes in what the students learn and how they may learn it [1]. The curriculum of higher education and the careers of the academic profession are transformed by new IT [2]. The knowledge can be delivered more effectively and efficiently than traditional methods. Both teachers and students should understand the changes and then benefit from the challenges. Developing and using IT may improve the understanding of knowledge and develop skills. This article discusses how IT can be used in medical education.

451.2 The Development of IT in Education

In 1980s, the research of IT was shifted from learning computers to computer aided instruction (CAI). Thus, many computer applications were developed in education [3]. Programs for drill and practice, instructions and simulations were available in the classroom. In 1990s, the use of computer in different forms increased extremely. Computer was applied to broader education field than just CAI and programming.

Two decades later, IT is still developing rapidly to create powerful learning environment. Compared to traditional passive learning styles, teachers can organize teaching process in new forms by using IT including spreadsheets, data acquisition and visualization [4]. Students can understand abstract concepts and complex relationships by using computer as a modeling, instruction and assessing tool. With the help of multimedia, the complicated processes can be visualized and manipulated. By combining text, image, sound, animation and video, the lifelike problems can be simulated. With the aid of new IT, teachers can stimulate them to reflect and give the feedback to help them solve problems in daily life. Computer programs can be developed to introduce concepts, theories and experiments in virtual settings. The self-learning methodologies based on computer programs can facilitate students to participate actively in learning [5]. Students can understand concepts easily and learn to perform experiments without long term practical experiences. Students also can learn knowledge outside school by self-directing and self-evaluation.

Recently, due to the falling cost of modern electronics and the pervasion of the worldwide web, networked laptops and mobile phones become general [6]. A number of information and software are available on the web, which can be used as complementary materials and tools in the courses [7].

451.3 The Status of IT in Medical Education

The education reform engendered by IT affects medical education with some unique aspects. The worldwide web is important in medical education. Many medical universities invest in extensive computer networks. Teachers can prepare the courses and transfer the knowledge efficiently by using IT with web.

The computer with a visual or aural component can be applied to teach abstract concepts and difficult topics effectively, such as histopathology, anatomy and heart sounds. Furthermore, a step-through program with adjacent frames linked to a database is developed to represent the learning process in clinical settings. The problem-oriented learning and clinical reasoning models are straight forward and student-centered [6]. Students can call up information of the case promptly with a complete record including their responses. Moreover, the high-power workstations can simulate the virtual-reality interaction to improve surgery skills. For example, haptics coupled with algorithms can be used to describe the tissue deformation.

The life-long learning process is important for medical profession due to the standards of licensing institution and the requirement for quality health care. However, the teachers have less time with the advances in medicine and the changes in health care delivery. Thus, e-learning becomes popular to deliver knowledge in a flexible and innovative way [8]. The on-line education providers and websites increase dramatically. Many physicians earn the Continuing Medical Education (CME) credits through online courses [9]. They can acquire and share medicine and product information by professional association communications on internet [10].

451.4 The Challenge of IT in Medical Education

The increasing role of IT in modern medical education brings both opportunities and challenges. Easily access to computers and the web makes learning through the internet available. However, fostering IT acceptance among some teachers remains a challenge because they received less training in it [11]. Acceptance of new IT will be hindered by teachers with increasing demands of research workload at stringent time but.

It is crucial to manipulate the mobile-learning platform with a planning strategy. Computers are seldom used to teach the body of knowledge, which should be embedded within the course and supported by the content. It is necessary to develop programs that permit effective interaction between teachers and students. Furthermore, the information on the internet is overwhelming, due to their unstructured and mixed nature. The use of IT in medical education should be developed in the right direction. Both teachers and students should learn how to use it effectively.

With less assessment on the benefits of the training, IT is only a supplement method and cannot replace the traditional teaching methods. For instance, no additional benefit was recorded in training venous catheter placement with distorted information and unexplained science phenomena. Compared to e-learning education of health care staff, classroom-based education is useful to enhance the skills by actual experience [12].

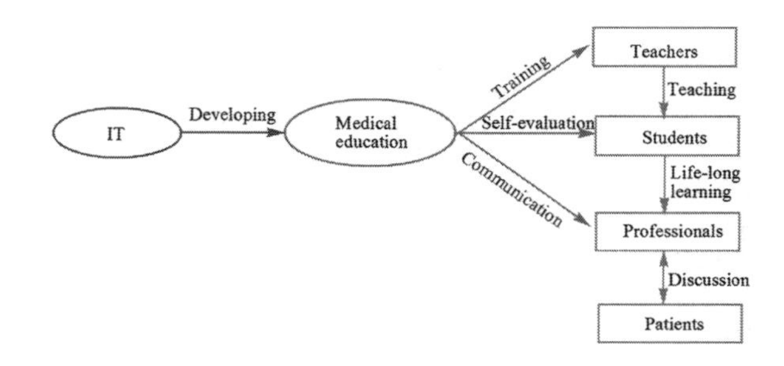

Fig. 451.1 Developing IT in medical education

451.5 The Promise of IT in Medical Education

There are potential impacts and benefits on medical education with the development of IT. The new IT can improve the teaching and learning environment. For instance, special teaching programs can provide opportunities for the orientation and development of gifted students [13]. It also can be designed to introduce new concepts based on the knowledge that students have acquired.

IT is helpful to construct the multidisciplinary and interdisciplinary curriculum. For example, medical physics needs correlation with molecular biology, computational biology, biochemistry, mathematics and technology [14]. A medical physicist needs a multidisciplinary vision of physics, biomedicine, bioengineering, sociology, psychology and philosophy.

In China, medical education is in the period of transformation. IT including PowerPoint and Microsoft Excel has been widely used in courses. For example, in the experiment of the saponification of ethyl acetate, the progress of the second order reaction can be followed by measuring the conductivity [15]. However, analysis of the results through experience formula is complex. In order to process the experimental data, the linear and nonlinear fitting methods can be performed in Microsoft Excel. The rate constant can be easily calculated with better correlation coefficient. The Arrhenius activation energy of the reaction also can be determined conveniently.

Chinese curricula call for extensive revision and reform, because the structure and content have not changed for nearly 40 years [16]. We should develop IT in medical education to train teachers, to teach students and to help professionals (Fig. 451.1). In the end, the patients will benefit from that system. Therefore, there is a great deal to do in developing IT in medical education both in China and other countries.

Acknowledgments The authors would like to acknowledge Zhongwei Zhao for help with the English expression. This work was supported by Funding of PHR(IHLB) (3500-11250509; 3500-1125062201), Funds of Beijing Education Commission (PXM2013-014226-07-000001; PXM2013-014226-07-000025) and Foundation of President of Capital Medical University (13JYY26; 13JYY30).

References

1. Van Dusen GC (1997) The virtual campus: technology and reform in higher education. ASHE-ERIC higher education report. George Washington University, Washington, DC
2. Baldwin RG (1998) Technology's impact on faculty life and work. New Dir Teach Learn 76:7–21
3. Volman M, van Eck E (2001) Gender equity and information technology in education: the second decade. Rev Edu Res 71(4):613–634
4. Chiu M-H, Wu H-K (2009) The roles of multimedia in the teaching and learning of the triplet relationship in chemistry. Multiple representations in chemical education. Springer, pp. 251–283
5. Sánchez JM, Hidalgo M, Salvadó V (2007) VALORA: a PC program for the self learning of acid base titrations. INTED2007 proceedings international technology, education and development conference
6. Ward JP, Gordon J, Field MJ, et al (2001) Communication and information technology in medical education. Lancet 357(9258):792–796
7. Ruedas-Rama MJ, Orte A (2011) Using text-to-speech generated audio files for learning chemistry in higher education. Eurasian J Phys Chem Edu 4(1):65–77
8. Ruiz JG, Mintzer MJ, Leipzig RM (2006) The impact of e-learning in medical education. Acad Med 81(3):207–212
9. de Silva N, Kulasekera GU (2013) Learner evaluation of an online continuing medical education course for general practitioners. Sri Lanka J Bio-Med Inform 3(3):65–74
10. Casebeer L, Bennett N, Kristofco R et al (2002) Physician internet medical information seeking and on-line continuing education use patterns. J Contin Educ Health Prof 22(1):33–42
11. Hu PJ-H, Clark TH, Ma WW (2003) Examining technology acceptance by school teachers: a longitudinal study. Inf Manage 41(2):227–241
12. Pulsford D, Jackson G, O'Brien T et al (2013) Classroom-based and distance learning education and training courses in end-of-life care for health and social care staff: a systematic review. Palliat Med 27(3):221–235
13. Kelemen G (2010) A personalized model design for gifted children'education. Procedia-Social and Behav Sci 2(2):3981–3987
14. Whitehead C (2013) Scientist or science-stuffed? Discourses of science in North American medical education. Med Educ 47(1):26–32
15. Xiang M, Zeng X, Zai S, et al (2004) Application of non-linear fitting capability of Excel in processing experiment data of ethyl acetate saponification. J Southwest Univ Natl 30(1):16–20
16. Sherer R, Dong H, Yunfeng Z et al (2013) Medical education reform in Wuhan University, China: a preliminary report of an International collaboration. Teach Learn Med 25(2):148–154

Chapter 452
The Comparison of Fetal ECG Extraction Methods

Zhongliang Luo, Jingguo Dai and Zhuohua Duan

Abstract Fetal Electrocardiogram (fetal ECG) can reflects the tiny change in the potential of fetal heart activity cycle, which has become an main means for prenatal maternal and fetal safety. It has important theoretical significance and practical value to get a clear fetal electrocardiogram and improve the performance of fetal ECG extraction. In this paper, three typical fetal ECG extraction methods is studied, i.e., artificial neural networks, blind signal separation and adaptive filtering method. The results show that blind signal separation method is a relatively better extraction method for fetal ECG extraction, this method combined with empirical mode decomposition (EMD) denoising technology, it can get clearer fetal ECG.

Keywords Fetal ECG · Blind sources separation · Adaptive filtering · Empirical mode decomposition

452.1 Introduction

The fetal ECG as an objective index to judge the safety status of fetus in mother, which can reflect important information for instant changes in fetal heart and fetal health status [1–3]. Currently, the fetal ECG acquisition method is mainly from fetal scalp electrode method and maternal abdominal skin electrode one [3]. The former method is obtained directly through the fetal surface maternity, having high signal-to-noise ratio, its waveform is stable and clear. But it can not be repeated to detect and vulnerable to infect the fetus. The latter one is an effective non-invasive way, as is shown in Fig. 452.1, which is extracted from pregnant women body

Z. Luo (✉) · J. Dai · Z. Duan
School of Computer Science, Shaoguan University, Shaoguan, China
e-mail: luozl66@126.com

S. Li et al. (eds.), *Frontier and Future Development of Information Technology in Medicine and Education*, Lecture Notes in Electrical Engineering 269,
DOI: 10.1007/978-94-007-7618-0_452, © Springer Science+Business Media Dordrecht 2014

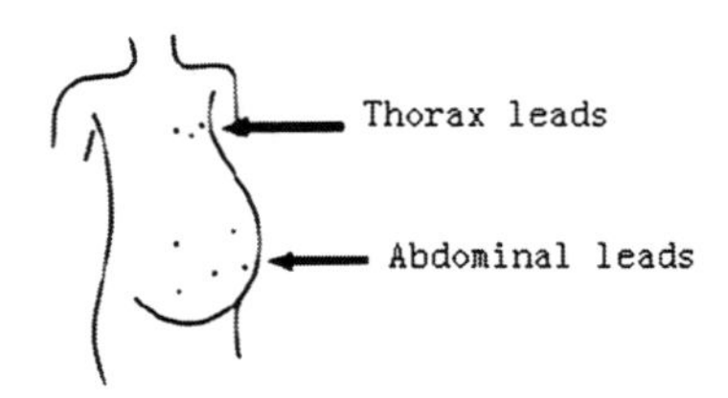

Fig. 452.1 Signal acquired from non-invasive way

surface, the fetal ECG can be used repeatedly in the prenatal care by health workers and welcomed by pregnant women, but the acquired signal contains more interfering signal, such as electromyography noise, power line interference, baseline wandering and so on. Lots of experiments show that the Fetal ECG fluctuates fast and weak, however, the maternal ECG fluctuates slow and strong. Therefore, it is a challenging item in the field of biomedical signal processing and analysis, so an effective method to extract fetal ECG from maternal abdominal signal is need to study.

Many scholars proposed a number of fetal ECG extraction methods to obtain pure fetal ECG. There are many extraction methods for non-invasive way, such as artificial neural network [1, 2], matched filtering method [2], blind signal separation method [1, 3, 4], adaptive filtering method [1, 2], support vector machines [5].

452.2 The Illustration of Typical Fetal ECG Extraction Method

452.2.1 Introduction Artificial Neural Network

In 2004, Camps-Valls [5] applied dynamic neural networks to extract fetal ECG signal, X. J. Pu obtained a clear fetal ECG by neural network method with radial basis function (RBF) [5], it has three steps: (1) initialize the training data, (2) training RBF neural network, (3) extracting fetal ECG .

In 2005 and 2007, Assaleh extracted to clear fetal ECG by successively using a polynomial neural network and adaptive neuro-fuzzy inference system (ANFIS) [5], greatly accelerating speed of network learning, as is shown in Fig. 452.2.

452.2.2 Blind Source Separation Method

The process of blind source separation, which separates source signal from a number of observation mixed-signal, recovery source signals that can not be directly observed. Using the prior of signal characteristics to extract focus signal, it

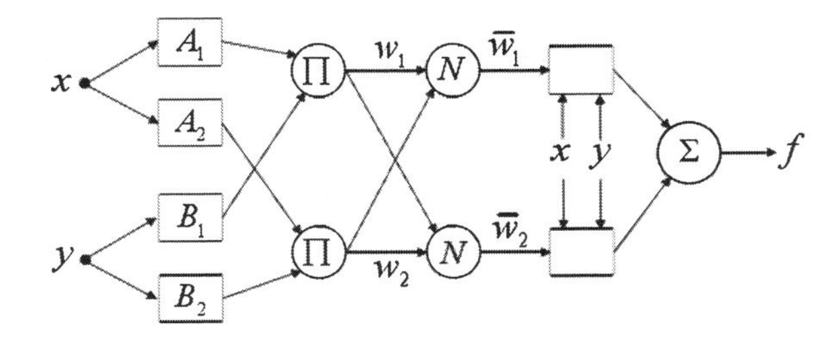

Fig. 452.2 The structure of ANFIS

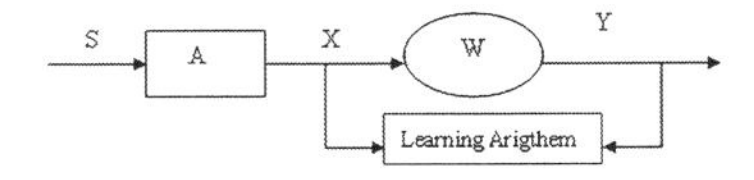

Fig. 452.3 Blind signal separation method

can save lots of computation time and CPU resources, thus get faster processing speed. The separation principle as is shown in Fig. 452.3, where S is the source signal vector, A is the hybrid matrix (i.e. transmission channel), X is observed signals, W is the separating matrix, Y is the separated signal.

Every component is statistical independence, the observation vector can be got by the $m \times n$ order mixing matrix:

$$X(t) = AS(t) = [x_1(t), x_2(t), \ldots, x_m(t)]^T \tag{452.2}$$

using $X(t)$ to obtain separation matrix W, then

$$Y(t) = WX(t) \tag{452.3}$$

$Y(t)$ is an estimate of the source signal.

Currently, blind source separation algorithm main divides three kinds [1, 3, 4], i.e. independent component analysis (ICA) algorithm, the information entropy maximizing method and nonlinear principal component analysis (PCA) algorithm.

452.2.3 Adaptive Filtering Method

Most cases, the acquired non-invasive ECG signal can not be guaranteed to absolutely smooth and constant statistical characteristics. Adaptive filter can ignore of the statistical properties unknown or slowly changing, and adjust its parameters to meet a certain standards.

In Fig. 452.4, $S(n)$ is the fetal ECG signal, $N(n)$ includes maternal ECG signal and other interference, reference input $X(n)$ acquired from the mother's chest. It is assumed that the $d(n)$ is unrelated between fetal ECG and maternal ECG, but the chest signal and maternal ECG signal of abdomen mixed signal is related in some way. The system achieve the best output by constantly adjust the adaptive filter weights, and obtain clear fetal ECG $S(n)$ from $d(n)$.

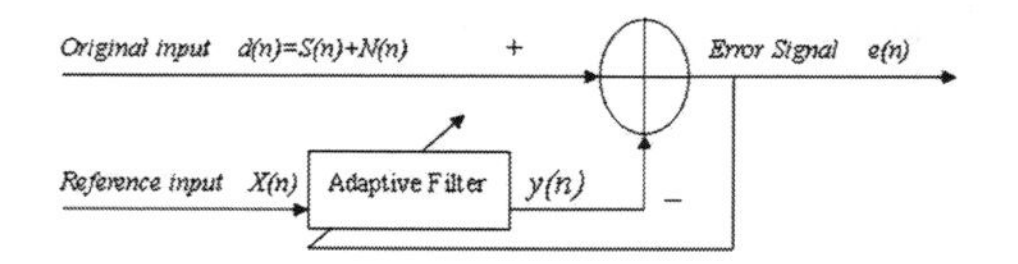

Fig. 452.4 Adaptive filter method

The main adaptive filtering includes [1, 2]: least mean square error (LMS), normalized least mean square error (NLMS) algorithm and the recursive least squares (RLS) algorithm. LMS process is as follows:

$$e(n) = d(n) - y(n) = d(n) - X^T(n)W(n) \tag{452.4}$$

$$y(n) = X^T(n)W(n) \tag{452.5}$$

$$W(n+1) = W(n) + 2\mu e(n)X(n) \tag{452.6}$$

where $W(n)$ presents weights vector of filter at time$n$, $\mu$is step factor.

452.3 The Experimental Results and Discussion

The experimental data obtained from Dalsy database [13]. The recorded data are acquired from maternal body surface by electrodes. The later three channels recorded maternal chest signal and the former five-channel recording maternal abdominal signal, it is a mixed-signal of the maternal ECG and fetal ECG. The sampling frequency is 250 Hz, record time is 10 s and it acquired 2500 data for each channel, as is shown in Fig. 452.5.

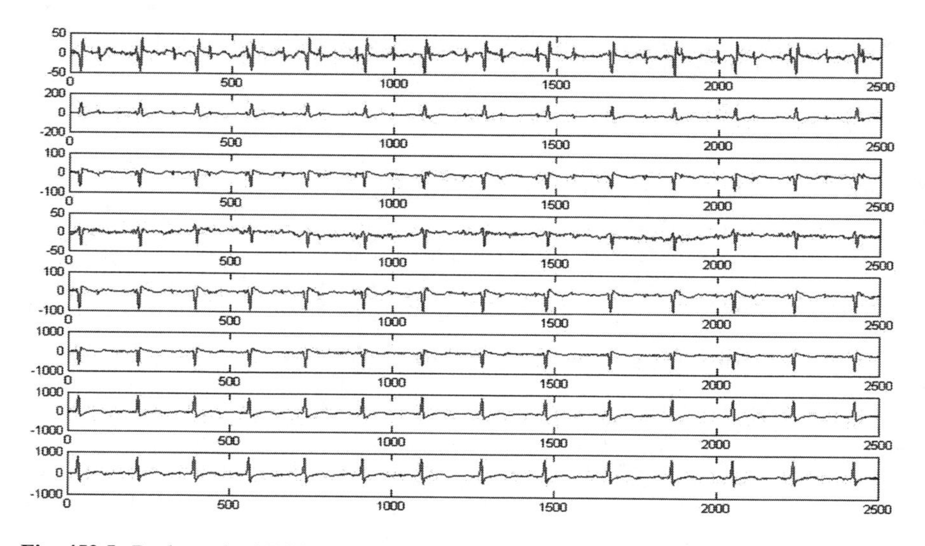

Fig. 452.5 Real acquired ECG data

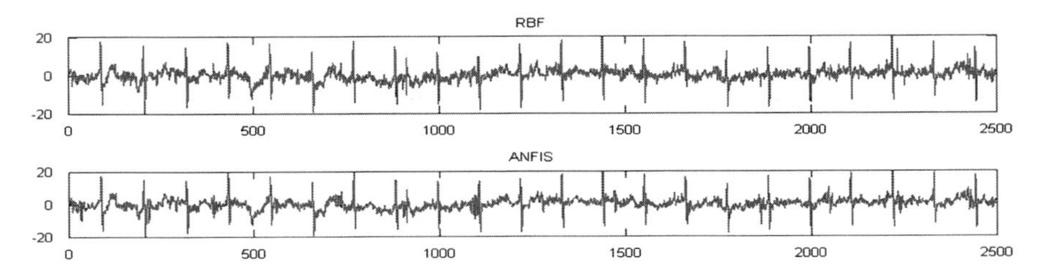

Fig. 452.6 The fetal ECG extracted from artificial neural network algorithm

During the Fetal ECG extraction process, it took the former five channels signal as original input and the later three as reference input. In order to verify the validity of algorithm, it uses three kinds algorithm test on the actual ECG data.

As can be seen from Figs. 452.6 452.7 to 452.8, the three methods can obtain Fetal ECG. Extraction method based on artificial neural networks only need two leads record maternal chest and abdomen ECG, taking the chest ECG as reference signal. It has better performance for extracting fetal ECG from the mixed ECG signal, even if the SNR of fetal- maternal ECG is lower. Based on RBF, most maternal ECG component in the mixed signal is suppressed, however, there is a little maternal ECG component still exist in fetal ECG.

The LMS algorithm is simple, robust and easy to implement, which widely used in practical. However, its performance less than RLS, such as clarity, stability and filtering effect and its convergence rate is quite slow.

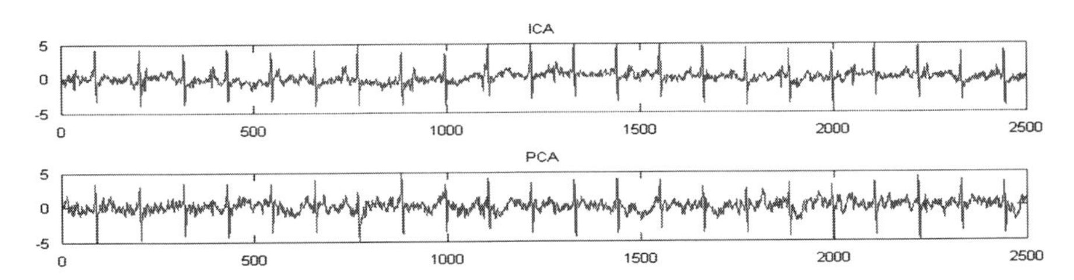

Fig. 452.7 The fetal ECG extracted from blind source separation

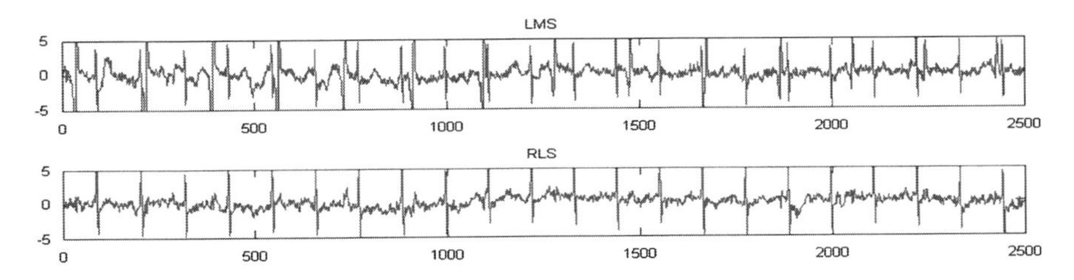

Fig. 452.8 The fetal ECG extracted from adaptive filter algorithm

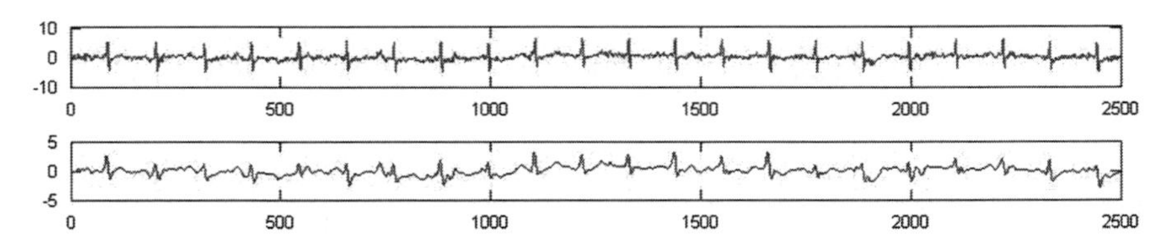

Fig. 452.9 Results of using blind source separating and EMD denoising

Generally, using the ICA algorithm, its final result will different when the signal adopts different measure. Entropy maximization method requires output spread in the hypercube as uniformly as possible. However, it separates signal based on orthogonal when separation using non-linear PCA algorithm.

Comparing the three methods from clarity and stable, blind source separating method is best. In order to get a clearer fetal ECG signal, the extracted fetal ECG need suppress noise with denosing method, as is shown in Fig. 452.9. Thus, it help doctors make the right judgments.

452.4 Conclusion

Three typical extraction methods are introduced in this paper. These methods can extract a better fetal ECG, especially, blind signal separation combined with EMD method obtained clearer fetal ECG, the results indicate its feasibility, which has potential clinical application. In practical application, it may achieve better performance by combining with several better extraction algorithm.

References

1. Zhou ZH, YangKY (2012) Fetal electrocardiogram extraction and performance analysis. J Comput 7(11):2821–2828
2. Sheikh Algunaidi MM, Mohd Ali1 MA, Fokhrul Islam Md (2011) Comparative analysis of fetal electrocardiogram extraction techniques using system simulation. Int J Phys Sci 6(21):4952–4959
3. Zarzoso V, Nandi AK (2001) Noninvasive fetal electrocardiogram extraction blind separation versus adaptive noise cancellation. IEEE Trans Biomed Eng 48(1):12–18
4. Lee J, Park KL, Lee KJ (2005) Temporally constrained ICA-based fetal ECG separation. Electron Lett 41(21):1158–1160
5. Pu XJ, Zeng XP, Han L (2009) Extraction of fetal electrocardiogram signal using least squares support vector machines. J Electron Inf Technol 31(12):2941–2947
6. De Lathauwe L (2011) Database for identification of systems: fetal ECG data EAST/SISTAK. U. Leuven, Belgium [EB/OL]. http://www.esat.kuleuven.ac.be/sista/daisy

Chapter 453
Study on Evaluation Index System of Hotel Practice Base Based on Bias Analysis and Reliability and Validity Test

Changfeng Yin

Abstract The satisfaction degree with the hotel practice base not only embodies the quality of teaching, but also reflects the management level of hotel to some extent. Applying SPSS19.0 statistical software technology, by bias analysis and reliability and validity test, The paper makes analysis on the survey data about satisfaction degree with practice hotels for students of grades 2009 and 2010 majored in tourism management in Hefei University by means of mathematical models on reliability analysis, validity analysis and difference test etc. comes to the conclusion that University-enterprise cooperation has obtained the greatest satisfaction and Satisfaction degree of students has obtained the least satisfaction among the factors affecting the satisfaction with the practice base of students. In addition, the internship satisfaction of students varies greatly with hotels of different cooperation degrees, different levels of hotels and different departments.

Keywords Hotel · Practice base · Evaluation · Research · Bias analysis · Reliability · Validity test

As an essential link for practical teaching of tourism colleges, specialty practice enables the students to apply the theory to practical work, improve the professional skills and professional qualities of students, and deepen the understanding of professions and accumulation of practical experience so as to achieve the high-skilled talent training objectives of tourism colleges. Guided by the evaluation system of practice base, the selection of high-quality practice bases may enable the tourism colleges to make remarkable achievements in practical teaching; hotels with favorable internship experience may become the prime choices of students majored in tourism management; and practical work experience may cultivate the students majored in tourism management to be talents required by the hotels, thus to achieve the "triple-win" situation among the colleges, students and hotels.

C. Yin (✉)
Hefei University, Hefei City 230601 Anhui, China
e-mail: yin_chf2003@126.com

S. Li et al. (eds.), *Frontier and Future Development of Information Technology in Medicine and Education*, Lecture Notes in Electrical Engineering 269,
DOI: 10.1007/978-94-007-7618-0_453,

The paper carries out an evaluation research on the evaluation index system for hotel practice bases, which is of great significance for tourism colleges to select practice bases in a more scientific and reasonable way, establish a long-term and stable relations of cooperation with tourism enterprises and improve the practical abilities of the students majored in tourism management.

453.1 Questionnaire Design and Survey

453.1.1 Questionnaire Design

According to the training objectives of tourism management major and the requirements of practical teaching system, a preliminary evaluation index [1] has been proposed with reference to the previous research achievements combining with the practical teaching work in hotels over the years. A random survey was conducted for 51 students of grade 2010 majored in tourism management in Hefei University with practice bases located in cities including Hefei, Nanjing and Shanghai etc. from November to December of 2012, and a preliminary revision for the index system of hotel practice bases had been carried out according to the survey on the students. Afterwards, by means of interviews and discussion with middle and senior managers of the hotels as well as tourism experts and scholars repeatedly and taking the advices of each other, these proposed evaluation indexes were further divided into 5 primary indexes and 26 secondary indexes[2], including the degree of cooperation with the hotel B1 (listing C1, mutual cognition C2, internship arrangement C3, collaborative attitude C4 and communication degree C5), hotel hardware B2 (hotel humanization C6, ranking of hotel C7, hotel environment C8, hotel facilities C9 and safety facilities of the hotel C10), hotel software B3 (rules and regulations C11, management level C12, service level of the hotel C13, hotel enterprise culture C14, hotel brand C15 and hotel popularity C16), student satisfaction B4 (hotel accommodation and meals C17, internship allowance in hotel C18, hotel trainings C19, internship position arrangement C20, job achievement C21 and interpersonal relationships in hotel C22), hotel location B5 (city location C23, city grading C24, city image C25 and regional advantages C26). In addition, the questionnaire design for this study will be performed based on the evaluation indexes of the hotel practice base, and index design will be conducted from the aspects of student and expert evaluation. The option design for questions applies the Likert five-point scale to indicate 5 grades of "Very satisfied, Satisfied, Average, Dissatisfied and Very dissatisfied" with "5, 4, 3, 2 and 1" respectively [3].

453.1.2 *Questionnaire Survey*

The author has conducted a questionnaire survey for the undergraduates of grades 2009 and 2010 majored in tourism management in Hefei University from January to May of 2013. The questionnaires were issued and recovered by means of phone, QQ and E-mail etc. As the issuing of questionnaires was targeted to special groups of people, the recovery rate was relatively high.

453.2 Questionnaire Analysis

453.2.1 *Reliability Analysis*

Reliability refers to the consistency, stability and credibility of the test results. The internal consistency is generally applied to indicate the reliability of this test. The higher the reliability coefficient is, the more consistent, stable and reliable the test results will be. The paper will measure the Cronbach and Alpha reliability coefficients at various dimensions [4]. Reliability analysis for internship satisfaction scale is carried out through SPSS19.0 with the summarized results shown in the following Table 453.1.

As shown in Table 453.1, the overall reliability of the scale is 0.937, the reliability of university-enterprise cooperation degree is 0.802, the reliability of hotel hardware is 0.821, the reliability of hotel software is 0.724, the reliability of student satisfaction is 0.793, and the reliability of hotel location is 0.913. All the above reliability coefficients are greater than 0.70, which conforms to the judgment of scholar Deville's (1991) et al. that the minimum reliability of scale shall not be less than 0.70. It also suggests that the scale built in this study has shown a favorable reliability level with internal consistency.

453.2.2 *Validity Analysis*

Validity refers to the degree of object measurement accuracy by means of measuring tools or methods [5]. The validity of index selection scale for practice base

Tab 453.1 Questionnaire reliability analysis

	Overall satisfaction	Cooperation degree	Hotel hardware	Hotel software	Student satisfaction	Hotel location
Number of questions	48	10	8	8	9	13
Alpha	0.937	0.802	0.821	0.724	0.793	0.913

is mainly analyzed from two aspects, one is content validity, and the other is Construct validity. From content validity, the validity in this study is revised from expert interviews and student testing on the basis of the analysis on pertinent literature. It is formed through strict revision programs. Therefore, it can be assumed that the structure and item selection of the questionnaire have good sense of content validity. Generally, factor analysis need to be performed for construct validity. The calculated KMO value of the questionnaire is 0.942 which is close to 1; the Chi square value is 8016.104, the degree of freedom is 1107.012 and the significance probability is less than 0.01, passing the Bartlett test. Therefore, it is suitable for factor analysis. See Table 453.2 for detailed information:

Perform factor analysis for all the items applying the exploratory factor analysis, extract common factors applying Principal Component Analysis and perform orthogonal rotation processing for common factors combining the varimax method in orthogonal rotation in order to extract the factors with the eigenvalue of greater than 1. Through repetitive extraction, it is found that there are 5 common factors with the eigenvalue of greater than 1. The results are shown in Table 453.3.

As shown in Table 453.3, all the Eigen values of the five factors are greater than 1, and the variance contribution reaches 79.52 %. This indicates that the questionnaire is of favorable construct validity, and the above five factors can be applies in this study.

453.2.3 Mean Satisfaction Analysis on Evaluation Index System of Hotel Practice Base

In this paper, SPSS19.0 software is applied to perform measurement analysis on the independent variables and dependent variables with the interval measurement scale, thus to obtain the maximum value, minimum value, mean value and standard deviation etc. each satisfaction index. Among them, the mean value of overall satisfaction as well as the mean satisfaction for each index of the hotel base arranged randomly. The results are shown in Table 453.4.

As shown in Table 453.4, the overall satisfaction of interns with the practice base, satisfaction with university-enterprise cooperation degree, hotel hardware index, hotel software index, internship satisfaction of students and satisfaction with hotel location are 2.910, 3.015, 2.733, 2.614 and 2.850 respectively. These values are all greater than 2.5, but most of them are less than 3. That is, the satisfaction degree of students falls in between "Average" and "Satisfied". The

Tab 453.2 KMO and Bartlett's test

Kaiser -Meyer–Olkin measure of sampling adequacy	Bartlett's test of sphericity	
	Approx.	Chi square df Sig.
0.942	8016.104	1107 .012

Tab 453.3 Analysis results on satisfaction factors of practice base

Item description	Eigen value	Accumulated variance contribution
Cooperation degree of both parties	3.87	43.03 %
Hotel hardware	4.91	52.12 %
Hotel software	6.07	66.34 %
Student satisfaction	7.38	75.05 %
Hotel location	10.05	79.52

Tab 453.4 Statistical analysis of satisfaction on practice base

Item description	N	Minimum	Maximum	Mean value	Standard deviation	Variance
Overall index satisfaction	183	1.87	3.83	2.910	0.437	0.216
Cooperation degree of both parties	183	1.73	3.71	3.015	0.514	0.271
Hotel hardware index	183	1.71	3.26	2.841	0.612	0.261
Hotel software index	183	1.62	3.57	2.733	0.710	0.342
Student satisfaction	183	1.53	4.02	2.614	0.654	0.513
Hotel location	183	1.68	3.86	2.850	0.700	0.460

table also shows that the interns are most satisfied with the item "University-enterprise cooperation" with the mean value of 3.015; and they are most dissatisfied with "Student satisfaction" with the mean value of 2.614.

453.2.4 *Difference Test*

In order to get a better understanding of the impact of different cooperation degree, hotels at different star levels and different practice departments upon internship satisfaction, a variation analysis is performed for the questionnaire. The above factors are analyzed and compared applying the one-way analysis of variance in SPSS19.0. The results are as follows:

As shown in Tables 453.5, 453.6 and 453.7, the significance level for different internship cooperation degrees, different hotel hardware levels, different hotel software levels and different hotel locations is 0.000, which is less than 0.05. This indicates that significant differences exist at different internship cooperation degrees, different hotel hardware levels, different hotel software levels and different hotel locations, as follows:

Tab 453.5 Variance analysis on cooperation degree and internship satisfaction

	Quadratic sum	df	Mean square	F	Significance
Inter-group	4.357	4	1.482	7.851	0.000
Intra-group	35.712	177	0.217		
Total	40.069	181			

Tab 453.6 Variance analysis on internship satisfaction of hotels at different star levels

	Quadratic sum	df	Mean square	F	Significance
Inter-group	5.825	3	2.902	15.251	0.000
Intra-group	34.244	178	0.201		
Total	40.069	181			

As shown in Table 453.8, the mean differences of internship satisfaction between Close and Close & Close and Average cooperation with the practice hotel are 0.2567 and 0.3102 respectively, which are less than 0.05. This indicates that the satisfaction degrees between Close and Close & Close and Average cooperation with the practice hotel vary significantly.

As shown in Table 453.9, the mean differences of internship satisfaction between hotels of Five star and Four star & Five star and other star levels are 0.3604 and 0.4215 respectively with the corresponding significance levels of 0.000 and 0.023. These values are all less than 0.05. This indicates that internship

Tab 453.7 Variance analysis on internship satisfaction of different practice departments

	Quadratic sum	df	Mean square	F	Significance
Inter-group	6.084	3	3.001	16.012	0.000
Intra-group	33.985	178	0.198		
Total	40.069	181			

Tab. 453. 8 variance analysis on internship satisfaction at different cooperation degrees

Practice hotel	Practice hotel	Mean difference	Significance
Close	Close	0.2567	0.000
Close	Average	0.3102	0.002
Average	Average	0.2124	0.213

Tab. 453. 9 Difference analysis on internship satisfaction of hotels at different star levels

Star level of hotel	Star level of hotel	Mean difference	Significance
Five Star	Four Star	0.3604	0.000
Five Star	Others	0.4215	0.023
Four Star	Others	0.6123	0. 421

Tab 453.10 Variance analysis on satisfaction degree of different practice departments

Practice department	Practice department	Mean difference	Significance
Catering	Lobby	0.2541	0.003
Catering	Guest room	0.3214	0.001
Lobby	Guest room	−0.0234	0.761
Guest room	Others	−0.0324	0.345

satisfaction degrees between hotels of Five star and Four star & Five star and other star levels vary significantly.

As shown in Table 453.10, the mean differences of internship satisfaction between Catering and Lobby and Catering and Guest room are 0.2541 and 0.3214 respectively with the corresponding significance levels of 0.003 and 0.001. These values are all less than 0.05. This indicates that satisfaction degrees between Catering and Lobby and Catering and Guest room vary significantly.

453.3 Research Conclusions

First, the overall satisfaction of interns with the practice base, satisfaction with university enterprise cooperation degree, hotel hardware index, hotel software index, internship satisfaction of students and satisfaction with hotel location are 2.910, 3.015, 2.733, 2.614 and 2.850 respectively. These values are all greater than 2.5, but most of them are less than 3. That is, the satisfaction degree of students falls in between "Average" and "Satisfied". This indicates that the satisfaction degree with hotel practice base is at a relatively lower level. It is further needed to strengthen the development and research on the practice base, improve the construction of hotel practice bases, create a better internship environment for interns and improve the practicing quality of tourism management major.

Second, in the evaluation index system for all the hotel practice bases of tourism management major, the interns are most satisfied with the item "University-enterprise cooperation" with the mean value of 3.015; and they are most dissatisfied with "Student satisfaction" with the mean value of 2.614. This indicates that the hotel practice bases are less concerned about the practice of interns and fail to improve the internship satisfaction of intern students from the perspective of interns so as to improve the motivation them, strengthen the proper guidance intern students and improve the practice effect. Internship training and guidance need to be strengthened constantly in the future to improve the practice effect of intern students.

Third, the satisfaction degree of students practicing in five-star hotels is significantly greater than that of students practicing in hotels at other star levels. This indicates that the five-star hotels are quite consistent with student expectations. And the hardware or software facilities of five-star hotels are significantly better than the hotels at other levels.

Fourth, the internship satisfaction of students practicing in the catering and guest room departments is significantly lower than that of students practicing in other departments. This has a lot to do with the working environment, workload, working hours and work content of the two departments.

Acknowledgments Key project of Teaching and Research funded by Anhui Provincial Education Department (2012jyxm472); project of Teaching and Research funded by Hefei University.

References

1. He L (2009/12) Survey and analysis: satisfaction degree of hotel-management trainees in training base of higher vocational schools. Vocat Educ Res
2. Liu F (2010/3) A survey of hotel majors' satisfaction with their hotel practice. Sinkiang Vocat Educ Res
3. Guo Y (2011/2) Constitution and evaluation of evaluating indicator system of off-campus internship base for hotel management major. J Zhongzhou Univ
4. Yao X (2010/12) Tourism undergraduate internship system evaluation and empirical research. Tourism Forum
5. Li D (2007/35) Selection and evaluation of hotel practice base for tourism management major. Sci Technol Inf

Chapter 454
Improvement on Emergency Medical Service System Based on Class Analysis on Global Four Cases

Zhe Li and Feng Hai

Abstract Different kinds of extreme incidents and catastrophes around world have given Emergency Medical Service System (EMSS) tremendous challenges, especially in details on IT, structural and operational levels. And it makes how to rethink and improve the problems in emergency rescue to be of urgent theoretical and practical significance. First, this chapter revealed specific deficiencies exposed from three countries' EMSS in three typical cases. Furthermore, this chapter focused on further typology model, measure evaluation and extraction of basic elements, using vector clustering method. In addition, the chapter demonstrated common elements in an evaluation model, with discussion on national rescue framework of China and problems found in Wenchuan earthquake. Lastly, this chapter presented the latent issues that should be avoid and improved in emergency relief and corresponding suggestions, both on structural and operational levels.

Keywords EMSS · Rescue · Disaster medicine

454.1 Introduction

In the past decade, terrible accidental incidents and natural disasters have been keeping occurrence one by one such as the Asian Tsunami in 2001, Rita and Wilma in 2005, 2013 Sichuan Yaan earthquake, etc. These extreme events posed

Z. Li (✉) · F. Hai
Economics and Management School, Wuhan University, Wuhan 430072, China
e-mail: leetets@sina.com

S. Li et al. (eds.), *Frontier and Future Development of Information Technology in Medicine and Education*, Lecture Notes in Electrical Engineering 269,
DOI: 10.1007/978-94-007-7618-0_454,

Table 454.1 .

Nation	US	Japan	Haiti	China
Land area size level	Large	Small	Small	Large
Economic level	Developed	Developed	Undeveloped	Developing
Disaster name	Katrina	Tohoku	Port-au-Prince	Wenchua
Time of occurrence	Aug 2005	Mar 2011	Jan 2010	May 2008
Affected area	233,098 km^2	561 km^2	30 km^2	130,000 km^2
Number of death	1,833	15,843	500,000	69,227
Economic losses	$108 billion	$235 billion	$ 1billion	$113 billion

serious challenges to (EMSS)[1] [1] and recovery operations of relief to those impacted disaster sites. According to the past research, relatively rear of them concentrated on view from the IT, structure and operation of the system. Therefore, the rethinking and improving on the process of emergency rescue is extremely important and has strategic significance of necessity for many countries to improve their performance on relief disaster medicine.

454.2 Methodology

454.2.1 Cases Selection

This chapter selected four countries and their cases, based on two considerations:

1 The diversity of the EMSS levels due to their different geographical attributes and economic development levels;
2 These cases are typical and representative catastrophes in recent years around world. Table 454.1 represents the caparison of major statistical data[2] among four catastrophes.

454.2.2 Data Collection and Classification

Based on these cases, through 891 pieces of information from related materials, media reports, documentation, official data, interviews and record collection (due to language capability, all collected materials were all written in English or Chinese, and did not include materials of other languages.), the authors made

[1] An Emergency Medical Service (EMS) can be defined as "a comprehensive system which provides the arrangements of personnel, facilities and equipment for the effective, coordinated and timely delivery of health and safety services to victims of sudden illness or injury.".

[2] Data collected from wikipedia.org.

Table 454.2 .

Vector A	Vector A	Vector A
A subclass: [BD]	A subclass: [BD]	A subclass: [PD]
Uncontrollable random factors, hard to improve	System factors, non-majeure, easy to improve	System factors, non-majeure, easy to improve
B subclass: [O]	B subclass: [Ss]	B subclass: [So]
Vector B	Vector B	Vector B

screening and extraction 454 valid pieces of information regarding Emergency Medical Service.

454.2.3 Vector and Classes Setting

Set two class vectors for the clustering combination: time vector A and emergency rescue objective and subjective factors vector B. Then code their subclasses: A has two subclasses: before-disaster preparation [BD] and post-disaster response [PD]; B contains three subclasses: devastation and the unpredictability of disasters (objective factor) [O], emergency medical system structure (subjective factor) [Ss], emergency rescue operation (subjective factor) [So]. As shown in Table 454.2, these two categories have a certain degree of Subclass mapping relationship: from the time vector [BD] class usually maps [O] and [Ss] while [PD] class usually corresponds to [So]. Due to most of the [O] class issues are more likely uncontrollable risks from random factors, in addition, also more difficult to improve or avoid within a short period of time in emergency EMSS activities. Pragmatically, [BD]–[Ss] and [PD]–[So] should be given more attention with regard to emergency EMSS.

454.3 Results

According to the data collection and classification above, after merging and filtering some repetitive information, specific medical rescue problems in Katrina, Tohoku and Haiti are respectively shown in Tables 454.3, 454.4 and 454.5.

The authors took equal weight basis on type of problem for preliminary qualitative and quantitative analysis. The proportions of the ingredients for each case are shown in Table 454.6.

As the tables shown, if in the assumption to exclude the share of ingredients of random factors [O], in the case of Katrina, the issues in operational aspects is relatively equal to the ones in system and architecture with the former slightly conspicuousness. As for Tohoku, the more prominent issues reflected in the emergency medical services operational level relatively rather than ones caused by

Table 454.3 .

Type of the problem root	Specific problem representation
Unpredictability of disaster (objective aspects)	a. The unmet tremendous demand of materials and services in affected areas [2]
	b. Invalid and insufficient pre-disaster prediction and preparation
	e. The damage of infrastructure led extra obstacles for the rescue and coordination
System structure of emergency rescue system (subjective aspects)	c. IT system of state level and federal level are not well integrated [3]
	d. The instability of key coordinating organization and lack of sufficient staff training
Operation of EMSS (Subjective aspects)	h. Lack of planning on management and distribution of in kind donations
	g. Failure of follow-up on supply, inefficiency of distribution and operation
	F. Inaccessibility on tracking and positioning of relief materials and medical supplies

Table 454.4 .

Phenomena of the problems	Type
b. The terminal medical supply distribution lacked well preparedness for the compound disaster [4]	Pre-disaster
c. The transport routing design was in lack of sufficient flexibility in the face of nuclear radiation [5]	Preparation
d. Lack of understanding for the intensity of disaster and the details of preparedness was not well deployed.	
i. The lack of adequate personnel training target to post-disaster operation and practical experience to face such a compound disaster event.	
a. The function and hierarchy of emergency medical supply network node was not implemented as planned.	Post-disaster Response
e. The speed of the supplies flows did not well match the recovery speed of the transport facilities [6, 7]	
f. Invalid donation and excessive accumulation of low demand items took too much EMSS resources, resulting hamper for high demand medical supply inject into the affected areas [8]	
g. The allocation, deployment and placement of supply network nodes took a long time.	
h. Lack of sufficient cooperation between official agencies and local third-party EMSS companies to some extent reduced the efficiency of the medical services [9]	

its hierarchy. As a matter of fact, the stability of the emergency system architecture has a certain relationship with Nippon's over 150 years' development in the field of disaster relief. As for Port-au-Prince, the reason for evaluation [Ss] as N/A or 1/2 relies on: Haiti does not have complete national emergency medical response architecture, so this matter should not be estimated in the range of area

Table 454.5 .

Phenomena of problems	Types and attributes
A. The chaos, dispersed forces and lack of coordination of the international rescue in the golden week of rescue [10]	Coordination level, lack of coordination between the international relief organizations
B. The lack of the effective localization institutions' association for international disaster medicine groups [11]	Corporation level, International relief organizations and local medical rescue resources had poor integration and complementary
C. The basic resources for emergency relief activities in operational aspects failed to timely access.	Lack of access to the operational aspects of the basic elements for emergency rescue activities
D. The forecast of demand for life-sustaining staff and actual needs got large deviation [12]	Relief staff and victims both had increase demand of life-sustaining supplies related to the number increase

Table 454.6 .

A Class	A subclass: [BD]		A subclass:[PD]
Katrina	5(5/8)		3(3/8)
Tohoku	4(4/9)		5(5/9)
Port-au-Prince	2(1/2)		2(1/2)
B Class	B subclass:[O]	B subclass:[Ss]	B subclass:[So]
Katrina	3(3/8)	2(1/4)	3(3/8)
Tohoku	3(1/3)	1(1/9)	5(5/9)
Port-au-Prince	Negligible	N/A or 2(1/2)	2(1/2)
	Katrina	Tohoku	Port-au-Prince
A[BD]	0.625	0.444	0.5
A[PD]	0.375	0.556	0.5
B[O]	0.375	0.333	0
B[Ss]	0.25	0.111	0.5
B[So]	0.375	0.556	0.5

[Ss]. Yet if with the consideration that dependent on foreign aid agencies in Haiti as [Ss], the value for this nominal is 1/2. Causes of the problems in Haiti is more due to coordination among external aid organizations and collaboration between external aid organizations and local organizations, thus its [So] problems are basically results or characterizations of its [Ss].

Based on the above analysis, the authors extracted four frequently occurring elements which is shown in Table 454.7.

Table 454.7 .

A :[BD]	B:[Ss]	Staff training
		EMSS network design (PODs layout, IT systems integration)
A:[PD]	B:[So]	Management of medical service materials (excessive aggregation of donation, priority classification confusion)
		Vertical and horizontal synergies among emergency aid organizations (organizations' cooperation with local resources, coordination among multi-organizations)

Table 454.8 .

Pros	Quasi-military operation			Medical supply assignment
				Information exchange in IT system
				System coordination.
Cons	[BD]	[Ss]	Network design	Inadequate inventory of National emergency and imbalance of medical material reserves structure [13]
	[PD]	[So]	Synergies among organizations	Low degree of integration between emergency rescue system body and civil medical rescue resources and utilization
			Management of medical materials	Improper management in low demand-high volume donations and waste in emergency EMSS resources

454.4 Discussions

As China's national emergency medical service management system improvement and gradual accumulation of experience in fight against major disasters, the emergency relief has also made significant progress, but from a more detailed operational level, there is still something need to be concerned and improved. Taking Wenchuan as an example, according to the data collection and classification in part 2, specific pros and cons in Wenchuan is shown in Table 454.8.

As shown above, three Cons can be grouped into three out of four frequently occurring elements which are extracted by vector clustering method based on the cases of United States, Japan and Haiti. Thus, it is again validated that the four categories common elements have high frequency in the operation of emergency Rescue, through the case of China.

454.5 Conclusion

By vector clustering method, though in-depth case analysis based on the EMSS frameworks and operations of the system of four countries, the authors proposed specific suggestions for improvement in emergency rescue operation:

1. Strengthen the training of medical rescue personnel at all levels. Microscopically, the operational principal of any emergency relief system are people with professional knowledge, experience, skills and characters which finally affect the rescue effect. The day-to-day training is a systematic process, and is gradually step-by-step penetrated. Once the overall level of the personnel within the system is promoted, the efficiency of EMSS will be systematically improved.
2. Improve the information coordination and collaboration among the organizational elements of the medical service system. As rescue organizations in the system often have different backgrounds and division of labor, the vertical corporation and horizontal coordination are particularly important. Therefore, the harmony among organizational elements of the system, the system will get better resource integration and optimization.
3. Clarify the roles and tasks of aid organizations in system-level. The basis of these synergies are the roles and tasks of each organization and system's identification and cognition. As for EMSS network node sets, the external organizations should focus more on the management of central medical material reserves and transit nodes, while the resource-localized organizations should more concentrate on the work of the local medical services distribution.
4. Identify medical supply materials needs priority, reasonable manages the rescue staff, maximize the utilization of limited inventory and distribution resources. In accordance with a lot similar actual cases, the top four most needed supplies are water, food, blood and other medical supplies.

References

1. Moore L (1999) Measuring quality and effectiveness of prehospital EMS. Prehosp Emerg Care 3(4):325–331
2. House US (2006) A failure of initiative, final report of the selected bipartisan committee to investigate the preparation for and response to Hurricane Katrina, U.S. House of Representatives, p 343
3. Destro L, Holguín-Veras J (2011) Material convergence and its determinants: The case of Hurricane Katrina. Transportation research Record
4. DHS (2006) A performance review of FEMA's disaster management activities in response to Hurricane Katrina. Department of Homeland Security, office of the inspector general, 2006
5. The Journal of Commerce (2011) Maersk ships to avoid Japanese radiation zone, Japan container ports face some radiation risk, german ocean carriers avoid Tokyo, Yokohama
6. The great east Japan earthquake (117th report): Outline, MILT official web site, http://www.mlit.go.jp/common/000138154.pdf
7. Daily Yomiuri (2011) 6 days on govt still looking for aid supply plan
8. Fritz CE, Mathewson JH (1957) Convergent behavior: A disaster control problem, special report for the committee on disaster studies, in disaster study. National Academy of Sciences, Washington DC
9. MLIT response and measure, data of the current survey on construction statistics, MLIT official Website, http://www.mlit.go.jp/toukeijouhou/chojou/stat-e.htm, http://www.mlit.go.jp/page/kanbo01_hy_001411.html

10. In Quake's Wake, Haiti Faces Leadership Void, New York Times http://www.nytimes.com/2010/02/01/world/americas/01haiti.html?scp=1&sq=haiti+earthquake+preval&st=nyt. Accessed 31 Jan 2010
11. Obstacles to Recovery in Haiti May Prove Daunting Beyond Other Disasters, New York Times, http://www.nytimes.com/2010/01/23/world/americas/23haiti.html?pagewanted=1. Accessed 22 Jan 2010
12. Dynes R, Quarantelli E Kreps G (1972) A perspective on disaster planning, Report Series #11
13. Tingqin Z (2009) Natural disasters from the earthquake emergency logistics and distribution. Econ Res Guide 9:p131–p132

Chapter 455
Educational Data Mining for Problem Identification

Sylvia Encheva

Abstract Students face a number of difficulties studying mathematics on all educational levels. Data mining techniques applied on educational data can allow better understanding of the large amount of challenges students meet taking mathematical courses. Many researches focus on investigating various factors causing exam failure or even drop out. They often refer to study anxiety as being one of the serious reasons for students failure in mathematics. We believe that application of methods from market basket analysis can assist for identifying students, experiencing significant difficulties in their studies.

Keywords Data mining · Problem identification · Learning

455.1 Introduction

Students usually face a number of difficulties studying mathematics on all educational levels. Data mining techniques applied on educational data can allow better understanding of the vast amount of challenges students meet taking mathematical courses. Whether educational data is taken from students' use of interactive learning environments, computer-supported collaborative learning, or administrative data from schools and universities, it often has multiple levels of meaningful hierarchy, which often need to be determined by properties in the data itself, rather than in advance [1].

Study anxiety investigated in [2–4] among many others, turns out to be one of the serious reasons for students failure in mathematics. Other works focus on investigating various factors causing exam failure or even drop out. A detailed

S. Encheva (✉)
Stord/Haugesund University College, Bjørnsong 45, 5528 Haugesund, Norway
e-mail: sbe@hsh.no

S. Li et al. (eds.), *Frontier and Future Development of Information Technology in Medicine and Education*, Lecture Notes in Electrical Engineering 269,
DOI: 10.1007/978-94-007-7618-0_455,

examination of different subsets of collected educational data is in the main focus of this work. Exploiting methods from the area of market basket analysis on such data is very helpful for discovering learners who experiencing significant difficulties in their studies. Mining association rules is a part of the market basket techniques [5] and [6]. Algorithms for fast discovery of association rules have been presented in [7–10]. Association rules have applications in different fields such as market basket analysis [11], medical research [12], web clickstream analysis [13], and census data [14]. The complexity of mining frequent itemsets is exponential and algorithms for finding frequent sets have been developed by many authors such as [15] and [16].

455.2 Data Mining

Let $D = \{t_1, t_2, \ldots, t_n\}$ be a relational database of n tuples (or transactions) with a set of binary attributes (or items) $I = \{I_1, I_2, \ldots, I_m\}$; each transaction t in D can be considered as a subset of I, $t[I_j] = 1$ if $I_j \in t$, and $t[I_j] = 0$ if $I_j \notin t$ $(j = 1, 2, \ldots, m)$ [17]. An association rule is of the form: $X \Rightarrow Y$, where X and Y are two disjoint nonempty subsets of I (itemsets). Support and confidence for rule $X \Rightarrow Y$ are defined as $supp(X \Rightarrow Y) = \frac{|D_{X \cup Y}|}{|D|}$ and $conf(X \Rightarrow Y) = \frac{|D_{X \cup Y}|}{|D_X|}$ respectively, where $|D|$ is the number of tuples in D, $|D_X|$ is the number of tuples in D that contain X and (hence) $|D_{X \cup Y}|$ is the number of tuples in D that contain both X and Y. Also, we define the support of itemset X as $supp(X) = \frac{|D_X|}{|D|}$; clearly $supp(X \Rightarrow Y) = supp(X \cup Y)$. A valid association rule is a rule with support and confidence greater than given thresholds.

Positive, negative and irrelevant examples of association rules are shown in [18]. Degree of implications are discussed in (see e.g. [19]).

Educational Data Mining is discussed in details in [20]. It is an emerging discipline, concerned with developing methods for exploring the unique types of data that come from educational settings, and using those methods to better understand students, and the settings which they learn in, [1]. Educational Data Mining accommodates both existing and new approaches that build upon techniques from a combination of areas, including but not limited to statistics, psychometrics, machine learning, information retrieval, recommender systems and scientific computing [21].

Students failure in mathematics has been raising serious concerns among educators for a large number of years, [22]. Our work is an attempt to find dependences between students' results from already taken mathematical courses, midterm evaluations and final outcomes. Once some patterns or clusters are found, they will be used in future work to support new students in their studies.

As an illustration of the idea we take real data derived from results of 274 students placed in seventeen sets according to gender and background. Our findings are summarized in a concept lattice shown in Fig. 455.1 where the following

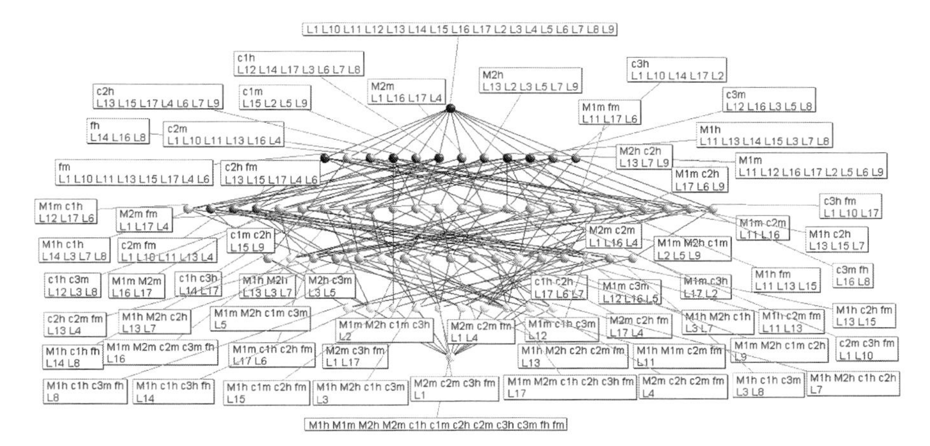

Fig. 455.1 Concept lattice

abbreviations are used: L1, L2, …, L17—sets of learners (students), C1, C2, C3—courses they have taken before, M1, M2—mid term evaluations, F—final outcome, where 'm' indicates middle level of presentation and 'h'—high level of presentation.

Interesting association rules are derived from the collected data, f. ex.: middle level of outcome of course C2 implies middle level of the final outcome with support 30 % and confidence 84 %; high level of outcome of course C2 implies middle level of the final outcome with support 29 % and confidence 71 %.

455.3 Conclusion

The presented work shows how useful data mining techniques taken from market basket analysis can be for avoiding the potential failure of a student. Further work is required for additional tuning of mid term evaluations and conclusions drawn thereafter. An important question that might be of additional interest is related to the degrees to which qualities of lectures and supplementary learning materials predetermine exam results.

References

1. http://www.educationaldatamining.org/
2. Erden M, Akgul S (2010) Predictive power of mathematics anxiety and perceived social support from teacher for primary students' mathematics achievement. J Theory Pract Educ 6(1):3–16

3. Idris N (2006) Exploring the effect of ti-84 plus on achievement and anxiety in mathematics. Eurasia J Math Sci Technol Educ 2(3):1–13
4. Ma X, Xu J (2003) The causal ordering of mathematics anxiety and mathematics achievement a longitudinal panel analysis. J Adolesc 27(2):165–179
5. Agrawal R, Imielinski T, and Swami A (1993) Mining association rules between sets of items in large databases. In: Proceedings of ACM SIGMOD international conference on management of data, Washington, DC, USA, pp 207–221
6. Agrawal R, Srikant R (1994) Fast algorithm for mining association rules. In: Proceedings of the 20th very large data base conference, Santiago, Chile, pp 487–489
7. Agrawal R, Mannila H, Srikant R, Toivonen H, Verkamo AI, (1996) Fast discovery of association rules. In: Uthurusamy F, Piatetsky-Shapiro G, Smyth P (eds) Advances in knowledge discovery of association rules, MIT Press, Cambridge, pp 307–328
8. Pasquier N, Bastide T, Taouil R, Lakhal L (1999) Efficient mining of association rules using closed item set lattices. J Inf Syst 24(1):25–46
9. Zaki MJ (2000) Generating non-redundant association rules. In: Proceedings of the 6th ACM SIGKDD international conference on knowledge discovery and data mining, Boston, USA, pp 34–43
10. Zaki MJ, Hsiao C-J (2002) CHARM: an efficient algorithm for closed itemset mining. In: Proceedings of the 2nd SIAM international conference on data mining, Arlington, VA, USA, pp 34–43
11. Brin S, Motwani R, Ullmann J D, and Tsur S (1997) Dynamic itemset counting and implication rules for market basket data. In: Proceedings of the ACM SIGKDD international conference on management of data, Tuscon, AZ, USA, pp 255–264
12. Delgado M, Sanchez D, Martin-Bautista MJ, Vila MA (2001) Mining association rules with improved semantics in medical databases. Artif Intell Med 21(1–3):241–245
13. Sweiger M, Madsen M R, Langston J, Howard Lombard H (2002) Clickstream data warehousing. John Wiley and Sons, Hoboken
14. Malerba D, Lisi FA, Appice A, Sblendorio F (2002) Mining spatial association rules in census data: a relational approach. In: Proceedings of the ECML/PKDD'02 workshop on mining official data, University Printing House, Helsinki, pp 80–93
15. Bastide T, Taouil R, Pasquier N, Stumme G, Lakhal L (2000) Mining frequent patterns with counting inference. In: SIGKDD explorations, special issue on scalable algorithms, 2(2): 71–80
16. Carpineto C, Romano G (2004) Concept data analysis: theory and applications. John Wiley and Sons, New York
17. Yan P, Chen G (2004) Mining positive and negative fuzzy association rules, KES 2004. Lecture Notes in Artificial Intelligence, vol 3213. Springer, Berlin, pp 270–276
18. Dubois D, Hüllermeier E, Prade H (2003) A note on quality measures for fuzzy association rules. Lect Notes Artif Intell 2715:346–353
19. De Cock M, Cornelis C, Kerre EE (2005) Elicitation of fuzzy association rules from positive and negative examples. Fuzzy Sets Syst 149(1):73–85
20. Baker K (2010) Data Mining for Education. In: McGaw B, Peterson P, Baker E (eds) International encyclopedia of education, 3rd edn, vol 7. Elsevier, Oxford, pp 112–118
21. Romero C, Ventura S, Pechenizkiy M, Baker RSJ (2011) Handbook of educational data mining. Taylor and Francis Group, London
22. Osburn WJ (1925) Ten reasons why pupils fail in mathematics. Math Teacher 18(4):234–238

Chapter 456
Statistics Experiment Base on Excel in Statistics Education: Taking Zhejiang Shuren University as Example

Wenjie Li, Yitao Wang and Guowei Wan

Abstract With the development of computer, analysis of statistical data becomes more simple, convenient and accurate. Therefore computer prompts statistics popularization. So, it is urgent to build Statistics experiment in Statistics teaching. This chapter discusses the statistics experiment teaching system based on Excel and also investigates the teaching effect.

Keywords Excel · Statistics experiment · Statistics education

456.1 Introduction

Statistics is one of the core courses in economics and management majors. It develops the students' ability to solve specific problems by using statistical methods and statistical information. However, teaching effect of statistics is not good for non-statistics major students. For weak mathematics, the students feel that the statistical concept is abstract and the formula is very complex. At last, many students lose their interest in learning statistics. The phenomenon is more serious in the Third Degree College in China. However, experimental course can help students solve difficulties in study statistics. Because statistics experiment combines the actual data, statistical methods, statistical analysis tools and related background knowledge together, it can help the students understand the concepts and methods of statistics. This chapter discusses the statistics experiment teaching system based on Excel.

W. Li (✉) · Y. Wang · G. Wan
School of Management, Zhejiang Shuren University, 310015 Hangzhou, China
e-mail: lwenjie@163.com

S. Li et al. (eds.), *Frontier and Future Development of Information Technology in Medicine and Education*, Lecture Notes in Electrical Engineering 269,
DOI: 10.1007/978-94-007-7618-0_456,

456.2 Application of Excel in Statistics Experiment

456.2.1 Design of Teaching Process in Statistics Experiment

456.2.1.1 Teaching Purpose of Statistics Experiment

The purpose of statistics experiment is to enhance students' ability in statistical application. So, statistics experiment need combine the statistical software with statistics contents. Students should use statistical software to help them finish many statistics work: data input, descriptive statistics analysis, drawing statistical charts, parameter estimation, hypothesis testing, analysis of variance, correlation and regression.

456.2.1.2 Contents of Statistics Experiment

According to purpose of statistics experiment and actual teaching situation, we designed reasonable statistics experiment teaching contents in Zhejiang Shuren University (Table 456.1). We hope students can solve statistical problems by course training.

456.2.1.3 Organization and Guidance of Statistics Experiment

Statistics experiment should be carried on strictly in teaching plan. Before experimental course, students are divided into several project teams. Every task for them includes the survey project, the survey questionnaire, data input, data analysis and survey report. All the work should be done by students themselves. In the

Table 456.1 Content and period assignation of statistics experiment

Serial number	Experiment project	Experiment contents	Hours
1	Data input	Understanding data structure and input	2
2	Data handling	Data filter, data classification, data Pivot table	2
3	Descriptive analysis	Calculation the mean, median, mode, range, standard deviation	2
4	Graphical techniques	Drawing chart and figure	2
5	Inference analysis	Parameter estimation and hypothesis test	2
6	Cross Tabulations	Cross tab and Chi square test	2
7	ANOV	Analysis of variance	2
8	Regression analysis	Calculating correlation coefficient and regression analysis	2

experimental process, every student must fill out test records and test report. After the experiment, the teacher should evaluate the students' training score based on their test cases and make a summary.

456.2.2 Excel Application in Statistics Experiment

456.2.2.1 Advantages and Disadvantages of Excel in Statistics Experiment

SPSS, SAS, Eviews, Minitab and Excel are commonly used in statistics. SPSS, SAS, Eviews, Minitab are considered as professional statistical software. The students need specialized training before they use them. So they are not suitable for the students of non-statistical majors. But as office software, Excel provides strong statistics function to meet basic statistics needs. At the same time, students are familiar with Excel before learning statistics. The points above are main advantages for application in statistics experiment.

Excel should be applied throughout the whole statistics course, in order to improve the students' statistical ability. But Excel is only used in general statistical analysis. If students meet some complex statistic problems, they have to use other professional statistical software.

456.2.2.2 The Statistical Function of Excel

The statistical function of Excel is mainly shown in three aspects: graph functions, statistical functions and data analysis tools. We mainly introduce three statistical functions in the experimental teaching.

1. Graph function

Excel consists of 14 types of graphics, including column charts, bar charts, line charts etc. Moreover, Excel chart has better visual effect. Statistical chart is mainly used in descriptive analysis. A good cartogram makes the statistics obvious, so charting method is basic statistics method. In the experimental course, teacher demonstrates and explains the statistical charts in detail through specific cases, such as bar charts, scatter plots, statistical statements, to enable students to master the charting method.

2. Statistical functions

Besides mathematical functions and logic functions, Excel provides a lot of statistical functions, such as AVERAGE (mean), CONFIDENCE (confidence interval) and COV (covariance) function etc. The application of statistical function is very extensive. Statistical function can not only be calculated descriptive statistics, such as to calculate the arithmetic mean using AVERAGE function, calculate the harmonic mean using ARMEAN function, calculates the median using MEDIAN, sample standard deviation calculation using STDEV, but also can be inferred the critical value by using NORMSDIST, TINV, CHIINV, FINV function.

In experiment teaching, the teacher should introduce the definition function format, function parameters, the meaning of the output, and the use of methods in order to help student master the statistical function.

3. Data analysis tools

In the Excel data analysis tool library, there are 19 kinds of data analysis tools. Most methods in statistics, such as descriptive statistics, histogram, hypothesis testing, analysis of variance, correlation and regression, can be found in Excel data analysis tools. So, how to use the data analysis tools is the key point in statistics experiment.

456.3 Teaching Results of Statistics Experiment Based on Excel

With application of Excel, students become more interested and focused in statistics course. The effect in teaching statistics and students' statistical application ability has improved since statistics experiment. The following questionnaire survey shows the result of statistics experiment in Zhejiang Shuren University.

1. Participants' basic information

In this statistics educational survey, we investigate total 177 students from school of management, who finished statistics course just now. Because their majors are all financial management, the rate of female students accounted is 68.4 %, which is significantly higher than male students' 31.6 %. Students have deferent subject background in their high school stage, the proportion of liberal arts is 49.7 % and science is 50.3 %. All students are sophomore and have not foundation of probability theory (see Table 456.2).

2. The effect evaluation of statistical experiment

About effect evaluation of statistical experiment, the survey shows students who think the effect of statistical experiments is very good accounted for only

Table 456.2 Participants' basic information

Gender	Arts	Science	Total
Male	15	41	56
Female	73	48	121
Total	88	89	177

Tab 456.3 Evaluation of statistical experiment

Evaluation	Frequency	Percentage	Cumulative percentage
Very good	65	36.7	36.7
Good	67	37.9	74.6
Normal	30	16.9	91.5
Bad	2	1.1	92.7
Very bad	13	7.3	100

Tab 456.4 Suggestions for improvement statistics education

Suggestions	Frequency	Percentage	Cumulative percentage
Increasing the experiment teaching	65	36.7	36.7
Adding case teaching	67	37.9	74.6
To increase exercise	30	16.9	91.5
Increase the hours	2	1.1	92.7
Don't need	13	7.3	100

9.6 %, good level accounted for 52 %, normal level is 31.1 % (Table 456.3). We can find that most students approve of statistics experiment, but there are still space to improve this experiment in Zhejiang Shuren University.

3. Suggestions for improving statistics education

On Suggestions for improving statistics education, Students suggest enhancing experiment teaching and case teaching methods accounted for 36.7 and 37.9 %, which shows that the statistics experiment teaching and case teaching, have been recognized by the students (Table 456.4).

456.4 Conclusions

In this chapter, we discuss how to design statistics experiment based on Excel by taking Zhejiang Shuren University as an example. We also point out some advantages and disadvantages of Excel in statistics experiment. Finally, we find that most students approve of Statistics experiment by statistics survey. There is still a lot of work for the teachers to do in order to make the experiment much more effective.

References

1. Feng S (2004) Institutions of higher learning and some suggestions on statistics construction in China university. Stat Res 52–54
2. Jia J (2006) Statistics. Tsinghua University press, Beijing

3. Sun F, LI Y (2011) Application of Excel in the teaching of principle of statistics. J Liaoning Tech Univ (Soc Sci Ed) 216–218
4. Wu Z (2011) About mathematics experiment on probability and statistics based on Excel. J Qin Zhou Univ 5–8
5. Niu C (2012) The statistical software experimental teaching of mathematical statistics in statistics major. Gansu Sci Technol 76–78

Chapter 457
Simulating the Space Deep Brain Stimulations Using a Biophysical Model

Yingyuan Chen, Fei Su, Jiang Wang, Xile Wei and Bin Deng

Abstract In this paper, A computational biophysical model of basal ganglia (BG) thalamic (TC) network is introduced to assess the influence of space deep brain stimulation (DBS) on motor symptoms of Parkinson's disease (PD). In PD state, the firing of globus pallidus in pars interna (GPi) is burstlike and synchronized. If the standard DBS current is applied, the tonic rhythm output of GPi could restore the TC relay properties. Under the consideration of space stimulation, the firing patterns of BG-TC network are similar to the standard DBS. These results demonstrate that the single-compartmental, conductance-based network model can simulate space electrical stimulation into the brain.

Keywords Parkinson's disease (PD) · Deep brain stimulation (DBS) · Space stimulation · Basal ganglia thalamic network

457.1 Introduction

Deep brain stimulation (DBS) has become an efficient therapy for Parkinson disease (PD) in recent years (3 4 5).The therapeutic effects are remarkable and can improve PD motor symptoms, but the mechanism for DBS is unknown [1]. In current

This work is supported by the National Natural Science Foundation of China (Grant No. 61072012 and 61172009), the Young Scientists Fund of the National Natural Science Foundation of China (Grant Nos. 61104032), and the China Postdoctoral Science Foundation (Grant No. 2012M510750).

Y. Chen · F. Su · J. Wang · X. Wei · B. Deng
School of Electrical and Automation Eng, Tianjin University, Tianjin 300072, People's Republic of China
e-mail: jiangwang@tju.edu.cn

S. Li et al. (eds.), *Frontier and Future Development of Information Technology in Medicine and Education*, Lecture Notes in Electrical Engineering 269,
DOI: 10.1007/978-94-007-7618-0_457,

application,DBS is implemented by an implanted pulse generator that delivers an ongoing stream of high frequency current pulse [2], stimulation is always on, the stimulator batteries have to be replaced surgically every 3–5 years for PD patients [3], which causes a great damage to the patients. So it is essential to optimize the DBS waveform pattern, but efforts are hampered, due to the unknown mechanism of DBS and its clinical efficacy. There is a complex relationship between DBS parameters (amplitude, frequency, duration) and their therapeutic effects [4]. Many previous studies have focused their attention on frequency and found a replaceable low frequency compared with the standard stimulus waveform [3]. But they always assume the DBS amplitude to be a constant, in practice, the stimulus amplitude applied to every neuron may be different, because their distance to the stimulus electrode is different. Besides, if lower average amplitudes can performance as good as or even better than their high amplitudes counterparts, their use would prolong the life of stimulator batteries.

Rubin and Terman [1] make the hypothesis that DBS works by replacing pathologically rhythmic basal ganglia output with tonic, high frequency firing. In this paper, we use the BG-TC network model proposed by Rubin and Terman [1] to simulate the space electrical stimulation applied to STN neurons. First, we generate data under healthy, PD and PD with DBS conditions. Then we construct a space DBS waveform according to the distance from each STN neuron to the stimulation electrode. We find that this DBS paradigm can restore both pathological activity of GPi and the thalamic relay fidelity.

457.2 Model and Methods

The basal ganglia thalamic network model is composed by 16 STN cells, 16 Gpe cells, 16 GPi cells and 2 TC cells, respectively. They are linked by excitatory and inhibitory synaptic currents and are subjected to external currents input, as depicted in Fig. 457.1.

The membrane potential of BG-TC network neurons is described as:

$$\begin{aligned}
C_m \frac{dv_{Th}}{dt} &= -I_L - I_{Na} - I_K - I_T - I_{Gi\to Th} + I_{SM} \\
C_m \frac{dv_{Sn}}{dt} &= -I_L - I_{Na} - I_K - I_T - I_{Ca} - I_{AHP} - I_{Ge\to Sn} + I_{DBS} \\
C_m \frac{dv_{Ge}}{dt} &= -I_L - I_{Na} - I_K - I_T - I_{Ca} - I_{AHP} - I_{Sn\to Ge} - I_{Ge\to Ge} + I_{Ge}
\end{aligned} \tag{457.1}$$

It is determined by a HH-type equation. I_L is the leakage current. I_K is the potassium current. I_{Na} is the sodium current. I_T is a low-threshold T-type Ca^{2+} current. I_{AHP} is a Ca^{2+} activated, voltage-independent afterhyper-polarization K^+ current. I_{SM} is the sensorimotor input to the TC cells. I_{Ge} is a constant and represents input from striatum.

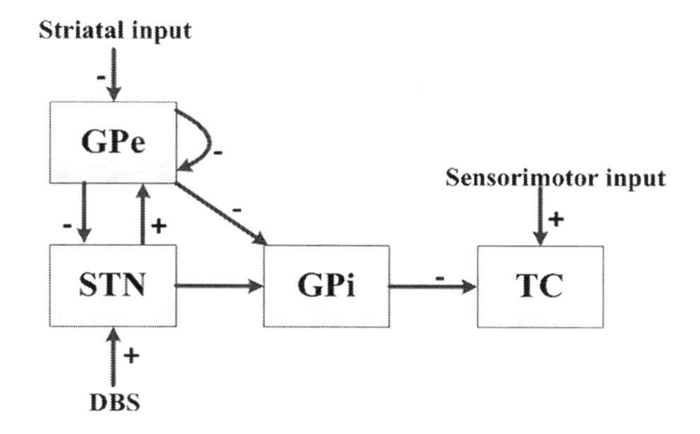

Fig. 457.1 The synaptic connection between BG network and TC. + means excitatory synaptic connection between neurons, and – means inhibitory connection

The stimulation applied to STN neurons is modeled as a square-wave pulse train, described by,

$$I^{j}_{DBS} = \theta_j i_D H\left(\sin\left(\frac{2\pi t}{\rho_D}\right)\right)\left(1 - H\left(\sin\left(\frac{2\pi(t+\delta_D)}{\rho_D}\right)\right)\right) \tag{457.2}$$

Here, $\theta_j \in [0,1]$is a weight term which indicates the distance from the stimulation electrode to the jth STN neuron, i_D, ρ_D, δ_D is the amplitude, period and duration of stimulation pulse, respectively. H is a Heaviside step function. Note that δ_D is set to be 0.6 ms, ρ_D is set to be 6 ms in all simulations.

Synaptic current $I_{\alpha\to\beta}$ from α cell to β cell is described as:

$$I_{\alpha\to\beta} = g_{\alpha\to\beta}\left[V_\beta - E_{\alpha\to\beta}\right]\sum_j s^j_\alpha \tag{457.3}$$

Here, $g_{\alpha\to\beta}$ means the maximal synaptic conductance between presynaptic neuron α and postsynaptic neuron β. $E_{\alpha\to\beta}$ means the synaptic reversal potential. $\sum_j s^j_\alpha$ means the sum of synaptic conductance over presynaptic cells j.

The sensorimotor input is modeled as a pulse train. To quantify our detection, We define Rel to measure the reliability of thalamic neurons responding to sensorimotor inputs.

$$\mathrm{Re}l_j = 1 - \frac{b+c}{n},\ j = 1,2 \tag{457.4}$$

Here n is the number of sensorimotor inputs, which equals to the sum of these three types of spikes. b is the number of false spikes and c is the number of missed spikes. Subscript j denotes the jth thalamic neuron. This definition equals to the error index of Rubin and Terman [1] and it's defined by Feng et al. [5].

457.3 Results

457.3.1 BG Network Under Healthy and PD Condition

We adjust I_{app} and $g_{GPe \to GPe}$ to simulate the BG network in the healthy state. As depicted in Fig. 3.2a, we see the GPi activity is irregular and uncorrelated, TC neuron is able to transmit sensorimotor signals accurately. Then we increase the value of I_{app} and decrease the value of $g_{GPe \to GPe}$ to achieve a PD condition. As Fig. 3.1b shows, in PD condition, the GPi neurons fire bursts and are synchronous under the subpopulations of neurons. Under this condition, the TC neuron can't relay sensorimotor input faithfully.

457.3.2 PD BG Network with Standard and Space DBS

In real clinical application of DBS, each stimulated STN neuron can't receive the same stimulus amplitude, because their distance to the electrode is different. In order to illustrate this qualitatively, we simulate each STN to different stimulus amplitude, so the weight term θ_j is different in STN neurons to represent the distance from STN neuron to the stimulator electrode. We assume the site of the stimulator electrode is in the central of STN neurons, the weights for each neuron are chosen from a uniform distribution. In order to make the two TC cells receive similar synaptic input, we give the symmetric weights to 16 STN neurons, as described in Fig. 3.3.

Figure 3.2c shows the BG network activity when STN cells are applied to this kind of more practical stimulation. The nice thing is that besides the restoration of TC reliability, the firing activity of GPi neurons are closer to the normal state. Dorval 2009 refers that the ideal DBS may be one that rather than forcing regular GPi activity, restores GPi activity to the healthy condition [6]. So this space DBS we used is closer to the ideal DBS.

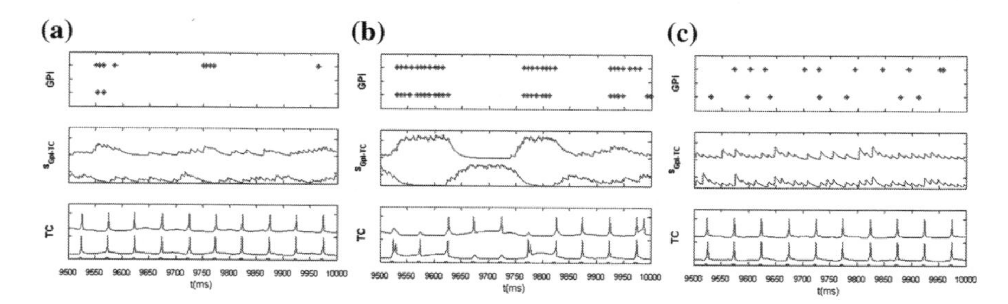

Fig. 457.2 The GPi firing activity, synaptic input from GPi to TC and TC firing activity under healthy (*a*), PD (*b*) and standard and space DBS (*c*) condition

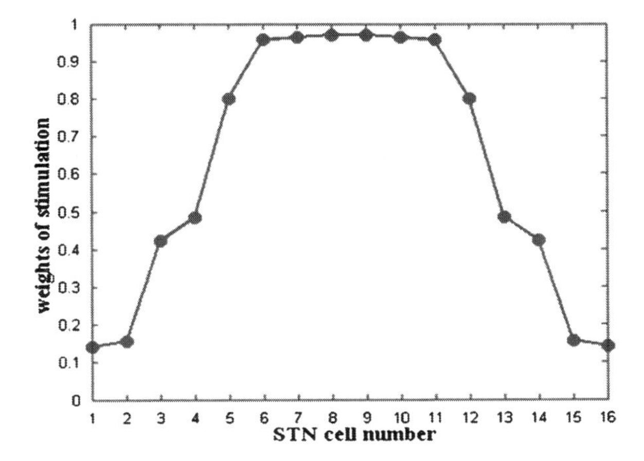

Fig. 457.2 The amplitude weight of DBS for each STN neuron. The value of DBS amplitude applied for each neuron is its weight multiply by 200 pA/μm^2

457.4 Conclusion

In this paper, we use a biophysical model of the BG thalamic network, based on the previous work. We tuned the model parameters to generate healthy, PD and DBS data for analyzing. The standard DBS applied to STN is the same as Rubin and Terman [7], but the space DBS are different. We find that the phasic bursting activity of GPi neurons is diminished and TC relay reliability is restored.

In order to make our model research closer to clinical application, we use the RT model to simulate the effect of space varying DBS waveform based on the STN neurons distance from the DBS electrode. After analyzing the BG activity, we find a nice thing, some GPi neurons firing activity are closer to the healthy state, besides the TC reliability is restored too. This work makes a contribution to study the mechanism of DBS more accurately.

References

1. Rubin JE, Terman D (2004) High frequency stimulation of the subthalamic nucleus eliminates pathological thalamic rhythmicity in a computational model. JCoN 16(3):211–235
2. Guo Y, Rubin JE, McIntyre CC, Vitek JL, Terman D (2008) Thalamocortical relay fidelity varies across subthalamic nucleus deep brain stimulation protocols in a data driven computational model. J Neurophysiol 99:1477–1492
3. Agarwal R, Sarma SV (2012) The effects of DBS patterns on basal ganglia activity and thalamic relay:a computational study. J Comput Neurosci 33:151-167
4. Feng XJ, Greenwald B, Rabitz H, Shea-Brown E, Kosut R (2007) Toward closed-loop optimization of deep brain stimulation for Parkinson's disease: concepts and lessons from a computational model. J Neural Eng b4:L14–L21
5. Feng XJ, Brown ES, Greenwald B, Kosut RL, Rabitz H (2007) Optimal deep brain stimulation of the subthalamic nucleus–a computational study. J Comput Neurosci 23(3):265–282

6. Dorval AD, Panjwani N, Qi RY, Grill WM (2009) Deep brain stimulation that abolishes parkinsonian activity in basalganglia improves thalamic relay fidelity in a computational circuit. In: 31st annual international conference of the IEEE EMBS Minneapolis, Minnesota, USA, 2–6 Sept 2009
7. Terman D, Rubin JE, Yew AC (2002) Activity patterns in a model for the subthalamopallidal network of the basal ganglia. J Neurosci 22(7):2963–2976
8. Schiff SJ(2010) Towards model-based control of Parkinson's disease. Phil Trans R Soc A, 368:2269-2308

Chapter 458
Strategy and Analysis of Emotional Education into the Cooperative Learning in Microcomputers Teaching

Dongxing Wang

Abstract Cooperative learning emphasizes the unity and uses all positive factors to let the leaner be integrated into the team in order to improve themselves together. If we integrate the emotional education into the cooperative learning that would not only help to study and explore the truth continually, but also be conducive to heritage the university spirit of absorbing everything and cooperating with everything. This is a kind of ideal situation of cooperative learning. So in microcomputer teaching, we use the above method which is also an efficient way to carry out the moral education in college. From the analysis of the present situation of emotion education, this paper puts forward a strategy of integrating the emotional education into the cooperative learning in microcomputer teaching, and the result shows that the effect of the strategy implementation is good, which provides the good reference for the related teaching.

Keywords Cooperative learning · Microcomputer · Emotional education

458.1 Analysis of Present Situation of Lack of Emotional Education in Microcomputer Teaching

With the help of multimedia technology and network technology to carry out the cooperative learning on microcomputer is a optimizing way of cooperative learning; it is superior to the traditional media education in the sharing resources, student interactions, and teacher student interactions and so far [1]. It integrates a variety of information by use of network which is very convenient for the education, but at the same time, obviously has the tendency of neglecting emotional education.

D. Wang (✉)
Institute of Computer Science, Daqing Normal University, 1,63712 DaQing, China
e-mail: cnwindy02@163.com

S. Li et al. (eds.), *Frontier and Future Development of Information Technology in Medicine and Education*, Lecture Notes in Electrical Engineering 269,
DOI: 10.1007/978-94-007-7618-0_458,

458.1.1 The Current Situation Analysis

Most of the cooperative learning in microcomputer teaching just uses network technology to carry out" text content moving", and publish some textual notification or teaching exercise etc. Undoubtedly, this" movement" is cold and lack of emotion. This is bound to arouse students' antipathy; when they face the computer screen, they could not have any interest, and thus will not have a good learning effect. Of course, the kind of this movement is an extreme phenomenon; in fact people would process the teaching resources properly, but if there is no certain theoretical guidance and the elaborate teaching design, the developed teaching resources still cannot achieve the expected goal of optimizing teaching.

458.1.2 The Reasons for Lack of Emotional Education

There are many reasons for the absence of emotional education in microcomputer teaching, such as: the character of network, the traditional concepts of education, education content and teaching resources development.

458.1.2.1 The Reasons of the Network

Everything has two sides, the network is also so. It brings people great convenience at the same time, also expose its weakness. If the lack degree of the emotional education in network environment is not given the corresponding attention, it is difficult for us to imagine the status that the network education will develop into [2].

458.1.2.2 The Lack of Emotion in Education Concept

Along with the development of the modern industry and science, scientism gradually gets his guidance position in the education field. By the guide of it, the emotion layer in the education field languishing, purely developing cognitive education, neglecting the emotional cultivating, the cognitive theory and the rationalism get the education circles [3]. The cognitive theory and rationalism mainly displays that its ultimate goal of education is to train the students to be the talents with the high technology and the high intelligence. Therefore the education pays more attention to how to impart knowledge, improve people's intelligence, but despise emotional care for the students.

458.1.2.3 The Lack of Emotion in Education Content

Because the science focuses on the fact, the systematic scientific knowledge, theory, and the occupation skills are regarded as the main education content. But the human values, ideal, sentiment and so on became a subsidiary. In fact, the learning process can be divided into two interrelated areas: cognitive domain and emotional domain, the former including perceiving and analyzing the information in order to acquire the new knowledge; the latter including feeling and emotional control in order to obtain affection experience and evaluation. Modern education, especially cooperative learning in network environment should not be "getting the half, at the cost of the other half of the education". So we cannot put emphasis on cognition, and neglect emotion; or put emphasis on science, and neglect moral education.

458.2 The Emotion Care Measures

During the traditional teaching design, the teaching content is carried out only from the cognitive domain, but in this cooperative learning, we mainly process the factors from the emotional domain.

In the cooperative learning, let students solve the problem by the way of the game or task. During this period, let the students gradually be confident and full of sense of responsibility and other positive emotions.

Constructing collaborative learning mode with the aid of the CSCW, the students could collaborate with each other in a virtual learning environment [4].

458.3 Emotional Strategies of Improving Cooperative Learning Ability in Microcomputer Teaching

458.3.1 Pay Attention to Social Skill of Cooperative Learning

In learning process, the students' cooperative skills should be developed. First, by the net, arranging proper situation let the students carry on a planned collaborative practice, so that everyone can express and listen fluently. Secondly, encourage students to practice the cooperative skill in real life continuously. Finally, teachers should make a positive evaluation on cooperative skills [5].

458.3.2 Optimize the Cooperative Method and Grouping Strategy

Firstly, we should building the network platform. Secondly, display the works in the platform which could turn the competition among individuals into the teams' competition in cooperative learning. In the process, the cooperative mechanism and the cooperation system is adjusted and optimized. The method is as follows.

458.3.2.1 Proper Grouping

Let's group according to the principle of being heterogeneous in the same team and homogeneity in the different teams. There are generally 4-6 students in a team. Let the students cooperate in the same team and compete among the teams, thus forming a good cooperative and competitive environment [6].

458.3.2.2 Setting Clear Division of Responsibilities

Every student of the team should have a defined job and affords the corresponding responsibility. The division of the work is determined according to their characteristics and specialty. The team set the leader, programmers and program testers etc. Also according to the teaching needs, let students take their turns on playing different roles.

458.3.2.3 Setting clear targets

Before cooperative learning, let the students make clear the problems to be solved, set the target, start thinking around the target and express their opinions, and then improve cooperative study effect. Set the proper problems according which has a certain degree of difficulty, and could be solved by students' hard work.

458.3.3 Grasp the Opportunity to Carry Out Cooperative Learning in Microcomputer Teaching

The implementation of cooperative learning in microcomputer teaching not only needs teachers' consent, but also needs the course and the students' consent. When the students' thinking is hindered, the team members have different opinions, and the answers of the questions diversify, the cooperative learning should be carry out which should be integrated into the emotional education factors and at the same time, the teachers should timely grasp the opportunities to teach students according to the situation.

458.4 Conclusion

Using cooperative learning in microcomputer teaching can help to carry out cognitive learning, but it need systematically be supplemented into emotional education factors. The feedback of teaching effect and the questionnaire survey showed that: 100 % of the students like cooperative learning with the emotional education in microcomputer teaching, and have a greater harvest. 95 % of the students hope to get more moral education in microcomputer classes, 93 % of the students accept and are in favor of integrating the emotional education into cooperative learning in microcomputer homework. The evaluation results showed that: cooperative learning with the emotional education in microcomputer teaching well completed the cognitive education and emotional education double teaching targets.

Acknowledgments The studies were funded by Heilongjiang High Education Reform Project (JGZ201201005) and Heilongjiang High Education Reform Project: the construction and research of the teaching mode of the guiding learning in "Microcomputer Principle" lessons and the reform project: Teaching reform research of the embedded course in application-oriented college.

References

1. Qin G (2007) Theories of cooperative learning and its essence. Heilongjiang Researches on Higher Education
2. Liu J, Zhong Z (2010) Lack of sensation in on-line teaching and countermeasure. China Distance Education
3. Lin Y (2002) On engaging college students in cooperative learning. J Guangdong Univ Technol
4. Chafe Allison Computer Technology and Cooperative Learning. http://www.cdli.ca/achafe/maj-index.html
5. Johnson DW, Johnson RT (2009) Cooperative learning and social interdependence theory. http://www.co-operation.org/pages/SIT.html
6. Xie Z, Xu Q, Wang X (2009) Problems and countermeasures in collaborative learning. J Zhejiang Wanli Univ

Chapter 459
Construction and Practice of Network Platform for Training of GPs

Gang Liu, Guochun Xiang, Heqing Huang, Junsheng Ji, Hong Chen, Haitao Guo, Biyuan Li, You Li, Guangqiong Liu, Zegui Li and Kehou Wang

Abstract Insufficiency of qualified general practitioners (GPs) has hindered the development of the health service in China. To accelerate the training of GP, we built the first information platform for them and created the stereo mode of the network by combining base training with our standardized GP base. The transfer training has been offered to tens of thousands of GPs throughout the country. Therefore, the conflict between the need for GPs and the longer periods of training cycle will be effectively alleviated.

Keywords GP · Information training · Network platform

General practice emphasizes the patient-centered, family-oriented, community-based, and prevention-oriented health care. When people's health was effectively improved, the best cost-effectiveness of the medical service and health benefits would be obtained by the *"six-in-one"* service which is consisted of the prevention, medical treatment, care, rehabilitation, health education and maternity [1–3]. Therefore, the establishment of general practitioner (GP) system will play a positive role in promoting reform in China's medical and health system. However, the training of GPs is still in its initial stage [4–6], because the shortage of qualified GPs has hindered the development of community health service in China [7].

To accelerate the training of GP, China's State Council issued *The Guidance on Establishing a General Practitioner System* in July 2011 and called for training over 300,000 community GPs till 2020, so that the situation of the "visiting doctors being difficult and expensive" might be alleviated. Facing the huge gaps for GP posts, the first network platform of online education for GPs (http//

G. Liu (✉) · G. Xiang · H. Huang · J. Ji · H. Chen · H. Guo · B. Li · Y. Li · G. Liu · Z. Li
Southwest Hospital, The Third Military Medical University, 29 Gaotangyan street, 400038 Shapingba, Chongqing, China
e-mail: liugang6399@sohu.com

K. Wang
Chongqing Yuanqiu Company for Science and Technology, 400038 Chongqing, China

S. Li et al. (eds.), *Frontier and Future Development of Information Technology in Medicine and Education*, Lecture Notes in Electrical Engineering 269,
DOI: 10.1007/978-94-007-7618-0_459, © Springer Science+Business Media Dordrecht 2014

www.gpes.com.cn) and its software resource library have been constructed on the basis of the army network course by our hospital and Chongqing Yuanqiu Company for Science and Technology since 2008 to provide a convenient web platform for the online training of GPs. It has offered the transfer training opportunities over time and space to tens of thousands of GPs from community and army through our practice in the past 4 years. Therefore, the conflict between the need for GPs and the longer periods of training will be effectively alleviated.

459.1 Construction of Network Platform for GPs

459.1.1 Development of Hardware and Software for Platform

There is an Entity-datacenter of hardware and the software systems on the online education training network for GPs (http//www.gpes.com.cn) [8], and the hardware-data center is consisted of three high-performance servers, two IP-SAN behind the servers and the total storage volume over 20 TB, and the network mirror is achieved. Its key techniques are processing resources in depth by using OCR, correcting links of knowledge using self-developed thesaurus, and all-round display for the same knowledge point. Software system framework is an external website-"an online education training network for GPs" released on the hardware system. We designed and constructed eight database systems including the autonomous learning, disease diagnosis and treatment, online examination, preventive health care, health education, counseling, maternity and online communication. These 8 databases are in meshed links and are efficiently interacted to obtain good results.

459.1.2 Construction and Application of the Autonomous Learning System

There are six open network classrooms in the autonomous learning system. They were designed based on the six-in-one service of GPs. They are the clinical medicine, preventive care, mental health, rehabilitation and physical therapy, health education, and prenatal and postnatal care, respectively. According to the standard for GP training issued by the Ministry of Health, the twenty online courses including introduction to general practice, internal medicine, surgery, rehabilitation medicine, clinical counseling, and so on were offered in these virtual classrooms. The functional databases of the network teaching materials, the video tutorials, the homework exercises and tests, and the interactive communication were constructed for each course. Over ten thousands of students have taken our online classes since the construction of the six virtual classrooms, with 68,551 students participating in the network Diagnostics course and 15,865 of them took it. Because the course is rich in resources, well-illustrated, fully-equipped, it will provide a good self-learning and self-testing platform to students.

459.1.3 Construction and Application of the Diagnosis and Treatment System

Disease diagnosis and treatment system is a first large multimedia medical database for the clinical diagnosis and treatment. It is also one of the unique and highlighted databases in the platform. Nine functional modules are designed and constructed in the system, including: (1) the disease database for over 14,000 common diseases, (2) the clinical symptom database for over 6,000 common clinical symptoms, (3) the Chinese Medicine database, (4) the disease research database, (5) the database for the laboratory examination, (6) the drug database, (7) the clinical path database, (8) the standard operational database, (9) the database of clinical teaching resource. The users could query through various ways and means in these linked databases. For example, the visitors are accessible to a full-service approach including the theoretical knowledge, the diagnosis and differential diagnosis, the laboratory examination, the principles of treatment and medication, and the good clinical operations by inputting the disease names or clinical symptoms of disease. It could help doctors to improve their working efficiency and become a convenient "online encyclopedia of medicine" for them.

459.1.4 Construction and Application of the Online Medical Examination System

The online medical examination system is practical and powerful, and it is easy to operate database in this network system. More than 1 million questions exist in the database which covers twenty network courses for the general practice training, as well as the professional title examination and the licensing examinations for doctors and nurses. Every test has two function modules which are the online exercises and online tests. The system could ensure thousands of students to take online examination at the same time.

459.1.5 Construction and Application of the Maternity System

The maternity system was directly set up under the maternity virtual classroom. Besides the courses of Obstetrics and Gynaecology as well as Pediatrics for the

GPs, it also includes the genetic health promotion and education, prepregnancy genetic engineering, use of pregnancy rational drug, the screening for birth defects and progress in the field at home and abroad.

459.1.6 Construction and Application of the Online Communication System

The modules of the network communication, questions and answers, exchanges and discussions between teachers and students, and the latest progress have been designed and constructed in the online communication system. It also has several other modules such as the online consultation by academic experts and cases of online discussion in the system.

459.1.7 Construction and Application of the Counseling System

There are ten database modules in the counseling system. They are psychological knowledge, psychological disorders, psychological measurement, psychological diagnostics, psychological consultation, psychological therapy, case study, clinical psychology, psychological research and psychological test. Through online training, the GPs could understand the basics of psychological counseling, the early identification and diagnosis of common psychological obstacles, and the treatment methods and principles of psychological disorders. Meanwhile, the counseling system could provide the mental health counseling to young people to help them grow to be experienced GPs.

459.1.8 Construction and Application of the Health Education System

The system was developed on the basis of scientific basic knowledge of health education, covering good physical health, the mental health, the social and moral health. It could also provide the health consultation of the longevity and wellness to the old people in addition to GP training.

459.1.9 Construction and Application of the Preventive Health Care System

This database includes two modules. One is the disease prevention and the other is the health care. The module of disease prevention includes the prevention knowledge for the epidemic diseases and the chronic non-communicable diseases, in which the tertiary prevention included in the database is consisted of the early diagnosis, preventive treatment and rehabilitation measures. The system can be used as not only a training platform for students but also the health consultation platform for publics.

459.2 Construction of Online Training Mode for GPs

459.2.1 Mode Construction by Online Training in Combination with Base Training

We have built a general practice training base in our hospital to cooperate with online training for GPs. The training base would be responsible for the simulated training and departmental rotation, where the theory learning is largely based on the network training and the practical teaching is based on the hospital training. The two could be well fused, cross penetrating, and complementing each other. We have taken two types of projects of the post training and the transfer training of GPs. The "5 + 3" training project was performed in the post training for GPs. The trainees were required to complete undergraduate education for 5 years and would be trained for 3 years. The project of the transfer training was for the doctors from the community. The training content includes the theory of general medicine, the emergency and treatment of common diseases, and the chronic disease prevention and control. The training tools are the network teaching and base practice.

459.2.2 Construction of Scheduled and Random online Training

We have built a new training mode for GPs. It includes the scheduled online training for the post training and the random online training for the transfer training. The students meeting for scheduled online training was asked to enter the standardized training track in hospital. According to the schedule for three years, they should finish all required courses through the online learning and then begin to practice rotation after registration. For most GPs from the community, they would take the project of the random online training according to their individual needs. That is to say, they could take classes, participate in discussions and receive appraisal at random online. Therefore, the scheduled online training is suitable for the position requirements, while the random online training based on self needs would be based on the online training.

In summary, our online training system for GP will fulfill the following purposes. Firstly, the teaching ideas of student-centered and teacher-led would eventually come true through the self-learning based on the individual needs. Secondly, the high quality teaching resources from the universities would be developed and the education effect might be improved. Thirdly, the problem of the educational resources scarcity in remote areas can be effectively solved so that the community doctors in remote areas can also receive the good education. The problem of the imbalanced development of education would be resolved. Fourthly, our online training system would meet community doctors' personalized needs for further medicine, and reflect innovation of teaching methods and self-learning. Fifthly, the concepts and contents of general practice should be more popular in China, and let the public know that GPs are doctors of a high level of professional career and new medical talents, so that the doctors' professional identity and social status would be improved. Along with the further development of the online training system, our platform would be expected to become the lifelong education station for GPs, the lecture hall for famous doctors, the health consultants for the people and the medical guide for patients. Thereby, it would become a professional network platform to meet the needs of the public health and the society.

References

1. Simonella L, Marks G, Sanderson K et al (2006) Cost-effectiveness of current and optimal treatment for adult asthma. Intern Med J 36:244–250
2. Qian N, Du XP (2004) Comparation of training for family doctors between the University of WISCONSIN medical school and the Beijing capital Medical University. Chin J GPs 3:385–389
3. Wu Y, Huang ZJ (2009) Similarity and its enlightenment of medical education in Britain, Germany, the United States and France. China High Med Educ 23:421–425
4. Wang L, Du YP (2011) Comparison and discussion on the general practice service model in China and In the United Kingdom. Clin Educ Gen Pract 9:241–244
5. Ji JS, Liu G, Chen H, et al (2012) Overview of GPs training abroad and the enlighten about domestic training of GPs. Chin J GPs 11:217–222
6. Campbell JL, Carter M, Davey A et al (2013) Accessing primary care: a simulated patient study. Br J Gen Pract 63:171–176
7. Lu ZX (2011) Current analysis and construction concept for teaching staff in general practice in China. Clin Educ Gen Pract 9:121–124
8. Zhou LX, Liu G, Ji JS et al (2012) The construction and preliminary practice of the distance education network platform for GPs. China Med Educ Technol 26:276–279

Chapter 460
Research on the Construction of Regional Medical Information Service Platform

Qun Wang, Chuang Ma, Yong Yu and Gen Zhu

Abstract With the development of communication technology and information networks, The new medical service mode is regional health information platform construction and application. Through the establishment of a service platform based on the regional synergy of medical information, the hospital can not only obtain real-time two-way referral service platform, online booking, telephone booking, public health electronic files and other regional collaborative health care information, and also the referral hospital for public information, admissions information, the appointment online registration information is uploaded to the server, to improve the level of the National Health service is of great significance.

Keywords Regional Medical service platform · SOA · HL7 · Appointment register

---

Q. Wang · G. Zhu
The Institute of Public Administration, Hubei University of Medicine,
ShiYan, HuBei Province, China
e-mail: yymcc@qq.com

C. Ma
Computer Technology and Software Engineering,
WuHan Vocational and Technical College, WuHan, HuBei Province, China
e-mail: Mac@e21.edu.cn

Y. Yu (✉)
Center of Health Administration and Development Studies,
Hubei University of Medicine, ShiYan, HuBei Province, China
e-mail: Andyook@21cn.com

S. Li et al. (eds.), *Frontier and Future Development of Information Technology in Medicine and Education*, Lecture Notes in Electrical Engineering 269,
DOI: 10.1007/978-94-007-7618-0_460,

460.1 Introduction

With the improvement of social and material conditions and people's living standards, the demand for health care, emergency services exponentially increases; chronic common diseases frequently occurring younger Extension Trend, one of the health services and health care a higher demand. So, In a city or region need to establish a set of standardized, social, digital, networked medical, health and epidemic prevention and information sharing system to meet the health needs of the modern. Levels of medical institutions and hospitals How to realize internal medical resources sharing, inter-agency interoperability, each hospital must solve the problem. Therefore, the hospital must establish a regional medical service platform used to implement two-way referral network or telephone appointment with registration, query and other functions of public health information.

460.2 Status of the Regional Health Information Service Platform

Domestic regional medical late development from the 1980s began to gradually carry out the research and construction of the hospital information system has made significant progress, in varying degrees, all medical institutions to carry out the construction of medical information, the initial establishment of the hospital information system, radiology department information systems, image transmission and storage system, clinical information systems and medical information systems. However, these information systems among independent medical information in the region can not be effectively shared. The survey found that, in the process of regionalization of medical information systems, there is the following question:

Lack of integration between systems, data can not be shared and exchanged between the system and the system. Achieved the regionalization of medical information, but various medical institutions, medical information systems from different manufacturers, the data can not be shared in various systems, the formation of a "information island". Information data of the patients during the treatment can not be mutually transmission and access to, resulting in a waste of resources of medical information, and can not reduce health care costs. Meanwhile, can not be guaranteed the performance and stability of the system. Regional medical information sharing and collaboration platform is a distributed heterogeneous systems, need to have a good mechanism to realize the exchange and sharing of data, but also to ensure that the real-time data access and network security, and therefore need to study the data storage mode and network design [1].

460.3 The Objectives and Significance of the Platform

Medical information regionalization is not only the needs of medical institutions, but also the National health care reform, has important significance for building regional health information sharing and collaboration platform for patients, physicians, hospitals, health care industry as well as government.

The establishment of the platform will greatly improve the province health information system, to improve the public health information system in our province, to improve the province prediction of early warning and analysis capabilities, relying on the platform to achieve the establishment of the health of residents file, build rural and community health information network platform to improve the level of primary health care institutions, from medical technology guidance, continuing medical education. Promoting at all levels of primary hospital information construction platform network information technology, to promote cooperation in large urban hospitals and the community, grassroots health service institutions, to accelerate efficient interaction of all levels of medical service agencies information to improve the level of health care and efficiency of the primary health care sector.

Establishment of the medical information network platform as the core of the health of residents file, the patient in the treatment process can reduce the repetitive inspection saving medical treatment costs can be a greater degree the people to see a doctor is difficult and expensive, and between urban and rural health care resource allocation seriously uneven. Doctor can access to patient information across agencies, to reduce the rate of misdiagnosis, and can provide services such as teleconsultation. Hospitals can improve the level of management. Government departments can share data analysis provide strong regulatory system and the system for the medical industry, reduce medical risk.

Establishment of the good regional health information network platform not only from the server to obtain public way referral online reservation record, and stored in the HIS system, but also the public success in hospital admissions and referral information online appointment status information uploaded to the system. Medical information network platform to achieve the public in various medical institutions diagnosis and treatment information (between hospitals, between hospitals and community among communities) full sharing and exchange, including electronic prescriptions, electronic application form, electronic reports, electronic medical instruments. Through the referral and two-way services, online or by phone appointment function, the entire area of personal health data integration and business integration, shared with the configuration of health resources, in order to achieve the true sense of the regional collaborative medical.

460.4 Design of the Regional Medical Information Service Platform

Regional medical information service platform is related to the field of computer and medical technology and specifications, such as SOA, Web Service and other key technologies and HL7, IHE, DICOM and other medical norms, brief as follows:

460.4.1 Structure of the Platform System

Regional medical information service platform is based on the medical information resources in heterogeneous, distributed, and a large amount of data, highly dynamic characteristics of distributed heterogeneous systems. Service-oriented architecture SOA is a model of component-based thinking, is a software design approach, it will be the entire application system functional modules encapsulated into services, data exchange and transfer services through a unified interface. SOA is mainly implemented through Web Services, it is a platform-independent use interface connection services technology, the use of XML technology, including networking or Internet services provided, the request, calling the various different heterogeneous system integration.HL7 (Medical information exchange standards) is the 1987 HL7 organization built on ISO Layer 7 application layer on an international medical information exchange standards used to regulate the transmission of data between different applications of information systems in the medical field standard protocols [2].

The overall software architecture of the platform is the idea of SOA-based architecture, service registration, service integration, service provider collaboration mode to achieve the collaboration between the regional medical business. The platform is divided into three subsystems: the regional medical basis of information systems, regional health thematic information systems, regional health information system, the three major subsystems through service-oriented architecture ideas interoperability [3]. Regional Medical thematic information systems based on the basis of a regional medical information system, covering medical information systems for the medical field and related business sector is the source of the data. The subsystem major business system can be shared data services through the regional medical infrastructure information system to register for other business sectors to find and use. Individual business units can take advantage of basic services in the regional medical infrastructure information systems integration services, the encapsulation of sensitive data.

460.4.2 Function of the Platform System

In order to achieve the medical resources shared within the medical institutions at all levels, inter-agency interoperability, regional health information service platform has at least the following functions.

Portal login functionality, the different user groups depending on the permissions you can access different information and use different functions. The user group can be divided into public, doctors, nurses, medical technicians, medical administrators, researchers, system administrators [4].

Medical Service functions, medical resources queries, feature specialist hospital, renowned experts, large equipment, medical items, costs, and other inquiries. Online or telephone registration and appointment, the patient via the online registration, appointment of experts.

Health education for patients, such as providing health education promotional materials, publicity clinic time, vaccination schedules, etc.

Clinical service functions: doctors can access to hospital outpatient and inpatient electronic medical records and community electronic health records. Application consultation between the hospital can provide incurable diseases, approving the transfer of medical records, scheduling, billing, remote consultation, ask consultation comments transmission.

Management services functions, medical safety events, medical malpractice incident reports. The online dynamic query and reporting services for hospital operating statistics, to provide outpatient and emergency services, hospital and surgical volume of business, the bed occupancy rate, the amount of health insurance business, medical expenses such as query, the hospital managers to grasp the various hospitals situation.

460.5 Outlook

Through the establishment of a service platform based on the regional synergy of medical information, the hospital can not only obtain real-time two-way referral service platform, online booking, telephone booking, public health electronic files and other regional collaborative health care information, and also the referral hospital for public information, admissions information the appointment online registration information is uploaded to the server. Timely medical services personnel can obtain the necessary information to support high-quality medical services, which is of great significance to improve the National Health service.

Acknowledgments Project Funds: Supported by Key Research Center for Humanities and social sciences in Hubei Province, Hubei University of Medicine (2011B004)

References

1. Zhamng BO, Song RH (2011) Distributed web services-based information retrieval mechanism. Software Gui:76–78
2. Xu HF, Wang WP (2007) Based information exchange platform between the HL7. Web Serv Reg Med Inst Res 24(3):88–98
3. Wan Y (2012) Regional medical information sharing collaborative platform technology research and application. Cent South Univ
4. Li XP (2012) Regional medical information sharing platform construction. J Med Informatics (5)

Chapter 461
Study on the Application of Simulation Technology in the Medical Teaching

Yong Yu, Xiaolin Chen, Qun Wang and Gen Zhu

Abstract With the progress of society and the rapid development of medical technology, the rights and self-protection awareness of the patients is gradually increased, traditional clinical practice teaching mode gradually restricted, and the continuous development of medical simulation technology is getting the favour of clinical medical education. This paper through studies the status of clinical teaching and clinical medical education mode, introduces the classification of medical simulation technology to analyze the advantages of medical simulation technology, and pointed out the problems that needed attention in the medical simulation technology, in order to push forward the reform of the traditional medical education to cultivate high quality of medical personnel.

Keywords Medical simulation · Medical education · Simulation technology · Clinical medicine · Standardized patients

Y. Yu
Center of Health Administration and Development Studies,
Hubei University of Medicine, ShiYan, Hubei Province, China
e-mail: yymcs@qq.com

X. Chen · Q. Wang (✉) · G. Zhu
The Institute of Public Administration, Hubei University of Medicine,
ShiYan, Hubei Province, China
e-mail: Andyook@21cn.com

X. Chen
e-mail: hbmu@21cn.com

G. Zhu
e-mail: hbmu@21cn.com

S. Li et al. (eds.), *Frontier and Future Development of Information Technology in Medicine and Education*, Lecture Notes in Electrical Engineering 269,
DOI: 10.1007/978-94-007-7618-0_461,

461.1 Introduction

Medicine is a high risk service industry, involves a lot of social ethical and legal issues, but medical education is not only the implementation of the teaching of the theory of knowledge, also requires students to practice clinical teaching, so the students must have a solid theoretical foundation, and solid clinical application capabilities. The best learning object for Medical students is a patient or real human, but patient rights and self-protection awareness gradually increased. Fewer are willing to let student internships, restricting the development of clinical teaching career. At a time, the growing popularity of computer simulation and simulation techniques, more in line with the humane care of medical simulation teaching applications are becoming the dominant way of clinical medicine practice teaching. Medical simulation teaching in medical education practice has a broad application prospects, more scientific and humane teaching and assessment tools to cultivate students agility, correct judgment, and comprehensively improve clinical decision-making ability of the students and nursing skills, thus effectively reduce the occurrence of medical malpractice and disputes in the clinical work vigorously to enhance the quality of clinical teaching has an important role in promoting the development of medical simulation teaching [1].

461.2 Medical Simulation Technology in the Teaching

The Shortage of teaching resources has become the most prominent difficulties in Medical Education. With the regionalization of health resources, the positioning of the functions of hospitals at the clinical practice of teaching resources become more shortages, greatly reducing the opportunities for students to clinical practice. Patients rights protection consciousness to strengthen, have the right to refuse the teaching demonstration. Without first obtaining the consent of the patients and their families in the case, let the students contact with patients, causing pain and discomfort to the patient. Due to the limitations of the traditional model of medical education, medical schools use the following clinical medicine education mode.

"Problem-based learning" (PBL) is commonly used in international medical education, medical education research hotspot [2].

Standardized patient (SP) teaching methods, also known as simulated patients, standardized patients or patient guidance, normal people or patients with mild non-medical work, after a standard systematic training, accurate performance in patients with clinical signs and symptoms, realistically replicate real clinical situations, play patients, three functions act as assessment and teaching guide.

Medical Simulation Technology is mainly relying on high-tech medical simulation products include advanced simulation, simulation training. The combination of computer technology and clinical anatomy, the creation of a body three-dimensional model of the all-digital and biophysics characteristics of the computer model, the effective realization of the human form and function of digital description directly to modern medicine, teaching, research, and application will simulation practice conditions indispensable basic skills can operate on the model.

461.3 Classification of Medical Simulation Technology

Medical simulation technology along with the development of medicine throughout the grounds with the modern advances in technology continue to penetrate to the field of medical education, medical simulation technology gradually become parts of a five types for low to high, basic anatomy model, the local functional training model, computer-aided model, virtual training system, physiological driven simulation system.

The basis of anatomical models shows the anatomy or pathology anatomical structure of the model. This type of model is mainly used in teaching. The use of anatomical teaching model based on the boring theoretical study becomes vivid, easy to understand. It also can assist in the teaching of anatomy, physiology and pathology, and other basic medical disciplines.

The local functional training model provides simulation of partial function of one or more of the body, or of one or more medical operation simulation allows students to understand a local function, to get training in a medical procedure, a cleavage of a single training. Main physical diagnosis applications trainees and interns learning and preclinical learning.

Computer-aided model [3] is a part or a variety of medical operations, and computer software to combine the model, to achieve the control of one or a series of procedure through the computer software, in a certain extent on the combination of a set of separate functional training, so that students can get a complete medical treatment process from the training.

Virtual training system [4] is another direction for the development of high-end analog technology. This system through the software to create a virtual patient environment and condition, the operator through a computer screen to see the anatomical structure of the human internal to hear the voice of the reaction of the patient, the same time, by acting on the electronic hardware carrier of the "force feedback" technique, actually feel in the medical procedure which various tactile information. Virtual training system of computer software and electronic hardware carrier of perfect combination, medical operations in the visual, auditory and tactile integrated applications in the three disciplines of training and continuing education of doctors.

Physiological driven simulation system or the full simulation system technically belongs to the most high-end analog system, is the most complete in the world today, it brings students closest to the reality of class true feelings, it gathers physiological functional operation of portable software and knowledge of the system, through technology integration and digital models of the use of computer software features a comprehensive simulation of the entire health care environment, including the patient, the condition and treatment of the environment. The analog system has the same shape with people, such as breathing, heartbeat, pulse, blink signs can be connected to the normal monitoring equipment, ventilators, anesthesia machines and diagnostic equipment to simulate the complete treatment process. Such models can be applied in various stages of clinical teaching, comprehensive, real analog of the health care environment.

461.4 The Advantage of Medical Simulation Technology

Medical simulation technology in clinical skills training has the following advantages:

Time convenience: Students do not have to wait until the patient comes to training, training simulation system can be completely in accordance with the arrangements for the teachers and students of the time.

Repeatability: Students can simulation system can repeatedly practice it to perfection. Adjust degree: all types of difficulty and the stage of the training can be carried out in an analog system.

Rare case of learning: Usually a lot of disease incidence is relatively low, the junior doctors are more difficult to see, the use of the analog system can be trained to deal with this unusual but potentially serious nature cases;.

No risk: When using the analog system, capable of it as a real patients, students can go wrong, but is harmless to the patient.

Can record and playback: The training process can be recorded through a variety of ways, including the camera device or system that comes complete training students and teachers can be watched or inspection records, discussion and evaluation, is helpful to find advantages and failure.

Team collaboration: Learning exchanges with the common treatment of patients develop their team spirit of collaboration.

The standardization of training: Student can according to set procedures to standardized the training, in strict accordance with the requirements of the practice, plays a key role in clinical practice in the late.

461.5 Problems of Medical Simulation Technology in Practical Use

Although medical simulation technology has many advantages, but the medical simulation teaching system also has some problems in the practical use.

Just copying standard textbooks through simulated medical record and often, encountering in the actual clinical work is not so typical, in practice still has limitations in its complexity and diversification.

Simulation teaching depends on the designer's clinical experience, theory and practice, which is impossible to exceed our understanding level, but also may affected practice effect due to the designer's incomplete consideration. Therefore, the simulation of medical education have higher requirements for teachers, the choice of analog products also need to consider the product after-sales, as well as upgrading and maintenance.

Medical simulation education in China promote a slower speed, analog equipment expensive prices, regional development imbalances, in various regions of the teaching content have some differences, the teachers need to design their own cases and teaching process, due in case design may be more integrated into the clinical nursing knowledge and nursing skills into teaching, the simulation system must be pre-run to ensure the effectiveness of teaching.

Before simulation teaching training must have sufficient knowledge of base and clinical, or they will not get the desired results. "Theoretical lectures + sub-technical exercises + comprehensive simulation drills + video analysis summarizes + assessment and evaluation + clinical practice" mode can be used for training. First explain the basic theoretical knowledge, simulations and training teachers for the operation of the contents of the teaching demonstration, and then let the students as a group, the breakdown of technical exercises, repeatedly stressed that the standard operating practices in the practice of the process of steps and clear operation ideas and the spirit of teamwork, the final analysis of the video analog operation, error correction, allowing students enhance the memory. After through comprehensive assessment of the evaluation, the students have mastered the basic skills to some extent, students can enter the clinical practice and patient contact, to further improve the comprehensive clinical skills of medical students, to ease the contradiction between the clinical teaching and patient so as to achieve good teaching effect.

In short, how to play the advantages of medical simulation education, promote the reform of the traditional medical education is to train high-quality medical personnel still need we to continue to study and explore.

Acknowledgments Project Funds: Supported by Key Research Center for Humanities and social sciences in Hubei Province, Hubei University of Medicine (2011B004) and Hubei University of Medicine Research project (2011020).

References

1. Jian L (2004) Medical simulation and medical education. Chin Hosp Jul:73–74
2. Yu YX (2004) Modern medical simulation center classification and planning. Chin Hosp Aug:76–78
3. Krapichler C et al (1998) Computation methods programs. Biomed 56(1):65–742
4. Burdea GC, Coiffet P (2003) Virtual real technology. Wiley, new Jersey, p 6
5. Bing WH (2001) Virtual reality technology—retrospect and prospect. Comput Eng Appl :48–52
6. Zheng GY (2005) Talk about the development of medical simulation technology. Chin Med Educ Technol 19(6)

Chapter 462
Desynchronization of Morris: Lecar Network via Robust Adaptive Artificial Neural Network

Yingyuan Chen, Jiang Wang, Xile Wei, Bin Deng, Haitao Yu, Fei Su and Ge Li

Abstract This paper has presented a robust adaptive artificial neural network (ANN) method to desynchronize a network composed of Morris–Lecar (M–L) neuron model. During the whole process of desynchronizing the network, the robust adaptive controllers play the roles of synchronizing a selected neuron in the network and a reference neuron, and desynchronizing the network with desired phase differences generated by constructing the difference between the output curve of the reference neuron and the shifted output curve of the reference neuron with desired phase difference. The method is robust and can be applied in Deep Brain Stimulation (DBS) therapies.

Keywords Desynchronization · Morris–Lecar network · Artificial neural network · Phase shifting

462.1 Introduction

Synchronization, which is a universal phenomenon in coupled nonlinear systems [1], exists and plays an important role in the nervous system [2]. Experimental evidence demonstrates that synchronous neuronal oscillations underlie many

This work is supported by the National Natural Science Foundation of China (Grant No. 61072012 and 61172009), the Young Scientists Fund of the National Natural Science Foundation of China (Grant Nos. 61104032), and the China Postdoctoral Science Foundation (Grant No. 2012M510750).

Y. Chen · J. Wang (✉) · X. Wei · B. Deng · H. Yu · F. Su · G. Li
School of Electrical and Automation Eng, Tianjin University,
300072 Tianjin, People's Republic of China
e-mail: jiangwang@tju.edu.cn

S. Li et al. (eds.), *Frontier and Future Development of Information Technology in Medicine and Education*, Lecture Notes in Electrical Engineering 269,
DOI: 10.1007/978-94-007-7618-0_462, © Springer Science+Business Media Dordrecht 2014

cortical processes [3–5]. However, unnecessary synchronization in neural system may cause some neuron diseases. Researches have shown that synchronization of neurons in neural system is a main cause of Parkinson disease [6–8]. So it is required to develop some desynchronization methods to avoid the effect of these unnecessary synchronization phenomena in neural system.

Many researchers have developed variety of methods to desynchronize abnormal synchronized neural network which can be used as electrical stimulation therapies in recent few years [9–12]. However, most of the existed methods may change the firing patterns during the process of desynchronizing neurons, or may be greatly affected by the changed parameters and external stimulus of the neuron. In this paper, we use controllers composed of adaptive artificial neural networks (ANNs) and robust controller to desynchronization a Morris–Lecar [13] network with desired phase differences. Taking a neuron which can produce the desired firing pattern in the synchronized network or from the other area of neural system as a reference neuron, a desired phase difference signal can be generated by the reference neuron and the delay component. Using the generated phase difference signal, a robust adaptive ANN controller is designed and added on each neuron to make neurons in the abnormal network produce the same phase difference signal as the desired phase differences. The simulation results demonstrate the robustness and effectiveness of the proposed control method.

462.2 Model and Methods

The system composed of two single Morris–Lecar neurons [13] can be described as:

$$\begin{cases} C_m\dot{X}_m = I_{extm} - \bar{g}_{Ca}M_{\infty m}(X_m - V_{Ca}) - (\bar{g}_K N_m + \bar{g}_{KS}S_m)(X_m - V_K) - g_L(X_m - V_L) \\ \dot{N}_m = \varphi_N \dfrac{N_{\infty m} - N_m}{\tau_{Nm}} \\ \dot{S}_m = \varphi_S \dfrac{S_{\infty m} - S_m}{\tau_{Sm}} \\ C_m\dot{X}_s = I_{exts} - \bar{g}_{Ca}M_{\infty s}(X_s - V_{Ca}) - (\bar{g}_K N_s + \bar{g}_{KS}S_s)(X_s - V_K) - g_L(X_s - V_L) + u \\ \dot{N}_s = \varphi_N \dfrac{N_{\infty s} - N_s}{\tau_{Ns}} \\ \dot{S}_s = \varphi_S \dfrac{S_{\infty s} - S_s}{\tau_{ss}} \end{cases} \tag{462.1}$$

where u is the adaptive robust ANN controller, neuron with subscript m (m-neuron in the following text) is considered as the reference neuron, and neuron with subscript s(s-neuron in the following text) is required to show the same character as the m-neuron. In this paper, the synapse is considered as electrical synapse (also called gap-junctions).

The error system of Eq. (462.1) is defined as:

$$\begin{cases} \dot{e}_X = X_m - X_s \\ \dot{e}_N = N_m - N_s \\ \dot{e}_S = M_m - M_s \end{cases} \tag{462.2}$$

and the Lyapunov function of the system can be written as:

$$V = \frac{1}{2}e_X^2 + \frac{1}{2}e_N^2 + \frac{1}{2}e_S^2 \tag{462.3}$$

Assume that our controller u is effective enough to ensure $e_V = 0$, then the other state variables will satisfy:

$$\dot{e}_y = \dot{y}_m - \dot{y}_s = \varphi_y\left(\frac{y_{\infty m} - y_m}{\tau_{ym}} - \frac{y_{\infty s} - y_s}{\tau_{ys}}\right) = -\varphi_y\frac{e_y}{\tau_{ym}} \tag{462.4}$$

where $y = N, S$. Then the derivate of Lyapunov function can be written as:

$$\dot{V} = e_V\dot{e}_V + e_N\dot{e}_N + e_S\dot{e}_S = -\varphi_N\frac{e_N^2}{\tau_{Nm}} - \varphi_S\frac{e_S^2}{\tau_{Sm}} \leq 0 \tag{462.5}$$

which means the error system will be stable as long as the controller make the error of two membrane potentials of the two neuron achieve zero. So we just need to add a 1-order controller on the membrane potential subsystem of s-neuron to make two M–L neurons achieve synchronization.

The parameters of Morris–Lecar models in the following simulations is set as $C_m = 20$, $g_{Ca} = 4$, $g_K = 8$, $g_L = 2$, $g_{KS} = 0.5$, $V_{Ca} = 120$, $V_K = -80$, $V_L = -60$, $V_1 = -1.2$, $V_2 = 18$, $V_3 = 12$, $V_4 = 17.4$, $V_5 = -25$, $V_6 = 10$, $\varphi_N = 0.22$, $\varphi_S = 0.001$. The input current I_{exti} of each neuron ranges from $I_{exti} = 48 \sim 52$. The 3-dimensional Morris–Lecar model can display spiking and bursting firing pattern under a constant external stimulus (Fig. 462.1).

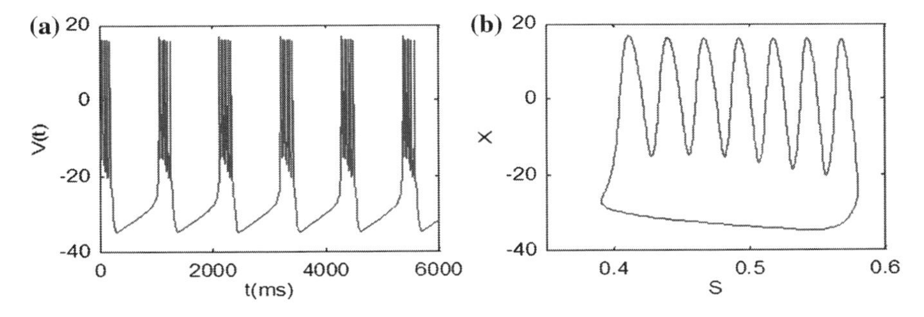

Fig. 462.1 **a** The bursting of Morris–Lecar neuron model, **b** the phase portrait

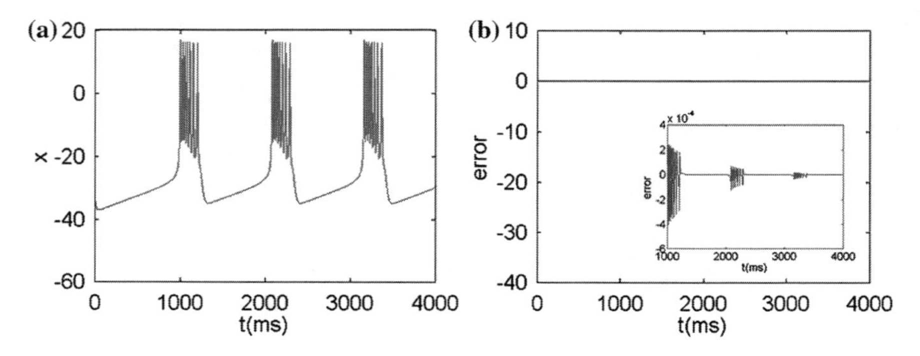

Fig. 462.2 Synchronizing a neuron in Morris–Lecar network and the reference neuron with the robust adaptive ANN controller. **a** The membrane potentials of the two neurons, **b** the error between the two neuron

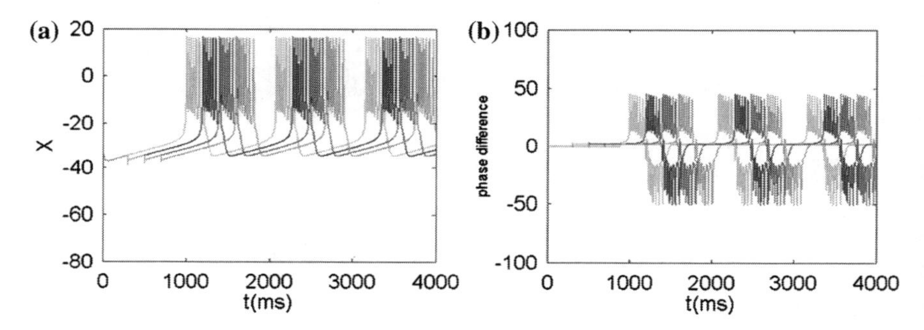

Fig. 462.3 Desynchronizing the synchronized M–L network with the robust adaptive ANN controller. **a** The membrane potentials of four neurons in this network, **b** the phase differences between these neurons and their neighbor neurons

462.3 Results

In this section, numerical simulations are carried out for the desynchronization of the Morris–Lecar network via the robust adaptive ANN controller. Assume that the coupling strength of synapses between neurons in the network is highly strengthened because of some unknown disturbance, and Gaussian white noise is introduced in the ion channels of each neuron. Under the effect of disturbances in ion channels and synapses, the spikes produced by neurons in the network achieve phase synchronization, which may lead to Parkinson disease or abnormal tremor in neural systems. To solve this problem, we use the robust adaptive ANN controller to desynchronize the ill-state network.

As mentioned above, we first select one neuron in the synchronized M–L network to make this neuron and the reference neuron achieve synchronization. Figure 462.2 shows the effect of the synchronization controller. From the simulation result, we can see that the abnormal hub neuron in the ill network achieve complete synchronization with the reference neuron.

Then we will desynchronize each neuron in the abnormal synchronized network with the reference phase difference generated by the reference neuron. Figure 462.3a shows the desynchronization effect of the robust adaptive ANN controller. Figure 462.3b shows the dynamics of the differences between every two neighbor neurons in the desynchronized network. It is easy to see that our method can accurately desynchronize a network with a desired phase difference.

462.4 Conclusion

In this paper, desynchronization of Morris–Lecar networks via the robust adaptive ANN controller has been studied. The method consists of two parts during the process of desynchronizing a network. First one of the neurons in the network is synchronized with the reference neuron which can produce normal desired output via robust adaptive ANN synchronization controller, then other neurons in the network is desynchronized by the robust adaptive ANN desynchronization controllers with the reference phase difference generated by the output of the reference neuron and the output of that neuron with a proper time delay. According to the Lyapunov stability theorem, the proposed controller ensures stable synchronization between the reference neuron and the one chosen in the synchronized network, or stable synchronization between the reference phase difference and real error differences between every two neurons in the process of desynchronizing the network. Moreover, one can decide the character of the neurons in the network by choosing different reference neurons with different desired characters. The control scheme is robust to the approximate errors, ionic channel noise and disturbance. The simulation results have demonstrated the efficiency of the proposed control method.

References

1. Kurths J, Pikovsky A, Rosenblum M (2001) Synchronization: a universal concept in nonlinear science. Cambridge University Press, Cambridge
2. Womelsdorf T, Fries P (2007) The role of neuronal synchronization in selective attention. Curr Opin Neurobiol 17(2):154–160
3. Gray C M, Konig P, Engel A K, Singer W (1989) Oscillatory responses in cat visual cortex exhibit inter-columnar synchronization which reflects global stimulus properties. Nature 338:334–337
4. Steriade M, McCormick DA, Sejnowski TJ (1993) Halamocortical oscillations in the sleeping and aroused brain. Science 262:679–685
5. Roelfsema PR, Engel AK, Singer W (1997) Visuomotor integration is associated with zero time-lag synchronization among cortical areas. Nature 385:157–161

6. Edwards R, Beuter A (1999) Parkinsonian tremor and simplification in network dynamics. Bull Math Biol 51:157–177
7. Schiff S J (2010) Towards model-based control of Parkinson's disease. Phil Trans R Soc A 368:2269–2308
8. So RQ, Kent AR, Grill WM (2012) Relative contributions of local cell and passing fiber activation and silencing to changes in thalamic fidelity during deep brain stimulation and lesioning: a computational modeling study. J Comput Neurosci 32:499–519
9. Hauptmann C, Popovych O, Tass PA (2005) Delayed feedback control of synchronization in locally coupled neuronal networks. Neurocomputing 65–66:759–767
10. Hauptmann C, Popovych O, Tass PA (2007) Demand-controlled desynchronization of oscillatory networks by means of a multisite delayed feedback stimulation. Comput Visual Sci 10:71–78
11. Popovych O, Hauptmann C, Tass PA (2005) Effective desynchronization by nonlinear delayed feedback. Phys Rev Lett 94:164102
12. Hauptmann C, Popovych O, Tass PA (2005) Effectively desynchronizing deep brain stimulation based on a coordinated delayed feedback stimulation via several sites: a computational study. Biol Cybern 93:463–470
13. Morris C, Lecar H (1981) Voltage oscillations in the barnacle giant muscle fiber. Biophys J 35(1):193–213

Chapter 463
Building and Sharing of Information Resources in Radio and TV Universities Libraries Under Network Environment

Liu Juan and Wang Jing-na

Abstract This paper introduces the status of Radio and TV University Libraries, expatiates the changes of information resources construction and put forward the ways to realize building and sharing of information resources in Radio and TV Universities Libraries under network environment.

Keywords Library · Information resources · Building and sharing

463.1 The Status and Meaning of Radio and TV Universities Libraries' Resource Building

463.1.1 The Status of Resource Building

463.1.1.1 Each Library Is Fiercely Independent, Repetitive Resource Construction

As one of the most basic elements for digital library construction, digital resources establish the foundation for digital library to develop information service, its construction directly influences the using effect of digital library. The library, as Radio and TV Universities' (hereafter referred to as RTVUs) resource center, cultural center, learning center and service center, is an important part of university's teaching-supporting service system, whose resource construction should adhere to the required reader-oriented and offer targeted, applicable resource to readers. At

L. Juan (✉) · W. Jing-na (✉)
Shaanxi Radio and TV University, Xi'an 710119 Shaanxi, China
e-mail: 270617839@qq.com

W. Jing-na
e-mail: 417292017@qq.com

S. Li et al. (eds.), *Frontier and Future Development of Information Technology in Medicine and Education*, Lecture Notes in Electrical Engineering 269,
DOI: 10.1007/978-94-007-7618-0_463,

present, RTVUs' digital resources consists mainly purchased commerce databases and self-built characteristic databases, however, because of lacking unified planning, each RTVUs is basically independent, these purchased commerce databases are mostly repetitive and self-built databases are almost same, which consumes a lot of manpower and money, finally readers can't obtain more information resources under the condition of insufficient funds investment.

463.1.1.2 Low Personnel Quality, Outdated Service

Traditional library built service relationship between librarian and reader via book. Their duties are to preserve book, process the data and borrow book. Library work was called a simple "borrowing and returning" without any technical content. With the rapid development of network and appearance of various digital technologies, library's connotation and denotation have undergone earth-shaking change. Librarian has to complete service to readers through network, which requires certainly high-quality librarian not only to be information science expert but also the professional mastered advanced computer technology and certain English skills. However, there exist structural forms of personnel imbalance, low-quality librarian and outdated service now in RTVUs libraries, which fails to meet requirements of modern digital library.

463.1.1.3 Poor Technology and Data Standardization

RTVUs started late on digital library, lagging in technology, and poor standardization of digital resources construction without unification, its self-built resources adopted mostly low-tech scanning technology which digitalize simply information resources, can't retrieve, classify and analyze information, much less higher level of information mining and processing. Moreover, image format file takes up large space and scanning effect is poor, which go against the management and utilization of digital library. Now the digital resources of RTVUs libraries have isomerization and diversity features to make many digital resources incompatible, much less sharing. Reader must shift the system to use different database, causing the difficulty of readers to use resources and bring inconvenience for managing digital resources at the same time.

463.1.2 The Meaning of Building and Sharing of Information Resources in RTVUs Libraries

With the information age arrival, that network technology continuous renewal has decided the developing trend of future library is to implement building and sharing of information resources. RTVUs libraries' service is relatively backward relative to social libraries because of late and low starting and poorer ability to collect literature resources. The imbalance of regular users and areas, a lower utilization of current collection that hugely wasted the information resources. So unified planning, multi-azimuth, multi-channel, three-dimensional co-construct and share reasonably information resources, which is a key way to solve RTVUs libraries' present paradox and its efforts direction. Owing to modern open and distance education's particularity on teaching, management and service mode, library service also has particularity.

463.2 The Changing of Information Resource Building for RTVUs Libraries

463.2.1 The Changing of Operation Idea

RTVUs is a higher school which develop distance education with modern information technology. The formation of the network environment promoted environmental change of RTVUs library which do not collect, sort book magazine materials any more. The information service of library is a composite of many objective conditions and strength including collection information resources system, various technical means and service modes so that make RTVUs libraries's information resource construction work change from printed information to electronic information from printed information, from internal to internal and external equal value, to realize the communication and cooperation of the online information and resource sharing. Subitems in a list should use the "subitem" style.

463.2.1.1 From Entity to Virtual Library

Since network became library's operating platform, a lot of the information is stored in the computer, created a series of information resources retrieval mechanism, information transfer and service mode. The work object of library no longer exists in complete entity, then formed virtual library.

463.2.1.2 From "Walled" to "No Wall"

With the development network technology, RTVUs libraries under network environment not only offer information retrieval to teachers and students, but also offer broader and faster information service to distance education students vis network.

463.2.1.3 From Isolated to Network

Network environment aids the foundation for networking among several libraries, which brings convenient to distance learners and improve greatly the degree of information resource building and sharing under network environment.

463.2.2 The Changing of Information Resources Structure

The literature information resource location of RTVUs libraries is broader under network environment. Entity collection resources and online information resources together make up the resource base of RTVUs libraries information service. So collection information resources are divided into two parts: one is entity collection including printed literature, electronic literature such as tape, optical disk and floppy disk, etc.; two is virtual collection, i.e. network information resources. Entity collection and virtual collection each other are closely related and inseparable. Network environment changes the single collection idea. Collections transferred from single printed literature to variety of media literature, the literature information resource structure changed from static to dynamic.

463.2.3 The Changing of Librarians' Quality Requirements

Network environment asks librarian to adjust knowledge structure, improve service quality, become information guide and network exchange hand, as well choose information in huge information flow to help readers open the door of information resources, make full use of information retrieval ways and methods, achieving rapid inquiry information and maximum meet all readers' information requirements.

463.3 The Ways to Achieve Building and Sharing of Information Resources in RTVUs Libraries

463.3.1 Shift Ideas to Coordinate the Organization

To realize the building and sharing of information resources in RTVUs system must rely on library work committee of RTVUs allover the country. Several libraries formed a authority management organization to plan, design and implement building and sharing scheme of the network literature information resources. Practically, optimize organizational structure, improve operation mechanism, set standard, build a new mode of literature information resources development and utilization which has highly developed ability, adapt to the market economy system's industrialization, networked and socialization. Meanwhile, this organization must clear the right and obligation among these libraries and be Responsible for the organization and coordination in the process of the construction. In addition, each library should build up the idea that building information resources together can share them together.

463.3.2 Strengthen the Standardization and Normalization of Literature Resources Inside the Library

Database construction is the foundation of realizing literature information sharing. Standardization must throughout the each link of the building and sharing of information resources, apply scientific classification and indexing tool to deal with the data standardly. To guarantee quality and maximum realize resource sharing. RTVUs libraries urge to formulate unified standards of the database to realize information resources sharing. Macro-control database construction must develop reasonably and orderly the characteristic resource base of each grassroot RTUV librariy under unified standard framework.

463.3.3 Strengthen the Construction of Each Provincial Libraries' Collections

Each provincial RTVU should strengthen its own collection of information construction. Distribute collection proportion scientifically according to different disciplines, levels, carrier types. According the characteristics of distance education students of RTVU and collection features to transform accumulated characteristic literature resources to digital resources and service online. Apply the flowing information resources to complement and rich collections to make sure RTVU teachers and students obtain their library's literature information resources and digital information resources most conveniently and efficiently. Reach a certain literature supporting ratio and upload some featured resources to the website of CRTVU for nationwide RTVU libraries to use.

463.3.4 Pay Attention to Personnel Training, Strengthen the Technical Team Building

The building and sharing of RTVU libraries resources need a batch of professionals who have suitable idea, ability, knowledge structure and technological level. RTVU libraries should put training technical personnel in the first place. The building and sharing of literature information resources are intelligence development and technological development, it raises new and higher requirements to librarian. Librarian not only master library and information professional knowledge, but also modern information processing technology. Meanwhile, speed up the construction of the digital library, build public digital library for nationwide RTVU system's resource service, realize the building and sharing of RTVU system libraries' literature information resources to make it become digital literature information resources' guarantee system of modern open and distance education.

463.4 Conclusion

Under the network environment, RTVUs libraries need to set up correct concept of document resources sharing, standard the safeguards of library information resources building and sharing system, strengthen the characteristic construction of the network information resources and cultivate a new generation of literature information management personnel. Only in this way, the building and sharing of information resources in RTVUs libraries can improve further, not only can avoid repeated construction of information resources, but also solve the documents' fund shortage problem. Meanwhile, it can enable collection resources to sustainable development.

References

1. Liang W (2011) Construction status and development strategy of RTVUs digital library—a case study of Guizhou Radio and TV University Library. J Heilongjiang College Edu 6:197–199
2. Wang Y (2010) The discussion on the construction and sharing of RTVUs library information resource under the network environment. Manag Technol SME 10:274
3. Zhou Y (2005) The construction and sharing of university library information resource under the network environment. J Libr Tribune 4:109–112
4. Ge X (2002) The construction strategies of network information resources in RTVUs library—to build the protective system for online information resources. J Mod Inf 8:118–119

Chapter 464
Research on Network Information Resources Integration Services in Medicine Library

Zhang Li-min

Abstract The paper discusses the types and characteristics of medical network information resources, analyzes the necessity, tools and three methods of medical network information resources integration, and probes into the development direction of medical library information resources integration.

Keywords Hospital library · Medical informatics · Digital resource integration

Information Integration is based on information development trend. Which management processes can achieve optimal allocation of resources and broaden the application areas of information resources and maximizing the value of mining information by information resources ordering and sharing under leadership of organization. Library information's resources integration is the demand from mass to personalize. It is also user-oriented information services inevitable result of development. Clinical medicine has a very rich source of information from internet. However, recourse is too large, too fasting increased and too scattered disorderly to start searching by users. The integration of information resources can fully develop and use diverse information resources. It can supply proactive, comprehensive, systematic, high-quality service which extend and promote the library service to a high level.

Z. Li-min (✉)
Shaanxi Radio and TV University, Xi'an, Shaanxi, China
e-mail: yay386@163.com

S. Li et al. (eds.), *Frontier and Future Development of Information Technology in Medicine and Education*, Lecture Notes in Electrical Engineering 269,
DOI: 10.1007/978-94-007-7618-0_464,

464.1 Medical Information Resources Online

464.1.1 Electronic Publication Resources

Lectronic journals and electronic book is the preferred source of information. Most of the medical journals and electronic books has been the realized of electronization and networked for reading and browsing convenient.

464.1.2 Medical Database Resources

International common medical database: Embase, Medline (PubMed), Cochrane library, etc. National common database resources: China HowNet (CNKI), Wanfang, VIP, etc. They are collected much information source. There are many kinds of domestic and foreign patent, standard database which also collected a lot of medical information resources.

464.1.3 Medical Industry Resources

Including the association/society, university departments, research institutes and other organizations. Medical authorities and academic organization website information are reliable. The academic quality of the sites are very high. It can also be got international conference information and the world's leading academic groups and medical-related meetings organized by the exchange of operational information and academic which can be used as accumulate professional information browsing tools.

464.2 Library Information Resources Integration Tools

Integration of information resources is not only the digital resources together, but also involves the information description, organization, processing, sorting, searching, service and other aspects. All these need corresponding technical support. The author thinks that considering the following kinds of digital resources integration tools:

464.2.1 Resource Integration Based on OPAC

Information resource integration based on OPAC is a kind of resource integration solutions. It based on OPAC, on library integrated management system, fully occupies library bibliographic data resources, and on this basis, through the functional extension and implementation of other of the integration of information resources. Can pass to MARC cataloging to integrate electronic books, electronic journals and OPAC system, and provide hyperlinks in the OPAC system function, so that readers in the OPAC system retrieval to the required electronic books and electronic journals at the same time open full text directly.

464.2.2 SFX Technology

SFX is Ghent university, Belgium, H. Fort Sam, put forward by the research group headed by a uniform resource locator based on open (open URL) standard context related reference link system. As academic information navigation in the network environment and discovery tool, it passed a strong link service for academic information users. Librarians by linking knowledge base configuration directly participate in the management of the resources link, can provide the reader with the use of more fluid and more convenient alternative.

464.2.3 Web Services Technology

Last century network through the "static data (HTML)", "dynamic data" (ASP, JSP, CGI, ISAP), "application service" (such as n-tier architecture) era, in the network application service should be a Web service. Once pushed on Web Service that is widely admired in the industry; Multilayer distributed system is a database application system development trend. Web Service in addition to publishing capabilities with business logic processing functions, are more powerful programming and automatic processing functions.

464.3 Medical Network Information Resource Integration Model

In recent years, various types of integrated approach has been brought out from both domestic and international study and practical application.

According to the specific object and process of different, network resources can be divided into four kinds of cyber source integration:

464.3.1 Based on OPAC Integration

Interlibrary collection of books can be achieved with the integration of CD with the book, e-book collection of books and the integration of collections and Electronic Journal of integration. Based on the integration of information resources OPAC integration of resources belonging to a solution. It is based on the OPAC, relying on the integrated library management system, fully occupied Bibliography data resources, on this basis, through extensions, to achieve the integration of other sources of information. MARC catalogung will be available through e-books, e-journals into OPAC retrieval system, and in the OPAC system provides hyperlinks functionality so readers OPAC system to retrieve the desired e-book or e-journals at the same time directly open text. However, integration of resources based OPAC system of its links to resources are static, once the target resource has changed, the link will be updated maintenance points, which is a very large project, which will inevitably produce a lot of broken links.

464.3.2 Based on Resources Integration Navigation System

Navigation system is a resource library and a variety of networked digital resources to establish a URL navigation database, the platform offers a variety of entry, it can be alphabetical, by document type, by subject categories and other ways to be retrieved. Book navigation main journals, databases, navigation, institutions navigation key disciplines navigation, Medical News Resources Navigation, forums and expert blog navigation.

Subject Navigation is deeper domestic level network information resources development and utilization patterns. At present, many foreign medical professional societies and educational institutions have been established medical navigation libraries. Such as domestic Academy "National Science Digital Library Project" (CSDL) subproject life sciences medical information portal portal emphasized in the construction of resource availability, authority, stability, comprehensive and unique. China Academic Library and Information System (CALIC) according to the needs of each school key disciplines for overall planning and division of labour, organization construction of key disciplines Navigation Database Library, which houses medical resource navigation subdirectories.

464.3.3 Based on the Digital Resources Integration of Cross-Database Retrieval System

Medical information resources contained in multiple databases, resources for heterogeneous database integration and unified search, will greatly facilitate user access to information resources efficiency. In recent years, many libraries are conducting unified retrieval of heterogeneous data resources research, many software companies are developing similar systems. According to preliminary statistics, the domestic inputs used or being tested unified search platform has reached more than ten kinds. In library and information sector, Singh Tong Fang Hangmen text Database CNKI a "unified search technology" has been widely used, the journals, Hobo papers, conferences, patents, standards, newspapers and other database integration, to achieve a unified retrieval. Unified retrieval system in addressing the readers to search multiple electronic resources needs to be repeated many times login, retrieval issue, played a key role.

464.4 Library Information Resources Integration Direction

464.4.1 Improving the Information System and Carrying Out Comprehensive Information Service

It emphasizes the systematic design of information service, strengthens the survey and scientific decision-making, constantly promotes the subject coverage and data size of the digital resources of medical library, and provides all-around documental information service.

464.4.2 Keeping a Foothold on Hospitals and Serving the Clinic are the Theme of Information Service

Hospital library is the academic institution providing services for the treatment, teaching and scientific research of hospitals. It adopts modern electronic technology and network equipment, provides high-quality information services for readers and meets the continuously developing demands of hospitals.

464.4.3 Construction of High-Quality Literature Information with a Reasonable Team

The development of information technology has reduced to the necessity for the fundamental transformation of the methods and approaches of information services, while high-quality information services group is the most important factor. Librarians have to be possessed of the senses of mission and responsibility, and constantly promote their own levels of expertise, never stop to learn new theories and new technologies, and integrate themselves into the general environment of overall hospital works, meanwhile, they shall provide deep-seated information services with superb skills, so as to promote the effective utilization of medical information resources.

References

1. Dai H (2011) Library information resources construction resource integration. J Edu Teach Forum 34
2. Weng H, Yu X (2011) Strategies and direction of the information resources integration and information services integration viewed from current situation. J Library Info Service 19
3. Xing X, Ning G (2010) Library information resources integration model analysis. J Handan Polytechnic College 2

Chapter 465
Applied Research of Ultrasound Microbubble in Tumor-Transferred Lymph Node Imaging and Treatment

Xin Zhao and Guijie Li

Abstract The risk of cervical lymph nodal metastases is related to the stage and will significantly affect treatment of squamous cell carcinoma in tongue or cheek. Timely diagnosis and treatment of patients with metastatic lymph nodes of the neck is an important factor to improve survival rates. The advantage of ultrasound examination is non-invasive, so the indirect injection of lymphatic system has been put on the research agenda. This method is known as the organization injection, which means injecting colored injection into the space of tissues and organs. Ultrasound microbubbles injected into tissues can enhance local lymph nodes. Self-made Fluorocabon-filled surfactant contrast agent injected from primary cancer can turn into lymph tract and remarkably intense echoes of lymph node.

Keywords Ultrasound microbubble · Lymph nodes · Metastatic · Blood

465.1 Introduction

Cancer patients in the early stage are prone to have cervical lymph node transferred, which will greatly influence the prognosis, tumor stage division as well as the treatment. It is an important factor to improve the survival rate by diagnosing and treating cervical transferred lymph node promptly [1]. In recent years, researchers use ultrasonic tissue characterization to evaluate lesion tissues quantitatively. Ultrasound microbubble is injected into the general blood circulation through peripheral vein. By way of changing acoustic attenuation, sound velocity or enhancing backscatter, changing the interaction between sound waves and tissues enhances the blood echo signal in the examined area in order to realize

X. Zhao · G. Li (✉)
Department of Biological and Chemical Engineering, Chongqing University of Education, Xuefu Main Street 9, Nan'an District, Chongqing 400067, People's Republic of China
e-mail: foods@live.cn

S. Li et al. (eds.), *Frontier and Future Development of Information Technology in Medicine and Education*, Lecture Notes in Electrical Engineering 269,
DOI: 10.1007/978-94-007-7618-0_465,

obvious lymph node ultrasonography enhancing effect [2]. This provides scientific support for ultrasound noninvasive diagnosis of cancer-transferred lymph node and target treatment with ultrasound microbubble as the carrier of lymph node [3].

Apart from the size of lymph node, hardness and cervical type, the positive rate of traditional examination mainly depends on inspectors' experience. Skilled person can touch the superficial area (under the jaw) about 0.5 cm lymph nodes. While in the deeper parts (deep side of digastric muscle) they can touch only 1.0 cm-sized lymph nodes, with the missed diagnosis rate reaching to 20–30 %. In addition, the size of a few normal lymph nodes can be up to 2.0 cm, and false positive rate is 20 %. With the development of imaging examination and deepening understanding of cervical transverse sectional anatomy, the accuracy of cervical transferred lymph nodes imaging treatment was much improved. The sensitivity of physical palpation is 82.1 %, while CT 94.6 % and B-ultrasound 91.1 %, whose specificity is obviously higher than physical palpation and the imaging examination can find 28–75 % the occult metastatic lymph nodes [4]. In recent years, more and more researchers use ultrasonic tissue characterization to evaluate lesion tissues quantitatively. It usually takes video of ultrasound tissue characterization, that is, ultrasonographic echo intensity. At the same time, the combination of new ultrasound microbubble and second harmonic generation enhances the ultrasound imaging effect.

Since Gramiak first reported the application of ultrasound microbubble (UM) in 1968, the development of UM research has achieved rapid progress [5]. In recent years, researchers found that as the targeted microbubble can distinguish and combine from the level of molecular in lesions; it can produce special imaging in the targeted point, which will obviously improve the ultrasound diagnosis ability of early pathological changes [6]. At the same time, UM can become the carrier of medicines or therapeutic genes, by ultrasonic irradiation effect to achieve targeted lead-in and release. Targeted microbubble is the hot issue of ultrasound-contrast-agent research and attracts attention from many other medical areas [7]. Recently, research on UM contrast agent carrying drugs to the targeted tissue treatment has made and important application value has achieved in drug-carrying problem such as thrombolytic therapy and anti-tumor treatment [8].

465.2 Brief Introduction of UM

UM, discovered in recent years, is a kind of ultrasound contrast agent. By changing tissue ultrasonic characterization to produce contrast agent effect, it can be used in contrast imaging of human blood and organs [9]. The ideal new-type UM should possess the following characterizations, such as high scattering, low dispersion, low solubility, no biological activities, freely through the capillaries, the good organization contrast imaging, similar-sized microbubbles and the particle size of about 5 μm [10].

The constitution of UM: UM is made up of packed polyethylene gas and microbubble capsule. The gas of microbubble mainly includes air, sulfur hexafluoride gas, fluorine carbon gas, etc [11]. Because fluorine-containing gas belongs to inert gas, with the characterization of high relative molecular mass, poor solubility and dispersion in the blood and good stability, it can go through the pulmonary circulation and the microcirculation blood capillary network. It has been wildly used. The materials covering the microbubbles include human albumin, lipid, plasmatic acid, polymer, etc [12].

The principle of UM angiographic diagnosis: ultrasound microbubble is injected into the general blood circulation through peripheral vein. By way of changing acoustic attenuation, sound velocity or enhancing backscatter, changing the interaction between sound waves and tissues enhances the blood echo signal in the examined area. At the same time, because the uptake of contrast agent is different from normal tissue and lesion tissue, it can enhance the blood flow signal and obviously improve the signal-to-noise ratio, which will improve gray-scale imaging of tissues. The activity characterization of microbubble in the ultrasonic field is closely related to the microbubble's size, density, micro bubble shell, packed gas and so on, especially the sound pressure of incident sound waves [9].

465.3 The Targeting Effect and Therapeutic Effect of UM

The targeting of UM: nowadays, there are two main mechanisms which can achieve the purpose of targeted UM to specific molecular targeting, that is, passive targeting and active targeting. The passive targeting is through body inherent defense mechanism-phagocytes, mainly by the macrophages in the mononuclear macrophage system, with the help of opsonin, it can clear out the foreign body (UM). Experiments successfully show that protein and lipid UM can be adhered to venule endothelial cells of "inflammation" organization through activated leukocyte [13]. But because of the lack of high degree of specificity and targeting and low ability to combine, the use of passive targeting is limited in its application in targeting contrast ultrasound imaging.

Active targeting is realized by specializing ordinary UM with targeting ligands, such as monoclonal antibodies on the surface [14]. UM with targeting ligands no longer requires the leukocyte as media, but can directly combine with the venule endothelial cells of targeted issues or organs, or some materials of targeted molecular in the vein. Because the mechanism has the highly-specific and targeted characteristics, and avoids the damage to the UM by phagocytic cells, it is advanced and feasible in theory, making it become the core mechanism in the research and development of noninvasive targeted contrast ultrasonic imaging. Many experiments have proved this mechanism.

The cavitation of UM: microbubble containing gas will compress and expand under the action of ultrasonic wave. Under the action of a strong ultrasonic energy, the bubble will burst. Ultrasonic cavitation effect can lead to the increase permeability of tissue cell membrane, while UM can reduce the ultrasonic cavitation threshold and strengthen the cavitation effect. The "shock wave" produced by cavitation effect can make permeability of local capillaries and adjacent tissue cell membrane increased, which is good for the targeted UM with anti-tumor drugs or genes entering into the vascular gap, improving the tumor targeting function, and enhancing the transfection and expression of gene. Many scholars at home and abroad confirmed the existence of the above mechanism through experiments in vitro and in vivo [15].

The tumor-targeted UM mechanism: the mechanism of UM targeting for tumor therapy mainly manifested in promoting veins to produce angiogenesis factor and platelet in the tumor tissues. New tumor vascular endothelial expresses a lot of growth factor receptors and adhesive molecule receptor family, which are not only the targeting point of chemotherapeutic drugs, but also the targeting point of tumor-nourish vessel embolism treatment, as well as the target of targeting microbubble. Targeting UM with the corresponding ligand arrived at the tumor site, then through the low-frequency, high-energy ultrasonic irradiation, it can burst and release the drugs and produce shock wave, making cells to form sound hole in order to help kill or inhibit tumor drug or gene inside [16].

465.4 The Application of UM in Tumor Diagnosis and Treatment

The application of UM in tumor-transferred lymph node diagnosis and treatment: with the development of imaging examination, the accuracy of the ultrasound cervical lymph node diagnosis was increased. Color Doppler ultrasound can provide richer diagnosis information and further improve the sensitivity, specificity and accuracy of cervical transferred lymph nodes diagnosis. Deng et al. [17] found that after subcutaneous injection of ultrasound contrast agents, it can show the sentinel lymph node, as well as the sentinel lymph node metastases. Subcutaneous contrast sonography is more effective than the lymphoid flashing imaging. Yang et al. [18] found that injection of UM through tissue can reach the purpose of enhancing the lymphatic system contrast. Meanwhile, UM can be injected through planter subcutaneous injection and enter the lymphatic channel in order to achieve remarkable enhancement effect of lymph node.

Ultrasonic diagnosis and treatment of oral cancer transferred lymph nodes: oral cancer is very common in the world, which accounts for 25 % of total tumor incidence. Oral cancer is easy to transfer in the early stage, and its 5 year survival rate is low. In recent years, more and more researchers use ultrasonic tissue characterization to evaluate lesion tissues quantitatively. It usually takes video of ultrasound tissue characteri-zation, that is, ultrasonographic echo intensity. At the same time, the combination of new ultrasound microbubble and second harmonic generation enhances the ul-trasound imaging effect. Yang et al. [19]. using the UM sonograms echo intensity, found that UM angiography can clearly distinguish tumor metastasis, inflammatory and normal lymph nodes. It laid imaging foundation for the research on whether the oral cancer cervical lymph node transfers. In Pang's study [20], the dectection rate of metastatic lymph nodes and inflammatory lymph nodes was 61 % and 50 % before contrast-enhanced ultrasound imaging, while 82 % and 75 % after ultrasoun imaging. After ultrasoun imaging, the echo intensit of primary cancer and cervical metastatic lymph nodes was increased,there was significant difference.

References

1. Kademani D (2007) Oral cancer. Mayo Clin Proc 82:878–887
2. Tang MX, Mulvana H, Gauthier T et al (2011) Quantitative contrast-enhanced ultrasound imaging: a review of sources of variability. Interface Focus 1:520–539
3. Yasufuku K, Nakajima T, Motoori K et al (2006) Comparison of endobronchial ultrasound, positron emission tomography, and CT for lymph node staging of lung cancer. Chest 130:710–718
4. Wang WD, Luo JC, Qiu WL et al (1995) Computed tomography of the occult cervical lymph node metastasis in the malignant tumors of the head and neck. Chin J Radiol 8:543–546
5. Gramiak R, Shah PM (1968) Echocardiography of the aortic root. Investig Radiol 3:356–366
6. Salvatore V, Borghi A, Piscaglia F (2011) Contrast-enhanced ultrasound for liver imaging: recent advances. Curr Pharm Des 18:2236–2252
7. Rapoport N, Kennedy AM, Shea JE et al (2010) Ultrasonic nanotherapy of pancreatic cancer: lessons from ultrasound imaging. Mol Pharm 7:22–31
8. Frenkel V (2008) Ultrasound mediated delivery of drugs and genes to solid tumors. Adv Drug Deliv Rev 60:1193–1208
9. Ophir J, Parkerk J (1989) Contrast agents in diagnostic ultrasound. Ultrasound Med Biol 15:319
10. Borden MA, Kruse DE, Caskey CY et al (2005) Influence of Lipid Shell Physicochemical Properties on Ultrasound-Induced Microbubble Destruction. IEEE Trans Ultrason Ferroelectr Freq Control 52:1992–2002
11. Bloch SH, Wan MX, Dayton PA et al (2004) Optical observation of lipid- and polymer-shelled ultrasound microbubble contrast agents. Appl Phys Lett 84:631–634
12. Klibanov AL (2006) Microbubble contrast agents: targeted ultrasound imaging and ultrasound-assisted drug-delivery applications. Investig Radiol 41:354–362
13. Lindner JR, Song J, Christiansen J et al (2001) Ultrasound assessment of inflammation and renal tissue injury with microbubbles targeted to P-selectin. Circ 104:2107–2112
14. Weller GE, Lu E, Csikari MM et al (2003) Ultrasound imaging of acute cardiac transplant rejection with microbubbles targeted to intercellular adhesion molecule-1. Circ 108:218–224
15. Krasovitski B, Kimmel E (2001) Gas bubble pulsation in a semiconfined space subjected to ultrasound. J Acoust Soc Am 109:891–898
16. Skyba DM, Price RJ, Linka AZ et at (1998) Direct in vivo visualization of intravascular destruction of microbubbles by ultrasound and its local effects on tissue. Circ 98:290–293
17. Deng XD, Liu JB, Goldberg BB (2006) Experimental study in detecting sentinel lymph nodes by contrast-enhanced lymphatic ultrasonography. Shanghai Med Imaging 15:58–60
18. Yang CJ, Wang ZG, Ran HT et at (2005) Effect of self-made fluorocabon-filled surfactant ultrasound enhanced contrast agent in lymph nodes. Chin J Ultrasound Ed 21:417–419

19. Yang CJ, Wang ZG, Peng XQ et al (2006) Experimental study on ultrasound contrast agent enhancing images of inflammatory and metastatic lymph nodes of rabbits. Chin J Ultrasonography 15:142–145
20. Pang L, Qiu LH, Gao Z et al (2011) Experimental study on contrast-enhanced ultrasound imaging of metastatic lymph nodes of cheek carcinoma. J Clin Ultrasound Med 13:581–583

Chapter 466
The Examination of Landau-Lifshitz Pseudo-Tensor Under Physical Decomposition of Gravitational Field

Peng-Cheng Zhang, Jia Guo, Jun Zhao and Ben-Chao Zhu

Abstract Physical decomposition of gauge fields (including Abelian and non-Abelian fields) [1–3] have been widely accepted by most particle physics researchers. The authors also extended the approach to gravitational field and attacked the century-lasting problem of gravitational energy density [4]. Reference [4] gives a physical decomposition of affine connection, and raises a revisited way to compute traditional energy density formula. In this paper, we will adopt their decomposition to Landau-Lifshitz pseudo-tensor definition, and examine whether the results are reasonable or not.

Keywords Physical decomposition · Gravitational energy density · Landau-Lifshitz pseudo-tensor

466.1 Introduction

General relativity as a basic theory in physical has an awkward problem in defining energy-momentum tensor. There is still no general agreement on the definition of conserved quantities associated with gravitational field. In the past century, many researchers have made great efforts to find a "right" energy-momentum tensor, these attempts aimed at finding a quantity for describing distribution of energy-momentum due to matter, non-gravitational and gravitational fields only resulted in various energy-momentum complexes (like Einstein-Tolman, Landau-Lifshitz, Møller, Papapetrou Weinberg energy-momentum complex) [5]. The problems associated with energy-momentum complexes resulted in some researchers even abandoning the concept of energy-momentum localization in favor of the

P.-C. Zhang · J. Guo · J. Zhao · B.-C. Zhu (✉)
Department Mathematics and Physics, Hubei University of Medicine, Shiyan 442000 Hubei, China
e-mail: zbc@hust.edu.cn

S. Li et al. (eds.), *Frontier and Future Development of Information Technology in Medicine and Education*, Lecture Notes in Electrical Engineering 269,
DOI: 10.1007/978-94-007-7618-0_466,

alternative concept of quasi-localization [5]. (Throughout this paper we use the convention that summation occurs over dummy indices, Greek indices take values from 0 to 3 and Latin indices values from 1 to 3).

In general relativity, Einstein aimed to hold the conservation law in the form of $\frac{\partial}{\partial x^{\mu}}(\sqrt{-g}(T_{\nu}^{\mu}+t_{\nu}^{\mu}))=0$ (where T_{ν}^{μ} representing the stress energy density of matter, $g=Det|g^{\mu\nu}|$, $g^{\mu\nu}$ denotes the metric tensor of the curved space-time). Einstein firstly gave the expression of t_{ν}^{μ}. The quantity t_{ν}^{μ} as representing the stress energy density of gravitation is the homogeneous quadratic in the first derivatives of the metric tensor and thus it is obviously not a tensor. Furthermore, Einstein's energy-momentum $t^{\mu\nu}(t^{\mu\nu}=g^{\mu\rho}t_{\rho}^{\nu})$ is not symmetric in its indices, thus Landau and Lifshitz modified $t^{\mu\nu}$ to be:

$$
\begin{aligned}
t^{\mu\nu}=\frac{1}{16\pi G}[&(2\Gamma_{\alpha\beta}^{\sigma}\Gamma_{\sigma\rho}^{\rho}-\Gamma_{\alpha\rho}^{\sigma}\Gamma_{\beta\sigma}^{\rho}-\Gamma_{\alpha\sigma}^{\sigma}\Gamma_{\beta\rho}^{\rho})(g^{\mu\alpha}g^{\nu\beta}-g^{\mu\nu}g^{\alpha\beta})\\
&+g^{\mu\alpha}g^{\beta\sigma}(\Gamma_{\alpha\rho}^{\nu}\Gamma_{\beta\sigma}^{\rho}+\Gamma_{\beta\sigma}^{\nu}\Gamma_{\alpha\rho}^{\rho}-\Gamma_{\sigma\rho}^{\nu}\Gamma_{\alpha\beta}^{\rho}-\Gamma_{\alpha\beta}^{\nu}\Gamma_{\sigma\rho}^{\rho})\\
&+g^{\nu\alpha}g^{\beta\sigma}(\Gamma_{\alpha\rho}^{\mu}\Gamma_{\beta\sigma}^{\rho}+\Gamma_{\beta\sigma}^{\mu}\Gamma_{\alpha\rho}^{\rho}-\Gamma_{\sigma\rho}^{\mu}\Gamma_{\alpha\beta}^{\rho}-\Gamma_{\alpha\beta}^{\mu}\Gamma_{\sigma\rho}^{\rho})\\
&+g^{\alpha\beta}g^{\sigma\rho}(\Gamma_{\alpha\sigma}^{\mu}\Gamma_{\beta\rho}^{\nu}-\Gamma_{\alpha\beta}^{\mu}\Gamma_{\rho\sigma}^{\nu})
\end{aligned}
\tag{466.1}
$$

This expression does give right symmetry of μ and ν. But Landau-Lifshitz did not overcome all shortcomings of Einstein's energy-momentum complex. So that some others like Møller, Papapetrou, Weinberg also gave their own definitions of energy-momentum complex of gravitational field [5]. This awkward problem is still an open question for us.

466.2 The Physical Decomposition of Gravitational Field

Gauge invariance is the most elegant and efficient principle for constructing interactions in the present field theories of physics. Theoretically, gauge field theory requires all field equations should be gauge invariant, but the key obstacle to constructing all physical quantities gauge invariantly is the inevitable involvement of gauge field with their ordinary derivatives, which are all intrinsically gauge dependent. The idea in Refs. [1, 2] is to decompose the gauge field: $A_{\mu}=\hat{A}_{\mu}+\bar{A}_{\mu}$. The aim is that $\hat{A}_{\mu}$ will be a physical term which is gauge-covariant and always vanishes in the vacuum, and the $\bar{A}_{\mu}$ is a pure-gauge term which solely carries (particularly, it does not contribute to electric or magnetic field strength), if we replace A_{μ} with $\hat{A}_{\mu}$ and the ordinary derivative with the pure-gauge covariant derivative constructed with $\bar{A}_{\mu}$ instead of A_{μ}, we will surely reduce a gauge-dependent quantity to be a gauge-independent [1, 2]. The physical decomposition of gauge fields (including Abelian and non-Abelian fields) [1–3] have been widely accepted by most particle physics researchers.

The Einstein's gravitational theory has a deep analogy with the non-Abelian gauge theory. The gauge invariance of gravitational theory refers to general covariance under arbitrary coordinate transformation. In gravitational theory, the covariant Riemann curvature tensor, $R^{\rho}_{\sigma\mu\nu}$ which is a true tensor and always zero in an intrinsically flat space-time, is built out of the non-covariant connection $\Gamma^{\rho}_{\sigma\mu}$, which can be made non-zero in an intrinsically flat space-time by using curvilinear coordinates. This property is the reason why gravitational energy density in the traditional pseudo-tensor constructions meaningless. Analogous to the physical decomposition of the gauge field, we can write $\Gamma^{\rho}_{\sigma\mu} = \bar{\Gamma}^{\rho}_{\sigma\mu} + \hat{\Gamma}^{\rho}_{\sigma\mu}$, the physical term $\hat{\Gamma}^{\rho}_{\sigma\mu}$ always vanishes as does curved tensor $R^{\rho}_{\sigma\mu\nu}$ in an intrinsically flat space-time, the pure-geometric term $\bar{\Gamma}^{\rho}_{\sigma\mu}$ gives zero curved tensor and solely carries gauge freedom in coordinates transformation. In Ref. [4] we have demonstrated that the separation $\Gamma^{\rho}_{\sigma\mu} = \bar{\Gamma}^{\rho}_{\sigma\mu} + \hat{\Gamma}^{\rho}_{\sigma\mu}$ in general relativity has the same effect as the separation $A_{\mu} = \hat{A}_{\mu} + \bar{A}_{\mu}$ in gauge fields, that is to say,

$$\bar{R}^{\rho}_{\sigma\mu\nu} = \partial_{\mu}\bar{\Gamma}^{\rho}_{\sigma\nu} - \partial_{\nu}\bar{\Gamma}^{\rho}_{\sigma\mu} + \bar{\Gamma}^{\rho}_{\beta\mu}\bar{\Gamma}^{\beta}_{\sigma\nu} - \bar{\Gamma}^{\rho}_{\beta\nu}\bar{\Gamma}^{\beta}_{\sigma\mu} = 0 \tag{466.2}$$

$$\bar{D}_i\hat{\Gamma}^{\rho}_{\sigma i} = \partial_i\hat{\Gamma}^{\rho}_{\sigma i} + \bar{\Gamma}^{\rho}_{i\alpha}\hat{\Gamma}^{\alpha}_{\sigma i} - \bar{\Gamma}^{\alpha}_{i\sigma}\hat{\Gamma}^{\rho}_{\alpha i} - \bar{\Gamma}^{\alpha}_{ii}\hat{\Gamma}^{\rho}_{\sigma\alpha} = 0 \tag{466.3}$$

Reference [4] also gave the idea to calculate a physically meaningful energy density of the gravitational field. For a finite and weak gravitational system, we can use vanishing boundary values, and apply perturbative expansions for both $\hat{\Gamma}^{\rho}_{\sigma\mu}$ and $\bar{\Gamma}^{\rho}_{\sigma\mu}$:

$$\bar{\Gamma}^{\rho}_{\sigma i} = \partial_i\partial_k^{-2}\partial_j\Gamma^{\rho}_{\sigma j} + higher\ \ order\ \ terms \tag{466.4}$$

$$\bar{\Gamma}^{\rho}_{\sigma 0} = \int_{\infty}^{x} dx^i\partial_0\bar{\Gamma}^{\rho}_{\sigma i} + higher\ \ order\ \ terms \tag{466.5}$$

If a coordinate gives non-zero $\bar{\Gamma}^{\rho}_{\sigma\mu}$, it means that it contains spurious gravitational effect, and one should not use the pseudo-tensor formula directly. But these pseudo-tensor formulas can be ungraded to be physical ones just simply replacing the full affine connection $\Gamma^{\rho}_{\sigma\mu}$ with the physical affine connection $\hat{\Gamma}^{\rho}_{\sigma\mu} = \Gamma^{\rho}_{\sigma\mu} - \bar{\Gamma}^{\rho}_{\sigma\mu}$.

466.3 The Examination of Landau-Lifshitz Pseudo-Tensor

We are now in the position to examine whether Eqs.(466.4) and (466.5) are valid in calculating energy density of space-time or not. Here now, we just discuss the simplest Schwarzschild solution in weak approximate:

$$ds^2 = (1 - \frac{2m}{r})dt^2 - (1 + \frac{2m}{r})(dx^2 + dy^2 + dz^2) \tag{466.6}$$

The non-zero affine connections are:

$$\Gamma^0_{01} = \frac{mx_1}{r^2(r-2m)} \quad \Gamma^0_{02} = \frac{mx_2}{r^2(r-2m)} \quad \Gamma^0_{03} = \frac{mx_3}{r^2(r-2m)} \tag{466.7}$$

$$\Gamma^1_{11} = \Gamma^2_{12} = \Gamma^3_{13} = -\Gamma^1_{22} = -\Gamma^1_{33} = -\Gamma^1_{00} = -\frac{mx_1}{r^2(r+2m)} \tag{466.8}$$

$$\Gamma^2_{22} = \Gamma^3_{23} = \Gamma^1_{12} = -\Gamma^2_{11} = -\Gamma^2_{33} = -\Gamma^2_{00} = -\frac{mx_2}{r^2(r+2m)} \tag{466.9}$$

$$\Gamma^3_{33} = \Gamma^2_{23} = \Gamma^1_{13} = -\Gamma^3_{11} = -\Gamma^3_{22} = -\Gamma^3_{00} = -\frac{mx_3}{r^2(r+2m)} \tag{466.10}$$

By using Eqs. (466.1) and (466.7–466.10), the energy density of Landau-Lifshitz pseudo-tensor in Schwarzschild solution is:

$$\begin{aligned}
t^{00} &= \frac{1}{16\pi G}[(2\Gamma^\sigma_{\alpha\beta}\Gamma^\rho_{\sigma\rho} - \Gamma^\sigma_{\alpha\rho}\Gamma^\rho_{\beta\sigma} - \Gamma^\sigma_{\alpha\sigma}\Gamma^\rho_{\beta\rho})(g^{0\alpha}g^{0\beta} - g^{00}g^{\alpha\beta}) \\
&\quad + 2g^{0\alpha}g^{\beta\sigma}(\Gamma^0_{\alpha\rho}\Gamma^\rho_{\beta\sigma} + \Gamma^0_{\beta\sigma}\Gamma^\rho_{\alpha\rho} - \Gamma^0_{\sigma\rho}\Gamma^\rho_{\alpha\beta} - \Gamma^0_{\alpha\beta}\Gamma^\rho_{\sigma\rho}) \\
&\quad + g^{\alpha\beta}g^{\sigma\rho}(\Gamma^0_{\alpha\sigma}\Gamma^0_{\beta\rho} - \Gamma^0_{\alpha\beta}\Gamma^0_{\rho\sigma})] \\
\Rightarrow t^{00} &= \frac{g^{00}g^{11}}{8\pi G}[(\Gamma^1_{11}\Gamma^0_{10} + \Gamma^2_{22}\Gamma^0_{20} + \Gamma^3_{33}\Gamma^0_{30}) + 7(\Gamma^1_{11}\Gamma^1_{11} + \Gamma^2_{22}\Gamma^2_{22} + \Gamma^3_{33}\Gamma^3_{33})] \\
&= -\frac{m^2}{4\pi G}\frac{3r - 8m}{(r+2m)^3(r-2m)^2}
\end{aligned} \tag{466.11}$$

The above discussion tells us that the quantity t^{00} is not reasonable because it contains spurious gravitational effect. The true gauge-independent energy density is $\hat{t}^{00}$

$$\begin{aligned}
\hat{t}^{00} &= \frac{g^{00}g^{11}}{8\pi G}[(\hat{\Gamma}^1_{11}\hat{\Gamma}^0_{10} + \hat{\Gamma}^2_{22}\hat{\Gamma}^0_{20} + \hat{\Gamma}^3_{33}\hat{\Gamma}^0_{30}) + 7(\hat{\Gamma}^1_{11}\hat{\Gamma}^1_{11} + \hat{\Gamma}^2_{22}\hat{\Gamma}^2_{22} + \hat{\Gamma}^3_{33}\hat{\Gamma}^3_{33})] \\
&= \frac{g^{00}g^{11}}{8\pi G}\{[(\Gamma^1_{11} - \bar{\Gamma}^1_{11})(\Gamma^0_{10} - \bar{\Gamma}^0_{10}) + (\Gamma^2_{22} - \bar{\Gamma}^2_{22})(\Gamma^0_{20} - \bar{\Gamma}^0_{20}) \\
&\quad + (\Gamma^3_{33} - \bar{\Gamma}^3_{33})(\Gamma^0_{30} - \bar{\Gamma}^0_{30})] + 7[(\Gamma^1_{11} - \bar{\Gamma}^1_{11})^2 + (\Gamma^2_{22} - \bar{\Gamma}^2_{22})^2 + (\Gamma^3_{33} - \bar{\Gamma}^3_{33})^2]\}
\end{aligned} \tag{466.12}$$

Here, we replace the full affine connection $\Gamma^\rho_{\sigma\mu}$ with the physical affine connection $\hat{\Gamma}^\rho_{\sigma\mu} = \Gamma^\rho_{\sigma\mu} - \bar{\Gamma}^\rho_{\sigma\mu}$ and use Eq. (466.4) to calculate $\bar{\Gamma}^\rho_{\sigma\mu}$ in the first order:

$\bar{\Gamma}^{\rho}_{\sigma i} = \partial_i \partial_k^{-2} \partial_j \Gamma^{\rho}_{\sigma j}$, $\bar{\Gamma}^{\rho}_{\sigma 0} = \int_{\infty}^{x} dx^i \partial_0 \bar{\Gamma}^{\rho}_{\sigma i}$. Equation (466.7) tells us $\bar{\Gamma}^{\rho}_{\sigma 0} = \int_{\infty}^{x} dx^i \partial_0$ $\bar{\Gamma}^{\rho}_{\sigma i} = 0$. Finally, we get:

$$\begin{aligned} \hat{t}^{00} = & \frac{g^{00} g^{11}}{8\pi G} [(\hat{\Gamma}^1_{11} \hat{\Gamma}^0_{10} + \hat{\Gamma}^2_{22} \hat{\Gamma}^0_{20} + \hat{\Gamma}^3_{33} \hat{\Gamma}^0_{30}) \\ & + 7(\hat{\Gamma}^1_{11} \hat{\Gamma}^1_{11} + \hat{\Gamma}^2_{22} \hat{\Gamma}^2_{22} + \hat{\Gamma}^3_{33} \hat{\Gamma}^3_{33})] \\ & = -\frac{7m^2}{8\pi G} \frac{(r - 2m)}{(r + 2m)^5} \end{aligned} \tag{466.13}$$

466.4 Conclusions

1. There are various types of the energy–momentum pseudo-tensor. None of them gave reasonable physical meaning energy density [5], but if one adopted our decomposition of affine connection $\hat{\Gamma}^{\rho}_{\sigma\mu} = \Gamma^{\rho}_{\sigma\mu} - \bar{\Gamma}^{\rho}_{\sigma\mu}$, it is true that the unreasonable energy density of different definitions can be easily reduced to be reasonable one. Comparing with Eq. (466.11), our result Eq. (466.12) shows the same algorithms. This is not a surprised conclusion, because although we replace the full affine connection with the physical affine connection, the dimension of these two affine connection is not changed any more. Our result is different with previous work by numerical value, which means the contribution from geometry.
2. The energy density of Landau-Lifshitz pseudo-tensor in Schwarzschild solution $\hat{t}^{00} < t^{00}$, this is a rather successful representation of our decomposition, because we have eliminated the pure-gauge term $\bar{\Gamma}^{\rho}_{\sigma\mu}$, so that we have eliminated the spurious gravitational effect in Schwarzschild solution. There is no need simulated experimental since there is not only one definition of gravitational field energy-momentum tensor. The best possible experiment to check the physical decomposition of gravitational field must rely on the space observation experiment out of the earth.
3. Although the $\hat{t}^{00}$ is more close to the truth physical energy density, the negative property of $\hat{t}^{00}$ (because the Landau-Lifshitz energy-momentum pseudo-tensor is negative) told us the truth definition for energy-momentum is still not like what Landau-Lifshitz had done.
4. Finally, we remark that in this paper we have restricted our discussions and calculations to the weak-field approximation. It is a non-trivial work to define gauge invariant energy density of strong gravitational field and also leaves for future studying.

References

1. Chen XS, Lü XF, Sun WM, Wang F, Gold-man T (2008) Phys Rev Lett 100:232002
2. Chen XS, Sun WM, Lü XF, Wang F, Gold-man T (2009) Phys Rev Lett 103:062001
3. Liang W-F, Wu M, Liu H, Chen X-S (2008) Chin Phys Lett 25(12):4227
4. Chen X-S, Zhu B-C (2011) Physical decomposition of the gauge and gravitational fields. Phys Rev D 83:084006
5. Xulu SS (2003) The energy-momentum problem. Gen Relat 2003-5-11 http://xxx.itp.cn/abs/hep-th/0308070

Chapter 467
Exploring of the Integration Design Method of Rectal Prolapse TCM Clinical Pathway System

Zhihui Huang

Abstract This paper advocates the use of expert system and evidence-based medicine in the traditional Chinese medicine (TCM) clinical pathway system. It proposes an intelligent multi-agent reconfigurable system to cope with a dynamic traditional Chinese medicine environment where support the rectal prolapse clinical pathways system application integration in the face of the clinical medical decision-making existing more uncertainty field. An integration design method of rectal prolapse TCM clinical pathway system is through the use of design rules which are based on empirical and theoretical knowledge. Based on case reasoning medical expert system for improvement and regulating rectal prolapse clinical pathway system are presented. The relationship between the design for clinical path information system and expert system and analysis of system reliability growth test platform is discussed.

Keywords Clinical pathway system integration · Expert system · TCM surgery

467.1 Introduction

TCM clinical pathway (CP-TCM) is based on evidence-based medicine, purpose on the expected therapeutic effect and cost control, standardize the medical service, clear and definite doctor and nurse clinical workflow reduce delayed rehabilitation and waste of resources, draw up a procedured and standardized diagnosis plan which measure up to strict work order and accurate time requirements, so that patients receive optimal medical care service.

Z. Huang (✉)
Fujian University of Traditional Chinese Medicine, 1 Huatuo Road, Fuzhou, Fujian, China
e-mail: mrhuangzhihui@163.com

S. Li et al. (eds.), *Frontier and Future Development of Information Technology in Medicine and Education*, Lecture Notes in Electrical Engineering 269,
DOI: 10.1007/978-94-007-7618-0_467,

Rectal prolapse is refers to the anal canal, rectum mucous membrane, rectal full-thickness, even part of the sigmoid colon downward shift, emerge or don't emerge outside the anus of a disease, which is one of the refractory diseases of anus bowel division. Name of disease of TCM is named rectocele. According to evidence-based medicine and clinical epidemiology method, the implementation of clinical pathway of TCM not only can realize orderly and effective hospital medical service, to control the quality of the diagnosis and treatment funds, but also can solve the doctor of TCM clinical evaluation standard short of precise, randomized controlled trial the lack of enough samples and calculation basis, and many other complex problems. Gabriel [1] proposed clinical pathway decision support information technology, it adopt knowledge-based clinical pathway information system that is content different structure. Inokuchi [2] created a online analytical processing system, that applicate existing knowledge and interactive clinical decision intelligence (CDI) systems. Rani [3] extracted clinical information (CI) from medical documents, extracted extract relations and channel information unstructured text. Chen [4] established a feasibility evaluation method to assess traditional Chiniese medicine clinical pathway. Wang Jialiang [5], Liu Jianping [6] created evidence-based TCM clinical research method. Alexander [7] proposed that evidence-based TCM clinical method is feasible, point out that the TCM quality control is a precondition for clinical trial reliability.

In the field of medical application of Expert system (ES) began feigenbaum development of Expert system in 1965, university of Pittsburgh in 1982, Miller developed a medical Internist-1 computer aided diagnosis system, the knowledge base contains 572 kinds of diseases, more than 4,500 kinds of symptoms [6]; Developed at harvard medical school in 1991 DX-PLAIN system contains 2,200 kinds of diseases, and more than 5,000 kinds of symptoms. Abas [7] put forward a kind of original knowledge ontology such as clinical decision support system (CDSS) in acute postoperative pain management (APPM) applicationt. Gabriel [2] of clinical path decision support information is proposed in this paper, it can satisfy different structure based on knowledge base of the clinical path information system. James [8] put forward a kind of imitating cerebellum functions of a cortical cell CCU model, it can through the planning, implementation target and control the behavior of the purpose. Astrom [9] proposed the modeling design expert system with particular emphasis on technology and the thinking mode transformation.

467.2 Evidence-Based TCM Clinical Pathway System Architecture

Evidence-based traditional Chinese medicine clinical pathway system architecture(ECPS-TCM)can be divided into four main sub system modules: Evidence-based TCM sub system, TCM expert sub system, clinical pathway management sub system, reconfigurable quality evaluation sub system. As shown in Fig. 467.1, at top of the system is expert system module and evidence-based medicine system module, act a guide and evidence-based part in system implementation. Bottom of system is realization method to clinical pathway system function. Establishment of evidence-based and expert system that must need to evaluate system from beginning to end. Therefore, setting up a reconfigurable system quality control module, that each subsystem module through information interaction constitutes a network. The system embodies the principle of "taking patient as the center" management concept, standardizing medical behaviors, establishing mechanisms for system reliability growth, continuous meliorating improve medical measures, putting an end to measures with a haphazard and error, improving the quality of health care, reduce medical cost. Expert system and medical resource database that according famous TCM case to finishing, extraction and induction, realizing TCM expert database that is efficient, accurate, thoughtful, quick to promote precious and scarce medical expert knowledge and experience.

1. Based on case reasoning medical expert system. Established by the method of evidence-based medicine for hospital clinical characteristics of clinical path, at the same time need to find other type original rectal prolapse clinical pathway

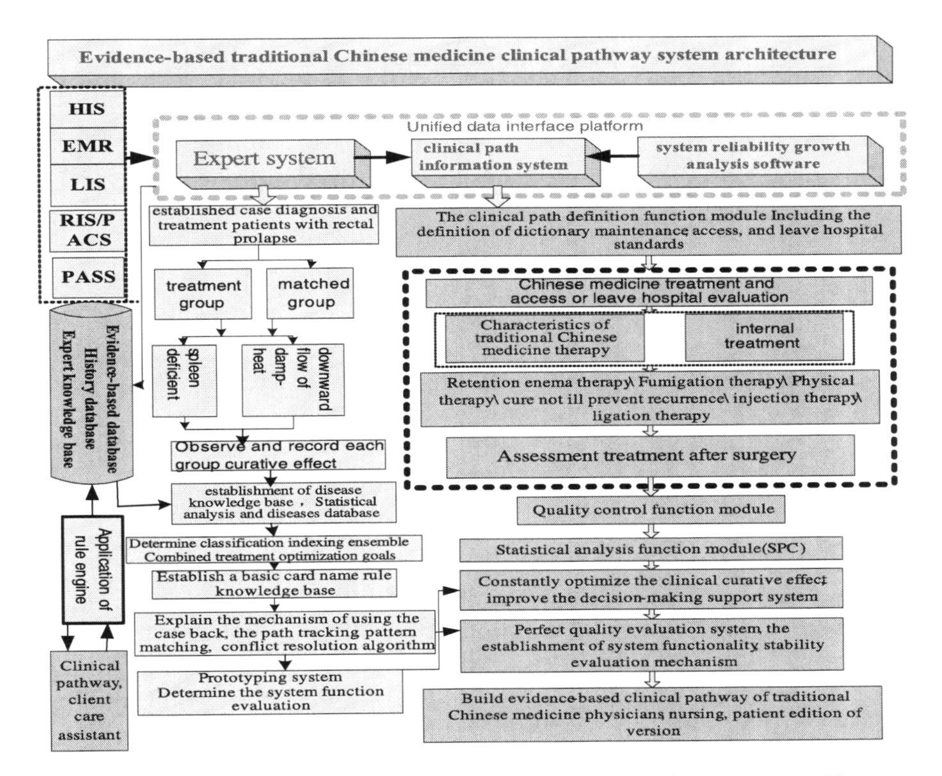

Fig. 467.1 Evidence-based traditional Chinese medicine clinical pathway system architecture

implementation process of related clinical evidence, targeted for disease diagnosis and treatment means to the kinds of interventions involved and the type of evidence, which is incorporated into the clinical pathway, and provide evidence for the process.
2. In the face of the clinical medical decision-making existing more uncertainty field, such as in the knowledge base premise and conclusion, reasoning, take the appropriate regulating mechanism, to design a kind of strong adaptability, wide application, association function, automatic learning, improvement the storage function, quickly set up and efficiently retrieve large medical record repository synchronization mechanism of similar cases.
3. The design of object-oriented system model to support the clinical pathways giant system application integration. Design a distributed object system network to support the activity in real time. Design clinical pathway system workflow model to support a variety of clinical diagnosis and treatment quality control strategy, realize the path control.
4. Based on clinical path information system and expert system, the analysis of system reliability growth test platform is established. The entire life cycle of a clinical pathway system at various stages to evaluate the reliability of the factors analysis, put forward a rectal prolapse clinical pathway of TCM system reliability growth test planning model. As shown in Fig. 467.1.

467.3 Based on Multi Agent Clinical Pathway Structure System

Evidence-based TCM clinical pathway is a kind of distributed complex system. This is an agile intelligent system commingles multi agent organization structure, such as, doctors agent, nursing agent, patients agent. To some extent, they could made the local decision and utilize certain function independently, And complete the medical system task through mutual cooperation. The structure of agent is consisting of execution module, decision-making module, information processing module and Knowledge Base Nursing center and doctor agent interact and receive information and inferential results which is from decision support module (knowledge base database accessed) applied to patients. Nursing center agent execution module according to the doctor agent decision module obtains the decision to execute a predefined operation. Processing module is responsible for the perception and the received information to preliminary processing, handling and storage, information exchange requires a doctor and nurse workstations and electronic patient cases, achieve the full integration of the hospital medical information by a continuous information flow. As shown in Fig. 467.2. It seeks to continue the optimization of the entire traditional Chinese medicine clinical pathway, not a single solution to a clinical disease problem.

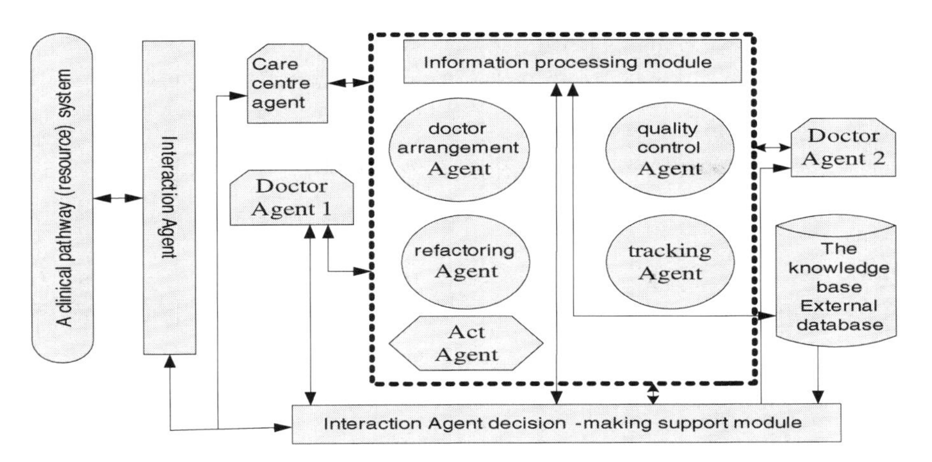

Fig. 467.2 TCM clinical pathway information system agent support module model

TCM clinical pathway system is a multi agent, distributed artificial intelligence system, it has overcome the time and space, resources and functions limitations of a single intelligent systems, has an open, parallel, distributed, assistance and fault tolerance and other advantages.

467.4 Reconfigurable Clinical Pathway Quality Control System and Data Analysis Model

Control system, which comprises three main functional modules: ① control parameters selected module, include key characteristic parameters of selected prescription drugs and determine the error factors that impact these key characteristic parameter, its output is the object and parameters which you want to monitor during the clinical pathway. ② data analyse module, through layout from clinical pathway of physician, nursing, patient versions, get layers of various types of information, upload to Statistical Process Control module (spc); spc module monitoring the status of the system and patient care quality characteristics, analysis of the fluctuations in the clinical process, if find abnormal conditions then will spread to the Statistical Process Diagnosis & Maintenance (SPD &M)module; ③ SPD &M module diagnoses the abnormal condition on the SPC module, given the pathway of adjustment and maintenance recommendations.

In addition, in order to realize precise control on the process of diagnosis and treatment, utilization of system reliability growth analysis test, study on weak links of system, analysis of main factors affecting the quality characteristic parameters, critical quality parameters for disease treatment and parameters which impacts obtain these characteristics, aiming at every key processes to establish quality control nodes, thus guiding physicians and nursing take the correct pathway and method. The system will employ a Bayesian network, clustering analysis, heuristic search algorithms and mathematical statistics and other theories, analysis on the associated control parameters and the evolution of the quality control node network dynamic behavior, thus achieve correlation analysis among pathway, dynamic tracking of quality information etc.

467.5 Conclusion

Clinical path theory adopts industrial engineering standardization principles, takes human, financial, material and other factors, involved in the workflow process with scientific, standardized, eliminating the unreasonable error action and useless, thus greatly improve the efficiency of the process. Not only the study can solve the rectal prolapse TCM evidence-based medical evidence, also from expert system extract TCM treatment of rectal prolapse of the best diagnosis and treatment scheme, so as to improve the characteristics of TCM and curative effect, to reduce the patients' medical costs, and for other diseases TCM clinical pathway research and promotion providing scientific basis.

References

1. Gabriel R, Lux T (2010) Modelling and decision support of clinical pathways. In: Kostkova P (ed) Electronic healthcare-second international ICST conference, vol 27. ehealth, Istanbul, pp 147–154
2. Inokuchi A, Takeda K, Inaoka N, Wakao F, MedTAKMI-CDI (2007) Interactive knowledge discovery for clinical decision intelligence. IBM Syst J 46(1):115–133
3. Rani P, Reddy R, Mathur D, Bandyopadhyay S, Laha (2011) A compositional information extraction methodology from medical reports. In: 2011, database systems for advanced applications-16th international conference, DASFAA 2011, Proceedings, vol 6588(2), pp 400–412
4. Chen B, Lin D, Kong C et al (2011) Establishment and preliminary assessment of traditional chinese medical clinical pathway for cervical spondylotic radiculopathy. J Guangzhou Univ Tradit Chin Med 02
5. Newsham AC et al (2011) Development of an advanced database for clinical trials integrated with an electronic patient record system. Comput Biol Med 41(8):575–586
6. Miller RA, Pople HE, Myers JD (1982) Internist-I: an ex-perimental computer-based diagnostic consultant for general internal medicine. N Engl J Med 307(8):468–476
7. Abas H, Mohd Y, Mohd N, Shahrul A (2011) The application of ontology in a clinical decision support system for acute postoperative pain management. In: 2011 international conference on semantic technology and information retrieval, STAIR, pp 106–112
8. Albus JS (2010) A model of computation and representation in the brain. Inf Sci 180(9):1519–1554
9. Åström KJ (2011) A perspective on modeling and simulation of complex dynamical systems. In: Proceedings of SPIE 8336, integrated modeling of complex optomechanical systems, vol 8336

Author Index

S. Li et al. (eds.), *Frontier and Future Development of Information Technology in Medicine and Education*, Lecture Notes in Electrical Engineering 269,
DOI: 10.1007/978-94-007-7618-0, © Springer Science+Business Media Dordrecht 2014

J

K

L

M

X